Health and Social Justice

Health and Social Justice

*Politics, Ideology, and Inequity in the
Distribution of Disease*

Richard Hofrichter

Editor

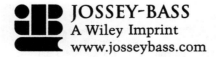

JOSSEY-BASS
A Wiley Imprint
www.josseybass.com

Published by Jossey-Bass
A Wiley Imprint
989 Market Street, San Francisco, CA 94103-1741   www.josseybass.com

Jossey-Bass books and products are available through most bookstores. To contact Jossey-Bass directly call our Customer Care Department within the U.S. at 800-956-7739, outside the U.S. at 317-572-3986 or fax 317-572-4002.

Jossey-Bass also publishes its books in a variety of electronic formats. Some content that appears in print may not be available in electronic books.

Library of Congress Cataloging-in-Publication Data
Health and social justice : politics, ideology, and inequity in the distribution of disease / Richard Hofrichter, editor.—
1st ed.
p. ; cm.
Includes bibliographical references and index.
ISBN 0-7879-6733-5 (alk. paper)
1. Social medicine. 2. Social justice. 3. Equality—Health aspects. 4. Health—Social aspects. 5. Public health—Social aspects. 6. Social status—Health aspects. 7. Economic status—Health aspects. [DNLM: 1. Public Health. 2. Socioeconomic Factors. 3. Public Policy. WA 30 H43453 2003] I. Hofrichter, Richard.
RA418.H388 2003
362.1'042—dc22
2003016408

Printed in the United States of America
FIRST EDITION
PB Printing 10 9 8 7 6 5 4 3 2 1

CONTENTS

SOURCES

Part One

Chapter 1: Previously unpublished.

Chapter 2: Previously unpublished.

Chapter 3: James House and David Williams, "Understanding and Reducing Socioeconomic and Racial/Ethnic Disparities in Health," in *Promoting Health: Intervention Strategies from Social and Behavioral Research,* Brian D. Smedley and Leonard S. Syme, eds., Washington, D.C.: National Academy Press, 2000. © National Academy Press. Reprinted with permission.

Chapter 4: Piroska Ostlin, Asha George, and Gita Sen, "Gender, Health and Equity: The Intersections," in *Challenging Inequities in Health,* Timothy Evans, and others, eds., New York: Oxford University Press, 2001. © 2001 by the Rockefeller Foundation. Used by permission of Oxford University Press, Inc.

Chapter 5: John Gershman, Alec Irwin, and Aaron Shakow, "Getting A Grip on the Global Economy: Health Outcomes and the Decoding of Development Discourse," excerpted and heavily edited and revised from Chapters 2 and 3 in

Dying for Growth: Global Inequality and the Health of the Poor, Jim Yong Kim, Joyce Millen, Alec Irwin, and John Gershman, eds., Monroe, Maine: Common Courage Press, 2000. Used by permission.

Chapter 6: Vincente Navarro and Leiyu Shi, "The Political Context of Social Inequalities and Health," *International Journal of Health Services,* 31(1): 1–21, 2001. © Baywood Publishing Company, Inc., Amityville, NY. Reprinted by permission.

Chapter 7: John Lynch, George Davey Smith, George A. Kaplan, and James S. House, "Income Inequality and Mortality: Importance to Health of Individual Income, Psychosocial Environment, or Material Conditions," *British Medical Journal,* Apr 29; 320:1200–1204, 2000. © British Medical Journal. Reprinted with permission.

Chapter 8: Juliana Maantay, "Zoning, Equity, and Public Health," *American Journal of Public Health,* Jul; 91(7):1033–1041, 2001. © American Public Health Association. Reprinted by permission.

Chapter 9: Sarah Kuhn and John Wooding, "The Changing Structure of Work in the United States: The Implications for Health and Welfare," in *Work, Health and Environment: Old Problems, New Solutions,* Charles Levenstein and John Wooding, eds., New York: Guilford Press, 1997. © Guilford Press. Reprinted by permission.

Part Two

Chapter 10: Dan E. Beauchamp, "Public Health as Social Justice: Ideology of Market Imperatives," *Inquiry,* Mar; Vol. 13, 1976. Reprinted by permission.

Chapter 11: Carles Muntaner, John Lynch, and George Davey Smith, "Social Capital and the Third Way in Public Health," *Critical Public Health,* 10(2), 2000. © Taylor & Francis, http://www.tandf.co.uk/journals. Reprinted by permission.

Chapter 12: Previously unpublished.

Chapter 13: Alexandra Bambas and Juan Antonio Casas, "Assessing Equity In Health: Conceptual Criteria," in *Equity and Health: Views From the Pan American Sanitary Bureau.* Washington, D.C.: Pan American Health Organization, 2001. To obtain more information about PAHO Publications, write to Pan American Health Organization, Publications Program, 525 Twenty-third Street, NW, Washington, DC 20037; Fax (202) 338-0869; email paho@pmds.com; Internet http://publications.paho.org.

Chapter 14: David Coburn, "Income Inequality, Social Cohesion, and the Health Status of Populations: The Role of Neoliberalism," *Social Science & Medicine,* Vol. 51: 135–146, 2000. © Elsevier Science. Reprinted by permission.

Chapter 15: John Lynch, "Income Inequality and Health: Expanding the Debate," *Social Science & Medicine,* Vol. 51: 1001–1005, 2000. © Elsevier Science. Reprinted by permission.

Chapter 16: Richard Levins, "Is Capitalism a Disease?: The Crisis in U.S. Public Health," *Monthly Review,* Sept; 51(4):8–33, 2000. Reprinted by permission.

Chapter 17: Jennie Popay, Gareth Williams, Carol Thomas, and Anthony Gatrell, "Theorising Inequalities in Health: The Place of Lay Knowledge," in *The Sociology of Health Inequalities,* Mel Bartley, David Blane, and George Davey Smith, eds., Oxford: Blackwell Publishers, 1998. Reprinted by permission.

Chapter 18: Dennis Raphael and Toba Bryant, "The Limitations of Population Health as a Model for a New Public Health," *Health Promotion International,* 17(2), 2002. © Oxford University Press. Reprinted by permission.

Chapter 19: Nancy Krieger, "Theories for Social Epidemiology in the 21st Century: An Ecosocial Perspective," *International Journal of Epidemiology,* Vol. 30: 668–677, 2001. © Oxford University Press. Reprinted by permission.

Part Three

Chapter 20: Previously unpublished.

Chapter 21: Previously unpublished.

Chapter 22: Nancy Moss, "Socioeconomic Disparities in Health in the US: An Agenda for Action," *Social Science & Medicine,* Vol. 51: 1627–1638, 2000. © Elsevier Science. Reprinted by permission.

Chapter 23: Hilary Graham, "From Science to Policy: Options for Reducing Health Inequalities," in *Poverty, Inequality and Health: An International Perspective,* David Leon and Gill Walt, eds., Oxford: Oxford University Press, 2001. © Oxford University Press. Reprinted by permission.

Chapter 24: Arline T. Geronimus, "Addressing Structural Influences on the Health of Urban Populations," *American Journal of Public Health,* 90(6): 867–872, 2000. © American Public Health Association. Reprinted by permission.

ACKNOWLEDGMENTS

This book was made possible through many months of dialogue with friends and colleagues who offered their time and effort in reviewing the introduction and outline for the book. Many thanks to Julie Barnet, Grigsby Hubbard, Nancy Meyer, Carles Muntaner, and Dennis Raphael.

A good deal of thanks is in order as well to those who engaged in many insightful discussions about health inequities, including Rajiv Bhatia, Margy Heldring, Barbara Krimgold, Vincent Lafronza, Mary Northridge, Elaine O'Keefe, Ngozi Oleru, Adewale Troutman, Teresa Wall, and Larry Wallack.

Thanks to my editor at Jossey-Bass, Andy Pasternack, who provided a great deal of guidance and support along the way, and to Seth Schwartz, who organized the logistics and kept me on schedule.

Finally, I owe a great debt and special thanks to Ruth Etzel, not only for reviewing the manuscript, but also for her ongoing support, encouragement, and many ideas throughout the project.

R.H.

PREFACE

What does social justice have to do with health? I became interested in editing a book focusing on this question because of two concerns. The first concern is that the United States spends more on health than any nation yet continues to have some of the poorest health outcomes in the industrialized world. The distribution of health outcomes is extremely uneven across population groups according to class, race, and gender. The second concern is the way in which our society treats social and economic injustices as problems to be managed instead of transforming the power relations and rules that give rise to those injustices. Although the knowledge that social and economic inequality produces inequities in health status has long been available, policymakers avoid their root causes. Contemporary approaches in the health professions provide fairly narrow frames of reference directed primarily at service delivery.

In recent years, new efforts have been initiated to explore, in a limited way, some of the underlying conditions that generate inequalities in health and well-being. But discussions about the conditions necessary for producing health and well-being often ignore analysis of the political conflicts that might suggest why some population groups are healthier than others.

PURPOSE OF THE BOOK

Health and Social Justice, a collection of reprinted and new articles, assembles a broad range of contributors in different fields, including sociology, epidemiology, public health, ecology, politics, organizing, and advocacy in order to explore particular political and ideological aspects of health inequities among different population groups. Its purpose is to extend public debate about the ways in which the sources of health inequities derive from injustices associated with class, race, and gender relations and to encourage questioning of contemporary approaches, in theory and practice, in addressing them. It presents many different strands of recent progressive analysis of the political issues surrounding inequalities in health and offers innovative ideas for action and research.

The central theme of the book is that creating health equity requires a coherent strategy that addresses social and economic inequality, as well as the ideologies that support and sustain it. A major assumption for many of the contributors is that imbalances in political power and the institutions that maintain those power relations are primarily responsible for producing inequities, apart from other uncertainties and immeasurable factors. Controlling the definition of health has important implications for choosing among competing approaches to create and sustain healthy communities. Eliminating health inequities is important as a matter of social justice because health is an asset and a resource critical to human development, beneficial to society overall.

Taking as a given much of the research documenting the strong relationship between social and economic inequality and health inequities, the book's authors examine the issues and conflicts underlying the sources of those inequities. By drawing attention to the priorities, ideologies, and values embedded in political choices, it challenges assumptions about the definition of health as well as assumptions about how to achieve equity in health outcomes. For example, recent research on health inequities suggests that enhanced social services or other interventions aimed primarily at effects cannot eliminate the sources of health inequities.

The contributors to this book provide the context, research, methods, and frameworks that allow us to rethink how we might create health equity or at least overcome barriers to achieving it. Most take for granted the relevance of structural determinants of health in examining disease causation and the requirements for well-being more generally. For them, health is a dynamic concept, broadly defined, emphasizing quality of life and the exercise of physical and social capacities.

ORGANIZATION OF THE BOOK

Three broadly linked themes organize the work in three parts. The chapters in the first part, "Social Forces Exacerbating Health Inequities," concern the influence of economic, political, and social forces that cause health inequities, primarily in the United States and Canada, with some focus on international issues that transcend borders. Dennis Raphael provides a summary of the social determinants of health. James House and David Williams focus on the role of racism in generating inequalities in health, and Piroska Östlin, Asha George, and Gita Sen examine the effects of gender discrimination. John Gershman, Alec Irwin, and Aaron Shakow explore the global connections among growth, poverty, and health inequity, followed by Vincente Navarro and Leiyu Shi's consideration of how the character of political institutions in a society contribute to health disparities. John Lynch, George Davey Smith, George Kaplan, and James House evaluate the role of income and material conditions as they affect health outcomes, while Julianna Maantay homes in on the effects of zoning and land use decisions. Finally, Sarah Kuhn and John Wooding examine the way in which workplace conditions and the organization of work influence health. These chapters cover only a small number of specific major determinants of health, but the analyses contained in them demonstrate the strong relation between social and economic inequality and inequities among and within particular population groups. This relationship, often ignored and often associated with structural and institutional factors, has been known for a long time.

The chapters in Part Two, "Theory, Ideology, and Politics: Critical Perspectives," involve an exploration of key ideologies and paradigms that limit coordinated public action and obscure underlying causes. Prevailing paradigms essentially depoliticize the social conflict surrounding the issue, distracting attention from structural sources of inequity. Contributors analyze how the perspectives, assumptions, and methodologies in epidemiology and society reflect values and power relations that determine choices made about how to confront health inequities.

Dan Beauchamp begins by demonstrating the intimate connection between public health and social justice and how market values often dominate over collective needs for well-being. Carles Muntaner, John Lynch, and George Davey Smith then critique the concept of social capital and psychosocial factors in seeking to explain health inequities. Paula Braveman follows with an examination of the politics of methodology and its ideological implications for public policy. Alexandra Bambas and Juan Antonio Casas, demonstrating the importance of categories of analysis and language, provide precise definitions of health inequity and criteria for its identification. The chapter by David Coburn shows how the market-oriented political doctrine of neoliberalism finds affinity with recent theories of income inequality and social cohesion as an explanation of poor health status and how this leads to ignoring the broader social context of health inequalities. Following on this analysis, John Lynch demonstrates the need to look beyond income inequality as an explanation of health inequalities to larger political, cultural, economic, and historical factors. In a critique of assumptions within epidemiology and Western science that have limited the ability to cope with the emergence of new diseases and the reemergence of old ones, Richard Levins investigates the connection among disease, the changing ecosystem, and inequities within the social order of capitalism. Jennie Popay, Gareth Williams, Carol Thomas, and Anthony Gatrell present a theoretical framework for considering the role of lay knowledge in inequalities research that would more effectively link social structure to human agency. Dennis Raphael and Toba Bryant explore the ideological implications of population health as a model for public health, criticizing its lack of a values base and inattention to social structures as determinants of health. Finally, Nancy Krieger, seeking better approaches to explaining population patterns of health, well-being, and disease, argues for more adequate theorization within social epidemiology to link biology and the material world.

The chapters in Part Three, "Strategies: Perspectives on Social Policy and Practice," center on actions that could eliminate health inequities, locally and nationally, based on principles of social justice and emphasizing root causes. Dennis Raphael reviews approaches to influence the social determinants of health. Ronald Labonte analyzes the consequences of globalization and offers a framework for assessing its impact on health, particularly as related to increased poverty, income inequality, and environmental sustainability. Nancy Moss evaluates strategies drawn from the European experience, among others, aimed at health inequities. Relying on international experiences, Hillary Graham examines three policy choices to reduce inequalities, emphasizing income redistribution, improvements in employment opportunities, and publicly funded welfare services. Based on a structural analysis and recent research on race and class, Arline Geronimus proposes principles for action and research in an urban environment. At the level of practice, Rajiv Bhatia provides case studies involving challenges faced by a local public health agency in seeking to act on health inequities. Gavin Kearney discusses similar issues at the state level in Minnesota. Finally, Lawrence Wallack offers a detailed analysis of the importance of the mass media in influencing the conceptualization of public health issues.

Concepts and ideas expressed throughout overlap within the different parts of the book. What connects the three parts is the way the outcomes of political struggles—whether about the definition of health or about the nature of effective public policy—influence the health and well-being of population groups.

This book will be of value to anyone with an interest in the sources of inequalities in health, both material and ideological, and in seeking political strategies that might address them. Thus the book will be useful for health practitioners and social epidemiologists, organizers and activists. In the classroom, *Health and Social Justice* provides a supplement to the literature that analyzes the research findings in this field, as well as a counterpoint to the more mainstream theories that underlie the analysis. Students in schools of public health, environmental sociology, health policy, medical sociology, environmental sociology, and political science will find the book useful in numerous ways: to identify the social determinants of health—social and economic conditions that improve community health; to examine the political implications of differing paradigms and perspectives used to explain health inequities; and to explore alternative strategies for eliminating health inequities. Readers will find that the contributors suggest possibilities for social change that go well beyond remediation.

August 2003

Richard Hofrichter
Washington, D.C.

THE CONTRIBUTORS

The Editor

Richard Hofrichter is a writer and social critic. He is the editor of *Reclaiming the Environmental Debate: The Politics of Health in a Toxic Culture* (MIT Press, 2000) and *Toxic Struggles: The Theory and Practice of Environmental Justice* (University of Utah Press, [1993] 2002), as well as the author of *Neighborhood Justice in Capitalist Society: The Expansion of the Informal State* (Greenwood Press, 1987). He received a doctorate in politics from the City University of New York in 1983.

The Authors

Alexandra Bambas is the coordinator of the Global Equity Gauge Alliance, based in Durban, South Africa. After receiving a master of public health degree from the University of Texas and a doctorate in medical humanities from the University of Texas Medical Branch, she worked on issues of health equity with the Division of Health and Human Development at the Pan American Health Organization. Her area of expertise is ethics in public health policy, and she is especially interested in the process of developing effective advocacy arguments for health equity in different cultures and contexts.

Dan E. Beauchamp is an emeritus professor at the State University of New York, Albany, School of Public Health. His most recent publications are *New Ethics for the Public's Health* (edited with Bonnie Steinbock; Oxford University Press, 1999) and *The Health of the Republic: Epidemics, Medicine, and Moralism as Challenges to Democracy* (Temple University Press, 1988). In his retirement, he is serving his second term as the mayor of Bisbee, Arizona, a former mining town located near the U.S.-Mexico border.

Rajiv Bhatia is director of occupational and environmental health in the San Francisco Department of Public Health. He is also assistant clinical professor of medicine at the University of California, San Francisco. His experience reflects medicine, epidemiology, environmental policy and decision making, and program implementation and evaluation. His current research focuses on the health effects of pesticides; social, instrumental, and institutional barriers to healthy indoor environments; and the economic effectiveness of supportive housing for homeless individuals. He is also investigating and applying model approaches for participatory decision analysis in social and environmental policy through the integration of participatory research and health impact assessment. He serves on the boards of the Pesticide Action Network and the Sambhavna Trust in Bhopal, India, and is chair of the Health and Social Justice Committee for the National Association of County and City Health Officials.

Paula A. Braveman, M.D., M.P.H., is professor of family and community medicine and director of the Center on Social Disparities in Health at the University of California, San Francisco. She is recognized for her research on social inequalities in health and her active leadership in bringing attention to this field in the United States and internationally. A member of the Institute of Medicine, she has studied socioeconomic and racial/ethnic inequalities in maternal and infant health and policies to reduce the disparities for over two decades.

Toba Bryant is a postdoctoral fellow at the Centre for Health Studies at York University in Toronto, Canada. Her doctoral thesis examined how housing and health activists used different forms of knowledge to influence policy development during the "Common Sense Revolution" in Ontario. She is currently investigating how the ideological stances of government policymakers shape state receptivity to the theoretical concepts and demonstrated importance of the social determinants of health. Her recent publications have been concerned with the policy change process, hospital restructuring in Ontario, population health, and the quality of life of Toronto's seniors as revealed through a participatory policy process.

Juan Antonio Casas is the senior external relations officer of the World Health Organization Office for the European Union. He is a medical doctor with a master's degree in social medicine and public health and has worked for twenty-five years in academic and technical cooperation activities in international health with UNICEF and the Pan American/World Health Organization in Central America and the Caribbean and in the PAHO/WHO regional office in Washington as director of the Division of Health and Human Development.

David Coburn is a professor in the Department of Public Health Sciences, University of Toronto, Canada. His interests have focused on work and health, health occupations and professions, and the political economy of health and health care. He is coeditor of the reader *Health and Canadian Society* (University of Toronto Press, 1998) and coauthor of *Medicine, Nursing, and the State* (Garamond Press, 1999). His most recent publication on health inequalities is "Beyond the Income Inequality Hypothesis: Class, Neo-Liberalism and Health Inequalities" (*Social Science and Medicine*, 2003).

George Davey Smith is a professor of clinical epidemiology in the Department of Social Medicine at the University of Bristol in England. He was a member of the noise terrorism outfit Scum Auxiliary in the early 1980s, but since commercial and critical success eluded that group, he has since worked as a social epidemiologist. His research interests include inequalities in health and the long-term effects of early-life influences on health in adulthood. He is the author of numerous articles and books, including coeditor, with Mel Bartley and David Blane, of *The Sociology of Health Inequalities* (Blackwell, 1998).

Anthony Gatrell is professor of geography of health at Lancaster University in England and also director of the Institute for Health Research. His research interests are in geographical epidemiology and health inequalities. His most recent book is *Geographies of Health* (Blackwell, 2002).

Asha George has an M.Sc. from the Harvard School of Public Health. As a Research Fellow at the Harvard Center for Population and Development Studies, she coordinated research on gender and health that resulted in a variety of publications, including *Engendering International Health: The Challenge of Equity* coedited with Gita Sen and Piroska Östlin. She currently works as a Research Consultant at the Indian Institute of Management, Bangalore, India, while being a doctoral candidate at the Institute of Development Studies, Sussex University. Her field research focuses on health care delivery in rural, northern Karnataka from a perspective that combines public sector accountability with reproductive health and health systems analysis. She is an Editorial Advisory Board member for the journal *Reproductive Health Matters*.

Arline T. Geronimus is professor of health behavior and health education senior research scientist at the Population Studies Center, Institute for Social Research, University of Michigan. She is also affiliated with the Center for Research on Ethnicity, Culture and Health. She has also served on NIH study sections and worked with the U.S. Civil Rights Commission, the Federal Reserve Bank of New York, and the Aspen Institute's Roundtable on Comprehensive Community Initiatives to revitalize American cities. She developed an analytical framework known as "weathering" that posits that the health of African Americans is subject to early health deterioration as a consequence of social exclusion.

John Gershman is codirector of Foreign Policy in Focus and the Interhemispheric Resource Center's Global Affairs Program and Outside the U.S./South-North dialogue projects. The center is located in Silver City, New Mexico. He holds a master's degree in political science from the University of California, Berkeley, where he is currently a doctoral candidate. He is also an adjunct professor of public administration at New York University's Robert F. Wagner School for Public Service. Prior to working at the Interhemispheric Resource Center, he was a research fellow at the Institute for Health and Social Justice in Cambridge, Massachusetts, and policy director at Food First/The Institute for Food and Development Policy, in Oakland, California.

Hillary Graham is director of the Economic and Social Research Council's Health Variations Programme, a five-year research program concerned with advancing understanding of socioeconomic inequalities in health. Her background is in sociology and social policy, and she has held research and training posts spanning both disciplines. She is the author of numerous articles and books and editor of *Understanding Health Inequalities* (Open University Press, 2000).

James S. House is a senior research scientist and former director of the Survey Research Center at the Institute for Social Research, as well as professor of sociology and former chair of the Department of Sociology at the University of Michigan. He received his Ph.D. in social psychology from the University of Michigan in 1972. His research has focused on the role of social and psychological factors in the etiology and course of health and illness, currently emphasizing the role of psychosocial factors in explaining social inequalities in health and the way health changes with age. He is an elected member of the American Academy of Arts and Sciences and the Institute of Medicine of the National Academies of Science, author of *Work Stress and Social Support* (1981), coeditor of *Aging, Health Behaviors, and Health Outcomes* (1992) and *Sociological Perspectives on Social Psychology* (1995), and an associate editor (for health entries) of the *International Encyclopedia of the Social and Behavioral Sciences* (2001).

Alec Irwin is a research associate at Partners in Health, Boston. Previously, he taught in the Religion Department at Amherst College. He coedited *Dying for Growth* and is coauthor, with Dorothy Fallows and Joyce Millen, of *Global AIDS: Myths and Facts* (South End Press, 2003).

George A. Kaplan is professor and chair of the Department of Epidemiology in the School of Public Health; a senior research scientist at the Institute for Social Research; and director of the Michigan Initiative on Inequalities in Health, the Michigan Interdisciplinary Center on Social Inequalities, Mind, and Body, and the Center for Social Epidemiology and Population Health—all at the University of Michigan. He is also an associate in the Population Health Program of the Canadian Institute for Advanced Research. He also directs the newly formed Robert Wood Johnson Foundation Health and Society Scholars Program at the University of Michigan. Among his recent honors are membership in the Institute of Medicine and election to the presidency of the Society for Epidemiologic Research. He has published over two hundred papers on the role of behavioral, social, psychological, and socioeconomic factors in disease prevention and health promotion.

Gavin Kearney is the director of research and programs at the Institute on Race and Poverty at the University of Minnesota Law School. He was a member of the Social Conditions and Health Action Team, which produced the *Call to Action* report, and subsequently served on the Minnesota Health Improvement Partnership's Health Impact Assessment Action Team. He holds a J.D. degree from the University of Minnesota Law School.

Nancy Krieger is an associate professor in the Department of Health and Social Behavior the Harvard School of Public Health in Boston. She is coeditor, with Elizabeth Fee, of *Women's Health, Politics, and Power: Essays on Sex/Gender, Medicine and Public Health* (Baywood Press, 1994) and the author of dozens of empirical studies and theoretical articles on epidemiological issues related to understanding and analyzing social inequalities in health, past and present, especially in relation to social class, racism, race/ethnicity, gender, and sexuality.

Sarah Kuhn is an associate professor in the Department of Regional Economic and Social Development at the University of Massachusetts in Lowell. The author of several articles and monographs on information technology professionals, the computerized workplace, and the reform of technical education, she is also a principal investigator of Project TechForce, a National Science Foundation–funded study of women and men in the software and Internet industry in Massachusetts. She served on the National Research Council's Workforce Needs in Information Technology committee and helped draft the committee's report, *Building a*

Workforce for the Information Economy (National Academy Press, 2001). She was a fellow at the Radcliffe Public Policy Center, Radcliffe Institute for Advanced Study, Harvard University, in 2000–2001.

Ronald Labonte is director of the Saskatchewan Population Health and Evaluation Research Unit; a professor at the University of Saskatchewan and at the University of Regina; and a member of the International Union for Health Promotion and Education's Advocacy Working Group. He also consults on the links among globalization, trade, and health for the World Health Organization. He is a coauthor of *Fatal Indifference: The G8 and Global Health* (University of Capetown Press, 2003). He is also a member of the steering committee for the Canadian Coalition for Global Health Research, a new organization dedicated to closing the "10/90" gap in global health research—the fact that more than 90 percent of health research goes into problems affecting fewer than 10 percent of the planet's wealthier citizens.

Richard Levins teaches human ecology at the Harvard School of Public Health in Boston and is on the advisory boards of the River Watch Network and the International Society for Ecosystem Health. He is the author of *Evolution in Changing Environments* (Princeton University Press, 1968) and coauthor, with Richard Lewontin, of *The Dialectical Biologist* (Harvard University Press, 1986).

John W. Lynch is an associate professor in the Department of Epidemiology, School of Public Health, at the University of Michigan. He has joint appointments at the Center for Human Growth and Development, the Institute for Social Research, and the Center for Research on Ethnicity, Culture and Health. His research investigates how life course processes acting at multiple levels in different birth cohorts affect overall levels and the social distribution of different components of population health. In addition to his U.S.-based research interests, he has research collaborations in Australia, Brazil, Britain, Canada, Denmark, Finland, Norway, and Sweden.

Juliana A. Maantay is an associate professor of urban and environmental geography at Lehman College, City University of New York, and director of Lehman's Geographical Information Science (GISc) program. She has more than two decades' experience as an urban and environmental planner and policy analyst and has been active in environmental justice research and advocacy for the past ten years. Her recent research on environmental justice has been published in the *American Journal of Public Health, Environmental Health Perspectives,* and the *Journal of Law, Medicine, and Ethics.* She is the author of *GIS for the Urban Environment* (Environmental Systems Research Institute Press, 2003). She holds a doctorate in environmental geography from Rutgers University, a master's degree in urban planning from New York University, and a master's degree in geographic information systems from Hunter College/CUNY.

Nancy E. Moss is Program Officer for the Global Network for Women's and Children's Health Research in the Center for Research on Mothers and Children at the National Institute of Child Health and Human Development, Rockville, Maryland. She is a social demographer and has devoted much of her career to research on the ethnic, social, economic, and cultural factors affecting risk behavior, morbidity, and mortality in women's, children's, and adolescent health, with a special emphasis on Latinas. She has also served as lead investigator in studies examining the effects of state and national health policies and programs on the health of women and children. During the 1990s, she participated in numerous activities calling attention to the need for improved socioeconomic measures and data. Her current work looks at the interaction of gender and socioeconomic context among African American and Latina women and Latino adolescents' perspectives on neighborhood characteristics.

Carles Muntaner is a professor in the Department of Behavioral and Community Health at the University of Maryland's School of Nursing and in the Department of Epidemiology and Preventive Medicine at the university's School of Medicine. Since the 1980s, his research has been focusing on the role of social class, racism, work organization, and political factors in shaping social inequalities in health.

Vincente Navarro is a professor of health and public policy, sociology, and policy studies at the Johns Hopkins University in Baltimore and professor of political and social sciences at the Universidad Pompeu Fabra in Spain. He is founder and editor in chief of the *International Journal of Health Services* and has written extensively on health and public policy themes. He recently edited the first volume of *The Political Economy of Social Inequalities: Consequences for Health and Quality of Life* (Baywood Press, 2000).

Piroska Östlin is a social epidemiologist with a Ph.D. in Medical Science from the University of Uppsala in Sweden. Currently, she is Research Manager at the Swedish National Institute of Public Health and Adjunct Senior Lecturer in Public Health at the Karolinska Institute, Department of International Health. Her research concerns methodological problems in occupational epidemiology, as well as the significance of the work environment on women's and men's health. She was formerly secretary of the National Public Health Commission, where she was responsible for defining national public health targets and suggesting strategies to reduce social inequalities in health between different segments of the Swedish society. She is coeditor, with Gita Sen and Asha

George, of *Engendering International Health: The Challenge of Equity* (MIT Press, 2002), and coeditor with Maria Danielsson, Finn Diderichesen, Annika Harenstam, and Gudrun Lundberg of *Gender Inequalities in Health: A Swedish Perspective* (Harvard University Press, 2002).

Jennie Popay is professor of sociology and public health at the Institute for Health Research at the University of Lancaster and has more than three decades of experience in the health and social policy fields, where she has published widely. Her research interests include gender and social class, inequalities in health, and the sociology of knowledge, with particular reference to the relationship between lay and professional knowledge in the sphere of public health. Recent publications include the edited collections *Dilemmas in Health Care* (with Basiro Davey; Open University Press, 1993), *Researching the People's Health* (with Gareth Williams; Routledge, 1994), and *Men, Gender Divisions, and Welfare* (with Jeff Hearn and Jeanette Edwards; Routledge, 1998).

Dennis Raphael is an associate professor at the School of Health Policy and Management and a member of the Atkinson Faculty of Liberal and Professional Studies at York University in Toronto, Canada. A native of New York City, he was trained in human development and education. The most recent of his more than one hundred scientific publications have focused on the health effects of income inequality and poverty, the quality of life of communities and individuals, and the impact of governmental decisions on North Americans' health and well-being.

Gita Sen is Sir Ratan Tata Chair Professor at the Indian Institute of Management in Bangalore, India, and adjunct professor of population and international health at the Faculty of Public Health, Harvard University. She is a member of the Global Advisory Committee on Health Research of the World Health Organization. She also works with a number of nongovernmental organizations and other institutions in a consultative or advisory capacity. Her publications include *Engendering International Health: The Challenge of Equity* (MIT Press, 2002), *Women's Empowerment and Demographic Processes: Moving Beyond Cairo* (Oxford University Press, 2000), and *Population Policies Reconsidered: Health, Empowerment, and Rights* (Harvard Center for Population and Development Studies, 1994). She received the Volvo Environment Prize from the Volvo Foundation in 1994 and honorary doctorates from the University of East Anglia in 1998 and from the Karolinska Institute in 2003.

Aaron Shakow is a research affiliate at the Institute for Health and Social Justice. A historian by training, his work has focused on the transnational spread of health and development policy as sociopolitical phenomena, with special emphasis on Latin America and the Middle East. Since 1997, he has worked with the medical nonprofit Partners in Health as a grantwriter and public relations specialist. He is currently a doctoral candidate in the Department of History at Harvard University, focusing on the drug trade between Europe and the Ottoman Empire in the seventeenth and eighteenth centuries.

Leiyu Shi is an associate professor in the Department of Health Policy and Management at Johns Hopkins School of Public Health and codirector of Johns Hopkins Primary Care Policy Center for the Underserved Populations. His research focuses on primary care, health disparities, and vulnerable populations. He has conducted extensive studies on the association between primary care and health outcomes, particularly on the role of primary care in mediating the adverse impact of income inequality on health outcomes. He is also well known for his extensive research on the nation's vulnerable populations, in particular community health centers that serve vulnerable populations, including their sustainability, provider recruitment and retention experiences, financial performance, experience under managed care, quality of primary care, and disparities in care and health.

Carol Thomas is a senior lecturer on the sociology of health and illness in the Institute for Health Research at Lancaster University in England. Her research interests are disability studies, cancer and palliative care, and women's health. She is the author of *Female Forms: Experiencing and Understanding Disability* (Buckingham: Open University Press, 1999).

Lawrence Wallack is professor and director of the School of Community Health, College of Urban and Public Affairs, Portland State University, Portland, Oregon, and emeritus professor of public health at the University of California, Berkeley. In 1993, he was the founding director of the Berkeley Media Studies Group, an organization conducting research and training in the use of media to promote healthy public policies. He is one of the primary architects of media advocacy—an innovative approach to working with mass media to advance public health. He has published extensively and lectures frequently on the news media and public health policy issues. He is the principal author of *News for a Change: An Advocate's Guide to Working with the Media* (Sage, 1999) and *Media Advocacy and Public Health: Power for Prevention* (Sage, 1993). He is also coeditor of *Mass Media and Public Health: Complexities and Conflicts* (Sage, 1990).

David R. Williams is professor of sociology, a faculty associate in the African American Mental Health Research Center, and a senior research scientist at the Institute for Social Research, University of Michigan, Ann Arbor. His extensive research focuses on the socioeconomic status and health of the African American population. His publications have examined how psychosocial factors—ranging from stress, racism, and social support to psychological behaviors—are linked to social status and may affect socioeconomic and racial variation in health.

Gareth Williams is professor of sociology and deputy director of the Public Health Research and Resource Centre at the University of Salford in England. He has published extensively in sociological and health journals and is coauthor of *Understanding Rheumatoid Arthritis* (Routledge, 1996) and *Markets and Networks* (Open University Press, 1996) and coeditor of *Challenging Medicine* (Routledge, 1994) and *Researching the People's Health* (Routledge, 1994).

John Wooding is professor of political science and provost of the University of Massachusetts, Lowell. He has written extensively in the field of occupational and environmental health policy and is coeditor (with Charles Levenstein) of *Work, Health, and Environment: Old Problems, New Solutions* (Guilford Press, 1997) and coauthor (with Charles Levenstein) of *The Point of Production: The Political Economy of the Work Environment* (Guilford Press, 1999).

CHAPTER ONE

The Politics of Health Inequities

Contested Terrain

Richard Hofrichter

ven though mortality rates overall declined dramatically in the twentieth century and life expectancy increased, the United States nevertheless faces an increasing level of inequity in the health status and mortality of those with less material resources in relation to their social class, particularly in communities of color (Kawachi, Kennedy, and Wilkinson, 1999; Arno and Figueroa, 2000; LaVeist, 2002). For example, African Americans experience excess mortality and morbidity rates substantially higher than those for whites (National Center for Health Statistics, 2000; Williams, 1999). Differences in aggregate health status become inequitable when they are systemic and unjust, a result related to a lack of political power (Whitehead, 1987; Dahlgren and Whitehead, 1991; Evans and others, 2001; see also Chapter Twelve). That is, these patterned, persistent inequities (Beaglehole and Bonita, 1997; Bartley, Blane, and Davey Smith, 1998; Drever and Whitehead, 1977; Institute of Medicine, 2002) are due primarily to failed political struggles and power imbalances, not ad hoc events, individual failure, or the inevitable consequences of modern society. Material conditions such as poverty, inadequate housing, and excessive air pollution, generated by law, public policy, corporate decision making, and sometimes violence, produce and perpetuate health inequities. These conditions often derive from the institutional political and social power conferred by great inequalities of wealth (Callinicos, 2000; Halfon and Hochstein, 2002). Yet most discussions of health, whether in scholarship or the mass media, rarely touch on political

1

conflict. Health is usually about health of the individual, health care, behavior and lifestyles, or developments in medical research. Although equitable access to health care is necessary, it represents only a small part of the requirements necessary for eliminating health inequities (Beaglehole and Bonita, 1997). The United States, for example, is not investing to create the social and economic conditions for health (Arno and Figueroa, 2000). Yet historically, major advances in health status resulted from broad social reforms. These include actions such as the abolition of child labor, shortening of the working day, introduction of social security, reductions in the scale of poverty, improvements in the standard of living, and guaranteeing employment or at least a minimum wage, as well as efforts to improve sanitation, ensure safe food, and provide adequate housing. Improvements in living and working conditions led to reductions in deaths from major infectious diseases. Public health as a discipline arose as an organized response to the negative consequences of industrialization. Later, legislative developments such as the Social Security Act, the Clean Air Act, the Mine Safety Act, and the establishment of the Occupational Safety and Health Administration and Medicare were major steps that improved health for millions of people (Rose, 1992; Porter, 1999).

Although macro-level forces explain only part of a complex story of social structures, conditions, and events that influence health, they have generally been neglected until recently. Even less well examined is the part that power, politics, ideology, and conflict play in how those forces come to influence health and create inequities. Social conflicts involving inequalities continue to be displaced into the market or specializations within science, evading politics.

This chapter presents a framework for understanding and acting on health inequities. I begin by outlining major social, economic, and political forces that contribute to health inequities, explaining their connection through the concepts of class, race, gender, and social justice. I then consider the way in which contemporary ideologies that organize the social order limit critical thinking, thereby constraining effective action. The last part of the chapter offers suggestions for communicating and organizing more effectively to eliminate health inequities both within and outside of the health professions.

This is an opportune historical moment to examine inequities in health and well-being and to question the definition of health. As social and economic inequality widens dramatically and becomes impossible to ignore, the connection between the vulnerability of people who live on the margins and the importance of working together collectively as a community for the public good has become more salient, if unarticulated. A clearer picture is emerging of the relationship between community-level well-being, resources for basic infrastructure, economic equality, and good health (Institute of Medicine, 2002). Yet in the United States, the federal government continues to target diseases rather than health and redirects resources toward bioterrorism and military preparedness instead of the public health infrastructure (Altman, 2003).

Worldwide, growing social and economic inequality, a basic cause of inequalities in health status, is equally stark (Kim and others, 2000; United Nations Development Program, 1999; Beaglehole and Bonita, 1997; Wilkinson and Marmot, 1998). The richest two hundred people in the world have wealth equivalent to 41 percent of the world's population. About 20 percent of the world's population receives over 80 percent of domestic investment and global trade and income (United Nations Development Program, 1999). According to the World Health Organization, the gap between rich and poor within the industrialized countries, including the United States, is widening (Beaglehole and Bonita, 1997; Labonte, 1998; Wilkinson and Marmot, 1998; Arno and Figueroa, 2000; Callinicos, 2000).

Strikingly, in the United States, income and wealth inequality is greater than in any other industrialized country in the world (Ackerman, 2000; Kawachi, Kennedy, and Wilkinson, 1999; Wolff, 2002), wider than it has been for fifty years and continuing to deteriorate (Wolff, 2002; National Center for Health Statistics, 1998; Reich, 1997; Pappas and others, 1993; Madrick, 2002; Phillips, 2002; Pear, 2002; Krugman, 2002; Miringoff and Miringoff, 1999; Congressional Budget Office, 2001). A survey by the Federal Reserve Board in 2003 indicates a sharp rise in inequality, countering conventional notions about the boom years of the 1990s (Andrews, 2003). The share of wealth received by the wealthiest fifth of the population is greater than at any time since World War II (Wolff, 2002). Almost one-quarter of all children in the United States live in officially defined poverty (Danziger, Danziger, and Stern, 2000). In 2000, nearly one-fourth of the U.S. population earned poverty-level wages (Mishel, Bernstein, and Schmitt, 2001. Household net worth has declined dramatically since 1983 (Wolff, 2000). Tax rates for the wealthiest Americans also continue to decline as their wealth increases (Congressional Budget Office, 2001).

Great social costs arise from these inequities, including threats to economic development, democracy, quality of life, the exclusion of people from full participation in society, and the social well-being of the nation (Kawachi and Kennedy, 2002). Inequality limits people's freedom to develop their capacities and capabilities to the fullest (Sen, 1992). Countries with the most inequality often show signs of social disintegration, violence, and greater poverty (Wilkinson, 1996). Investments in infrastructure such as schools, transportation, and the environment tend to be lower in such societies. Economic growth and productivity gains have not led to better wages or more leisure time.

Serious health consequences result from these inequities, accumulating over the course of a lifetime (Davey Smith and others, 1997). They range from increased and unnecessary excess rates of mortality, morbidity, and psychological stress to reductions in economic productivity (Kuh and others, 2002). Even if people have access to the necessities of life, research shows that that may not be enough to participate fully in society, particularly in relation to things like access to adequate employment, adequate nutrition, modern communications technology, specialized training and skills, or health services (Kawachi and Kennedy, 2002). The most egalitarian countries in the world, not the richest, have the best health status (Wilkinson, 1996; Daniels, Kennedy, and Kawachi, 2000). In the United States, data show that states with greater inequality, such as Texas, Louisiana, Mississippi, New York, and West Virginia, have poorer health status than states with greater equality, such as Wisconsin, Utah, Minnesota, and Iowa (Miringoff, Miringoff, and Opdyke, 2001; see also Kaplan and others, 1996, and Kawachi and Kennedy, 2002).

Since the time of Rudolf Virchow, a public health pathologist, and sanitary reformer Edwin Chadwick in the nineteenth century, Western researchers and health professionals have understood the importance of the relationship between social class and mortality and morbidity (Hamlin, 1998; Sram and Ashton, 1998; Rosen, 1993; Porter, 1999; Antonovsky, 1967). A growing and significant body of research accumulated since the 1980s documents unequivocally that poverty, poor quality of life, and income inequality are principal causes of morbidity and mortality (Black and others, 1988; Acheson, 1998; Kawachi, Kennedy, and Wilkinson, 1999; Lynch and Kaplan, 1997; Kawachi, 2000; Kaplan and others, 1996; Wilkinson, 1996; Shaw, Dorling, and Davey Smith, 1999).[1] A wealth of data specifically demonstrate the relationship of racism to inequality in health status and the continuing high mortality rates of African Americans and other people of color, including Latinos and Native Americans, compared with other groups (Williams, 2000; Williams and Collins, 2002; Krieger and others, 1993; Waitzman and Smith, 1998; Northridge and Shepard, 1997). Moreover, health effects of socioeconomic status may be related not only to absolute levels of poverty or severe deprivation *but also to inequality itself* (Marmot and others, 1991). Individuals with relatively high socioeconomic status are less healthy than those with even higher status.

The particular macro-level pathways by which health inequities link to specific exposures are intricate. Establishing how given social contexts interact with multidimensional biological and psychological pathways to cause disease with any quantifiable certainty remains a challenge. These pathways are often tied to the way production and investment decisions, labor market policies, neighborhood and workplace conditions, and racism and sexism connect with individual histories. Essentially, social injustices become embodied in the individual as disease.

The relationships between class and racial inequality and the distribution of disease are gaining increasing attention. Beginning in the early 1990s, many organizations and government agencies initiated intensive action and dedicated resources toward the elimination of health inequities in Canada, Britain, Australia, Sweden, the Netherlands, and, to a lesser extent, the United States. In Britain, the health secretary called for a debate about the National Health

Service to "move away from a preoccupation with health service structures towards a concentration on improved health outcomes across the nation" and argued for "the biggest assault our country has ever seen on health disadvantage [to] start to break the link between poverty and ill health" (Department of Health, 2001). The Department of Health established national targets to reduce health inequalities within a larger policy agenda (Bull and Hamer, 2001). In Australia, the Health Inequalities Research Collaborative works with the federal government to enhance the evidence base across many disciplines and link it to the promotion of public policy, programs, and practice development. In Sweden, the National Public Health Committee proposed goals linked to social determinants of health, particularly full employment and reducing poverty (Östlin and Diderichsen, 2000); Diderichsen and others, 2001). In the Netherlands, the Dutch Ministry of Health conducts research designed to reduce socioeconomic inequities in health through comprehensive strategies with long-term goals (Mackenback and Stronks, 2002). Moreover, the World Health Organization (WHO; 2000) lent its support to minimizing health disparities.

In the United States, advances have been limited. In 2000, the U.S. Department of Health and Human Services established national health goals for 2010, including the elimination of health disparities and ways to assess them, although these goals remain largely symbolic and unprioritized. President Clinton signed into law the Minority Health and Health Disparities Research and Education Act of 2000, which established the National Center on Minority Health and Health Disparities at the National Institutes of Health. Although the Office of Minority Health in the Department of Health and Human Services hosted the National Leadership Summit on Eliminating Racial and Ethnic Disparities in Health in 2002 attended by more than two thousand people, little has come of it. It is conceivable that the attention by the federal government to health disparities reflects a desire to reduce expenditures for state-funded health care and not to transform society to eliminate the root causes of health inequities. The influential report *The Future of the Public's Health*, produced in 2002 by the Institute of Medicine, repeatedly stresses the importance of health inequities as leading to deterioration in population health. What may be done as a result remains to be seen, given the political climate and the reluctance to confront the political and economic interests that cause inequity. In Minnesota, one of the few states to initiate serious action to eliminate health inequities, the Department of Health in the late 1990s established the Minnesota Health Improvement Partnership Action Team on Social Conditions and Health (2001; see also Chapter Twenty-Six). This ongoing initiative seeks to identify action steps to address health disparities and increase analysis of the social conditions that affect health. Nonprofit public-interest organizations, academics in social epidemiology, and grassroots community groups represent some of the main sources that have been articulating bold visions, innovative theoretical perspectives, and strategies for action (see Chapter Nineteen and http://www.thepraxisproject.org). Some organizations may be counted as acting on health inequities even if they do not specifically identify their primary work as health-related.[2] As Nancy Krieger (2001b, p. 421) notes, "Novel investigations informed by the Civil Rights, women's, and other social movements have begun to analyze the health impact of non-economic as well as economic forms of racial discrimination and the ways in which these insults can be buffered or amplified by community characteristics."

This new attention offers possibilities for challenging the way in which many nations now address health inequities and rethinking the definition of a healthy society. It presents opportunities to investigate the role of social class, economic conditions, gender discrimination, and racism in perpetuating health inequality. Yet in the United States, the challenge is not being met. Policymakers often do not act, even with the knowledge that social and physical environments in which people live and work will significantly affect their health and well-being. I will examine why this issue is challenging for policymakers later in this chapter. But first I consider the social and political forces that cause health and health inequities. What makes one society healthier than another? Why do some groups of people historically have better health than other groups?

SOURCES OF THE INEQUITABLE DISTRIBUTION OF DISEASE

Robert Beaglehole and Ruth Bonita (1997, p. 4) note that "the foundations of health are common to all and include basic requirements such as adequate food, safe water, shelter, safety and hope. . . . These foundations have a more profound long-term effect on health status than the activities of the health system." Creating healthy populations depends on the organization of material conditions in everyday life. These conditions, often referred to as the social determinants of health, are deeply connected to the foundations of existence, to the entirety of economic and social life (Link and Phelan, 1995). They include such things as the quality and affordability of housing, level of employment and job insecurity, standard of living, income level, availability and quality of mass transportation, education, social services, crime rates, air and water quality, forms of economic development, racism, poverty, workplace conditions, and political equality. For example, without access to quality housing, education, a living wage, and mass transportation, many people not only become more vulnerable to stress and disease but are also more likely to lack access to resources that enable them to fulfill their capacities and experience well-being. These determinants influence health through biological and psychological pathways that affect individuals and may weaken community supports, thereby causing greater susceptibility to disease.

Social networks, educational systems, and family structure may affect the health of populations, although it remains difficult to quantify and segregate precisely the role of specific determinants. A strong organic link exists between the physical environment and ecosystem and the economic and social health of a community. As Robert Chernomas (1999, p. 17) comments, "the environment in which germs and genes travel is more important in determining disease than germs and genes themselves." Social environments, governed by particular structures of power and privilege, act to create differentials in health status. These disadvantages—interconnected, cumulative, and intergenerational— reduce the capacity for full participation in society.

Independent of individual behavior, the character of the political and economic system and of the ecosystem structure the possibilities for health and illness (McMichael, 2001; see also Chapter Sixteen). For example, a segregated community with high crime rates, low-paying jobs, high levels of pollution, deteriorating schools, one-party political dominance, and limited social supports is more likely than other communities to have many residents with poor health. Many diseases that contribute to inequalities have long histories. Contemporary research suggests that "differences in levels of health and well-being are affected by a dynamic interaction among biology, behavior, and the environment, an interaction that unfolds over the life course of individuals, families, and communities" (Smedley and Syme, 2000, p. 2).

No linear progression of causes can explain patterns of health inequities. The relationships are synergistic, and their sources remain embedded in major economic and social institutions, public policies, and infrastructural arrangements in given circumstances. In part they derive from historical relationships of power and property, racism, and gender discrimination. Income inequality by itself, for example, will not explain a great deal without an examination of relevant linkages with factors like racial segregation, educational opportunities, and the tax structure. This makes demonstrating causality difficult, although the general failure to invest in human development contributes to inequities in health outcomes.

Before highlighting the characteristics of specific determinants and policies that promote health inequalities, I present an overview of the links between major social determinants and the larger social order as a way to explain why social and economic inequality exists in the first place. Without such a context, it is difficult to identify effective strategies that do not rely on single-issue politics or an approach directed toward isolated phenomena instead of organized injustice.

CLASS, RACE, GENDER, AND HEALTH INEQUITY

The following framework, though brief and preliminary, suggests a way to explore core characteristics and dynamics of the social structure that link most determinants of health. Hierarchies of power considered through the lens of deeply embedded class, race, and gender relations provide the connections between these social and economic determinants, their distribution, and the basis of inequality more adequately than a determinant-by-determinant analysis. Such a theory seeks to explain the specific macro-level characteristics defining the organization of interests and privilege that lead to inequity.

Class relations, always affected by gender and race, contain an independent dynamic within each of the power structures that underlie them. However, for the purpose of linking social determinants of health within the dominant institutions of market relations that govern society on an unequal basis, we can say that racism and sexism are rooted in various forms of material exploitation. The social determinants of health must not be isolated as a list of subjects for "interventions." As Nancy Krieger (1993, p. 166) explains:

> What is not seen is the way in which the underlying structure of racial oppression and class exploitation—which are relationships among people, not between people and things—shape the "environments" of the groups created by these relations. [We must] see the causes of disease and the environment in which they exist as a historical product . . . constructed by society. . . . The same virus may cause pneumonia in blacks and whites alike, just as lead may cause the same physiologic damage—but why the death rate for flu and pneumonia and why blood lead levels are consistently higher in black as compared to white communities is not addressed. [We need a view that can] comprehend the all-important assemblage of features in black life.

Class

The concept of class—which here refers to social groups and their relationship to capital, labor, the labor process, property, and economic ownership—opens the possibilities for exploring the causes of social and economic inequality itself (see Scambler, 2002). Class analysis can show why inequality is not the impersonal, chance, or inevitable result of industrialization, modernization, technology, or the business cycle. It provides an explanation of social development. In class-based societies, people are systematically compelled to cede the surplus they produce to those who control the productive resources and private property. Class thereby reflects the content and processes that define the relations of a capitalist social order. How societies organize production and allocate resources and investments within a particular class formation will affect population health and the distribution of disease.

Carles Muntaner (2002) notes certain misunderstandings with respect to the relationship between class and health inequities and imbalances in political power:

> The recent growth of health disparities scholarship has not been accompanied by a parallel development in its key construct: social class. Rather, new research has kept the "social" in social inequalities to a minimum. . . . The typical pattern of relying on a single ordering of income does not tap into the social mechanisms that explain how individuals arrive at different levels of material resources. . . . By focusing on the properties of social positions rather than persons, power relations clash with the lay assumption that a person's social class reflects some intrinsic attribute. [p. 562]

Class analysis also provides an approach for exploring the continuing reproduction of health inequities, the relationship of health to major economic and political processes, and methods for evaluating strategies to eliminate health inequities, with an emphasis on progressive social change. Given that inequities in political power strongly affect social and economic inequity, what specific features of class power lead to social injustice?

Political power in capitalist societies is the result of antagonistic class interests between capital and labor, not general divisions among people. The outcome of the struggle between these class interests determines the production of society and the specific direction of social change. History is the process through which social change occurs. Class inequity derives not mainly from consumption or distribution but from production and property relations. It concerns the original appropriation of the surplus value created by labor, not advantages that arise from income or occupational status as a location in a generalized hierarchy (see, for example, Wood, 1995a). The concept of class, and its connection to a specific form of domination produced through historically structured social relations, helps explain why health inequities exist. It also suggests the need for structural changes to eliminate health inequities, rather than interventions or services to ameliorate the effects.

What are class antagonisms about? Erik Olin Wright (1994) relies on concepts of oppression and exploitation that are neither pejorative nor general. That is, exploitation has a precise and specific definition in a given social order such as capitalism. Thus he explains the connection to class: "Economic oppression can be defined as a situation in which three conditions are satisfied: (a) the material welfare of one group of people is causally related to the material deprivations of another, (b) the causal relation in (a) involves coercively enforced exclusion from access to productive resources, [and] (c) this exclusion in (b) is morally indictable" (p. 39). He further explains the particular nature of exploitation within capitalism by noting that "the material well-being of exploiters causally depends upon their ability to appropriate the fruits of labor of the exploited . . . [whereby] inequalities . . . are rooted in ownership of and control over productive resources. . . . The exploiter needs the [efforts of the] exploited" (pp. 39–40). The incessant drive to increase the rate of capital accumulation (that is, the unending quest for economic growth because of competition) by reducing labor costs and social investments creates inequities and uneven development, in part because of requirements associated with the need for flexible labor markets, secure infrastructural environments (the conditions and materials necessary for capital accumulation to occur), and increased levels of productivity. Accumulation depends on subjecting people to market imperatives and making them dependent on the market. Establishing these conditions, which are endlessly changing, requires constant negotiation. The class perspective demonstrates why reform and managerial approaches cannot resolve deep antagonisms that concern the conditions of existence. Increasing corporate globalization, however, may result in the expulsion of those already on the margins of society as more people become excluded from production and consumption.

Race

Racial and gendered structures of power and inequality profoundly influence health status because hierarchies of all kinds determine life chances and opportunities. As with class, various forms of racial and gender discrimination and oppression become embedded in social institutions, policies and cultural practices, rules, symbolic codes, and conditions in everyday life. The codings that occur in association with these identities often obscure their connection to class interests. Equally important, racial and gender relations influence class relations dialectically. This sometimes hinders identifying the primacy of one over the other.

Race is a constantly shifting category that is relatively new in human history. Like class, race involves historically constructed social relations that are constantly in flux (see, for example, Omi and Winant, 1993; Cooper and David, 1986). That is to say that although race has been viewed as both an ideology and a real condition based on experience, it is not fixed. The concept has been used as an ideology to justify political domination, exploitation, and exclusion, as well as a means to liberation by those seeking to forge collective identities that could motivate activism for change. Institutional racism, discussed in the next section, concerns practices that reinforce domination.

U.S. government policy demonstrates the many uses of race and ethnicity for political purposes, both in seeking to define or categorize people, as in the census, and in the distribution of resources. Equally important, government policy uses race in profiling individuals as suspects in crimes, determining who gets housing and educational subsidies, and setting other requirements for resource distribution that determine class position. A problem of race for epidemiology and addressing health inequities is not the confusion of racial differences in

health outcomes with biological and genetic differences but rather the failure
to recognize the effects of racism on health (LaVeist, 2002; Krieger, 1993;
Williams and Collins, 2002).

Gender

Gender is also an ideological social construct related to traditions, behaviors,
and relations between the sexes that establish a basis for moral and social life.
As such, it often functions as a vehicle for the systemic appropriation of reproduction, labor, and sexuality from women. Gender relations, which influence
the economy, vary historically and geographically, with no clear connection to
real sexual differences. Gender discrimination or sexism derives from relations
of domination and subordination connected to power imbalances (Barrett,
1980). Differentials in health outcomes between the sexes are more often attributable to sexism than to biological differences. Gender discrimination also
results from inequities in political representation, the division of labor, gender
segregation in labor markets, social stratification, and privatization within the
family, which limit women's access to resources available to men and within
different groups of women (Kawachi and others, 1999). Many government policies (welfare) and definitions (the family, mental health), implemented through
gendered rules and practices within predefined property relations and class positions, determine the nature of exploitation. But the power associated with patri-
archy transcends the question of roles and must be explored within a broader
"structural context of men's and women's lives" through the lens of the social
relations of gender (Annandale and Hunt, 2000, p. 22).

The division of labor along sexual lines, patterns of employment according
to gender, and changing household structures have often led women, particularly of low socioeconomic status, to be denied access to resources and advantages available to men, thereby creating systemic disadvantages that may limit
life chances and negatively influence health. Economic insecurity can lead to
psychosocial stress. Early parenthood creates special stresses for young and poor
women. Occupational segregation and limits on advancement help sustain economic inequities. At the same time, age and education differences play a role
in determining health outcomes that hinder the evaluation of their implications.

Transforming the debate about social and economic inequality and health
inequities suggests the usefulness of a framework to counter that of the market,
discussed later. Such a perspective, offering a basis for major social change,
would help clarify goals and objectives in determining what it means to achieve
health equity. It would also provide a basis for organizational and public policy
alternatives and identify methods to increase public awareness about the need
for new ways of thinking about realizing a healthy society and involving the
public as full participants in the process. I believe that a perspective grounded in
the values of social justice, at the root of public health, provides an adequate
basis for exploring the causes of health inequities and what to do about them.

OUTLINING A SOCIAL JUSTICE PERSPECTIVE

Disparities in health status among different population groups are unjust and inequitable because, as noted, they result from preventable, avoidable, systemic conditions and policies based on imbalances in political power. Without a perspective grounded in values of social justice, approaches to inequities in health will likely aim at symptoms, continuing to rely on cures, treatments, or individual interventions rather than transforming institutions that cause health inequities. While behavior clearly influences premature mortality and health, more basic ongoing socioeconomic conditions affect and condition behavior (Smedley and Syme, 2000). The process by which decisions about investment, labor market policies, taxation, and neighborhood development become linked with individual life histories strongly influences the pathways through which inequality develops.

Theories of disease causation and powerful ideologies such as individualism and the market limit critical thinking about the desirable means for confronting health inequities. A discourse based on social justice supports collective responsibility for achieving healthy communities; it also addresses the social and economic conditions at the core of health inequities.

The commitment to social justice is as old as Western political thought. Social justice has been an animating ideal of all modern democratic governments. Yet its meaning remains obscure, and theories put forward by political philosophers to explain it have often failed to capture the way many people think about it. Social justice is not a thing but rather an ongoing series of relationships that permeate everyday life. Social justice concerns the systematic treatment of people as members of a definable group, such as women or African Americans.

Historically, at least two features define the application of social justice: an opposition to inequality, based on recognition of common human interests, and support for democracy. First, social justice demands an equitable distribution of collective goods, institutional resources (such as social wealth), and life opportunities. Beyond distributional questions, Amartya Sen (1992) defines a just society as one that ensures the development and the capacities of all of its members. Second, social justice calls for democracy—the empowerment of all social members, along with democratic and transparent structures to promote social goals. This is another way of describing political equality.

Inequality in goods production and distribution, resources, and capacities is a negative consequence of unequal privilege, power, and exploitation. Race, class, and gender (along with a more recent addition, sexual identity) have historically been cited as the primary cleavage lines of social injustice. Equality, a goal of social justice, is more than a formal category such as equality before the law or equal opportunity. It is also more than an association with sectarian parties. According to Philip Green (1998), equality concerns "the systematic treatment of representative persons, viewed in the abstract as members and subjects of some organized social whole, rather than with the treatment of particular individuals with unique needs and interests" (p. 4). Achieving equality requires not merely redressing or ameliorating inequitable outcomes but creating a society that does not produce material inequality. Thus, beyond redistribution, it includes rethinking production and the conditions of production within a politics through which it becomes possible to articulate demands for social needs. Equality also means equalizing the circumstances over which people have no control and access to conditions that enable people to realize themselves however they wish. As Amartya Sen (1992) notes, the freedom to achieve through equal access to well-being with freely chosen goals is vastly different from equality of opportunity.

It is also useful to distinguish the concept of equality from equity. Equality refers to sameness, whereas equity refers to fairness. Our concern, as previously stated, is with differences in health status that are unjust. Phrased another way, the goal is to eliminate inequitable differences that systematically favor advantaged social groups. This might mean, for example, valuing communities, families, and the ecosystem over transnational corporations and their interests. Inequality tends to undermine democracy, the second feature of social justice.

Democracy has always depended on the willingness of ordinary people to participate, with or without the support of legal authorities, in social movements aimed at the collective empowerment of *whole classes of people*—women, minorities, workers, youth, the aged. It also depends on support for the social relations and political arrangements necessary to sustain and expand that power. Involving more than formal processes such as voting, it is defined through cooperation, not in the sense of acquiescence, but in relation to participation in all institutions that direct society and shape people's lives. These institutions include the family, schools, and businesses, as well as greater popular control over basic social decisions that determine what gets produced and distributed and for whom. Conventional uses of the term typically weaken the connection of democracy to class as well as the idea of popular power.

Democracy's roots in this regard derive from principles of inclusion rather than exclusion. In addition, democracy requires access to productive resources and the removal of barriers to economic well-being. Greater democracy means subjecting more issues and investment decisions to public decision making, expanding the political agenda. Democracy, a goal of social justice and not merely a means, is achievable only if equality, participation, and mutual respect are part of our institutions. In recent times, U.S. policy has denied social values in favor of market values, making it increasingly difficult to identify public forums and media willing to examine the importance of social justice to the development of a democratic society. Achieving social justice is about changing society so that claims for freedom, equality, and democracy receive adequate expression and so that the politics by which people pursue these goals gain acceptance as normal rather than exceptional and suspect. This sort of change depends on social solidarity, community, mutual reliance, and cooperation.

What has social justice to do with health? Nancy Krieger (1998) notes, "Social justice is the foundation of public health. . . . It is an assertion that reminds us that public health is indeed a public matter, that societal patterns of disease and death, of health and well-being, of bodily integrity and disintegration, intimately reflect the workings of the body politic for good or ill" (p. 1603; see also Sretzer, 1988). Ann Robertson (1998) reminds us that "attempts throughout the twentieth century to align public health with a social justice agenda reveal the persistence of the moral thrust of public health" (p. 1419). The International Society for Equity in Health's definition of health is "the absence of systematic and potentially remediable differences in one or more aspect of health across populations or population subgroups defined socially, economically, demographically or geographically" (Macinko and Starfield, 2002).

Broadly speaking, what principles might define the practice of social justice in the context of the public's health? According to Dan Beauchamp (1988), beyond the "abstract psychology of justice as fairness," we need to develop "shared loyalties to common institutions [that would] create popular solidarity based on political and communal loyalties stemming from the experience of common possession of shared institutions" (p. 24). In Beauchamp's view, "Public health stands for collective control over conditions affecting the common health" (p. 17). Acting on principles of social justice to assure health equity at the level of practice might begin with a commitment to social welfare, the well-being of all—or stated another way, a commitment to meet human need to eliminate health inequities as a priority and to equalize life chances. It would further involve an effort to expose and dramatize health inequities in a way that presents them not as individual and isolated problems but as *public* or *collective* issues.

Unfortunately, capitalist societies remain structured for inequality, through the division of labor, political and legal inequality, vast discrepancies in wealth, and hierarchical relations within the family. Beyond seeking to create more equitable government, communities must be able to choose actions that will enhance their capacities within institutions, as they exist. This means that the culture must become more supportive of equality. More important than redistributive justice is creating a society that is just in all of its basic structures, from production to the family.

SPECIFIC SOCIAL DETERMINANTS OR PROXIMATE SOURCES OF HEALTH INEQUITIES

Having concluded my brief consideration of class, race, and gender and the outlines of a perspective grounded in social justice, I now return to the description and implications of several major social determinants of health, recognizing the importance of their interconnectedness and their synergistic, dynamic character within particular social structural relations. They are proximate causes of health inequities within the larger social order of capitalism. Thus the intersection of decisions in land use planning, corporate development, hiring practices, and loan policies of banks, for example, can be connected to class interests, racism, gender discrimination, and health outcomes in a meaningful way. At the same time, compared with even thirty years ago, the determinants I shall discuss function in the context of a more insecure world with greater risks at every turn, less protections from the market, less social stability, and fewer institutions willing to address the disruptions to ordinary social life.

Inequality of Income and Wealth

Although income does not measure social welfare per se, less egalitarian societies with income inequalities have poorer overall health (Wilkinson, 1996). Research consistently demonstrates that inequality of income and wealth has a major impact on health outcomes, in connection with material deprivation, although it is not by itself a causal factor (Lynch and others, 1998). This is because lack of income limits access to resources related to the capacity to experience good health. Because lower-income people lack the ability to take advantage of the amenities, technologies, and conditions available to higher earners, social exclusion tends not only to marginalize the less well off but also to make them less healthy; they are in effect shut off from the prerequisites for good health. Political and cultural conditions and changing interpretations of what constitutes life's necessities thus play an important role in successful participation in society. Absence of control over social resources leads to changes in the built environment, such as suburban sprawl, which segregates people by income, thereby increasing social exclusion and limiting access to resources. High homicide rates, low birth weight, low high school graduation rates, and high unemployment rates are all linked to low income (Kaplan and others, 1996). As Kawachi and colleagues (1999) note, "The evidence shows . . . that the distribution of income among members of society matters as much for their health and well-being as does their absolute standard of living" (p. xi).

Inequality of wealth, or accumulated assets, is even more striking than the income gap (Wolff, 2002). People who are worse off, in terms of class, income, housing, education, and so on, have worse health. People who live in communities with extensive deprivation and deterioration can experience poor health, even when we control for individual disadvantage (Davey Smith and others, 1998). As Lynch and colleagues contend in Chapter Seven of this volume, "the effect of income inequality on health reflects a combination of negative exposures and lack of resources held by individuals, along with systematic underinvestment across a wide range of human, physical, health, and social infrastructure." Income inequality must be understood in relation to the multiple pathways or social contexts that affect individual outcomes. According to Wilkinson (1996), social disintegration is also directly related to high levels of economic inequality. As economic inequality increases, health declines (Raphael, 2000). Thus inequality itself is an issue, not just deprivation. The effects of social class on health and living in a stratified society suggest the need to eliminate inequalities, not merely increase income. This will become more apparent as wages continue to fall and the gap in wealth between rich and poor continues to increase.

Poverty and Deprivation

Perhaps the single most important determinant of ill health, long known, is absolute poverty, particularly as it relates to life expectancy, high infant mortality, and a wide range of diseases (Black and others, 1988). A significant body of research since the early 1980s documents clearly that poverty, poor quality of life, and low socioeconomic status are principal causes of morbidity and mortality, predisposing people to chronic disease in both the short and long term (U.S. Department of Health and Human Services, 1999; Kuh and Ben-Shlomo, 1997; Townsend, 2000). Poverty, a broad and multidimensional concept, is often a by-product of income and wealth inequality. The U.S. Census Bureau reported that the proportion of Americans living in poverty in 2001 had risen substantially since the previous census a decade earlier (Pear, 2002). Most live in families. In the United States, the data show a steady and substantial increase in the proportion of children in poverty since 1973. The poor have become a permanent class of people, even though the United States is one of the richest countries in the world with a rising life expectancy (but one that is still lower than that of Japan and all the nations of Western Europe; see Bagdikian, 2003).

Individuals at a socioeconomic disadvantage are more susceptible to death and disease, regardless of specific diseases, due to their greater exposure to the conditions that produce disease. A strong relationship exists between degree of economic inequality and child poverty (Kuh and Ben-Shlomo, 1997). These cumulative disadvantages occur within a historical legacy of socioeconomic and racial inequality. Poverty and correlated living conditions impose constraints on many aspects of everyday life that affect access to requisites for good health such as good nutrition, adequate housing, education, transportation, recreational facilities, and environmental conditions (Shaw, Dorling, and Davey

Smith, 1999; see also Pantazis and Gordon, 2000). Social and psychological effects of absolute poverty are also harmful. Uncertainty, lack of control over one's life, helplessness, chronic stress, anxiety, and depression all contribute to ill health and even death (Brunner and Marmot, 1999). Poor health can be a cause of poverty, and poverty can occur as a consequence of ill health. Given the economic chaos of recent years, as evidenced by increasing consumer debt, more people forced into relying on defined contribution benefit plans for their retirement, and the potential reorganization of Social Security as a social insurance system, we may expect increased stress and greater numbers of people slipping into poverty, thereby negatively affecting health outcomes and well-being.

Institutional Racism

Reliable data collected over the past two centuries consistently demonstrate that African Americans and many other people of color, including Native American and Latino populations, experience more illness and mortality than whites (Byrd and Clayton, 2002; Cooper and David, 1986; Krieger and others, 1993; National Center for Health Statistics, 2001; Vega and Amaro, 2002). Black Americans have a mortality rate 33 percent higher than whites; infant mortality is 2.4 times higher (see Chapter Three). These inequities are institutional to the extent that they arise from laws, policies, and restrictions on participation in decision making. They also result from efforts by the state to incorporate people of color into the dominant culture and stabilize the social order in ways that deny people's culture and history and otherwise constrain their lives. Institutions that reinforce these outcomes connect to a long history of social relations concerning racial policies, practices, and the analytical paradigms that seek to explain race and racism. Beyond economic circumstances, racism is a powerful force leading to persistent disadvantages in health outcomes (Krieger and others, 1993; Polednak, 1993. Thus even when we control for socioeconomic status, racial disparities in health remain, due to highly correlated factors such as segregation, economic disadvantage, and discrimination that affect life chances. David Williams (1998, p. 29) argues that "black-white differences in SES . . . are a direct result of the systemic implementation of institutional policies based on the premise of the inferiority of blacks and the need to avoid a social contract with them." The most basic type of group oppression, racism takes many forms, all of them restricting opportunities.

One example is evidence of the location of polluting industries in communities of color (Bullard, 1994; United Church of Christ, 1987; Center for Policy Alternatives, 1995). Another example concerns the discriminatory employment practices that have kept African American, Native American, Hispanic Americans, and other populations disproportionately at lower socioeconomic levels. Everything from segregated housing to discriminatory banking practices and poor-quality schools has cumulatively contributed to severe stress and unhealthy environments. In addition, people of color are more likely to experience police harassment and receive longer prison sentences than whites. In addition, racial prejudice itself is a force, collectively, for poorer health outcomes in many communities of color (Kennedy and others, 1999). Worse health outcomes occur at every level of income. Political power plays a crucial role in these results. The health status and living conditions of African Americans improved significantly in the 1960s and 1970s during the height of the civil rights movement, demonstrating the inverse relationship between advances in political power and a decline in mortality rates.

Gender Discrimination

Female poverty continues to rise in the United States, and the gender gap in after-tax median income is still relatively wide (Christopher and others, 2000). Extensive health inequities with respect to life expectancy, morbidity and mortality rates, maternal mortality rates, depression, and chronic conditions such as hypertension and diabetes exist among women, particularly African American women, regardless of socioeconomic status and race (Krieger and others, 1993). This suggests that interrelated conditions and experiences, including social status, working conditions, segregation, limited employment opportunities, and neighborhood safety, are important determinants of health inequities. Limited resources and multiple stressors in poor neighborhoods provide multiple pathways for ill health. As Arline Geronimus (2001, p. 133) notes, "American women in ethnically marginalized or economically disadvantaged populations have not enjoyed improved health or prolonged life in equal measure to those in more advantaged groups." She notes that this is especially true among African American women. Divorced and widowed women and those with child care responsibilities experience additional burdens, including gender discrimination in getting credit and gaining support from social service bureaucracies (Schulz, 2001). Violence against women has been associated with malnutrition (United Nations Children's Fund, 1998). Sexual harassment on the job, especially for low-income workers, generates further stresses related to health outcomes (Kawachi and others, 1999).

Corporate Globalization and Internationalization of Capital

Globalization is a "new logic and structure of rule," a form of sovereignty without boundaries, according to Michael Hardt and Antonio Negri in *Empire*. It places increasing control of speculative finance capital and the flow of the world's resources in the hands of large, unaccountable transnational corporations, thereby reducing the ability of national governments to influence economic practices (Hardt and Negri, 2000; see also Sassen, 1998; Amin, 1997; Petras and Veltmeyer, 2001). Subjecting people more forcefully to market imperatives for the purpose of expanding capital, globalization generates tremendous instability and inequality in communities all over the world (Kim and others, 2000). Markets governed by supranational institutions with their own rules, such as the World Trade Organization (WTO), come to dominate almost all aspects of social life, accentuating inequalities. Constant and rapid shifting of capital, resources, and jobs to locations of lowest production costs and cheap labor anywhere in the world, as well as the acceleration of global production, has led to the disintegration of communities, weakening of social institutions, higher unemployment, dislocation, insecurity, uneven development, and other stressors related to illness (Weisbrot and others, 2001).

Increasing social and economic inequalities through so-called free (not fair) trade policies and structural adjustment policies undermine the public's health in many ways, from the increased exportation of harmful products such as tobacco and toxic waste to the forced exportation of needed natural resources in developing countries (International Forum on Globalization, 2002; see Chapter Five). An endless and rapid investment-disinvestment cycle and the quest for economic growth and expanded markets with new forms of finance capital lead to the depletion of natural resources. The unlimited drive for growth also results in exploitative labor practices and destabilizes communities by reducing governments' ability to maintain a secure resource base to provide essential services that protect and improve health. Graham Scambler (2002) argues that growing inequities in health worldwide cannot be explained without reference to "the interlinked capital flows and fortunes of peoples from 'peripheral' nation-states in the Third World. . . . Greater transnational corporate penetration into nation-states in the Third World is associated with increased rates of infant mortality in those countries over time" (p. 155).

The vast resources and power of global corporations also enable them to limit governments' authority to enact protective labor, health, safety, and environmental laws by making countries compete with each other, and they shape national and international relations in many other ways without democratic accountability. Increases in international competition, and hence attempts to increase economic growth, reduce the bargaining power of labor and people with limited education. The benefits produced by corporate globalization tend to be unevenly distributed (see Chapter Five).

Degradation of the Environment and the Ecosystem: Disproportionate Burdens

While the ecosystem and nature have always been utilitarian objects for exploitation under capitalism, the current search for new markets and cost-cutting measures, along with the drive for endless economic growth, degrades the environment to a point that dangerously accelerates the destruction and depletion of ecosystems (Kovel, 2002). These changes in turn provide new opportunities for the development of infectious diseases and the return of old ones like tuberculosis and malaria. As Joel Kovel explains, "Malnutrition, unemployment, social alienation, systemic poisoning by chemical discharges, and the subtle effects of radioactive fallout and, indeed, of climatic change itself—all increase the likelihood that infections will take hold and become both lethal and pandemic" (p. 16). According to Tony McMichael (2001, p. xii), "Human economic activity on Earth's atmosphere, oceans, topsoil and biodiversity is weakening the planet's life-support systems," thereby increasing "risks for future populations." The limits of the planet's carrying capacity, coupled with more intensive extraction of material resources such as oil, gas, and coal and with the use of chemicals and toxic production processes, give rise to new health concerns that disproportionately affect poorer communities. The number of floods, droughts, and natural disasters appears to be increasing, with indications that human activities are a main cause, affecting the poor most severely (Kim and others, 2000).

As life's necessities, such as water and seeds, become privatized in an aggressively deregulated world economy, the result is severe environmental degradation, denoted by outcomes like unchecked global climate change, habitat destruction, deforestation, the loss of biodiversity, ozone depletion, and increased carbon dioxide emissions. Consequently, we can expect a disproportionate rise in cardiovascular disease, asthma, and premature death among people living under conditions where these effects are cumulative. Assaults on the ecosystem also destroy people's livelihoods, traditional cultural practices, and identities as their communities become subsumed into global modes of production (Tarbell and Arquette, 2000).

In the United States, the poor and communities of color are likely to experience a greater decline in their health and well-being than others, as they are exposed to a disproportionate share of environmental hazards such as lead and toxic waste and the associated risks (Bullard, 1994; Northridge and others, 2003). A study by James Boyce and colleagues (1999) suggests that power inequality is directly related to environmental degradation and therefore to the public's health.

Destruction of the Public Sector: Privatization, Deregulation, and the Elimination of Social Supports

In the twentieth century, the greatest reductions in inequality in health status occurred as a result of the introduction of major policy initiatives and legislation whereby the government accepted responsibility for the collective health of the nation (Rosen, 1993; Porter, 1999). Social supports and the productive use of resources matter much more than economic growth (Sen, 2001).

Typically, societies with weak social supports have higher rates of economic inequality (Wilkinson, 1996). We can expect that the reduction of the social wage will have negative effects on health status. Increases in inequality in health status have occurred when such initiatives and social reforms began to decline. Beginning with the Reagan administration, major reductions in expenditures on social programs and preventive services, along with a general attack on living standards, resulted in sharp increases in income inequality. These cutbacks also disrupted the organizational infrastructure that sustains political activism. As support for and investment in necessary infrastructure declines in the public sector—schools, mass transit, low-income housing—health risks increase (see Keating and Hertzman, 1999; Townson, 1999). Contemporary movements to privatize public health itself into separate parts opposes the demonstrated need for more unified systems approaches that are necessary to eliminate inequities (see Rhein and others, 2001). Reduced expenditures for public health programs and the misdirection of resources toward diseases rather than the conditions that produce disease will likely increase inequities further.

Reductions in social supports are not really about shrinking government in the name of efficiency but rather are a means to make people vulnerable and available for labor markets as cheap labor. The political goal in reducing the role of the public sector is to eliminate policies that protect people from the vagaries of the global market (Teeple, 2000). Coinciding with the elimination of social supports are attempts to apply market imperatives to an increasing proportion of the public sector and to end protective regulation (Beauchamp, 1988; Teeple, 2000). Examples include the campaign to privatize Social Security and Medicare, the press to convert health care more completely into a commodity, and industry efforts to control the earth's water supply. These actions are likely to increase health inequities.

Workplace Conditions and Employment

A strong connection exists between work and health, particularly given the relationship of work to family life and the well-being of communities, and the documented relationship between socioeconomic status and health (Amick and Lavis, 2000; see also Chapter Nine). In the United States, recent years have witnessed a decline in health and safety regulations for workers and a speedup in the pace of work, especially in the more dangerous industries and among the less skilled. But employment affects health apart from the specific character of the work process. Insecurity plays an important role in healthy outcomes, especially for groups without political power in the globalized, restructured economy. With rapidly changing patterns of employment and declining social supports that would guarantee income in new welfare provisions, increasing levels of stress exacerbate inequities among the most vulnerable in the population, increasing the potential for illness (Wilkinson and Marmot, 1998). Many employers reduce their full-time workforce, relying on temporary workers or contractors, often as a means to avoid paying benefits. Unemployment and chronic underemployment have a long association with serious health risks, including suicide, depression, violence, and alcohol abuse, particularly with continuing reductions in unemployment benefits (Dooley and others, 1996). Equally important for health is the level of control employees have over their work conditions. Those with less control, who tend to be in the lower social classes, have worse health outcomes—particularly with respect to cardiovascular and chronic diseases—as well as psychological problems and a greater opportunity in general for injuries and illness. And workers are losing more control in globalized labor markets, particularly where wages are lowest and unions are scarce. All of these features of work connect to the changing nature of global economic forces in a deregulated environment, including the division of labor, challenges to collective bargaining, increased exploitation, and the weakening of the labor movement in the United States.

Housing, Neighborhoods, and Land Use

Individual health risks are related to community health, residential location and density, characteristics and design of the built environment, and the uses of space (see Fullilove and Fullilove, 2000; Harvey, 1996; Fitzpatrick and La Gory, 2000). Yen and Syme (1999, p. 293) note that "areas have characteristics that are more than the sum of the individuals living in them. . . . [They] exhibit a patterned regularity of disease rates over time even though individuals come and go." Poor neighborhoods have multiple disadvantages affecting health (Northridge and others, 2003). Segregation (which influences access to employment and educational opportunities through isolation), substandard housing (a source of asthma and lead poisoning), overcrowding, failure to enforce housing regulations, lack of social services, deteriorating neighborhood conditions (crime, poor sanitation services, heavy traffic), discrimination in lending practices by banks reducing accessibility to affordable housing, and places where significant economic disinvestment occurs have been shown to contribute to inequities in health (Fitzpatrick and La Gory, 2000; Bashir, 2002). These forces and conditions parallel many health problems, from asthma, injury, and accidents to lead poisoning, heart disease, and psychosocial stress (Bashir, 2002). Infants, the poor, and the elderly are most at risk. Women living in low-income, minority communities are at greater risk for heart disease (Le Clere, Rodgers, and Peters, 1998). According to James Krieger and Donna Higgins (2002, p. 760), "Exposure to substandard housing is not evenly distributed across populations. People of color and people with low income are disproportionately affected." Spatial relations thus increase health risks, and the uses of space depend on highly politicized decisions.

The overall urban environment, and the process of urbanization itself, plays an important role in creating health disadvantages and a specific ecology of health or illness, particularly in conjunction with increasing levels of environmental pollution and toxic waste in locations with poor-quality housing (Northridge and

Shepard, 1997; see also Harvey, 1996). Thus land use and zoning decisions can determine who has access to necessities like clean air and mass transit, as well as education and support networks (Bullard, Johnson, and Torres, 2000; Mollenkopf, 1983). In New York City, for example, the location of most of the city's bus depots has been linked to increases in asthma rates for children in Harlem (Sclar and Northridge, 2001). Many of these conditions result from the outcomes of political battles over property rights and profit versus the public interest (Sclar and Northridge, 2001). Cities are particularly vulnerable to shifts of capital to more lucrative locations, as well as budget deficits resulting in uneven development, leading to stress and disorganization (see Harvey, 2001; Davis, 1990; Smith, 1984).

Weakening of Working-Class Power, Strengthening Power of Capital

An international study examining relationships between political variables and health indicators found a high correlation between working-class power and population health (Muntaner and others, 2002). Additional studies have found that more conservative governments worsen the health status of disadvantaged populations (Davey Smith and Dorling, 1996; Hicks and Swank, 1992). Political outcomes influence the distribution of investments in infrastructure and services that affect health. Levels of political participation can also affect morbidity and mortality rates (Kawachi and others, 1999).

Since 1973, the power of the working class and labor has been weakening in the United States. The deterritorialization of production, the decline of labor unions, and reduced voter turnout have contributed to this weakening, as well as the absence of any truly oppositional political party. In the United States, the federal government has increasingly come under greater control of well-financed corporations and wealthy individuals that make enormous monetary contributions to political campaigns (Phillips, 2002). These changes have given capitalist forces, investors, and owners of significant property an almost overwhelming edge in political power to act against the social well-being of the population. International treaties and new global institutions further enhance their power, as well as limits on the capacities of citizens to take protective legal action (see Chapter Five). Corporate policies and practices embodying capitalist power, apart from the specific effects of globalization, have negative consequences that generate health inequities for populations and individuals. These include, among many possibilities, economic disinvestment in poor communities, extensive layoffs, mass firings and restructuring, gentrification, targeting of industrial and toxic waste facilities in communities of color, elimination of protective regulatory structures, profiteering by drug companies seeking to maintain control of patents, financial speculation, use of dangerous technologies, restricting competition, shifting the tax burden to the less fortunate, tax subsidies to wealthy corporations, and failure to improve living conditions for farmworkers. Specific policies supported by capital to strengthen their position in relation to the work-force include failure to increase the minimum wage, reductions in unemployment compensation, elimination of health and safety regulations, weakening rights of labor to organize, and opposition to full employment and long-term job opportunities. All of these forces result in potential stresses and exposures leading to poorer health and well-being.

Both the unwillingness to invest in urban infrastructures and support for unproductive investments yielding short-term gain destabilize many economies. Concentration of wealth among fewer transnational corporations, driven by short-term financial gain, has led to a crisis of governance, limiting democracy. Economic concentration in the mass media reduces viewpoints critical of corporation actions. Corporate strategies, often intentionally designed to make populations vulnerable to labor markets, serve to reduce costs. Wage cuts, outsourcing, benefit reductions, and layoffs are some examples. They contrast with policies to invest in workers to increase productivity or to support community infrastructures.

Further Assaults on Democracy

Equity depends on democracy and accountability. Without political equality, economic equality becomes less realizable, further weakening the political power of ordinary citizens. Dan Beauchamp (1988, p. 135) remarks that "democratic discussion, with its creation of conflict and mass publics around health and safety issues, often . . . plays a key role in improving the public's health, setting the stage for . . . planned health education campaigns, changes in mass behaviors, and policy development, encouraging differing conceptions of problems." The history of public health in the United States is littered with battles between health authorities and business (Porter, 1999).

The United States, of course, was not founded as a democracy, since only white propertied men originally had political power. But today most elected officials, unduly swayed by corporations through huge contributions, take no action to reduce the extraordinary influence of wealth in the political system by those able to control resources and the mass media.

Antidemocratic trends, closely related to corporate globalization of finance capital, further diminish equal access to decision making over the basic forces that affect people's lives. In addition, many corporations narrowly define concepts of health and safety and the legitimate role of government in protecting the public. Moreover, the integration of news, public relations, and entertainment all constrict a true democratic process. Increased secrecy in government and rule through the WTO and other international institutions circumscribe public arenas for organized civic action. Accountability barely exists. Decisions about the development of technologies and products, the use of resources, and conditions in the workplace have profound implications for human development and health. The more they become private and beyond the reach of political and public authority, the weaker democracy becomes. Private interests then override public well-being. Addressing health inequities requires collective decision making and debate about fundamental features of society as a whole. The assaults on democratic institutions thus limit the kind of debate that would support necessary action to tackle health inequities.

IDEOLOGICAL OBSTACLES TO ELIMINATING HEALTH INEQUITIES: PARADIGMS AND POLITICS

In the mass media, very little public discussion occurs about root causes of health inequities and their consequences (Wallack and others, 1993, 1999; see also Chapter Twenty-Seven). With exceptions, few decision makers examine the relationship of inequalities in health status to racism or social, political, and economic inequality. None suggest the need for major political and economic transformations to eliminate health inequities. Many analysts and policymakers instead focus on symptoms and treatments, microanalysis of individual risk factors, and changing people's behavior and lifestyles, not conditions or places. They present options primarily through a biomedical model and remedial solutions, mostly associated with health care, rarely stressing social transformation.

What accounts for the lack of public attention to the processes that maintain and perpetuate social inequality that influence health inequities? Why is there no national debate? Why does government consider only ameliorative responses or limited regulation, rather than institutional transformations that would eliminate the causes of health inequities? At the simplest level, addressing the social determinants of health is made difficult because the phenomena are not especially observable. Achieving healthy communities is a process, not a measurable status. Measuring improvements in service delivery is certainly easier than achieving well-being in specific population groups. Many analysts still refuse to consider how people function as social beings in an ecological context (see Chapter Nineteen). In addition, governments mostly attend to single issues or "problems" through categorical programs for each that preclude a more integrated and comprehensive focus. They direct strategies to act on individuals, not communities, regions, or classes.

But perhaps most crucial in limiting the capacity to contest the root causes of inequality and expand public debate are various ideologies reflected in everyday life, based on hierarchies of power. Ideologies are systems of meaning and practice within a culture that guide the interpretation of everyday life. Embodied in social and political structures, they play an important role in legitimating and obscuring structures of political power associated with class, race, and gender (Metzaros, 1989; Deetz, 1992). They represent forms of social consciousness. Always in flux, contradictory, uncontrollable, and contested because of changing historical circumstances, they emerge from social relations and the conflicts within them. Capitalist ideologies exist mainly to contain conflict, neutralize or dissolve it, silence opposition, circumscribe alternative conceptions of society, mobilize consent, and otherwise legitimate inequality. Corporate public relations machinery and the mass media present the application of market relations to all aspects of social life as permanent and inevitable (Thompson, 1990). Counterideologies often develop from social movements and organizations resisting oppression. They may expose ideologies as arbitrary social constructions. But people concerned with security, family, and well-being constitute their own worldview. Dominant ideological discourses can become irrelevant to people's culture or lives. Ideologies are not necessarily the product of political strategy or direct class interests. Their character and content derive from the nature of the social relations that constitute a society. Thus free markets, contractual agreements, and individualism are capitalist ideologies, as are identities such as "consumers" (a label that ignores the role people play as producers of value and as citizens in a democracy). Why are ideologies important in discussions of health inequities? As Sylvia Tesh (1988, p. 154) observes:

> The politics of prevention is the struggle over the assignment of meaning to suspected causes of disease, for the political meaning that a causal statement acquires largely determines what kinds of prevention policies a society develops. Will "environmental hazards" bring to mind microparticles much like viruses and bacteria or uncontrollable industrial production? Will "occupational stress" come to mean terrible job conditions or tense workers? . . . Will the popular literature about unhealthy diets mainly discuss unscrupulous advertisers, or will it concentrate on inadequate health education? In short, will disease prevention policies place responsibility on individuals or on institutions and structures in the wider society?

Historical experience conditions consciousness that shapes the categories, concepts, and contexts for understanding health. Oppositional discourse always exists, produced by the particular oppressions of a given social order. But the ideas of certain interests tend to dominate in any particular moment; they condition the interpretations of the real and the possible. Thus the power of ideology lies in what is taken for granted.

Inequality often seems to occur as the result of natural economic forces. The separation of the political from the economic in liberal democracies conceals class interests and distorts the capacity to act and to articulate a plan of action outside of well-defined boundaries. A major feature of contemporary ideology with respect to health inequity is a refusal to recognize its systemic origins, roots, or logic, and therefore attempts to explore the relationship of political power to health inequities appear fruitless. In U.S. culture, a *political unconscious*—to misappropriate a term from Frederic Jameson (1981)— represses knowledge of our active participation in the production of inequality—an unwillingness to face the historical legacy, hidden realities, and political struggles that gave rise to and perpetuate inequity. Ideologies that limit the boundary of acceptable action and domesticate the struggles to address health inequities—in part by defining the nature of legitimate discourse and knowledge—have their roots, as noted, in class, race, and gender relations.

Many people are searching for better ways to present their vision of a more just and sustainable society and to stimulate robust public dialogues about central concerns in their lives. However, the space for and quality of public discourse is diminishing (McChesney, 1999; see also Deetz, 1992; Fraser, 1990; Ryan, 1989). The distribution of political power within the class structure creates systems of meaning, limiting critical inquiry by influencing the definition of issues, identities, what things mean, categories of analysis, what is desirable and possible, and common sense. Corporate public relations experts, economists, and pundits, mostly from conservative think tanks, dominate the mass media. The atrophy of imagination and the appropriation of culture often results in a further loss of meaning, the debasement of language, and the trivialization of public debate. Equally important, many voices have been effectively silenced or excluded from mainstream systems of representation. The struggles and suffering of those who experience inequities remain unarticulated. In addition, the discourse and practices of the health professions circumscribe national dialogue about confronting the social determinants of health, if inadvertently. Solutions to inequity, presented generally in medical or managerial terms, conceal injustices. Worse, new attacks are mounting against researchers engaged in the study and analysis of health inequities (see Muntaner and Gomez, 2002).

Given the urgency of investigating the elements of power beneath the surface of what otherwise appear to be inevitable and natural arrangements of human affairs in capitalist societies, several ideologies stand out that hinder full-scale debate on health inequities.

Interventions and Reform Versus Structural Systems Change

Interventions and reform refer to piecemeal, short-term actions, primarily through government policy, that respond only to the consequences or effects of inequality rather than to inequality itself while perpetuating the institutions that support it. Structural systems change requires deliberate long-term actions that lead, even if gradually, toward a transitional stage of development that addresses conditions to support health equity. That is, reforms may be effective if they are part of a comprehensive plan of action leading to broad change that eliminates the basic exploitations of the social order. As long as disadvantaged populations seek concessions while remaining in a subordinate position, reforms will fail and only perpetuate inequity.

Yet much of the debate and discourse on decreasing inequality remains focused not on causes but on access to health care and modification of individual behavior (see U.S. Department of Health and Human Services, 2000). Moreover, the reformist paradigm, by defining injustices as social problems in need of solutions, draws attention to features of the social environment that are least likely to effect permanent change. Supporters of remedial approaches tend to accept prevailing social conditions without exploring how they got that way. In traditional epidemiology, this is a result of certain features of clinical training and a professional perspective that takes the individual as the unit of analysis (Krieger, 1994; McMichael, 2001). It is also due to a discomfort with integrating political and social analysis. If we were back in the 1850s, the discussion to eliminate slavery would not emphasize best practices, model programs, or improvements in service delivery. Abolitionists identified slavery as a major institution of social injustice in American society and called for radical change.

The reformist perspective, seeking to absorb demands, leads only to limited policy choices and narrowly defined interventions unrelated to the scale and scope of the sources of inequity. It does little to prevent future inequities, as acting on their origins would. Options for change, in this view, rarely stress institutional failure. The potential for transforming community organizing, popular struggle, and the demonstration of responsibility for health inequities thereby becomes limited to programmatic and organizational issues about better service delivery or ways to educate the poor.

Individualism

Individualism, a powerful philosophy and practice in U.S. culture, limits the public space for social movement activism (Buechler, 2000). By transforming public issues into private matters of lifestyle, self-empowerment, and assertiveness, individualism precludes organized efforts to spur social change. It fits perfectly with a declining welfare state and also influences responses to health inequities (see Chapter Twenty). From this perspective, each person is self-interested and possessed of a fixed, competitive human nature. Everyone has choice and the potential for upward mobility through hard work—ignoring how we develop through the process of living in society (Tesh, 1988). Individualism presumes that individuals exist in parallel with society instead of being formed by society.

Individualism also supports a view that distrusts cooperative collective activity, situates people as isolated citizens, inhibits understanding the patterned nature of inequality, and looks to change individual behavior, not the conditions that give rise to inequalities. It represents, as Lawrence Wallack notes in Chapter Twenty-Seven, "one of the major barriers to collective action and a cornerstone of a market system that generates excess public health casualties." Individualism supports the belief that, as Ellen Wood (1995b, p. 6) notes, "there are no structured processes accessible to human knowledge." Individualism often leads to essentially blaming the victims of oppression for their own condition because of personal dysfunction. Moreover, individualism limits the ability to evaluate the social and historical dynamics of health and illness and leads to a greater emphasis on increasing social capital, social cohesion, and other psychosocial approaches, distorting connections to politics and power (Muntaner, Lynch, and Davey Smith, 2001).

The mass media almost always cover health as a personal issue, with emphasis on individual behavior, choice, and habits. Risks become personal risks, and health issues become medical issues. News coverage rarely presents stories about community health. Options, mainly posed in relation to fragmented policy, shun institutional critique (Lindbladh and others, 1998). Stories on health, as Lawrence Wallack suggests in Chapter Twenty-Seven, "communicate personal responsibility rather than social accountability." In his view, public health campaigns "are governed by the idea that people need more and better personal information to navigate a hazardous health environment rather than that people need skills to better participate in the public policy process to make the environment less hazardous." Journalists typically fail to *link* historical patterns associated with social conditions or the great shifts in wealth favoring the affluent and corporations to health outcomes. The crimes of the Enron Corporation represent an example of framing a problem to appear as the result of individual misconduct rather than institutional failure, ineffective laws and policies, or the pressures of short-term financial gain in a capitalist social order.

The individualist focus distracts critical thinking and eschews long-term approaches. For example, the stress on individual choice ignores the influences of the social environment that impose choices by offering only a limited set of alternatives. Thus the media typically encourage people to drink bottled water or place a filter on their sink in reaction to potential contamination in the water supply instead of participating in a planning process that would evaluate the health implications of economic activity that might cause illness. An example of the latter would include the development of health impact assessments prior to initiating a redevelopment project or redesign of a community.

The clinical tradition in medicine and medical research further conditions the individualist response. It promotes behavioral change and health education through personal responsibility rather than institutional change. As Lawrence Wallack indicates in Chapter Twenty-Seven, "Traditional behavioral-oriented media campaigns . . . have been limited . . . in part due to the failure of these campaigns to adequately integrate fundamental public health values related to social justice, participation, and social change." According to Dennis Raphael (2000, p. 194), "Most public health discourse and professional activity remains focused, with some notable exceptions, upon program delivery to low-income individuals identified as being at high risk for poor health outcomes." And as Graham Scambler (2002, p. 121) argues, "Medical discourse contributes to social control by reinforcing accommodation to a generally unchanged context." Competing concepts of health and health determinants regarding socioenvironmental versus lifestyle and medical explanations exacerbate conflicts among competing approaches to eliminating health inequities (McKinley and Marceau. 2000). Interestingly, a belief in the biological determinants of social reality is well suited to a politics seeking to avoid institutional change.

The Discourse of Markets and Economic Growth: Neoliberalism

The application of market-oriented discourse, with its emphasis on rational choices, prices, and risks, to health and the ecological system dominates contemporary analysis. Market discourse, guided by profitability, stresses the accumulation of capital and values such as efficiency over human need. Health inequities are interpreted as inevitable "externalities." The concept of the market, presented as the solution to almost all problems, excludes the possibility of an alternative social order. In this view, nothing exists outside the boundaries of markets, where all matter constitutes capital. Market perspectives assume that competition is more important than cooperation for achieving innovation. Although health, the ecosystem, and energy are not commodities like any others, thinking of health and well-being as commodities shapes ideas about the possibilities for ensuring healthy populations. For example, some people argue for a balance of interests in deciding whether millions of workers should experience pain and suffering because it might cost industry some profits to put ergonomic standards in place or that clean air should be a marketable good, traded with credits. Some economists seek to place a value on human life. Equally important is the way the language of economic growth and technological progress serves as a means to exclude politics by translating injustices, such as poverty, into social problems or private matters to be resolved by the natural result of impersonal market forces.

Market ideology not only separates the economic from the political—creating the impression that the market works outside of politics—but also portrays markets and the economy as disembodied, devoid of content, thereby obscuring exploitation within the class system. Externalizing markets as stable abstractions that work on their own through isolated individual decisions legitimates the failure to intervene in the economy on behalf of marginalized populations. It also leads to the depoliticization of basic issues about community health. Applying market criteria so broadly further supports the idea that capitalism is inevitable and permanent. Moreover, consumption replaces politics or at least serves as a distraction from politics. Shareholders become more important than ordinary citizens. Evidence suggests that policies directed primarily toward the creation of wealth and economic growth cannot reduce poverty (see Chapter Five). In the United States, economic growth often parallels inequality and deteriorating quality of life for many. Current indicators of social well-being—such as the gross domestic product, the Conference Board's consumer confidence reports, and the Dow Jones Industrial Average remain dominant measures in the media every day, often accepted uncritically. Regular presentation of indicators that would reflect public health concerns and social well-being—unemployment rates, air pollution levels, infant mortality rate—are absent (Miringoff and Miringoff, 1999).

Science and Epidemiology

Solutions to major chronic diseases are sometimes sought through new technologies, victory in the laboratory, or new medications. This belief in scientific progress and rationality often goes unchallenged. Scientific research, by itself, cannot address health inequities without political action, for many reasons. For one, the calculation of risk is difficult and essentially unmeasurable, indirect, and indeterminate for a whole range of conditions that are global in scope—chemical, nuclear, environmental, and rooted in historical injustices. Second, outcomes are not always quantifiable, particularly when developing long-term solutions focused on communities rather than individuals. Third, the phenomena are not directly observable. For example, the poor do worse on measures of health status, but why? What data are necessary to help rectify inequality, target policy, and redistribute resources? Health and wealth are closely associated, and measuring differences between social groups can help determine progress in reducing the gaps. Beyond the very basic descriptive data on health outcomes, better analytical techniques can explain more about the causal pathways that influence inequities. This includes identifying characteristics of communities, devising more accurate measures of racial and ethnic identity, and generating knowledge about the condition of the community infrastructure.

But there is a broader political issue: Whose questions define research agendas, particularly as they relate to population heath? Within what theoretical and methodological frame? (See Chapter Twelve.) Many people view science as a value-free discourse, uninfluenced by the culture in which it resides or the uses to which it is put. But science and policy remain inseparable; they are culturally based and related to social projects (Kuhn, 1962; Aronowitz, 1988; Harding, 1986). As Nancy Krieger (1993) argues, in the so-called environmental model, "individuals are harmed by inanimate objects, physical forces, or unfortunate social conditions (like poverty)—by things rather than people. That these objects or social circumstances are the creations of society is hidden by the veil of 'natural science'" (p. 165). The reliance on experts and technical expertise tends to obscure policy debates on broader questions about what constitutes legitimate knowledge, the relationship of knowledge to policy, and the objectives of so-called experts. Community-based researchers often rely on different methodologies that are more concerned with health effects and the impact of social conditions on culture than traditional scientists. In addition, the demand for proof of risk places on the defensive those seeking to challenge decisions, including decisions related to economic development, that may negatively influence the health status of given population groups.

The health professions, and the discipline of epidemiology in particular, often have a tendency to avoid both the study of structural social factors and involvement in social policy decisions (Wing, 2000). Of course, this is true of the social sciences more generally. Epidemiology is singled out only because of its deeper implication with health issues. As in most professions, critical influences on its own historical and political development, presuppositions, and epistemological traditions are often lacking (Shy, 1997; Wing, 2000; Yen and Syme, 1999; see also Chapter Nineteen). Until very recently, epidemiology as a discipline primarily emphasized risk factors, observed phenomena, and the agents of disease in methodological approaches focused on the body, not structured social relations (Berkman and Kawachi, 2000). Its theoretical paradigms, driven by the biomedical sciences, downplay the historical conditions and social context that make populations vulnerable, including class and racism (Wing, 2000). Many analysts still consider ill health mainly in relation to altered biochemical processes, lifestyles, or random events in the environment, devoid of social, economic, and cultural context.

Within the health community, debate continues on interpretation of the findings on health inequities and how to address the social determinants of health. Epidemiology has been generally ineffective in developing useful explanations to deal with social forces. Nancy Krieger (2001a, p. 44) comments, "Ignoring social determinants of social disparities in health precludes adequate explanations for actual changing population burdens of disease and death, thereby hampering efforts for prevention." And as Steve Wing (2000, p. 30) reminds us, "Populations . . . are not inherently defined as organized groups with unique histories involving economic, social, and ecological relationships. . . . Epidemiological studies [treat these factors] as individual attributes or exposure markers rather than as aspects of social and economic organization that provide the context for biopsychosocial development." Ideology plays an important role in epidemiology because data are a social product requiring interpretation, within a specific frame of values and theory of disease causation (Krieger, 1992). Powerful institutions often determine what concepts are appropriate for empirical research (Harding, 1986). For example, the United States does not publish health differentials by class or in ways that would draw attention to systemic outcomes necessary to protect the health of vulnerable populations (Krieger, 1992). The categories and variables addressed always express competing interpretations about the causes of disease.

How are scientific ideologies to be countered? It is not that science cannot tell us useful things. Questions, theories, and methods guide research, determined by institutions with agendas. As Stanley Aronowitz (1988, p. 341) indicates, "Truth is the critical exposition of the relations of humans to nature within a developing, historically mediated, context. . . . We can discover the external world as a product of the collective labor of centuries, not by observation, but by construction of . . . concepts that are contradictory to the certainty of the senses that only report the surfaces." Thus clearer articulation of the values guiding science is necessary to evaluate research goals and findings. As health inequities result from a clash of interests, the scientific world of prediction and control cannot resolve what is ultimately a political crisis.

Given the breadth and scope of the phenomena of health inequities and the political and ideological obstacles to generate support for social justice, I offer an outline for directing progressive energies.

SOCIAL CHANGE AND HEALTH INEQUITIES IN CAPITALIST SOCIETY: FUTURE DIRECTIONS

Health is a product of many social, political, and economic forces and institutions outside of health that produce risks for health and illness. The achievement of equity in health status is not about improving the management of disease or simply increasing resources. Realizing health requires cooperation and coalitions among disparate organizations and communities in a coordinated campaign against social and economic inequality, including the institutions that sustain it. Health inequities are not primarily the result of accidents of nature or individual pathology but result from long-standing conditions and injustice, often attributed to a particular regime of capital accumulation, racism, and sexism. Changing disease patterns are still primarily a function of changes in political power and processes of production, consumption, and distribution in a historically specific context.

The achievement of health equity cannot, in my view, be realized fully within the present capitalist market economy. A major objective must be to democratize rather than privatize more dimensions of production and social life. This does not mean relying on centralized government controls. Instead, it refers to greater public control over life's necessities. For example, with respect to economic redevelopment, communities ought to decide on the type and location of investment, based on needs and health considerations, rather than allowing developers to make these decisions.

What can be done to realize a more equitable society? Making major improvements in the health of vulnerable populations and anticipating future increases in health inequities depend on a clearly articulated agenda that directly addresses social and political inequality and the systems of power that sustain it. This agenda might include measures aimed at institutional change connected to conditions that give rise to disease patterns over time. For example, making strategic investments in the infrastructural conditions linked with population health throughout the life span and the social roots of suffering, premature death, and disability might be a good start. This would include ensuring resources for childhood development and education, affordable housing, clean air and water, and adequate income. Though it is necessary to engage in multiple struggles within the state, focusing on state power alone, without considering the forces arrayed by transnational capital, will limit transformation of social arrangements necessary to avoid endless remediation.

A preliminary challenge is to identify the requirements for confronting political interests and systems of rules that maintain those interests and to reclaim the political power that would make change possible. This is not an unrealistic or impossible objective if the direction of change is given priority over the speed of change. Effective reforms must lead to social transformation if they are not to perpetuate the cycle of inequity. That is, transformational reforms would address the social relations that generate inequity and the colonizing ideologies that make invisible the structures of exploitation that support those relations (see Gorz, 1973).

The remainder of this chapter explores, in a preliminary way, two things: public policy objectives that may support the elimination of health inequities and political strategies to achieve the objectives, with attention to reframing the debate by defining an appropriate narrative and organizing for change, including reclaiming the mission of public health within a social justice framework and aligning with and learning from the practice of social movements.

POLICY OBJECTIVES: OPPORTUNITIES AND LIMITATIONS

According to the Acheson Report, "All policies likely to have an impact on health should be evaluated in terms of the impact on health inequalities" (Acheson, 1998, p. xi). But policy effects are difficult to measure over time, particularly when seeking to change institutions and structures or improve the quality of life. Success is even more difficult to evaluate when seeking to narrow the gap between socioeconomic groups rather than making general improvements in health status. However, egalitarian policies are important, even if measurement is impossible. Investments and resources shift about the planet every day without justifying evidence on the effects or social consequences for health. Thus those seeking to protect and promote the health of particular groups should demand some leeway in making choices without perfect knowledge. In doing so, attention to the values that underlie policy and policy menus are critical, because the type and level of social change necessary are more comprehensive than policy list making would allow. Public policy affects the potential for health and illness in a variety of ways, positively and negatively. According to the Canadian Public Health Association (1996), "Policies shape how money, power and material resources flow through society and therefore affect the determinants of health. Advocating healthy public policies is the most important strategy we can use to act on the determinants of health. . . . Deficit reduction and private sector economic growth can be unhealthy for people. These policies may increase economic inequalities, environmental degradation, social intolerance, and violence."

Policy agendas, however, are part of a political strategy of different interests; for example, large landlords try to influence housing codes, automobile manufacturers try to limit safety features, polluting industries seek to limit regulations, and child advocacy groups lobby for public funding that invests in children. Who are the beneficiaries of public policy? A core theme of the policies categorized and listed here is to strengthen communities and, as Paula Braveman argues in Chapter Twelve, "to remove obstacles to achieving optimal health, giving the highest priority and devoting additional resources to removing obstacles for those with more barriers to health to begin with, because of underlying social disadvantage." The suggested sample of policy menus, mostly related to increased social investments, aims to generate security based on social citizenship. This includes, among other things, controlling the flow of capital and meeting basic social needs.

Recognizing the limits to what public policy can accomplish, the following suggested policy menus attempt to provide both social activists and policymakers with one element of a strategic approach to achieving health equity. Taken together, their purpose is to shift resources and power toward disadvantaged social populations.

Labor and Employment

It is important to ensure that labor is less subject to labor markets as a commodity and to the whim of employers seeking cheap labor. At the same time, the workplace must be made safer, healthier, and more democratic.

- Support labor market and workplace policies that consciously increase employment at a living wage.

- Increase the minimum wage and unemployment compensation.

- Support living-wage ordinances and campaigns to elevate the standard of living.

- Support pay equity.

- Create healthy working conditions.
- Support full-employment policies and the rights of workers.
- Support strong health and safety regulations, and expand long-term employment opportunities and training.

Public Investment in Children and Neighborhoods: Strengthening Communities

- Invest in children in order to eliminate childhood poverty and provide support throughout the course of life.
- Promote optimal childhood development in ways that can have lifelong consequences and reduce long-term risk, such as ensuring a proper diet and nutrition, providing early interventions, supporting high-quality public education, and abolishing child poverty to reduce infant mortality.
- Invest in public education, particularly teachers and school structures, as well as training.
- Invest in neighborhoods, public goods, and social infrastructure by revitalizing communities and offering increased access to social services.
- Create healthy and safe living conditions.
- Ensure adequate nutrition.
- Strengthen communities by developing employment policies that increase employment opportunities and training, facilitate networking and social interaction, and open new sources of access to investment capital.

Institutional Racism and Discrimination

- Enforce antidiscrimination laws.
- Support diversity in communities through zoning and land use laws that promote integration and low-income housing.
- Support an end to segregated housing and equitable distribution of social services.

Taxation

- Develop a more progressive tax system than the present one, which favors the well-off.
- Increase the amount and coverage of the earned-income credit.
- Tax capital gains at the same rate as wages.
- Eliminate subsidies for wealthy corporations, such as those in energy, agriculture, timber, and mining.
- Stop cutting taxes on the rich, and rescind recent tax cuts.

Income Supports

- Raise standards of living through cash or in-kind transfers and income supports.
- Provide adequate income maintenance and distribution policies and other social insurance systems.

Environmental Regulation

- Support full enforcement of laws, such as the Clean Air Act amendments, that seek to reduce pollution levels.
- Eliminate, not just regulate, certain forms of production and products that damage the ecosystem or cause global warming.

Social Services and Community Infrastructure

- Ensure equity in service delivery and access to services such as schools, transportation, libraries, and recreational facilities.
- Increase social spending on the social or public infrastructure and public goods to improve neighborhoods.

Housing and Land Use

- Eliminate land use and zoning regulations that have permitted the creation of sprawl.
- Ensure affordable, safe housing, and oppose the concentration of poor people in federal housing projects that segregate them.
- Create healthy living conditions, including safe and well-designed communities and homes.
- Support sustainable economic development.
- Oppose the locating of toxic waste facilities in communities of color.

Health Care

- Establish a system of health and health care institutions that is available to all.
- Integrate public health criteria into economic redevelopment and community development.

Trade

- Support fair and equitable global trade policies.
- Support a moratorium on the negotiation of new trade agreements.

Research, Data Collection, and Surveillance and Monitoring

- Support the appointment of a Council of Social Advisers to match the Council of Economic Advisers. (See Miringoff and Miringoff, 1999.)
- Support and develop health impact assessments for social and economic initiatives to evaluate the impact of programs, policies, and projects on the health of the population and to reveal possible inequalities.
- Support the collection of government data by class, investigate racism as a fundamental cause of ethnic inequities in health and its effects on health, and support the development and implementation of a health equity index to provide a core measure to focus public attention on health inequities.
- Develop effective ways of measuring and monitoring the impact on health inequities of policies and practices in housing, taxation, education, the health care system, and other aspects of society.

Democracy

- Support democratic control over major investment decisions
- Strengthen public participation in health decision making.
- Locally, create a systemic health planning process to form an integrated public health infrastructure with collaborative partnerships among the many agencies whose decisions affect the public's health.
- Support the chartering of corporations, and provide localities with more control over corporations.

Realizing these policies will not occur without long political struggles that involve both resistance to ongoing oppressions and strategies for shifting consciousness and building coalitions for social change. What are some possible avenues for transforming the dialogue and narratives used to debate the issue of health inequality? Let's look at a few.

REVITALIZING IMAGINATION AND REFRAMING THE DEBATE: IDEOLOGY AND CONSCIOUSNESS

A major obstacle to achieving equality in health status is a belief in its impossibility, based on a deeper belief that progressive social change is impossible. It is not. The contemporary system of political power is the result of struggle, not a natural order. Given the confusion and despair sometimes expressed about improving the quality of life for everyone, it is important to demonstrate the many ways in which people participate in struggles for social justice in everyday life. In order to transcend accommodation, it is necessary to overcome assumptions and the symbolic universe of the current order. Contingencies, resistance, and dreams for an expanded view of life, beyond the value of the market, are always present because ideologies are unstable, especially when they become detached from meaning in people's everyday lives. How can activists politicize health and health inequities within the realm of public debate, removed from the experts?

One approach is to envision a politics of emancipation, a positive view that seeks not only to overcome constraints to achieving a healthy society for everyone but also to imagine what life and work might look like without exploitation and with forms of democratic governance in support. Without a vision of a transformed reality and examples, historical or contemporary, achieving real social change becomes extremely limited. Transforming public consciousness about health inequities—why they matter and what to do about them—involves the ability to imagine and present a vision of a world without inequities, in part by making explicit the contradiction between the values expressed in the culture and the realities of how people live. Such a vision of a social economy of well-being would emphasize reciprocity and the old idea of the common good in place of market values. Dan Beauchamp (1988, p. 21) contends, "Alleviation of modern public health problems requires the reduction of risks that are faced by the community considered as a whole. . . . Preventive measures taken to reduce risks provide benefits that seem marginal when viewed from the standpoint of individuals considered privately." Eliminating health inequities will require reimagining the social order to expose and reject the myths, discourses, and practices that define social health (and wealth) and thereby expand the realm of legitimate debate. A critical discourse of resistance and possibility, linking many progressive interests, would support debate grounded in material realities. That is, the debate would shift away from treating the consequences of inequity and toward the fundamental injustices, institutions, practices, and conditions that cause and perpetuate health inequities. Such a discourse could invigorate action toward systemic change that would lead to a more equitable and more democratic social order.

The contesting and disruption of unquestioned concepts about health and well-being are important, particularly the idea that not everyone deserves to be healthy and that no collective action is necessary to establish the prerequisites for health equity and well-being. Bounded by a reformist paradigm, the contemporary dominant view of health refuses to recognize either real social divisions or the role of property and the conditions of production and its consequences. Opposing this view depends on embedding a discourse and practice about the collective, social, common dimensions of human existence in order to legitimate the idea of public control over a wider realm of social life associated with population health and reducing the unfettered role of capital.

One step in contesting current ideologies is to reconfigure the representation of health equity in order to highlight other systems of meaning that organize the world and raise questions now absent from current debates. Those systems of meaning would clarify common interests that unite people and ultimately create an agenda and a political project by showing the possibility of another kind of social reality. Making the case for social justice and equality as a value requires telling stories that highlight the features of a more equitable society. Such stories would include exposing the link between politics, science, and values. As Sylvia Tesh (1988, p. 3) comments, "I argue not that values be excised from science and from policy but that their inevitable presence be revealed and their worth be publicly discussed." An important objective, then, is to translate public health knowledge and outrage about inequities into issues of public concern.

Earlier I indicated some of the key ideological frames that limit critical thinking. Market ideology and the so-called invisible hand of the market provide some extraordinary excuses for decisions that harm human health. The mantra to reduce government in favor of the market does not suggest what form or principle of governance it opposes, nor does it allow for the interrogation of what true governance by the market means. It is important to explode the myth that there exists a private realm that is autonomous from public consequences and unaffected by corporate decisions. Invoking the precautionary principle is one method of taking the offensive. For example, the struggle to protect the public's health is often stymied by the request to prove with scientific evidence that harm will result from a given decision. Questioning the economic and political interests of the authorities who make decisions that affect the public's health can help reverse this way of thinking. Community residents might insist, for example, that developers provide proof demonstrating that no harm will result to the public's health from decisions regarding economic development, social programs, tax reductions, and capital investment.

Human need is another concept that often becomes absorbed into market ideology. Health is a requirement for active participation in the life of a community, not a marketable good. Thinking of health and well-being as a human need changes the focus away from seeking to measure the immeasurable and toward transformation of institutions (Robertson, 1998).

The individualist perspective, as noted earlier, frames issues as personal and disconnected from larger social factors. Yet the oppressions that afflict people are collective and systematic, based in a large array of institutions. Social change simply does not occur through sequential individual actions. The danger of nuclear waste or farms with contaminated cows transcends the world of individual risk. A necessary step is to reformulate and make salient the conditions for health and politicize its meaning more thoroughly in order to reveal that what appears as objective and neutral is in fact subjective and political. Recognizing health as a social concern and not only a human one is an important objective.

TAKING ACTION: RECLAIMING PUBLIC'S HEALTH'S MISSION AND PRACTICE—OPPORTUNITIES AND LIMITS

Today a disjunction exists between the ideals and goals of public health and the organization of its institutions. (See Chapter Twenty-Five.) That disjunction partly refers to a narrowing of focus on the technical as opposed to the political and losing the connection to social justice. As Elizabeth Fee notes in her introduction to George Rosen's *A History of Public Health* (1993, p. xxxviii), "When the history of public health is seen as a history of how populations experience health and illness, how social, economic, and political systems structure the possibilities for healthy or unhealthy lives, how societies create the preconditions for the production and transmission of disease, and how people, both as individuals and social groups, attempt to promote their own health or avoid illness, we find that public health history is not limited to the study of bureaucratic structures and institutions but pervades every aspect of social and cultural life."

Returning to the historical roots of public health means pursuing health equity through a social justice lens, beyond programs and interventions. This work entails developing a rights-based approach to public health, but one that sees health as a *social* and not merely an individual right. Proposing equity as a value to pursue supports the necessary redirection of social and political priorities and resources to address health inequities. It would also legitimate transcending remedial action in favor of more fundamental institutional change. The challenge for practitioners is to clarify the values that guide the work of public health within its broadest definition and to make a commitment to a collective idea of prevention. We can explore several areas of activity in public health practice that could influence the social determinants of health, assuming a supportive context in other relevant institutions directed at broad-based social change.

The discipline itself requires reorganization. Public health practice cannot advance without a more coherent philosophy and theory—one that links economics, ecology, geography, space and time, and philosophy of science. The study of health will always be an interdisciplinary undertaking, embedded in social processes and with awareness of a historical timeline that can determine its direction and progress. Given that the source of health depends on so many institutions, public health practice will require more permanent interagency and multidisciplinary coordination, recruiting, and cross-training in many subject areas. Many people perceive the location of public health practice as exclusively within designated health agencies, limited to the health professions. Making common cause with entities outside of the formal public health system means, for example, that health practitioners would work with agencies in economic development, land use, transportation, housing, and education, as well as community organizations. Health cannot be the responsibility of one organization; it must be a cooperative effort involving coalitions. A systematic approach to addressing patterns of risk in their social context, at the level of populations, suggests reconstituting the field of public health. That is, beyond forging partnerships and common cause with other public agencies, reorganization would lead to incorporating other disciplines, not merely partnering with them. Schools of public health would cross-train on environmental concerns, for example, to overcome endless specialization.

To improve the public's health and eliminate inequities in health outcomes, the theory, practice, and scope of work in the institution of public health require that attention be given to the broad range of social conditions, institutions, and structures that influence the quality of life. An expanded horizon generates action farther upstream toward addressing the prerequisites for population-based health. Health practitioners' involvement is crucial in activities such as city planning (to design cities to link work and home and reduce urban sprawl), economic redevelopment, and advocacy for public services, global climate change, and international trade.

Often heard in some public health circles is a complaint about the lack of resources or mandates to deal with health inequities, with an implication that social justice concerns are beyond the scope of public health practice. If public health practice is to return to the basic philosophy of social justice that constitutes its roots, then it must attend more forcefully to issues of social and economic inequality, because the conditions and systems of rule under which people live *produce* health. As Bernard Turnock (2001, p. 15) notes, "A critical challenge for public health as a social enterprise lies in overcoming the social and ethical barriers that prevent us from doing more with the tools already available to us. Extending the frontiers of science and knowledge may not be as useful for improving public health as shifting collective values . . . to act on what we already know. [Major public health successes] came through changes in social norms, rather than through bigger and better science." This may mean an explicit identification with goals of social justice and advocating for them, changing roles and expectations. Rethinking the work of public health toward prevention and system building recognizes that, for example, employment status, level of income, and quality of education are essential to the public's health.

Local public health agencies will need to exercise a greater leadership role. This involves seeking more decision-making authority and support for public policy at many levels directed at the elimination of health inequities. Agencies could collaboratively identify methods and incentives to give priority to the health impact of their activities and decisions. Moreover, popular engagement with public health issues facilitates community mobilization. Mobilization can in turn stimulate new demands or changes by addressing unacceptable conditions. Because the determinants of population health result primarily from conditions in the environment and not the individual, health professionals must support policies such as adequate and affordable housing, public transportation, reduction of sprawl, and a living wage, as well as those opposing discrimination.

A crucial element of leadership is the ability to relinquish control or power to the community by supporting its capacity for making decisions, similar to the way civilians hear evidence as jurors or determine actions based on competing scientific evidence. The field of popular epidemiology emerging in recent years could support grassroots approaches to community health (see Brown, 2000). These approaches consider disproportionate risks in exposure, for example, experienced by communities of color and low-income neighborhoods.

Public health must function as an expression of the community, as its representative seeking to advocate for social change that transforms the conditions that cause ill health. The issue demands political will, speaking out and building partnerships with those in need, and recognizing limited resources within rigid mandates in a conservative climate. Collaboration with and support of the community means an ongoing process of relationship building, dialogue, and cooperative action to address community health needs and issues, based on trust and reciprocity. That process can involve mobilizing resources, gathering information, generating major systems change, or influencing programs and practices associated with health inequities. A key element, however, requires engaging with the public in community decision making and information sharing around social change efforts beyond health protection and disease prevention. Collaboration may include larger community improvement issues or involvement in economic redevelopment policy because they relate to differentials in health status. The health agency and the community work together in planning, designing, implementing, and evaluating all activities. The level of community organization, resources, skills, and training affects collaboration because being heard takes money and resources. Local health authorities must help the community develop its resources and research skills, including obtaining assistance through the local bureaucracies. Investment in capacity building is crucial.

The health professions should work to acknowledge and reinforce the voices of those who experience injustices, emphasizing that they represent the shared experience of all people. Advocating for policies and change that give people more control over life circumstances, productive assets, production processes, and the labor process is essential. Advocates would also support ecologically sustainable development and the evaluation of development projects against criteria based on the protection of human health, ensuring the provision of basic needs such as jobs, good living and working conditions, safe housing, education, and social safety nets.

Communities and health practitioners are developing new decision-making tools for assessing the health impact of social and economic decisions, similar to the environmental impact statement (EIS), that may have a role in addressing health inequities. The health impact assessment (HIA) involves a process and procedures, with an ethical and moral element, for evaluating the effects of policies, programs, and projects on the range of forces that affect health and well-being. A major difference with the EIS is that the HIA is participatory and democratic in its development and implementation and typically incorporates equity in decision making as an objective. It responds to the need for evidence-based policymaking, but within a multidisciplinary model relying on qualitative and quantitative analysis (Scott-Samuel, 1998). Depending on who invokes its use, it has advantages and drawbacks. On the one hand, measures may not exist for structural influences on health. More important, the right to health and a decent standard of living should not have to be proved. On the other hand, the HIA reinforces a broader definition of health, involves the community in a public process, and potentially raises questions about health equity.

Public health practice can also engage in research that emphasizes the cumulative effects of poor social conditions (Davey Smith and others, 1997). Miringoff and Miringoff (1999) rightly argue for the frequent presentation and promotion of indicators that reflect public health concerns—unemployment rates, air pollution levels, infant mortality rate, child abuse, child poverty, homicide rates, access to affordable housing, weekly earnings, and so on, as well the links between social conditions and health. The annually calculated Fordham Index of Social Health (Miringoff, 1995), for example, relies on sixteen measures to provide an overall perspective of human welfare at each life stage. Using such measures or establishing a locally based "wellness" index requires promoting it in the media as a supplement to the endless array of economic indicators.

In addition, the pathogenic effects of social inequalities demand more research (Farmer, 1999). "By what mechanisms, precisely, do such noxious events and processes [racism, gender inequality, growing gap between rich and poor] become embodied as adverse health outcomes? Why are some at risk and others spared?" (p. 1492). The collection of data that focus on systemic outcomes is critical to an enterprise that seeks to eliminate health inequities. As Nancy Krieger (1992, p. 422) notes, "Keeping in mind that the information in U.S. data bases is actively collected, not passively discovered, we must therefore insist that all national vital statistics be reported stratified by gender-appropriate measures of social class, in combination with race/ethnicity and gender."

Health promotion is another arena for pursuing progressive change. Traditional health promotion emphasizes realizing healthy lives at the level of the individual, without stressing the need to alter economic, social, and ecological environments of populations with respect to the material disadvantages that people face in everyday life. Strategies would aim at removing or lowering risk for specific populations. For example, more attention would be given to critiquing the fast-food industry and countering its increasing ubiquity, which has extended even in hospitals. But improving health for everyone still leaves a gap. As Sally Macintyre (2000) observes, the rich are more likely to attend to and benefit from health promotion than the poor. "The capacity to benefit from individualized risk management or health education may be least among more disadvantaged people" (p. 1399).

Finally, to advance an agenda to eliminate health inequities, public health practitioners will have to communicate with a broader public more effectively, building a constituency. Lawrence Wallack and his colleagues (1993), in describing effective media advocacy, notes the importance of telling stories from the point of view of public health. These stories, in his view, must illustrate basic principles and values, describe the political context, express the mission of public health, and stress the "importance of community participation and self-determination as a strategy for change" (p. 3). This requires publicizing the relationship between inequities in health status, on the one hand, and social and economic inequality, on the other, translating the research in a way that the media can digest. Health professionals will need to explain why inequality is bad for health and show how everyone benefits from equality, using multiple avenues to articulate their ideas. Examples include developing campaigns, writing newspaper editorials, publishing in popular periodicals, developing seminars and workshops, and initiating speaking engagements. Public health needs to find its moral voice, expressing its values along with the factual information that provides legitimacy to its message. It needs to pressure the media to consider structural causes of health and illness and redirect attention to the social production of health.

Unclear at this moment is whether the contemporary system of public health, with its intellectual and resource constraints, can confront issues of health inequities at the level of populations without restructuring the scope of its work, the training of its workforce, and its analytical underpinnings. These changes will take political will and courage. But public health has allies in many disciplines if it chooses to work with them.

TAKING ACTION: STRENGTHENING SOCIAL MOVEMENTS

No great social change can occur without persistent pressure and struggle against a class-based society and the economic conditions it produces. Community residents must draft their own social agenda. The achievement of the right to vote, the minimum wage, Medicare, and desegregation of the schools took years of organizing, constituency building, and political will against entrenched institutions and the technologies that sustain them by people in social movements resisting the consequences of untamed capitalism and racism. In addition, the laws providing corporations with greater sovereignty than individuals, regressive taxation, zoning systems that support segregation, and tax subsidies for wealthy corporations also resulted from great collective organizing among the unions of capital, from chambers of commerce to industry associations and lobbying groups.

To enact and implement healthy public policy, the rarely heard voices will need to hold decision makers accountable for the public's health and the quality of their lives. Most social change addressing health inequalities does not emerge primarily from the professional health community. It derives from the experience of organized groups of people seeking to strengthen social movements to protect and improve their communities. They are challenging the causes of poor health directly through alliances, social mobilization, and coalition-building activities. Since the roots of ill health do not begin solely within their communities but are embedded in national and global policies associated with class, race, and gender discrimination, communities must strategize at all levels. This suggests uniting many social movements, with national and international links, similar to the civil rights, women's, and environmental justice movements in the United States or the movement for public health in the Victorian era in England. Beyond prevention and protection, the elimination of health inequities will depend on new forms of community activism. The challenge is to develop a common agenda among diverse cultural groups and organizations with differing identities but similar experiences, based on a commitment to social justice (Carlisle, 2000). It is therefore important not only to transcend identity politics, which facilitates a divide-and-conquer strategy, but also not to medicalize the issue of health inequities or create health movements. The latter cannot substitute for the identification of the common interests connected to social justice values that lead people to mobilize around the root causes of inequities more broadly (Scambler, 2002). Strong partnerships can address a much broader array of social needs and issues that affect health and well-being.

Although such an agenda may seem overwhelming, it can be pursued in small steps. These steps may lead in a different direction—toward major social transformations in the conditions of life that reduce inequalities, rather than only activities directed toward reform, regulation, technological advances, or advances in medical care that leave inequities in the social system untouched. These steps must aim at solutions that disturb political power relations. However, because the consequences of political power function everywhere in society, so must struggles for social justice and health justice be everywhere, not just within the realm of public policy or state institutions. Many locations, cultural practices, social institutions, and even personal relations remain sites of struggle for collective action to challenge health inequities, from universities and the mass media to workplaces and corporate boardrooms. The public health is a site of contestation that can challenge basic assumptions about what society and the future can be. The contributors to this book provide the context, the research, and the framework to rethink how we might achieve health equity by enabling people to create their own history.

Notes

1. Documentation of the relationship between health inequalities and income inequality was developed in the 1970s. See, for example, Wagstaff and Van Doorslaer (2000) and Bartley, Blane, and Davey Smith (1998). For a summary of research in the 1980s, see Feinstein (1993).

2. Two examples are the Labor Community Strategy Center, a multiracial, anticorporate think tank in Los Angeles, and the Association of Community Organizations and Reform Now (ACORN), a community organization of low- and moderate-income families in forty-five cities.

References

Acheson, D. *Independent Inquiry into Inequalities in Health.* London: Stationery Office, 1998.

Ackerman, F. "Overview." In F. Ackerman and others (eds.), *The Political Economy of Inequality.* Washington, D.C.: Island Press, 2000.

Altman, L. K., with O'Connor, A. "Threats and Responses: The Bioterrorism Threat." *New York Times,* January 5, 2003, p. 1.

Amick, B., and Lavis, J. "Labor Markets and Health: A Framework and Set of Applications." In A. Tarlov (ed.), *Society and Population Health.* New York: New Press, 2000.

Amin, S. *Capitalism in the Age of Globalization: The Management of Contemporary Society.* London: Zed Books, 1997.

Andrews, E. L. "Economic Inequality Grew in '90s Boom, Fed Reports." *New York Times,* January 23, 2003, p. 1.

Annandale, E., and Hunt, K. "Gender Inequalities in Health: Research at the Crossroads." In E. Annandale and K. Hunt (eds.), *Gender Inequalities in Health.* Buckingham, England: Open University Press, 2000.

Antonovsky, A. "Social Class, Life Expectancy, and Overall Mortality." *Milbank Quarterly,* 1967, *45,* 31–73.

Arno, P. S., and Figueroa, J. B. "The Social and Economic Determinants of Health." In J. Madrick (ed.), *Unconventional Wisdom: Alternative Perspectives on the New Economy.* New York: Century Foundation Press, 2000.

Aronowitz, S. *Science as Power: Discourse and Ideology in Modern Society.* Minneapolis: University of Minnesota Press, 1988.

Bagdikian, B. H. "A Secret in the News: The Country's Permanent Poor." [http://www.inequality.org/bagdikian2.html]. Accessed April 28, 2003.

Barrett, M. *Women's Oppression Today: Problems in Marxist Feminist Analysis.* New York: Verso, 1980.

Bartley, M., Blane, D., and Davey Smith, G. (eds.). *The Sociology of Health Inequalities.* Oxford: Blackwell, 1998.

Bashir, S. A. "Home Is Where the Harm Is: Inadequate Housing as a Public Health Crisis." *American Journal of Public Health,* 2002, *92,* 733–738.

Beaglehole, R., and Bonita, R. *Public Health at the Crossroads: Achievements and Prospects.* Cambridge: Cambridge University Press, 1997.

Beauchamp, D. E. *Health of the Republic: Epidemics, Medicine, and Moralism as Challenges to Democracy.* Philadelphia: Temple University Press, 1988.

Berkman, L. F., and Kawachi, I. (eds.). *Social Epidemiology.* New York: Oxford University Press, 2000.

Black, D., and others. *Inequalities in Health.* Harmondsworth. England: Penguin, 1988.

Boyce, J. K., and others. "Power Distribution, the Environment, and Public Health: A State-Level Analysis." *Ecological Economics,* 1999, *29,* 127–140.

Brown, P. "Popular Epidemiology and Toxic Waste Contamination: Lay and Professional Ways of Knowing. " In S. Kroll-Smith, P. Brown, and V. J. Gunter (eds.), *Illness and the Environment: A Reader in Contested Medicine.* New York: New York University Press, 2000.

Brunner, E., and Marmot, M. G. "Social Organization, Stress, and Health." In M. G. Marmot and R. G. Wilkinson (eds.), *Social Determinants of Health.* New York: Oxford University Press, 1999.

Buechler, S. M. *Social Movements in Advanced Capitalism: The Political Economy and Cultural Construction of Social Activism.* New York: Oxford University Press, 2000.

Bull, J., and Hamer, L. *Closing the Gap: Setting Local Targets to Reduce Health Inequalities.* London: National Health Service, London Development Agency, 2001.

Bullard, R. D. *Unequal Protection: Environmental Justice and Communities of Color.* San Francisco: Sierra Club Books, 1994.

Bullard, R. D., Johnson, G. S., and Torres, A. (eds.). *Sprawl City: Race, Politics, and Planning in Atlanta.* Washington, D.C.: Island Press, 2000.

Byrd, W. M., and Clayton, L. A. *An American Health Dilemma,* Vol. 2: *Race, Medicine and Health Care in the United States.* New York: Routledge, 2002.

Callinicos, A. *Equality.* Malden, Mass.: Blackwell, 2000.

Canadian Public Health Association. *Statement on Health Promotion.* Ottawa, Ontario: Canadian Public Health Association, 1996.

Carlisle, S. "Health Promotion, Advocacy, and Health Inequalities: A Conceptual Framework." *Health Promotion International,* 2000, *15,* 369–376.

Center for Policy Alternatives. *Toxic Waste and Race Revisited.* Washington, D.C.: Center for Policy Alternatives, 1995.

Chernomas, R. *The Social and Economic Causes of Disease."* Winnipeg, Manitoba: Canadian Centre for Policy Alternatives, May, 1999.

Christopher, K., and others. *Gender Inequality in Poverty in Affluent Nations: The Role of Single Motherhood and the State.* Chicago: Joint Center for Poverty Research, 2000.

Congressional Budget Office. *Historical Effective Tax Rates, 1979–1997.* (prelim. ed.) Washington, D.C.: U.S. Government Printing Office, 2001.

Cooper, R., and David, R. "The Biological Concept of Race and Its Application to Public Health and Epidemiology." *Journal of Health Politics, Policy and Law,* 1986, *11,* 97–116.

Dahlgren, G., and Whitehead, M. *Policies and Strategies to Promote Social Equality in Health.* Stockholm: Institute of Future Studies, 1991.

Daniels, N., Kennedy, B. P., and Kawachi, I. *Is Inequality Bad for Our Health?* Boston: Beacon Press, 2000.

Danziger, S., Danziger, S., and Stern, J. "The American Paradox: High Income and High Child Poverty." In F. Ackerman and others (eds.), *The Political Economy of Inequality.* Washington, D.C.: Island Press, 2000.

Davey Smith, G., and Dorling, D. "'I'm All Right John'. Voting Patterns and Mortality in England and Wales, 1981–92." *British Medical Journal,* 1996, *313,* 1573–1577.

Davey Smith, G., and others. "Lifetime Socioeconomic Position and Mortality: Prospective Observational Study." *British Medical Journal,* 1997, *314,* 547–552.

Davey Smith, G., and others. "Individual Social Class, Area-Based Deprivation, Cardiovascular Disease Risk Factors, and Mortality: The Renfrew and Paisley Study." *Journal of Epidemiology and Community Health,* 1998, *52,* 399–405.

Davis, M. *City of Quartz.* New York: Vintage Books, 1990.

Deetz, S. A. *Democracy in an Age of Corporate Colonization: Developments in Communication and the Politics of Everyday Life.* Albany: State University of New York Press, 1992.

Department of Health. "Milburn Urges Focus on Health Outcomes Particularly in Poorest Communities." Press release, London, November 1, 2001.

Diderichsen, F., and others. "Sweden and Britain: The Impact of Policy Context on Inequities in Health." In T. Evans and others (eds.), *Challenging Inequities in Health: From Ethics to Action.* New York: Oxford University Press, 2001.

Dooley, D., and others. "Health and Unemployment." *Annual Review of Public Health,* 1996, *17,* 449–465.

Drever, F., and Whitehead, M. *Health Inequalities.* London: Her Majesty's Stationery Office, 1977.

Evans, T., and others. "Introduction." In T. Evans and others (eds.), *Challenging Inequities in Health: From Ethics to Action.* New York: Oxford University Press, 2001.

Farmer, P. "Pathologies of Power: Rethinking Health and Human Rights." *American Journal of Public Health,* 1999, *89,* 1486–1496.

Fee, E. "Introduction: Public Health Past and Present: A Shared Social Vision." In G. Rosen, *A History of Public Health.* Baltimore: Johns Hopkins University Press, 1993.

Feinstein, J. S. "The Relationship Between Socioeconomic Status and Health: A Review of the Literature." *Milbank Quarterly,* 1993, *71,* 279–322.

Fitzpatrick, K., and La Gory, M. *Unhealthy Places: The Ecology of Risk in the Urban Landscape.* New York: Routledge, 2000.

Fraser, N. "Rethinking the Public Sphere: A Contribution to the Critique of Actually Existing Democracy." *Social Text,* 1990, *25–26,* 56–80.

Fullilove, M. T., and Fullilove, R. E., III. "Place Matters" In R. Hofrichter (ed.), *Reclaiming the Environmental Debate: The Politics of Health in a Toxic Culture.* Cambridge, Mass.: MIT Press, 2000.

Geronimus, A. T. "Understanding and Eliminating Inequalities in Women's Health in the United States: The Role of the Weathering Conceptual Framework." *Journal of the American Women's Medical Association,* 2001, *56,* 133-137.

Gorz, A. *Socialism and Revolution.* New York: Anchor Books, 1973.

Green, P. *Equality and Democracy.* New York: New Press, 1998.

Halfon, N., and Hochstein, M. "Life Course Health Development: An Integrated Framework for Developing Health, Policy, and Research." *Milbank Quarterly,* 2002, *80,* 433–479.

Hamlin, C. *Public Health and Social Justice in the Age of Chadwick: Britain, 1800–1854.* Cambridge University Press, 1998.

Harding, S. *The Science Question in Feminism.* (Ithaca, N.Y.: Cornell University Press, 1986.

Hardt, M., and Negri, A. *Empire.* Cambridge, Mass.: Harvard University Press, 2000.

Harvey, D. *Justice, Nature, and the Geography of Difference.* Malden, Mass.: Blackwell, 1996.

Harvey, D. *Spaces of Capital: Toward a Critical Geography.* New York: Routledge, 2001.

Hicks, A. M., and Swank, D. H. "Politics, Institutions, and Welfare Spending in Industrialized Democracies, 1960–1982." *American Political Science Review,* 1992, *86,* 658–674.

Institute of Medicine. *The Future of the Public's Health.* Washington, D.C.: National Academy Press, 2002.

International Forum on Globalization. *Alternatives to Economic Globalization.* San Francisco: Berrett-Koehler, 2002.

Jameson, F. *The Political Unconscious.* Ithaca, N.Y.: Cornell University Press, 1981.

Kaplan, J. R., and others. "Income Inequality and Mortality in the United States." *British Medical Journal,* 1996, *312,* 999–1003.

Kawachi, I. "Income Inequality and Health." In L. F. Berkman and I. Kawachi (eds.), *Social Epidemiology.* New York: Oxford University Press, 2000.

Kawachi, I., and Kennedy, B. P. *The Health of Nations: Why Inequality Is Bad for Your Health.* New York: New Press, 2002.

Kawachi, I, Kennedy, B. P., and Wilkinson, R. G. (eds.). *The Society and Population Health Reader,* Vol. 1: *Income Inequality and Health.* New York: New Press, 1999.

Kawachi, I., and others. "Women's Status and the Health of Women and Men: A View from the States." *Social Science and Medicine,* 1999, *48,* 21–32.

Keating, D. P., and Hertzman, C. (eds.). *Developmental Health and the Wealth of Nations: Social, Biological, and Educational Dynamics.* New York: Guilford Press, 1999.

Kennedy, B. P., and others. "(Dis)respect and Black Mortality." In I. Kawachi, B. P. Kennedy, and R. G. Wilkinson (eds.)., *The Society and Population Health Reader: Income Inequality and Health.* New York: New Press, 1999.

Kim, J. Y., and others (eds.). *Dying for Growth: Global Inequality and the Health of the Poor.* Monroe, Me.: Common Courage Press, 2000.

Kovel, J. *The Enemy of Nature: The End of the Capitalism or the End of the World?* London: Zed Books, 2002.

Krieger, J., and Higgins, D. L. "Housing and Health: Time Again for Public Health Action." *American Journal of Public Health,* 2002, *92,* 758-768.

Krieger, N. "The Making of Public Health Data: Paradigms, Politics, and Policy." *Journal of Public Health Policy,* 1992, *13,* 412–427.

Krieger, N. "The Health of Black Folk: Disease, Class, and Ideology in Science." In S. Harding (ed.), *The Racial Economy of Health.* Bloomington: Indiana University Press, 1993.

Krieger, N. "Epidemiology and the Web of Causation: Has Anyone Seen the Spider?" *Social Science and Medicine,* 1994, *39,* 887–903.

Krieger, N. "A Vision of Social Justice as the Foundation of Public Health: Commemorating 150 Years of the Spirit of 1848." *American Journal of Public Health,* 1998, *88,* 1603–1606.

Krieger, N. "Commentary: Society, Biology, and the Logic of Social Epidemiology." *International Journal of Epidemiology,* 2001a, *30,* 44-46.

Krieger, N. "The Ostrich, the Albatross, and Public Health: An Ecosocial Perspective— or Why an Explicit Focus on Health Consequences of Discrimination and Deprivation Is Vital for Good Science and Public Health Practice." *Public Health Reports,* 2001b, *116,* 419–423.

Krieger, N., and others. "Racism, Sexism, and Social Class: Implications for Studies of Health, Disease, and Well-Being." *American Journal of Preventive Medicine,* 1993, *9*(suppl. 6), 82–122.

Krugman, P. "For Richer: How the Permissive Capitalism Boom Destroyed American Equality." *New York Times Magazine,* October 20, 2002, p. 62.

Kuh, D., and Ben-Shlomo, Y. (eds.). *A Lifecourse Approach to Chronic Disease Epidemiology.* Oxford: Oxford University Press, 1997.

Kuh, D., and others. "Mortality in Adults Aged 25–54 Years Related to Socioeconomic Conditions in Childhood and Adulthood: Postwar Birth Cohort Study." *British Medical Journal,* 2002, *325,* 1076–1080.

Kuhn, T. *The Structure of Scientific Revolutions.* Chicago: University of Chicago Press, 1962.

Labonte, R. "Healthy Public Policy and the World Trade Organization: A Proposal for an International Health Presence in Future Trade/Investment Talks." *Health Promotion International,* 1998, *13,* 245–256.

LaVeist, T. A. "Segregation, Poverty, and Empowerment: Health Consequences of African Americans." In T. A. LaVeist (ed.), *Race, Ethnicity, and Health: A Public Health Reader.* San Francisco: Jossey-Bass, 2002.

Le Clere, F. B., Rodgers, R. G., and Peters, K. "Neighborhood Social Context and Racial Differences in Women's Health Disease Mortality." *Journal of Health and Social Behavior,* 1998, *39,* 91–107.

Lindbladh, E., and others. "Equity Is out of Fashion? An Essay on Autonomy and Health Policy in the Individualized Society." *Social Science and Medicine,* 1998, *46,* 1017–1025.

Link, B., and Phelan, J. "Social Conditions as Fundamental Causes of Disease." *Journal of Health and Social Behavior,* 1995 (special issue), 80–94.

Lynch, J. W., and Kaplan, G. A. "Understanding How Inequality in the Distribution of Income Affects Health." *Journal of Health Psychology,* 1997, *2,* 297–314.

Lynch, J. W., and others. "Income Inequality and Mortality in Metropolitan Areas of the United States." *American Journal of Public Health,* 1998, *88,* 1074–1080.

Macinko, J. A., and Starfield, B. "Annotated Bibliography on Equity in Health, 1980–2001." *International Journal for Equity in Health,* 2002, *1,* 1–50.

Macintyre, S. "Prevention and the Reduction of Health Inequalities." *British Medical Journal,* 2000, *320,* 1399–1400.

Mackenback, J., and Stronks, K. "A Strategy for Tackling Health Inequalities in the Netherlands." *British Medical Journal,* 2002, *325,* 1029–1032.

Madrick, J. "The Power of the Super Rich." *New York Review of Books,* July 18, 2002, pp. 25–27.

Marmot, M. G., and others. "Health Inequalities Among British Civil Servants: The Whitehall II Study." *Lancet,* 1991, *337,* 1387–1393.

McChesney, R. W. *Rich Media, Poor Democracy: Communication Politics in Dubious Times.* New York: New Press, 1999.

McKinley, J., and Marceau, L. D. "To Boldly Go . . ." *American Journal of Public Health,* 2000, *90,* 25–33.

McMichael, T. *Human Frontiers, Environments and Disease: Past Patterns, Uncertain Futures.* Cambridge: Cambridge University Press, 2001.

Metzaros, I. *The Power of Ideology.* New York: New York University Press, 1989.

Minnesota Health Improvement Partnership, Social Conditions and Health Action Team. *A Call to Action: Advancing Health for All Through Social and Economic Change.* Minneapolis: Minnesota Department of Health, 2001.

Miringoff, M. L. *1995 Index of Social Health: Monitoring the Social Well-Being of the Nation.* Tarrytown, N.Y.: Institute for Innovation in Social Policy, Fordham Graduate Center, 1995.

Miringoff, M. L., and Miringoff, L. *The Social Health of the Nation: How America Is Really Doing.* New York: Oxford University Press, 1999.

Miringoff, M. L., Miringoff, L., and Opdyke, S. *The Social Health of the States.* Tarrytown, N.Y.: Fordham Institute for Innovation in Social Policy, 2001.

Mishel, L., Bernstein, J., and Schmitt, J. *The State of Working America, 2000–2001.* Ithaca, N.Y.: Cornell University Press, 2001.

Mollenkopf, J. H. *The Contested City.* Princeton, N.J.: Princeton University Press, 1983.

Muntaner, C. "Power, Politics, and Social Class." *Journal of Epidemiology and Community Health,* 2002, *56,* 562.

Muntaner, C., and Gomez, M. B. "Anti-Egalitarianism: Legitimizing Myths, Racism, and 'Neo-McCarthyism' in Social Epidemiology and Public Health: A Review of Sally Satel's PC, M.D." *International Journal of Health Services,* 2002, *32,* 1–17.

Muntaner, C., Lynch, J. W., and Davey Smith, G. "Social Capital, Disorganized Communities, and the Third Way: Understanding the Retreat from Structural Inequalities in Epidemiology and Public Health." *International Journal of Health Services,* 2001, *31,* 213–237.

Muntaner, C., and others. "Economic Inequality, Working-Class Power, Social Capital, and Cause-Specific Mortality in Wealthy Countries." *International Journal of Health Services,* 2002, *32,* 629–656.

National Center for Health Statistics. *Health, United States, 1998.* Hyattsville, Md.: U.S. Department of Health and Human Services, 1998.

National Center for Health Statistics. *Health, United States, 2000, with Adolescent Chartbook.* Hyattsville, Md.: U.S. Department of Health and Human Services, 2000.

National Center for Health Statistics. *Health, United States, 2001, with Urban and Rural Health Chartbook.* Hyattsville, Md.: U.S. Department of Health and Human Services, 2001.

Northridge, M. E., and Shepard, P. M. "Environmental Racism and Public Health." *American Journal of Public Health,* 1997, *87,* 730–732.

Northridge, M. E., and others. "Environmental Equity and Health: Understanding Complexity and Moving Forward," *American Journal of Public Health,* 2003, *93,* 209–214.

Omi, M., and Winant, H. "On the Theoretical Status of the Concept of Race." In C. McCarthy and W. Crichlow (eds.), *Race and Representation in Education.* New York: Routledge, 1993.

Östlin, P., and Diderichsen, F. *Equality-Oriented National Strategy for Public Health in Sweden: A Case Study.* Brussels, Belgium: European Centre for Health Policy, 2000.

Pantazis, C., and Gordon, D. (eds.). *Tackling Inequalities: Where Are We Now and What Can Be Done?* Bristol, England: Policy Press, 2000.

Pappas, G., and others. "The Increasing Disparity Between Socioeconomic Groups in the United States." *New England Journal of Medicine,* 1993, *329,* 103–109.

Pear, R. "Number of People Living in Poverty Increases in U.S." *New York Times,* September 25, 2002, p. 1.

Petras, J., and Veltmeyer, H. *Globalization Unmasked: Imperialism in the 21st Century.* Halifax, Nova Scotia, Canada: Fernwood, 2001.

Phillips, K. *Wealth and Democracy: A Political History of the American Rich.* New York: Broadway Books, 2002.

Polednak, A. P. "Poverty, Residential Segregation, and Black/White Mortality Ratios in Urban Areas." *Journal of Health Care for the Poor and Underserved,* 1993, *4,* 363–373.

Porter, D. *Health, Civilization, and the State: A History of Public Health from Ancient to Modern Times.* New York: Routledge, 1999.

Raphael, D. "Health Inequities in Canada: Current Discourses and Implications for Public Health Action." *Critical Public Health,* 2000, *10,* 193–216.

Reich, R. "The Missing Options." *American Prospect,* 1997, *35,* 6–13.

Rhein, M., and others. *Advancing Community Public Health Systems in the 21st Century.* Washington, D.C.: National Association of County and City Health Officials, 2001.

Robertson, A. "Critical Reflections on the Politics of Need: Implications for Public Health." *Social Science and Medicine,* 1998, *47,* 1419–1430.

Rose, G. *The Strategy of Preventive Medicine.* Oxford: Oxford University Press, 1992.

Rosen, G. *A History of Public Health.* Baltimore: Johns Hopkins University Press, 1993.

Ryan, M. *Politics and Culture: Working Hypotheses for a Post-Revolutionary Society.* Baltimore: Johns Hopkins University Press, 1989.

Sassen, S. *Globalization and Its Discontents: Essays on the New Mobility of People and Money.* New York: New Press, 1998.

Scambler, G. *Health and Social Change: A Critical Theory.* Buckingham, England: Open University Press, 2002.

Schulz, A. "Social Context, Stressors, and Disparities in Women's Health." *Journal of the American Women's Medical Association,* 2001, *56,* 143–149.

Sclar, E., and Northridge, M. E. "Property, Politics, and Public Health." *American Journal of Public Health,* 2001, *91,* 1013–1015.

Scott-Samuel, A. "Health Impact Assessment: Theory into Practice." *Journal of Epidemiology and Community Health,* 1998, *52,* 704–705.

Sen, A. *Inequality Reexamined.* New York: Russell Sage Foundation, 1992.

Sen, A. "Economic Progress and Health." In D. Leon and G. Walt (eds.), *Poverty, Inequality, and Health: An International Perspective.* Oxford: Oxford University Press, 2001.

Shaw, M., Dorling, D., and Davey Smith, G. "Poverty, Social Exclusion, and Minorities." In M. G. Marmot and R. G. Wilkinson (eds.), *Social Determinants of Health.* New York: Oxford University Press, 1999.

Shy, C. M. "The Failure of Academic Epidemiology: Witness for the Prosecution." *American Journal of Epidemiology,* 1997, *145,* 479–484.

Smedley, B. D., and Syme, S. L. "Introduction." In B. D. Smedley and S. L. Syme (eds.), *Promoting Health: Intervention Strategies from Social and Behavioral Research.* Washington, D.C.: Institute of Medicine, National Academy of Sciences, 2000.

Smith, N. *Uneven Development*. Malden, Mass.: Blackwell, 1984.

Sram, I., and Ashton, J. "Millennium Report to Sir Edwin Chadwick." *British Medical Journal*, 1998, *317*, 592–596.

Sretzer, S. "The Importance of Social Intervention in Britain's Mortality Decline, c. 1850–1914: A Reinterpretation of the Role of Public Health." *Society for the Social History of Medicine*, 1988, *1*, 1–41.

Tarbell, A., and Arquette, M. "Akwesasne: A Native American Community's Resistance to Cultural and Environmental Damage." In R. Hofrichter (ed.), *Reclaiming the Environmental Debate: The Politics of Health in a Toxic Culture*. Cambridge, Mass.: MIT Press, 2000.

Teeple, G. *Globalization and the Decline of Social Reform: Into the Twenty-First Century*. Aurora, Ontario, Canada: Garamond Press, 2000).

Tesh, S. N. *Hidden Arguments: Political Ideology and Disease Prevention Policy*. New Brunswick, N.J.: Rutgers University Press, 1988.

Thompson, J. B. *Ideology and Modern Culture: Critical Social Theory in the Era of Mass Communication*. (Stanford, Calif.: Stanford University Press, 1990.

Townsend, P. "Ending World Poverty in the 21st Century." In C. Pantazis and D. Gordon (eds.), *Tackling Inequalities*. Bristol, England: Policy Press, 2000.

Townson, M. *Health and Wealth: How Social and Economic Factors Affect Our Well-Being*. Toronto, Ontario: Canadian Centre for Policy Alternatives, 1999.

Turnock, B. *Public Health: What It Is and How It Works*. (2nd ed.) Gaithersburg, Md.: Aspen, 2001.

U.S. Department of Health and Human Services. *Health, United States, 1998: Socioeconomic Status and Chartbook*. Washington, D.C.: U.S. Government Printing Office, 1999.

U.S. Department of Health and Human Services. *Healthy People 2010: Understanding and Improving Health*. (2nd ed.) Washington, D.C.: U.S. Government Printing Office, 2000.

United Church of Christ, Commission for Racial Justice. *Toxic Waste and Race in the United States: A National Report on the Socioeconomic Characteristics of Communities with Hazardous Waste Sites*. New York: United Church of Christ, 1987.

United Nations Children's Fund. *The State of the World's Children*. Oxford: Oxford University Press, 1998.

United Nations Development Program. *Human Development Report, 1999*. New York: United Nations, 1999.

Vega, W. A., and Amaro, H. "Latino Outlook: Good Health, Uncertain Prognosis." In T. A. LaVeist (ed.), *Race, Ethnicity, and Health: A Public Health Reader*. San Francisco: Jossey-Bass, 2002.

Wagstaff, A., and Van Doorslaer, E. "Income Inequality and Health: What Does the Literature Tell Us?" *Annual Review of Public Health*, 2000, *21*, 543–567.

Waitzman, N. J., and Smith, K. R. "Separate but Lethal: The Effects of Economic Segregation on Mortality in Metropolitan America." *Milbank Quarterly*, 1998, *78*, 341–373.

Wallack, L., and others. *Media Advocacy and Public Health: Power for Prevention.* Thousand Oaks, Calif.: Sage, 1993.

Wallack, L., and others. *News for a Change: An Advocate's Guide to Working with the Media.* Thousand Oaks, Calif.: Sage, 1999.

Weisbrot, M., and others. *The Scorecard on Globalization, 1980–2000: Twenty Years of Diminished Progress.* Washington, D.C.: Center for Economic and Policy Research, 2001.

Whitehead, M. *The Health Divide: Inequalities in Health in the 1980s.* London: Health Education Council, 1987.

Wilkinson, R. G. *Unhealthy Societies: The Afflictions of Inequality.* London: Routledge, 1996.

Wilkinson, R. G., and Marmot, M. G. (eds.). *Social Determinants of Health: The Solid Facts.* Copenhagen, Denmark: World Health Organization, 1998.

Williams, D. R. "African-American Health: The Role of the Social Environment," *Journal of Urban Health,* 1998, *75,* 300–321.

Williams, D. R. "Race, SES, and Health: The Added Effects of Racism and Discrimination," *Annals of the New York Academy of Sciences,* 1999, *896,* 173–178.

Williams, D. R. "Race and Health Issues in Kansas: Data, Issues, and Directions." In A. Tarlov and R. F. St. Peter (eds.), *The Society and Population Health Reader,* Vol. 2: *A State and Community Perspective.* New York: New Press, 2000.

Williams, D. R., and Collins, C. "U.S. Socioeconomic and Racial Differences in Health: Patterns and Explanations." In T. A. LaVeist (ed.), *Race, Ethnicity, and Health: A Public Health Reader.* San Francisco: Jossey-Bass, 2002.

Wing, S. "The Limits of Epidemiology." In S. Kroll-Smith, P. Brown, and V. J. Gunter (eds.), *Illness and the Environment: A Reader in Contested Medicine.* New York: New York University Press, 2000.

Wolff, E. N. *Recent Trends in Wealth Ownership, 1983–1998.* Working Paper no. 300. New York: Jerome Levy Institute, 2000.

Wolff, E. N. *Top Heavy: The Increasing Inequality of Wealth in America and What Can Be Done About It.* (expanded ed.) New York: New Press, 2002.

Wood, E. M. *Democracy Against Capitalism.* Cambridge: Cambridge University Press, 1995a.

Wood, E. M. "What Is the 'Postmodern' Agenda?" *Monthly Review,* 1995b, *47(3),* 1–12.

World Health Organization. *Health Systems: Improving Performance.* Geneva, Switzerland: World Health Organization, 2000.

Wright, E. O. *Interrogating Inequality: Essays on Class Analysis, Socialism, and Marxism.* New York: Verso, 1994.

Yen, I. H., and Syme, S. L. "The Social Environment and Health: A Discussion of the Epidemiologic Literature." *Annual Review of Public Health,* 1999, *20,* 287–308.

PART ONE

SOCIAL FORCES EXACERBATING HEALTH INEQUITIES

In this part of the book, contributors examine the political and social implications of specific determinants of health, including social class and income inequality, racism, gender discrimination, globalization, political institutions, zoning policy, and the work environment.

Dennis Raphael offers an overview of the role that social determinants of health play in influencing health. He emphasizes the effect of economic inequality and racial segregation in creating health inequities by creating poverty and weakening social support systems. Recommendations include the need to move from epidemiology to public health action through efforts to reverse the ongoing increase in economic inequality.

James S. House and David R. Williams examine what we already know and need to learn about reducing socioeconomic and racial/ethnic disparities in health. They provide an overview of the nature of both socioeconomic and racial/ethnic disparities and how the two are related. They then assess current understanding of the pathways or mechanisms by which the socioeconomic or racial/ethnic status of individuals affect their health and the implications of this understanding for taking action to reduce those disparities. Finally, they explore why and how communities and societies come to be stratified, how the resulting patterns affect people's health, and what can be done about it.

Piroska Östlin, Asha George, and Gita Sen illustrate the ways in which gender influences health inequalities. They describe the nature of gender and how it informs a health equity perspective. In addition, they evaluate how gender influences mortality and longevity, morbidity, health care, and medical research. Their final section evaluates policies that influence gender inequalities in health.

John Gershman, Alec Irwin, and Aaron Shakow investigate economic influences on health outcomes and health policy, with an emphasis on poverty, inequality, development, growth, and globalization. They consider how processes such as privatization, trade liberalization, and deregulation and the ideological assumptions of the discourse used to explain these concepts influence the health of poor communities.

Vincente Navarro and Leiyu Shi consider the influence of political forces such as political parties and their policies in determining the level of equality and inequality, the extent of the welfare state, the employment rate, and the level of population health. They demonstrate that political traditions committed to full employment and progressive redistributive policies improved the health of populations. Exploring political traditions in the advanced OECD countries from 1945 to 1980, they consider four areas: the major determinants of income inequalities, levels of public expenditure and coverage for health care, public services supporting families, and level of population health as measured by infant mortality.

Evaluating the conflicting evidence on various interpretations between income inequality and health, John Lynch, George Davey Smith, George A. Kaplan, and James S. House argue for a neomaterial perspective that considers systematic underinvestment across a wide range of human, physical, health, and social infrastructure in contemporary life.

Julianna A. Maantay evaluates the relationship of spatial inequalities to health inequities. Specifically, she explores ways in which zoning as a major land use planning tool has major implications for equity and public health. Because zoning determines land uses, health will be differentially affected in areas that permit greater environmental hazards. Relying on New York City as a case study, Maantay indicates that environmental hazards are concentrated in poor and minority neighborhoods because more affluent industrial areas and those with lower minority populations are rezoned for other uses.

Sarah Kuhn and John Wooding explore the way in which major transformations in the structure of work—due to phenomena like the expansion of global trade, foreign competition, the international division of labor, and the rapid movement of capital—influence the health and welfare of workers. They further argue that problems arising from these transformations have implications for health outside of the workplace.

CHAPTER TWO

A Society in Decline

The Political, Economic, and Social Determinants
of Health Inequalities in the United States

Dennis Raphael

In this chapter, I adopt a political economy perspective to consider how the concentration of wealth and power in the United States affects the overall health of Americans. Political decisions about how economic and other resources are distributed influence health by shaping the presence and quality of a number of social determinants of health. The relatively poor state of population health in the United States—including its profound health inequalities—results from a variety of political, economic, and social forces (Navarro, 2002; Bezruchka, 2001).

First I will review the current state of knowledge concerning the concentration of wealth and power in the United States and examine how these processes influence various social determinants of health, including the distribution of material resources, the social infrastructure, and communal aspects of civil society. The way in which factors interact to determine health helps explain why the United States has one of the worst population health profiles of any member nation in the Organization for Economic Cooperation and Development (OECD) (Raphael, 2000).

I will then compare population health, social determinants of health, and other indicators of societal functioning in the United States with those in other OECD nations. These political, economic, and social forces are creating a society whose civic institutions and population health profile are in decline (Raphael, 2000; Phillips, 2002; Putnam, 2000). I present various means of conceptualizing this process and conclude that improving the public's health requires an expanded concept of health (World Health Organization, 1986). This work will involve shifting focus away from traditional public health preoccupations with lifestyle and biomedical issues and adopting a political economy perspective (Raphael, 2001a). In Chapter 20 I also indicate the means by which those seeking to address the root causes of health inequities can act at various levels on the political, economic, and social forces that influence the quality of health determinants and work to counteract them. Through actions seeking to transform political, economic, and social institutions, ranging from political advocacy to community organizing, the process of reducing health inequalities and improving the population health of the nation can begin.

THE POLITICAL, ECONOMIC, AND SOCIAL DETERMINANTS OF HEALTH

An explosion of scholarship has increased understanding of how the health of a nation is determined by political, economic, and social forces (See Chapter Six; Auerbach and Krimgold, 2001; Wilkinson, 1996; Kawachi, Kennedy, and Wilkinson, 1999). The mediating processes between these forces and population health are various social determinants of health (Wilkinson and Marmot, 1998; Marmot and Wilkinson, 1999).

Before embarking on our examination of the social determinants of health, it is useful to define the terms we will be using.

Political economy is about how and why a society produces and distributes societal resources among its population in a certain way (Howlett and Ramesh, 1992). The perspective is helpful in understanding the roots of population health and health inequalities within a jurisdiction because it directs attention to the analysis of the political in addition to market relations.

Health refers to the health status of both individuals and communities. For individuals, health refers to the incidence of illness and premature death as well as the presence of physical, social, and personal resources that allow achievement of personal goals (World Health Organization, 1986). For communities, health refers to the presence of economic, social, and environmental structures that support the physical, psychological, and social well-being of community members (Davies and Kelly, 1993; Ashton, 1992).

Population health is primarily concerned with the societal or structural factors that determine the overall health of the population (Evans, Barer, and Marmor, 1994; Health Canada, 2001). The term takes various forms, but Health Canada (1998) has the most developed view, which builds on work by the Canadian Institute for Advanced Research. The Federal, Provincial, and Territorial Advisory Committee on Population Health (1994) defines it as follows:

"Population health refers to the health of a population as measured by health status indicators and as influenced by social, economic and physical environments, personal health practices, individual capacity and coping skills, human biology, early childhood development, and health services" (p. 1).

Social determinants of health are the economic and social conditions in a society that influence whether people stay healthy or become ill (Wilkinson and Marmot, 1998; Marmot and Wilkinson, 1999). Consensus is emerging about what constitutes these determinants, although less agreement exists concerning mechanisms by which they influence health and how these factors can be affected to improve health (Raphael, 2001a; Mutaner, Lynch, and Oates, 1999).

Economic inequality refers to the unequal distribution of income and wealth among residents in a nation, state or province, or locality (Wilkinson, 1996; Judge and Paterson, 2002). Overall distributions within a jurisdiction can be described through the Gini, Theil, or Robin Hood index or by indicators such as the percentage of overall income or wealth shared by a particular percentage of the population, such as the lower 50 percent of a nation, state, or municipality (Kennedy, Kawachi, and Prothrow-Stith, 1996; Kawachi and Kennedy, 1997a).

Support for social infrastructure refers to the percentage of revenues or gross domestic product (GDP) or the amount a jurisdiction allocates to social, health, or other social infrastructure (see Chapter Fifteen). Societal structures that support important life transitions are increasingly regarded as contributing to population health (Bartley, Blane, and Montgomery, 1997; Shaw and others, 1999).

Civil society refers to the organized arena outside of the formal state, consisting of property, economic, and other private relations (Bottomore, Harris, and Miliband, 1992). Politically engaged citizens, professional policy analysts, and associational networks such as unions and other social movements attempt to influence public policy decisions from their position in civil society (Bryant, 2002; Walt, 1994).

THE POLITICAL ECONOMY OF WEALTH AND INCOME INEQUALITIES

Political economy is about the relationships among the state, economy, and civil society (Howlett and Ramesh, 1992). As an area of inquiry, it provides insights that link specific disciplines such as political science, economics, and sociology. Some of the issues considered in the political economic perspective are the production and distribution of wealth, the relative political power of social classes such as capital and labor, and the extent to which society relies extensively on state production and distribution of resources versus market control of such activities. Navarro and Shi in Chapter Six provide an example of how this perspective informs understanding of population health differences among social democratic, Christian democratic, liberal, and ex-fascist OECD nations.

The specific aspects of political economy examined here are those of income and wealth distribution, support of social infrastructure, and support for activities associated with civil society. These areas are closely linked to the extensive literature on the social determinants of health that is informing current policy debates (Chapter Fourteen, Armstrong, Armstrong, and Coburn, 2001; Kawachi and Kennedy, 1997b; Davey Smith, 1996; Bryant and others, 2001). Before considering the political, economic, and social forces that influence population health, it is necessary to examine trends in the distribution of income, wealth, and other societal resources in the United States.

Increasing Income and Wealth Inequality in the United States

An unprecedented increase in income and wealth inequality has occurred in the United States over the past two decades (Wolff, 1995; Lardner, 2000). Former Secretary of Labor Robert Reich (1998, p. 1) observes: "Almost two decades ago, inequality of income, wealth, and opportunity in the United States began to widen, and today the gap is greater than at any time in living memory. All the rungs on the economic ladder are farther apart than they were a generation ago, and the space between them continues to spread."

In international comparisons such as the Luxembourg Income Study, "measures of social distance and overall inequality indicate that the United States has the most unequal distribution of adjusted household income among all 22 countries covered in the study" (Smeeding, 1998, p. 201). This analysis of income inequality in OECD countries found that "the United States, which had the most unequal income distribution in 1979, also had the most unequal distribution in 1994, with inequality growing rapidly through the mid 1990s" (p. 212). Most of the inequality is due to the lower living standards and wages of the least well off in American society: "American low-income families are at a distinct disadvantage compared with similarly situated families in other nations" (p. 201). The poor living conditions of low-income Americans result from low wages and low social spending by the national government.

Documentation of the growing gaps in income and wealth among Americans is widely available (Wolff, 1995; Collins, Hartman, and Sklar, 1999; Collins, Leondar-Wright, and Sklar, 1999; Miringoff and Miringoff, 1999; Freeman, 1998; Yellen, 1998). The recent report *Divided Decade: Economic Disparity at the Century's Turn* (Collins, Hartman, and Sklar, 1999) presents a striking contrast in the distribution of income growth between two recent periods of U.S. history, as shown in Table 2.1. By 1997, the top 1 percent of the U.S. population controlled 40 percent of American wealth. The top 5 percent controlled 62 percent of wealth. At the other end of the distribution, the lowest 40 percent of Americans controlled less than one-half of 1 percent of total wealth.

Table 2.1. Changes in U.S. Family Income, 1947–1979 and 1979–1998.

	Change in Family Income (%)	
Portion of Population	1947–1979	1979–1998
Bottom 20%	+ 116	–5
Next 20%	+ 100	+ 3
Middle 20%	+ 111	+ 8
Next 20%	+ 114	+ 15
Top 20%	+ 99	+ 38
Top 5%	+ 86	+ 64

Source: Collins, Hartman, and Sklar, 1999, p. 3.

Stock ownership is particularly unequal: the top 1 percent of Americans hold almost 48 percent of all stocks, while the bottom 80 percent have just 4 percent of all holdings (Mishel, Bernstein, and Boushey, 2003). This inequality is particularly important as the most recently proposed tax reductions are of particular benefit to stockholders (Citizens for Tax Justice, 2003).

Data from *Health, United States, 1998: Socioeconomic Status and Health Chartbook* (U.S. Department of Health and Human Services, 1998) document the role that race plays in these income and wealth inequalities. Median family income for white families in 1996 was $38,800; for black families, $23,500; and for Hispanic families, $25,000. The racial wealth gap however, is even more striking: in 1995, the median household net worth of white families was $61,000; that of black families, $7,400; and that of Hispanic families, $5,000 (Collins, Leondar-Wright, and Sklar, 1999). Financial worth excluding ownership of a residence was $18,100 for white families, $200 for black families, and $0 for Hispanic families. Poverty and racial composition is becoming even more concentrated in many American cities. The overall probability of an American black student having white classmates fell from 34.7 percent in 1989–1990 to 32.4 percent in 1997–1998 (Rosen, 2000). The increasing economic and racial segregation occurring in the United States has profound health implications (Waitzman and Smith, 1998; Badcock, 1984; Jackson and others, 2000).

Less Spending on Social Infrastructure

Reports by the Organization for Economic Cooperation and Development (2001) and the United Nations Development Program (2001) provide evidence of striking contrasts in expenditures in social infrastructure between the United States and other industrialized nations. The United States spends 33 percent of GDP on current general governmental expenditures, among the lowest of all OECD nations, and 16 percent of GDP on public social expenditures, also among the lowest of the OECD nations. The United States also spends significantly less on public education and social and health programs and provides less support in the form of unemployment insurance and welfare supports. (Smeeding, 1998; Rainwater and Smeeding, 1995; Raphael and Bryant, 2003) These deficits serve to heighten inequalities among Americans, with especially important effects on children (Lee and Burkam, 2002).

In the United States, less funding is available than in most OECD nations for public employment services and administration, labor market training, youth measures, and subsidized employment and measures for the disabled (Organization for Economic Cooperation and Development, 2001). Furthermore, the United States has one of the worst records in support of early childhood education and provision of child care and in supporting women in employment and child care roles (Raphael and Bryant, 2003; International Reform Monitor, 2002; Organization for Economic Cooperation and Development, 2000).This state has resulted in large part from a lack of resources due to profound tax reductions (to be explained shortly).

UNDERSTANDING THE FORCES DRIVING THESE DEVELOPMENTS

Mainstream economic and political analyses attempt to explain increasing income and wealth inequalities as reflecting the readjustment of market forces and changing family dynamics (Auerbach and Belous, 1998). However, research from a more critical perspective offers a rather less benign view of the forces that drive income and wealth inequalities and the weakening of social infrastructure and civil society. These views are considered next.

Decline of the Welfare State

Teeple (2000) regards increasing income and wealth inequalities and the weakening of social infrastructures in the United States and elsewhere as a result of the ascendance of concentrated monopoly capitalism and corporate globalization. Transnational corporations—many with home bases in the United States—actively apply their increasing power to oppose reforms associated with the welfare state to reduce labor costs.

Teeple defines the welfare state as "a capitalist society in which the state has intervened in the form of social policies, programs, standards, and regulations in order to mitigate class conflict and to provide for, answer, or accommodate certain social needs for which the capitalist mode of production in itself has no solution or makes no provision" (2000, p. 15).

The forces that led to the development of the welfare state at the end of World War II included strong national identities, the need to rebuild Western economies, the strength of national labor unions, the perceived threat of socialist alternatives, and a consensus for political compromise to avoid the boom-and-bust cycles of the economy. These forces led to policies that supported a more equitable distribution of income and wealth through social, economic, and political reforms such as progressive tax structures, as well as social programs and governmental structures that mitigated conflicts between business and labor, among other things.

These forces are now in decline. Since 1974, a fundamental change has occurred in the operation of national and global economics. The rise of transnational corporations that can easily shift investments around the globe puts pressure on nations to accede to demands for changes that reverse reforms associated with the welfare state.

International trade agreements are one way to weaken both national identities and nationally based labor unions. Trade is now international, but unions continue to be national. Businesses therefore have less need for political compromises among themselves, labor, and governments. The decline of the Soviet bloc and its diffuse threat of supporting working-class revolt has also removed incentives for businesses to compromise with employees and labor in general. Finally, the overall slowing of economic growth has reduced resources available for the welfare state. Increased concentration of corporate and media ownership helps ensure that justification for these changes, delivered in the form of neoliberal ideology, is now the dominant discourse related to political and economic processes (see Chapter Fourteen).

To illustrate, nationally based labor unions have little influence when the economies of nations become increasingly globalized. Labor demands in one nation simply cause companies to move elsewhere. Neoliberal political ideology serves the needs of global corporations attempting to maximize profits by weakening local legislation that ensures livable wages, workplace and environmental safety, and communal structures that support health. Every public service and communal structure is now seen as ripe for privatization. Social and economic conditions have deteriorated for the mass of citizens as national governments and more and more local governments either remain helpless to resist the power of transnational corporations or become complicit in these activities.

Indeed, Laxer (1998) argues that "everywhere in the world, multinational business has launched a frontal assault on the state" (p. 163), while others argue that the "deep-seated economic and social changes that have helped to erode the social contract—the predominant understandings about core economic and social relationships—that was built up during the post-war era" (Banting, Hoberg, and Simeon, 1997, p. 4) and that "the power of capital has been strengthened by threats to relocate if its demands for enhanced flexibility with regard to taxes, state regulation, and labor market policies are not met by policy-makers. The neoliberal political agenda has both shaped and been advanced by globalization" (McBride and Shields, 1997, p. 13).

Decline of Working-Class Power

Consistent with this approach is Zweig's analysis of class and power in the United States. Zweig (2000) argues that the 60 percent or more of Americans that constitute the working class in the United States have interests fundamentally at odds with the two hundred thousand or so individuals that serve on the governing boards of national-scale corporations. Zweig identifies how these corporations use their power and influence to weaken the institutions and services that support working-class Americans in their lives, thereby affecting their health and well-being.

Indeed, federal tax legislation over the past two decades has led to increasing income and wealth inequalities and served to remove revenues that would have been available to support social and health programs—key contributors to population health for the majority of Americans (Lardner, 2000; Terris, 1994; Johnston, 1997).

The Bush tax cuts of 2001 and the proposed ones for 2003 illustrate the influence that the wealthy and powerful have on federal legislation. Indeed, Robert McIntyre, director of Citizens for Tax Justice (2003, p. 1), states: "President Bush seems to have decided that the biggest problem facing America today is that the rich don't have enough money. If you agree with that odd diagnosis, then the president's tax plan is perfectly designed."

Analysis of the 2001 Bush $1.3 trillion in income tax cuts by Citizens for Tax Justice (2002) indicates that by 2010, fully 52 percent of the total tax cuts will go to the richest 1 percent of Americans. That is, of the total $234 billion in tax cuts scheduled for 2010, $121 billion will go to just 1.4 million taxpayers. Concerning the proposed 2003 tax reductions worth $674 billion, three-fifths of the proposed tax reductions would go to the wealthiest 10 percent of taxpayers.

Neoliberalism as a Justifying Discourse

Coburn considers in Chapter Fourteen how neoliberalism—through its emphasis on the market as the arbiter of societal values and resource allocations—serves to support these regressive political and economic forces. Furthermore, implementing neoliberal economic policies fosters income and wealth inequalities, weakens social infrastructure, dissipates social cohesion, and threatens civil society. I have written about how the one aspect of neoliberal ideology—the exaggerated emphasis on reducing taxes—directly benefits the wealthy and powerful and translates into both increasing economic inequality and the weakening of communal institutions that support civil society (Raphael, 2001a).

Indeed, in 1965, U.S. federal and state corporate taxes constituted 4.1 percent of GDP, which ranked third among OECD nations. By 2000, however, U.S. corporate income taxes were down to 2.5 percent of GDP, while among other OECD nations these taxes increased from 2.4 percent of GDP in 1975 to 3.4 percent in 2000. As a result, U.S. corporate taxes had dropped to twenty-second among the twenty-nine reporting OECD nations. In fiscal 2002, federal and state corporate taxes dropped further to 1.5 percent of GDP, less than every OECD nation except Iceland (Citizens for Tax Justice, 2003).

Threats to Civil Society

Debate persists as to whether increasing income inequality directly threatens population health by weakening social cohesion, social connectedness, or social capital (Chapter Fifteen; Mutaner, Lynch, and Oates, 1999; Kawachi and Kennedy, 1997b, 2002). The argument offered here is that increasing concentration of wealth and power—supported by increasing income inequality and the dominant societal discourse of neoliberalism—weakens both civil society and citizen commitment to communal structures associated with the welfare state. These weakened commitments on the part of the citizenry lead to two profound shifts in U.S. politics. The first is that members of civil society that oppose the concentration of wealth and power become increasingly marginalized and politically impotent. The second is that citizens become increasingly more likely to support political approaches that are fundamentally at odds with their objective self-interests. The end result of both processes is the weakening of opposition to increasing concentration of wealth and power, the weakening of the social determinants of health, and threats to population health. I shall consider each of these processes in turn.

The first key aspect is the weakening of civil society. Phillips (2002) outlines how U.S. democracy is directly threatened by the concentration of assets, growing inequality, and conspicuous consumption of the rich. Owing to mounting evidence of political corruption, the growing arrogance of global economic power, and the twisting of the U.S. tax code in the service of the wealthy and powerful, increasing numbers of citizen are coming to believe that governments are captive to the interests of the wealthy and powerful. Their perception of being able to influence governments dissipates. Many indicators of such alienation and declining interest in civil activity are in evidence, though explanations for the phenomena are in dispute (Putnam, 2000; Raphael, 2001a; Heying, 1995; Pollitt, 1996).

Phillips's analysis can be extended to explain increasing voter apathy among Americans and the increasing marginalization of many civil society voices that are opposed to the current political agenda. The public becomes less likely to hear these dissident voices and more likely to accept the dominant neoliberal discourse (McQuaig, 1998). People look for ways to maximize their immediate situation; are always receptive to tax reductions, no matter how meager they may be; and turn against those identified as a threat to their security: the ill, the poor, and the marginalized.

Concerning increasing acceptance of political directions at odds with fundamental self-interests, McQuaig (1993) describes the process by which citizen opinion is turned against the concept of entitlement as it applies to the public provision of goods and services. She uses the example of Canada's "child benefit" to explain how promoting the idea that the "wealthy banker's wife" was receiving the same benefit as the homeless, unemployed mother upon the birth of a child weakened public support for the benefit. The benefit was subsequently reduced to the point that what had been a strong material support for the great majority of Canadians virtually disappeared.

A similar process can be seen in the United States in the idea of school vouchers. Governments weaken the public school system through spending reductions to the point that parents become disillusioned with the system. They then demand the right to move their children to private schools, leaving the public system to wither on the vine. Kawachi and Kennedy (2002) provide similar examples with regard to citizens living in gated communities resenting paying taxes to support the community infrastructure outside their gates.

A final example of this process is the proposed elimination of the estate tax. This tax only affects the very wealthiest of Americans, yet its elimination is supported by an incredibly well organized campaign, which rails about the injustice of the "death tax." As a result, a surprising proportion of Americans across the income spectrum supports such regressive legislation (Brooks, 2003).

For Wilkinson (1996), this decline in commitment to communal structures is part of the process by which societies begin to disintegrate. These declining commitments are consistent with neomaterial explanations of the income inequality and population health relationships (Chapters Fourteen and Fifteen; Glyn and Miliband, 1994). Through these processes, the forces that threaten population health gain acceptance among their very victims.

These analyses are important given the burgeoning literature of the role that social determinants of health, such as income and wealth distribution, poverty, support for social infrastructure, and communal processes associated with civil society, play in population health and health inequalities (Auerbach and Krimgold, 2001; Kawachi, Kennedy, and Wilkinson, 1999; Shaw and others, 1999). The literature on social determinants of health, however, rarely considers the political and economic issues raised by a political economy analysis that explores shifting power relations (Poland and others, 1998; see also Chapter Eighteen).

THE IMPORTANCE OF THE SOCIAL DETERMINANTS OF HEALTH

Many of the profound improvements in health in the United States and other Western countries over the past century are not due to advances in medical and health care but rather to changes in the structures and distribution of resources in society (McKeown, 1976). To provide just one illustration, the public health community and the general public assume that the discoveries of the causes of infections diseases and means of immunizing children against them were responsible for much of the decline in mortality from common childhood diseases. Although these developments did support population health, improvements in general social conditions were most responsible for these advances (McKinlay and McKinlay, 1987). It is estimated 10 to 15 percent of increased longevity in Western nations since 1900 can be attributed to improved medical care (McKeown and Record, 1975; Kim and Moody, 1992).

More recently, public discourse has focused on the extent to which factors such as tobacco use, quality of diet, and physical activity are responsible for differences in the occurrence of ailments such heart disease, stroke, and cancer between and within nations (Nettleton, 1997; Nettleton and Bunton, 1995; Raphael, 2001b, 2002). But British studies of more than two decades ago found that most variation in health and disease among individuals could not be accounted for by these factors (Marmot and others, 1978). Similarly, studies in the United States reveal that behavioral risk factors account for a rather small proportion of variance in mortality rates when compared to income and education (Lantz and others, 1998; Roux and others, 2001; Feldman and others, 1989). The additional factors that predict illness and death include prerequisites for health, determinants of health, and social determinants of health.

The *Ottawa Charter for Health Promotion* (World Health Organization, 1986) identifies the *prerequisites for health* as peace, shelter, education, food, income, a stable ecosystem, sustainable resources, social justice, and equity. Health Canada (1998) accepted direction from the Canadian Institute for Advanced Research in outlining the *determinants of health* (only some of which are social determinants): income and social status, social support networks, education, employment and working conditions, physical and social environments, biology and genetic endowment, personal health practices and coping skills, healthy child development, and health services. A British working group identifies *social determinants of health* as social-class health gradient, stress, early life, social exclusion, work, unemployment, social support, addiction, food, and transport (Wilkinson and Marmot, 1998; Marmot and Wilkinson, 1999).

POVERTY, INCOME, AND WEALTH INEQUALITY AND POPULATION HEALTH IN INDUSTRIALIZED NATIONS

The focus in this chapter is on social determinants of health associated with the distribution of economic and other resources within jurisdictions. This leads to an initial consideration of poverty and its effects on individuals and communities. But the distribution of resources in a society is also associated with whether supports associated with social infrastructure are available to the population (Raphael, 2001a; Lynch and others, 2001).

Poverty and Its Effects on Health

Poverty is the most obvious manifestation of inequality in the distribution of economic and other resources and potentially the strongest determinant of health (Williamson and Reutter, 1999; Reutter, 1995; Reutter, Stewart, and Makwarimba, 2002). One by-product of unequal distributions of wealth is a greater number of poor people. Recent reanalysis of data from the Luxembourg Income Study found that the relationship between degree of income inequality within a nation—as measured by the Gini index—with child poverty for sixteen industrialized Western nations was strong, positive, and reliable ($r = .77$) (Raphael, 2001a). The United States has the highest levels of income and wealth inequality and the greatest level of child poverty among residents of these nations (Innocenti Research Centre, 2000).

Poverty can be considered in relation to absolute or relative material deprivation (Williamson and Reutter, 1999). Townsend (1979) provides compelling arguments for use of the latter concept, and international organizations and research studies favor the definition whereby families gaining less than 50 percent of a nation's median income are considered as living in poverty (see also Organization for Economic Cooperation and Development, 2001; United Nations Development Program, 2001). Statistics Canada sets low-income cutoffs—families spending more than 53 percent on basic necessities—to identify those living in "straitened circumstances" (Canadian Council on Social Development, 2001). This cutoff level is remarkably close to Canadians' views of what constitutes poverty. Because "poverty lines" in the United States are absurdly low (U.S. Department of Health and Human Services, 2002), I use internationally agreed definitions of poverty in this chapter (Bernstein, 2001; Bernstein, Brocht, and Spade-Aguilar, 2000).

The effects of poverty on health have been known since the nineteenth century, but interest was spurred by the publication in the United Kingdom of the Black and the Health Divide reports (Sram and Ashton, 1998; Black and Smith, 1992; Whiteside, 1992; Davey Smith, Dorling, and Shaw, 2001). These reports documented that individuals in the lowest employment groups are more likely than other wage earners to suffer from and die of a range of diseases and injuries at every stage of the life cycle. Differences in health occur across the socioeconomic range from professional practitioner to manual laborer.

Interest in poverty and its health effects continues unabated in the United Kingdom, and updates on health inequalities in Britain and means of addressing these are available (see, for example, Shaw and others, 1999; Benzeval, Judge, and Whitehead, 1995; Pantazis and Gordon, 2000; Acheson, 1998; Gordon and others, 1999). Indeed, British work in the area is the most advanced among industrialized nations and an excellent source of research ideas and potential policy solutions. Canadian research on the social determinants of health and means of addressing health inequalities resulting from these determinants is increasing (see Canadian Institute for Health Information, 2002; Raphael, Colman, and Labonte, 2003; Dunn, 2000; Dunn, Hargreaves, and Alex, 2002; Townson, 1999).

In 1998, a report of the U.S. Department of Health and Human Services documented the wide range of income-related health differences existing between poor and nonpoor children, adults, and older persons. In addition to many mortality and morbidity rate differences, differences are also seen for activity limitation among children and adults, as well as lifestyle factors such as cigarette smoking and overweight. To illustrate the magnitude of these income-related health differences, heart disease death rates for the periods 1979–1989 for Americans between the ages of twenty-five and sixty-four were 318 per 100,000 for individuals earning less than $10,000 a year; 251 for those earning $10,000 to $14,999; 142 for those earning $15,000 to $24,900; and 216 for those earning $25,000 or more. Similar findings occur for many other diseases. In addition, poverty has consequences with respect to performance in school, use of the health care system, and quality of attained employment. Poverty's effects on health can be direct, related to physical and mental illness resulting from absolute material deprivation, and indirect, involving psychological reactions to relative deprivation and feelings of powerlessness and lack of control over life situations (Benzeval and others, 2001; Brunner and Marmot, 1999; Wilkinson, 2001; Lynch, Kaplan, and Salonen, 1997).

Income Inequality and Population Health

The publication of Wilkinson's *Unhealthy Societies: The Afflictions of Inequality* (1996) stimulated interest in income inequality as an independent contributor to population health. Wilkinson assembled much of the research showing that societies with greater income inequality generally have higher mortality rates. For example, after decades of rapidly increasing economic inequality, the most well-off in Britain now have higher death rates among adults and infants than the least well-off in Sweden (Leon, Vagero, and Otterblad, 1992; Vagero and Lundberg, 1989). Wilkinson argued that degree of income inequality was the best variable to explain differences in life expectancy among residents of Western industrialized nations. Recent analyses of large data sets challenge this view, but even critics admit that the United States, with its tremendous gaps in income and wealth among its population, illustrates how growing economic inequality can lead to poor population health at the national, state, and municipal levels (Chapter Seven; Ross and others, 2000; Wolfson and others, 1999).

Degree of income inequality within each of the fifty U.S. states, rather than average state income, is the best predictor of overall mortality and general well-being among residents of these states (Kennedy and others, 1998; Kaplan and others, 1996). These effects are also seen for state homicide rates and other indicators of social health and well-being (Kawachi, Kennedy, and Wilkinson, 1999). Similar findings appear when considering municipal areas (Lynch and others, 1998). Average wealth and degree of income inequality are both related to health status of municipalities. These findings represent more than merely stating that these jurisdictions have a greater number of poor people. The findings indicate the presence of a carryover effect whereby even well-off people in unequal communities show greater evidence of illness and poor health, compared to those living in more equal communities.

These effects are profound. Differences in overall death rates between U.S. cities with low per capita income and high income inequality and those with high per capita income and low income inequality is 150 per 100,000 (Lynch and others, 1998). This difference is greater than the 1997 age-adjusted mortality rate from heart disease for all Americans. Findings like these led the *British Medical Journal* to editorialize: "What matters in determining mortality and health in a society is less the overall wealth of that society and more how evenly wealth is distributed. The more equally wealth is distributed, the better the health of that society" ("Big Idea," 1996, p. 985). As noted, this conclusion appears especially relevant to the United States and may explain not only differences among Americans but also why population health in the United States lags behind virtually all other OECD nations.

THREE EXPLANATIONS

Three main schools of thought attempt to explain why the United States falls short in population health: the materialist, neomaterialist, and social comparison approaches.

Materialist Approach: Poverty and Material Deprivation as Determinants of Population Health

The materialist explanation for the income inequality–population health relationship is based on the view that individuals are exposed to varying degrees of positive and negative influences over the course of their lifetimes. These exposures accumulate to produce either positive or negative health outcomes. The findings of stepped differences among social classes and income groups result because "the social structure is characterized by a finely graded scale of advantage and disadvantage, with individuals differing in terms of the length and level of their exposure to a particular factor and in terms of the number of factors to which they are exposed" (Shaw and others, 1999, p. 102).

In contrast to psychological arguments that differences in relative status lead to poor health, the materialist argument is that socioeconomic indicators such as income, wealth, educational attainment, and occupational group serve as indicators of material advantage that accumulate over the life span (Shaw and others, 1999; Davey Smith and Gordon, 2000; Davey Smith, Grunnell, and Ben-Shlomo, 2001; Davey Smith, Ben-Shlomo, and Lynch, 2002; Davey Smith and Hart, 2002). Material circumstances in early life are more potent predictors of later health than social position during adulthood (Lynch, Kaplan, and Salonen, 1997; Eriksson and others, 1999).

Benzeval, Judge, and Whitehead (1995) outline a triad of effects associated with material deprivation over the course of the life span. In addition to material deprivation related to greater exposure to health-threatening factors and fewer exposures to health-enhancing factors, poor people experience greater psychosocial stress. The fight-or-flight reaction—chronically elicited in response to continuing threats such as housing and food insecurity—becomes health-threatening through physiological processes such as weakening of the immune system, increased insulin resistance, and greater incidence of lipid disorders and other biomedical injuries (Brunner and Marmot, 1999). The third aspect of the materialist argument is how adoption of health-threatening behaviors occurs in response to material deprivation. The social and economic environments in which people live shape the behavioral risk factors of tobacco use, poor diet, and inactivity—associated with income level (Jarvis and Wardle, 1999). Stress produces tension-reducing behaviors such as carbohydrate-dense diets and tobacco and excessive alcohol use (Wilkinson, 1996; Stansfeld and Marmot, 2002).

Materialist arguments go a long way toward explaining the presence of large health inequalities in the United States and its relatively low level of overall population health. The United States has one of the highest rates of family and child poverty among the OECD nations (Rainwater and Smeeding, 1995). And as noted earlier, U.S. workers at the low end of the wage skills make far less than most low-end workers in European nations (Smeeding, 1998). These differences in material experience are aggravated by the weakening of social infrastructure that is an important aspect of the neomaterialist argument (see Chapter Fifteen).

Neomaterialist Approach: Material Deprivation and Weakened Social Infrastructure as Determinants of Population Health

Lynch and colleagues (Chapter Seven) note that jurisdictions that have inequitable income and wealth distributions invest fewer resources in public infrastructure. In the United States, for example, degree of income inequality at the state level is related to expenditure on public goods such as health insurance, social welfare, and supports for the unemployed and the disabled

(Kaplan and others, 1996). High-inequality U.S. states also spend less per capita on education and libraries. The neomaterialist view argues that "health inequalities result from the differential accumulation of exposures and experiences that have their sources in the material world" (Chapter Seven). In addition to the greater incidence of poverty that is typical of unequal jurisdictions, "the effect of income inequality on health reflects a combination of negative exposures and lack of resources held by individuals, along with systematic underinvestment across a wide range of human, physical, health, and social infrastructure" (p. 222 in this volume; see Chapter Fifteen).

The extent of material deprivation experienced by individuals is clearly related to the allocation of resources in a society or jurisdiction. There would appear to be no necessity that jurisdictions that tolerate wide economic inequalities would invest less resources in social infrastructure. But the evidence indicates that is the case when comparing the United States to other OECD nations (Organization for Economic Cooperation and Development, 2001).

One important way by which this happens is changing tax structures. In the United States, profound changes in the tax structure have favored the wealthy. Wealth inequality between rich and poor grows, and the money now unavailable to governments leads to less spending on education and social services. Such policies not only increase the number of poor people but also weaken the supports that allow poor people to function adequately in society. The United States spends less on social and health programs than most other OECD nations (Smeeding, 1998; Organization for Economic Cooperation and Development, 2001; United Nations Development Program, 2001). The neomaterialist framework is also clearly applicable for understanding the very poor population health profile of the United States.

Social Comparison Approach: Hierarchy and Social Distance as Determinants of Population Health

In volume 1 of *The Society and Population Health Reader, Income Inequality and Health*, Kawachi, Kennedy, and Wilkinson (1999) collected readings that emphasize what can be called the social comparison explanation of the income inequality–population health relationship. They argue that health effects related to income and wealth inequalities in the United States are not primarily due to material deprivation but rather to citizens' interpretations of their standings in the social hierarchy. The viewpoint is more fully outlined in Kawachi and Kennedy's *Health of Nations: Why Inequality Is Harmful to Your Health* (2002). In these works, two main mechanisms explain the relationship between economic inequality and poor population health.

At the individual level, psychosocial effects of hierarchy present in highly unequal societies are hypothesized to lead to stress and poor health. Through a process of psychosocial comparison, individuals come to experience ongoing feelings of shame, worthlessness, and envy. These perceptions have psychobiological concomitants that lead to poor health. They can also lead to behaviors to alleviate such feelings, such as overspending, taking on additional employment responsibilities that threaten health, or overeating and the use of alcohol and tobacco.

At the communal level, the widening and strengthening of hierarchy weakens social capital and social cohesion with effects that lead to poor health. Individuals become more distrusting and suspicious of others, weakening support for communal structures such as the education and social service systems and thereby reducing population health. These effects are clearly provoked by aspects of the material world, but the emphasis is on increased hierarchy, unfavorable social comparison, and a weakening of social capital as means by which economic inequality leads to poorer population health.

The social comparison view has been criticized as minimizing the profound effects on health of the material deprivation and material insecurity that many Americans increasingly experience (see Chapter Eleven). Indeed, Pearce and Davey Smith (2003, p. 122) argue that "intervening in communities to increase their social capital may be ineffective, create resentment, and overload community resources." Although proponents of the social cohesion or social capital approach such as Kawachi and Kennedy consider the political and ideological value systems associated with increasing income inequality, the approach may direct attention away from the political and economic forces that exacerbate income and wealth inequalities, weaken social infrastructure, and skew societal priorities. Even accepting that the processes of hierarchy and social dissolution contribute to poor population health, material aspects of society—such as those described in the materialist and neomaterialist approaches—are still the prime determinants of these processes.

A SOCIETY IN DECLINE

Not surprisingly, in statistical comparisons on the social determinants of health, the United States does poorly in relation to other OECD nations. In the following discussion, specific comparisons are made with Sweden (a nation with a social democratic tradition) and with Canada (a nation with both market and social democratic elements), which of course shares the North American continent with the United States (where a market orientation is predominant). A more extensive comparison of twenty-five indicators of social development among the United States, Sweden, and Canada is available (Jackson, 2002).

U.S. Population Health in Perspective

Table 2.2 shows average life expectancy, infant mortality rate, and heart disease mortality rates for the United States, Sweden, and Canada and the rankings for these nations among thirty OECD nations. The total number of OECD nations varies for comparisons as a function of data availability. Exhibit 2.1 provides a list of these OECD nations.

Table 2.2. Indicators of Population Health for
the United States, Sweden, and Canada, with OECD Ranks.

Indicator	United States	Rank	Sweden	Rank	Canada	Rank
Life expectancy at birth (years)	77.3	20/30	79.9	4/30	79.75	5/30
Infant mortality per 1,000 live births	6.7	24/30	3.4	1/30	5.0	16/30
Child injury per 100,000	14.1	23/26	5.2	1/26	9.7	18/26

Sources: Central Intelligence Agency, 2002; Innocenti Research Centre, 2000.

Despite spending a greater percentage of GDP (13.5 percent) on health care than any other OECD nation, the United States compares poorly in international health status comparisons: "For nearly all available outcome measures, the United States ranked near the bottom of the OECD countries in 1996, and the rate of improvement for most of the indicators has been slower than the median OECD country" (Anderson and Poullier, 1999, p. 6). Among thirty OECD nations, U.S. life expectancy ranks eighteenth for males and twentieth for females (Central Intelligence Agency, 2002; European Institute of Japanese Studies, 2002). Nations with lower life expectancy than the United States are Ireland, Denmark, Portugal, the Czech Republic, South Korea, Slovakia, Poland, Mexico, Hungary, and Turkey.

The United States also has a very high infant mortality rate and a high child injury mortality rate (Innocenti Research Centre, 2000; European Institute of Japanese Studies, 2002). The only OECD nations with a higher infant mortality rate than the United States are South Korea, Hungary, Slovakia, Poland, Mexico, and Turkey. Nations with higher child injury death rates are Portugal, Mexico, and South Korea.

Exhibit 2.1. OECD Nations Used in International Comparisons in This Chapter.

Australia	Denmark	Ireland	New Zealand	Spain
Austria	France	Italy	Norway	Sweden
Belgium	Germany	Japan	Poland	Switzerland
Canada	Greece	Luxembourg	Portugal	Turkey
Czech Republic	Hungary	Mexico	Slovakia	United Kingdom
Finland	Iceland	Netherlands	South Korea	United States

Social Determinants of Health

The United States compares unfavorably with OECD nations on most social indicators of population health (see Table 2.3). While having the second-highest gross domestic product per capita—only Luxembourg's is higher—the United States compares poorly on income distribution and child poverty rates and on public expenditure on social infrastructure. Even the U.S. unemployment rate is not among the top-ranked of OECD nations, and the United States has the dubious distinction of having the greatest proportion of low-paying jobs. Finally, unemployment benefits are among the lowest of any OECD nation as a percentage of average replacement value.

Signs of Disintegration

Wilkinson (1996) argues, as others do (Raphael, 2001a), that societies with high levels of income and wealth inequality show symptoms of social disintegration. The form that social disintegration takes in each society may be unique. In Britain, increasing economic inequality is associated with increased alcoholism,

Table 2.3. Various Social Determinants of Health
in the United States, Sweden, and Canada, with OECD Ranks.

Indicator	United States	Rank	Sweden	Rank	Canada	Rank
GDP per capita (U.S.$)	36,500	2/30	25,600	17/30	28,800	8/30
Income distribution (Gini)	34.5	18/21	23.0	3/21	28.5	13/21
Child poverty rate (%)	22.4	22/23	2.6	1/23	15.5	17/23
Unemployment rate (%)	4.8	12/30	4.9	13/30	7.2	21/30
Low-paid employment (%)	24	24/24	5	1/24	21	20/24
Unemployment benefit (%)	14	18/20	29	11/20	28	13/20
Public education spending (% of GDP)	5.2	12/28	6.8	1/28	5.4	10/28
Public social expenditure (% of GDP)	16	24/28	33	1/28	17	23/28
Public share of total health care expenditures (% of GDP)	45.0	28/29	84.3	4/29	69.4	22/29

Sources: Organization for Economic Cooperation and Development, 2001; European Institute of Japanese Studies, 2002.

higher crime rates, more deaths in roadway accidents, an increase in infectious diseases, poorer reading scores, increased drug offenses, decaying family functioning, and decreased voter turnout, among other tendencies (Wilkinson, 1996; see Chapter Fifteen). In the United States, income inequality among the fifty states is related to a series of indicators that may be seen as signs of social disintegration.

Degree of income inequality at the state level is related to levels of unemployment, proportion of the population incarcerated, use of income vouchers, food stamps, and proportion of population with no health insurance. Similar findings were reported for high school completion, reading and math proficiency, education spending, and library books per capita (Kaplan and others, 1996). Table 2.4 provides comparisons and rankings among OECD nations for the United States, Sweden, and Canada on some of these kinds of indicators.

The United States has the highest homicide rate among OECD nations (7.6 per 100,000 population; the next closest is Finland, with 3.3 per 100,000), and evidence is that the rates of decline experienced over the past few years are now reversing themselves. The United States also has the highest rate for incarceration of its citizens (546 per 100,000 population; the next closest is the Czech Republic, at 210 per 100,000). Motor vehicle death rates are high, and the United States does poorly in international literacy comparisons. The concept of social health offers further insights into why the United States is in social decline and how social conditions cause deteriorating health across population groups.

Table 2.4. Various Indicators of Social Disintegration for the United States, Sweden, and Canada, with OECD Ranks.

Indicator	United States	Rank	Sweden	Rank	Canada	Rank
Homicide rate per 100,000	7.6	26/26	1.2	12/26	1.4	17/26
Motor vehicle deaths per 100,000	15.3	22/26	4.9	1/26	9.3	10/26
Incarceration rates per 100,000	546	25/25	60	6/25	115	19/25
Reading scores	504	15/27	516	9/27	534	2/27
Mathematics scores	493	18/27	510	14/27	533	5/27
Science scores	499	14/27	512	10/27	529	5/27

Sources: Organization for Economic Cooperation and Development, 2001; European Institute of Japanese Studies, 2002.

Social Health

The Fordham Institute for Innovation in Social Policy has since 1990 reported overall U.S. national and state scores on its Index of Social Health (Miringoff and Miringoff, 1999). The index consists of sixteen indicators of health and well-being. Overall scores on the index have been declining in the United States since the mid-1970s even as GDP has increased. During the period 1970–1996, four indicators improved: infant mortality, high school dropouts, poverty among residents aged sixty-five and above, and life expectancy for residents aged sixty-five and above. However, on seven indicators, performance worsened: child abuse, child poverty, teenage suicide, number of health care uninsured, average weekly wages, inequality, and violent crime. Six indicators showed variable performance during the period: teenage drug use, teenage births, alcohol-related traffic fatalities, affordable housing, and unemployment. Canada's scores on this same index are noticeably higher than those for the United States.

Human and Social Development in the United States

It has been argued that these macro-level indicators become translated into poor population health through a variety of biological and psychosocial pathways. It is important to be able to show the mechanisms by which these factors "get under the skin" to influence health. Keating and Hertzman's *Developmental Health and the Wealth of Nations* (1999) provides a wealth of models and empirical findings that illuminate these processes. The high incidence of child poverty is important for understanding the poor population health profile of the United States (Innocenti Research Centre, 2000). The health issues associated with poverty are made worse by the lack of social infrastructure and supports for families. In a summary of the U.S. situation, Brooks-Gunn, Duncan, and Britto (1999, p. 122) comment:

> Income gradients during childhood are steeper in the United States than in Canada or the United Kingdom. First, . . . , more U.S. children are in deep poverty than in the two comparison nations. Second, the income disparities between the rich and poor and near poor are much larger in the United States than in Canada or the United Kingdom. Unless policies address these inequities . . . , it is likely that the SES gradient will remain steeper for U.S. children than for Canadian or British children, with the consequent risks for the developmental health of the American population.

Out of the Loop: U.S. Public Health Preoccupations

Considering the clear evidence that increasing economic inequality and the weakening of other social determinants of health lead to poor population health, how does the U.S. public health community consider these issues? Three frames of reference for considering these issues exist (Labonte, 1993; Labonte and Thompson, 1992). Biomedical approaches emphasize identification of high-risk groups, screening of one sort or another, and health care delivery. Behavioral approaches focus on high-risk attitudes and behaviors and programs to promote lifestyle changes. The socioenvironmental approach focuses on high-risk conditions and considers how individuals move to change them. Tesh (1990) argues that frames of reference are adopted on the basis of ideology and values rather than the available objective evidence. Current debates about the determinants of health are focused on the relative importance of personal and structural factors in determining health (Raphael, 2002). U.S. debate is dominated by biomedical and lifestyle discourse.

Until recently, the notion that income and wealth inequalities were public health issues was rarely heard in the United States (Auerbach, Krimgold, and Lefkowitz, 2000). Public health practice—with some exceptions—has been remarkably isolated for decades from developments in population health in Canada and elsewhere (Hertzman, 2001). While the Institute of Medicine's publication *The Future of the Public's Health in the 21st Century* (2002) raises issues about social determinants, efforts directed at root causes are primitive when compared to the theorization and activities that are under way in Canada, Europe, and elsewhere. The predominant approach to population health in the United States remains focused on behavioral change. Little notice is taken of developments outside the United States.

The U.S. public policy and public health communities must seriously consider and address the structural sources of increasing economic inequality and the deterioration of other social determinants of health. Whether such efforts can succeed in an era of increasing dominance by the corporate agenda remains an open question. In Chapter Twenty, I present developments in Europe and Canada that have resisted the corporate agenda and work toward reducing health inequalities and promoting population health.

References

Acheson, D. *Independent Inquiry into Inequalities in Health.* London: Stationary Office, 1998.

Anderson, G. R., and Poullier, J. "Health Spending, Access, and Outcomes: Trends in Industrialized Nations." *Health Affairs,* May-June 1999, pp. 178–192.

Armstrong, H., Armstrong, P., and Coburn, D. (eds.). *Unhealthy Times: The Political Economy of Health and Care in Canada.* Toronto: Oxford University Press, 2001.

Ashton, J. (ed.). Healthy Cities. Berkshire, England: Open University Press, 1992.

Auerbach, J. A., and Belous, R. (eds.), *The Inequality Paradox: Growth of Income Disparity.* Washington, D.C.: National Policy Association, 1998.

Auerbach, J. A., and Krimgold, B. (eds.). *Income, Socioeconomic Status, and Health: Exploring the Relationships*. Washington, D.C.: National Policy Association, 2001.

Auerbach, J. A., Krimgold, B., and Lefkowitz, B. *Improving Health: It Doesn't Take a Revolution*. Washington, D.C.: National Policy Association, 2000.

Badcock, B. *Unfairly Structured Cities*. Oxford: Blackwell, 1984.

Banting, K., Hoberg, G., and Simeon, R. (eds.). *Degrees of Freedom: Canada and the United States in a Changing World*. Montreal: Queens McGill University Press., 1997.

Bartley, M., Blane, D., and Montgomery, S. "Health and the Life Course: Why Safety Nets Matter." *British Medical Journal*, 1997, *314*, 1194–1196.

Benzeval, M., Judge, K., and Whitehead, M. *Tackling Inequalities in Health: An Agenda for Action*. London: Kings Fund, 1995.

Benzeval, M., and others. "Income and Health over the Lifecourse: Evidence and Policy Implications." In H. Graham (ed.), *Understanding Health Inequalities*. Berkshire, England: Open University Press, 2001.

Bernstein, J. *Let the War on the Poverty Line Commence*. New York: Foundation for Child Development, 2001.

Bernstein, J., Brocht, C., and Spade-Aguilar, M. *How Much Is Enough? Basic Family Budgets for Working Families*. Washington, D.C.: Economic Policy Institute, 2000.

Bezruchka, S. "Societal Hierarchy and the Health Olympics." *Canadian Medical Association Journal*, 2001, *164*, 1701–1703.

"The Big Idea." *British Medical Journal*, 1996, *312*, 985.

Black, D., and Smith, C. "The Black Report." In P. Townsend, N. Davidson, and M. Whitehead (eds.), *Inequalities in Health: The Black Report and the Health Divide*. New York: Viking Penguin, 1992.

Bottomore, T., Harris, L., and Miliband, R. (eds.). *The Dictionary of Marxist Thought*. Oxford: Blackwell, 1992.

Brooks, D. "The Triumph of Hope over Self-Interest." *New York Times*, January 13, 2003, p. 15.

Brooks-Gunn, J., Duncan, G. J., and Britto, P. R. "Are SES Gradients for Children Similar to Those for Adults? Achievement and Health of Children in the United States." In D. P. Keating and C. Hertzman (eds.), *Developmental Health and the Wealth of Nations: Social, Biological, and Educational Dynamics*. New York: Guilford Press, 1999.

Brunner, E., and Marmot, M. G. "Social Organization, Stress, and Health." In M. G. Marmot and R. G. Wilkinson (eds.), *Social Determinants of Health*. Oxford: Oxford University Press, 1999.

Bryant, T. "Role of Knowledge in Public Health and Health Promotion Policy Change." *Health Promotion International*, 2002, *17*, 89–98.

Bryant, T., and others. "Opening Up the Public Policy Analysis Process to the Public: Participatory Policy Research and Canadian Seniors' Quality of Life." *Canadian Review of Social Policy*, 2001, *48*, 35–67.

Canadian Council on Social Development. *Defining and Re-Defining Poverty: A CCSD Perspective.* Ottawa: Canadian Council on Social Development, 2001.

Canadian Institute for Health Information. *Charting the Course: A Pan-Canadian Consultation on Population and Public Health Priorities.* Ottawa: Canadian Institute for Health Information, 2002.

Central Intelligence Agency. *The World Factbook, 2002.* Washington, D.C.: Central Intelligence Agency, 2002.

Citizens for Tax Justice. "Year-by-Year Analysis of the Bush Tax Cuts Show Growing Tilt to the Very Rich." Press release. Washington, D.C.: Citizens for Tax Justice, June 12, 2002.

Citizens for Tax Justice. "Details of the Effects of the Bush 2003 Tax Cut Plan in 2003." Press release. Washington, D.C.: Citizens for Tax Justice, January 7, 2003.

Collins, C., Hartman, C., and Sklar, H. *Divided Decade: Economic Disparity at the Century's Turn.* Boston: United for a Fair Economy, 1999.

Collins, C., Leondar-Wright, B., and Sklar, H. *Shifting Fortunes: The Perils of the Growing American Wealth Gap.* Boston: United for a Fair Economy, 1999.

Davey Smith, G. "Income Inequality and Mortality: Why Are They Related?" *British Medical Journal,* 1996, *312,* 987–988.

Davey Smith, G., Ben-Shlomo, Y., and Lynch, J. W. "Life Course Approaches to Inequalities in Coronary Heart Disease Risk." In S. A. Stansfeld and M. G. Marmot (eds.), *Stress and the Heart: Psychosocial Pathways to Coronary Heart Disease.* London: BMJ Books, 2002.

Davey Smith, G., Dorling, D., and Shaw, M. (eds.), *Poverty, Inequality and Health in Britain, 1800–2000: A Reader.* Bristol, England: Policy Press, 2001.

Davey Smith, G., and Gordon, D. "Poverty Across the Life-Course and Health." In C. Pantazis and D. Gordon (eds.), *Tackling Inequalities: Where Are We Now and What Can Be Done?* Bristol, England: Policy Press, 2000.

Davey Smith, G., Grunnell, D., and Ben-Shlomo, Y. "Life-Course Approaches to Socioeconomic Differentials in Cause-Specific Adult Mortality." In D. Leon and G. Walt (eds.), *Poverty, Inequality, and Health: An International Perspective.* New York: Oxford University Press, 2001.

Davey Smith, G., and Hart, C. "Life-Course Approaches to Socioeconomic and Behavioral Influences on Cardiovascular Disease Mortality." *American Journal of Public Health,* 2002, *92,* 1295–1298.

Davies, J. K., and Kelly, M. P. *Healthy Cities: Research and Practice.* New York: Routledge, 1993.

Dunn, J. "Housing and Health Inequalities: Review and Prospects for Research." *Housing Studies,* 2000, *15,* 341–366.

Dunn, J., Hargreaves, S., and Alex, J. S. "Are Widening Income Inequalities Making Canada Less Healthy?" In Ontario Public Health Association, *The Health Determinants Partnership—Making Connections Project.* Montreal: Ontario Public Health Association, 2002.

Eriksson, J., and others. "Catch-Up Growth in Childhood and Death from Coronary Heart Disease: Longitudinal Study." *British Medical Journal,* 1999, *318,* 427–431.

European Institute of Japanese Studies. *Economic and Social Data Ranking, Developed Countries (OECD).* Stockholm: European Institute of Japanese Studies, 2002.

Evans, R. G., Barer, M. L., and Marmor, T. R. *Why Are Some People Healthy and Others Not? The Determinants of Health of Populations.* Hawthorne, N.Y.: Aldine de Gruyter, 1994.

Federal, Provincial, and Territorial Advisory Committee on Population Health. *Strategies for Population Health: Investing in the Health of Canadians.* Ottawa: Federal, Provincial, and Territorial Advisory Committee on Population Health, 1994.

Feldman, J. J., and others. "National Trends in Educational Differentials in Mortality." *American Journal of Epidemiology,* 1989, *129,* 919–933.

Freeman, R. B. "The Facts About Rising Economic Inequality." In J. A. Auerbach and R. Belous (eds.), *The Inequality Paradox: Growth of Income Disparity.* Washington, D.C.: National Policy Association, 1998.

Glyn, A., and Miliband, D. *Paying for Inequality: The Economic Cost of Social Injustice.* London: IPPR/Rivers Press, 1994.

Gordon, D., and others. *Inequalities in Health: The Evidence Presented to the Independent Inquiry into Inequalities in Health.* Bristol, England: Policy Press, 1999.

Health Canada. *Taking Action on Population Health: A Position Paper for Health Promotion and Programs Branch Staff.* Ottawa: Health Canada, 1998.

Health Canada. *The Population Health Template: Key Elements and Actions That Define a Population Health Approach.* Ottawa: Strategic Policy Directorate, Population and Public Health Branch, Health Canada, 2001.

Hertzman, C. "Population Health and Child Development: A View from Canada." In J. A. Auerbach and B. Krimgold (eds.), *Income, Socioeconomic Status, and Health: Exploring the Relationships.* Washington, D.C.: National Policy Association, 2001.

Heying, C. "Civic Elites and Corporate Delocalization: An Alternative Explanation for Declining Civic Engagement." *American Behavioral Scientist,* 1995, *40,* 656–667.

Howlett, M., and Ramesh, M. *The Political Economy of Canada.* Toronto: McClelland & Stewart, 1992.

Innocenti Research Centre. "A League Table of Child Poverty in Rich Nations." United Nations, 2000. [http://www.unicef-icdc.org/publications].

Institute of Medicine. *The Future of the Public's Health in the 21st Century.* Washington, D.C.: National Academies Press, 2002.

International Reform Monitor. *Social Policy, Labour Market Policy and Industrial Relations, Family Policy: United States.* Gutersloe, Germany: Bertelsmann Foundation, 2002.

Jackson, A. *Canada Beats USA—but Loses Gold to Sweden.* Ottawa: Canadian Council on Social Development, 2002.

Jackson, S. A., and others. "The Relation of Residential Segregation to All-Cause Mortality: A Study in Black and White." *American Journal of Public Health,* 2000, *90,* 615–617.

Jarvis, M. J., and Wardle, J. "Social Patterning of Individual Health Behaviours: The Case of Cigarette Smoking." In M. G. Marmot and R. G. Wilkinson (eds.), *Social Determinants of Health*. Oxford: Oxford University Press, 1999.

Johnston, D. "Taxes Are Cut, and the Rich Get Richer." *New York Times*, The Week in Review, October 5, 1997, p. 1.

Judge, K., and Paterson, I. *Poverty, Income Inequality and Health*. Glasgow, Scotland: Health Promotion Policy Unit, Department of Public Health, University of Glasgow, 2002.

Kaplan, G. A., and others. "Income Inequality and Mortality in the United States." *British Medical Journal*, 1996, *312*, 999–1003.

Kawachi, I., and Kennedy, B. P. "The Relationship of Income Inequality to Mortality: Does the Choice of Indicator Matter?" *Social Science and Medicine*, 1997a, *45*, 1121–1127.

Kawachi, I., and Kennedy, B. P. "Socioeconomic Determinants of Health: Health and Social Cohesion: Why Care About Income Inequality?" *British Medical Journal*, 1997b, *314*, 1037.

Kawachi, I., and Kennedy, B. P. *The Health of Nations: Why Inequality Is Harmful to Your Health*. New York: New Press, 2002.

Kawachi, I., Kennedy, B. P., and Wilkinson, R. G. (eds.). *The Society and Population Health Reader*, Vol. 1: *Income Inequality and Health*. New York: New Press, 1999.

Keating, D. P., and Hertzman, C. (eds.). *Developmental Health and the Wealth of Nations: Social, Biological and Educational Dynamics*. New York: Guilford Press, 1999.

Kennedy, B. P., Kawachi, I., and Prothrow-Stith, D. "Income Distribution and Mortality: Cross-Sectional Ecological Study of the Robin Hood Index in the United States." *British Medical Journal*, 1996, *312*, 1004–1007.

Kennedy, B. P., and others. "Income Distribution, Socioeconomic Status and Self-Rated Health in the United States: Multilevel Analysis." *British Medical Journal*, 1998, *317*, 917–921.

Kim, K. K., and Moody, P. M. "More Resources, Better Health? A Cross-National Study." *Social Science and Medicine*, 1992, *34*, 837–842.

Labonte, R. *Health Promotion and Empowerment: Practice Frameworks*. Toronto: Centre for Health Promotion and Participation, 1993.

Labonte, R., and Thompson, P. *Promoting Heart Health in Canada: A Focus on Health Inequalities*. Ottawa: Health Canada, 1992.

Lantz, P. M., and others. "Socioeconomic Factors, Health Behaviors, and Mortality." *Journal of the American Medical Association*, 1998, *279*, 1703–1708.

Lardner, J. "The Rich Get Richer: Why Those at the Top Are Leaving the Rest of Us Behind." *U.S. News and World Report*, February 21, 2000, pp. 38–43.

Laxer, J. *The Undeclared War: Class Conflict in the Age of Cyber-Capitalism*. New York: Viking Penguin, 1998.

Lee, V. E., and Burkam, D. T. *Inequality at the Starting Gate: Social Background Differences in Achievement as Children Begin School.* Washington, D.C.: Economic Policy Institute, 2002.

Leon, D. A., Vagero, D., and Otterblad, O. "Social Class Differences in Infant Mortality in Sweden: A Comparison with England and Wales." *British Medical Journal,* 1992, *305,* 687–691.

Lynch J. W., Kaplan, G. A., and Salonen, J. "Why Do Poor People Behave Poorly? Variation in Adult Health Behaviours and Psychosocial Characteristics by Stages of the Socioeconomic Lifecourse." *Social Science and Medicine,* 1997, *44,* 809–819.

Lynch, J. W., and others. "Income Inequality and Mortality in Metropolitan Areas of the United States." *American Journal of Public Health,* 1998, *88,* 1074–1080.

Lynch, J. W., and others. "Income Inequality, the Psychosocial Environment and Health: Comparisons of Wealthy Nations." *Lancet,* 2001, *358,* 194–200.

Marmot, M. G., and Wilkinson, R. G. *Social Determinants of Health.* Oxford: Oxford University Press, 1999.

Marmot, M. G., and others. "Employment Grade and Coronary Heart Disease in British Civil Servants." *Journal of Epidemiology and Community Health,* 1978, *32,* 244–249.

McBride, S., and Shields, J. *Dismantling a Nation: The Transition to Corporate Rule in Canada.* Halifax, Nova Scotia, Canada: Fernwood, 1997.

McKeown, T. *The Role of Medicine: Dream, Mirage or Nemesis.* London: Neufeld Provincial Hospitals Trust, 1976.

McKeown, T., and Record, R. G. "An Interpretation of the Decline in Mortality in England and Wales During the Twentieth Century." *Population Studies,* 1975, *29,* 391–422.

McKinlay, J., and McKinlay, S. M. "Medical Measures and the Decline of Mortality." In H. D. Schwartz (ed.), *Dominant Issues in Medical Sociology.* (2nd ed.) New York: Random House, 1987.

McQuaig, L. *The Wealthy Banker's Wife: The Assault on Equality in Canada.* Toronto: Penguin, 1993.

McQuaig, L. *The Cult of Impotence: Selling the Myth of Powerlessness in the Global Economy.* New York: Viking Penguin, 1998.

Miringoff, M., and Miringoff, M. L. *The Social Health of the Nation: How America Is Really Doing.* New York: Oxford University Press, 1999.

Mishel, L., Bernstein, J., and Boushey, B. *The State of Working America, 2002–2003.* Ithaca, N.Y.: Cornell University Press, 2003.

Mutaner, C., Lynch, J. W., and Oates, G. L. "The Social Class Determinants of Income Inequality and Social Cohesion." *International Journal of Health Services,* 1999, *29,* 699–732.

Navarro, V. (ed.). *The Political Economy of Social Inequalities: Consequences for Health and Quality of Life.* Amityville, N.Y.: Baywood Press, 2002.

Nettleton, S. "Surveillance, Health Promotion and the Formation of a Risk Identity." In M. Sidell and others (eds.), *Debates and Dilemmas in Promoting Health.* Berkshire, England: Open University Press, 1997.

Nettleton, S., and Bunton, R. "Sociological Critiques of Health Promotion." In R. Bunton, S. Nettleton, and R. Burrows (eds.), *The Sociology of Health Promotion: Critical Analyses of Consumption, Lifestyle, and Risk.* New York: Routledge, 1995.

Organization for Economic Cooperation and Development. *Early Childhood Education and Care Policy in United States.* Paris: Organization for Economic Cooperation and Development, 2000.

Organization for Economic Cooperation and Development. *Society at a Glance: OECD Social Indicators, 2001 Edition.* Paris: Organization for Economic Cooperation and Development, 2001.

Pantazis, C., and Gordon, D. (eds.), *Tackling Inequalities: Where Are We Now and What Can Be Done?* Bristol, England: Policy Press, 2000.

Pearce, N., and Davey Smith, G. "Is Social Capital the Key to Inequalities in Health?" *American Journal of Public Health,* 2003, *93,* 122–129.

Phillips, K. *Wealth and Democracy.* New York: Broadway Books, 2002.

Poland, B., and others. "Wealth, Equity, and Health Care: A Critique of a Population Health Perspective on the Determinants of Health." *Social Science and Medicine,* 1998, *46,* 785–798.

Pollitt, K. "For Whom the Ball Rolls." *Nation,* April 15, 1996, p. 9.

Putnam, R. *Bowling Alone: The Collapse and Revival of American Community.* New York: Simon & Schuster, 2000.

Rainwater, L., and Smeeding, T. M. "Doing Poorly: The Real Income of American Children in a Comparative Perspective." Working paper no. 127, Luxembourg Income Study, 1995. [http://www.lisproject.org/publications/liswps/127.pdf].

Raphael, D. "Health Inequities in the United States: Prospects and Solutions." *Journal of Public Health Policy,* 2000, *21,* 392–425.

Raphael, D. "From Increasing Poverty to Societal Disintegration: How Economic Inequality Affects the Health of Individuals and Communities." In H. Armstrong, P. Armstrong, and D. Coburn (eds.), *Unhealthy Times: The Political Economy of Health and Care in Canada.* Toronto: Oxford University Press, 2001a.

Raphael, D. *Inequality Is Bad for Our Hearts: Why Low Income and Social Exclusion Are Major Causes of Heart Disease in Canada.* Toronto: North York Heart Health Network, 2001b.

Raphael, D. *Social Justice Is Good for Our Hearts: Why Societal Factors—Not Lifestyles—Are Major Causes of Heart Disease in Canada and Elsewhere.* Toronto: Canada: Foundation for Research and Education, Centre for Social Justice, 2002.

Raphael, D., and Bryant, T. *The Quality of Women's Life in Canada.* Toronto: Centre for Health Studies, York University, 2003.

Raphael, D., Colman, R., and Labonte, R. *Income, Health and Disease in Canada: Current State of Knowledge, Information Gaps and Areas of Needed Inquiry.* Toronto: York University, 2003.

Reich, R. B. "The Inequality Paradox." In J. A. Auerbach and R. Belous (eds.), *The Inequality Paradox: Growth of Income Disparity.* Washington, D.C.: National Policy Association, 1998.

Reutter, L. "Poverty and Health: Implications for Public Health." *Canadian Journal of Public Health,* 1995, *86,* 149–151.

Reutter, L., Stewart, M., and Makwarimba, E. "Poverty and Its Effects: 'Insider' and 'Outsider' Perspectives." Paper presented at the Eighth International Qualitative Health Research Conference, Banff, Alberta, Canada, April 5, 2002.

Rosen, J. "The Lost Promise of School Integration." *New York Times,* Week in Review, April 2, 2000, p. 1.

Ross, N. A., and others. "Relation Between Income Inequality and Mortality in Canada and in the United States: Cross-Sectional Assessment Using Census Data and Vital Statistics." *British Medical Journal,* 2000, *320,* 898–902.

Roux, A., and others. "Neighborhood of Residence and Incidence of Coronary Heart Disease." *New England Journal of Medicine,* 2001, *345,* 99–106.

Shaw, M., and others. *The Widening Gap: Health Inequalities and Policy in Britain.* Bristol, England: Policy Press, 1999.

Smeeding, T. M. "U.S. Income Inequality in a Cross-National Perspective: Why Are We So Different?" In J. A. Auerbach and R. Belous (eds.), *The Inequality Paradox: Growth of Income Disparity.* Washington, D.C.: National Policy Association, 1998.

Sram, I., and Ashton, I. "Millennium Report to Sir Edwin Chadwick." *British Medical Journal,* 1998, *317,* 592–596.

Stansfeld, S. A., and Marmot, M. G. (eds.). *Stress and the Heart: Psychosocial Pathways to Coronary Heart Disease.* London: BMJ Books, 2002.

Teeple, G. *Globalization and the Decline of Social Reform.* Aurora, Ontario, Canada: Garamond Press, 2000.

Terris, M. "Determinants of Health: A Progressive Political Platform." *Journal of Public Health Policy,* 1994, *15,* 5–17.

Tesh, S. *Hidden Arguments: Political Ideology and Disease Prevention Policy.* New Brunswick, N.J.: Rutgers University Press, 1990.

Townsend, P. *Poverty in the United Kingdom: A Survey of Household Resources and Standards of Living.* Berkeley: University of California Press, 1979.

Townson, M. *Health and Wealth: How Socio-Economic Factors Affect Our Well-Being.* Ottawa: Canadian Centre for Policy Alternatives, 1999.

U.S. Department of Health and Human Services. *Health, United States, 1998: Socioeconomic Status and Health Chartbook.* Washington, D.C.: U.S. Department of Health and Human Services, 1998.

U.S. Department of Health and Human Services. *The 2002 HHS Poverty Guidelines.* Washington, D.C.: U.S. Department of Health and Human Services, 2002.

United Nations Development Program. *Human Development Report, 2001: Making New Technologies Work for Human Development.* Geneva, Switzerland: United Nations Development Program, 2001.

Vagero, D., and Lundberg, O. "Health Inequalities in Britain and Sweden." *Lancet,* 1989, *2,* 35–36.

Waitzman, N. J., and Smith, K. R. "Separate but Lethal: The Effects of Economic Segregation on Mortality in Metropolitan America." *Milbank Quarterly,* 1998, *76,* 341–373.

Walt, G. *Health Policy: An Introduction to Process and Power.* London: Zed Books, 1994.

Whiteside, M. "The Health Divide." In P. Townsend, N. Davidson, and M. Whitehead (eds.), *Inequalities in Health: The Black Report and the Health Divide.* New York: Viking Penguin, 1992.

Wilkinson, R. G. *Unhealthy Societies: The Afflictions of Inequality.* New York: Routledge, 1996.

Wilkinson, R. G. *Mind the Gap: Hierarchies, Health and Human Evolution.* London: Weidenfeld & Nicolson, 2001.

Wilkinson, R. G., and Marmot, M. G. (eds.). *Social Determinants of Health: The Solid Facts.* Copenhagen, Denmark: World Health Organization, 1998.

Williamson, D. L., and Reutter, L. "Measuring Poverty: Implications for the Health of Canadians." *Health Promotion International,* 1999, *14,* 355–364.

Wolff, E. *Top Heavy: The Increasing Inequality of Wealth in America and What Can Be Done About It.* New York: New Press, 1995.

Wolfson, M., and others. "Relation Between Income Inequality and Mortality: Empirical Demonstration: Diminishing Returns to Aggregate Level Studies—Two Pathways, but How Much Do They Diverge?" *British Medical Journal,* 1999, *319,* 953–957.

World Health Organization. *Ottawa Charter for Health Promotion.* Geneva, Switzerland: World Health Organization, 1986.

Yellen, C. "Trends in Income Inequality." In J. A. Auerbach and R. Belous (eds.), *The Inequality Paradox: Growth of Income Disparity.* Washington, D.C.: National Policy Association, 1998.

Zweig, M. *The Working-Class Majority: America's Best Kept Secret.* Ithaca, N.Y.: Cornell University Press, 2000.

CHAPTER THREE

Understanding and Reducing Socioeconomic and Racial/Ethnic Disparities in Health

James S. House
David R. Williams

The burgeoning literatures on socioeconomic and racial/ethnic disparities in health establish that such disparities are *large, persistent,* and even *increasing* in the United States and other developed countries, most notably the United Kingdom (Marmot, Kogevinas, and Elston, 1987; Preston and Haines, 1991; Adler et al., 1993; Pappas et al., 1993; Evans, Barer, and Marmor, 1994; Williams and Collins, 1995). Differences across socioeconomic and racial/ethnic groups or combinations thereof range up to ten or more years in life expectancy and twenty or more years in the age at which significant limitations in functional health are first experienced (House et al., 1990, 1994; see Table 3.1). Both within and across countries, individuals with the most advantaged socioeconomic and racial/ethnic status are experiencing levels of health and longevity that increasingly approach the current biologically attainable maxima. Thus, the major opportunity for improving the health of human populations in

---

This chapter was prepared for the symposium "Capitalizing on Social Science and Behavioral Research to Improve the Public's Health," the Institute of Medicine and the Commission on Behavioral and Social Sciences and Education of the National Research Council, Atlanta, Georgia, Feb. 2–3, 2000. This work has been supported by a Robert Wood Johnson Foundation Investigators in Health Policy Research Award (JSH) and by a grant from the National Institute of Mental Health and the John D. and Catherine T. MacArthur Foundation Research Network on Socioeconomic Status and Health (DRW). We are indebted to Debbie Fitch for her work in preparing the manuscript, references, figures, and table.

the United States and most other societies lies in improving the longevity and health of those of below-average socioeconomic or racial/ethnic status.

Accordingly, the reduction of socioeconomic and racial/ethnic disparities in health has been identified by the U.S. Public Health Service and the National Institutes of Health as a major priority for public health practice and research in the first decade of the twenty-first century (U.S. Department of Health and Human Services, 1999; Varmus, 1999). This will involve some combination of either reducing the degree to which disparities in socioeconomic and racial/ethnic status are converted into health disparities or reducing the extent of socioeconomic or racial/ethnic disparities themselves. This will further entail understanding both (1) the psychosocial and biomedical pathways that translate socioeconomic and racial/ethnic disparities into disparities in health, and (2) the broader social, cultural, economic, and political processes that determine the nature and extent of socioeconomic and racial/ethnic disparities in our society, and the ways in which individuals become distributed across socioeconomic levels and defined into racial/ethnic groups.

This chapter seeks to elucidate what we already know and need yet to learn about reducing socioeconomic and racial/ethnic disparities in health. We first provide a brief overview of the nature of both socioeconomic and racial/ethnic disparities in health and how they are related to each other. Second, we assess current understanding of the pathways or mechanisms by which the socioeconomic or racial/ethnic status of individuals affects their health and the implications of this understanding for reducing socioeconomic and racial/ethnic disparities in health. Third, we explore what is known about how and why communities and societies come to be stratified both socioeconomically and in terms

Table 3.1. United States Life Expectancy at Age Forty-Five by Family Income (in 1980 Dollars).

Family Income	Females			Males		
	White	Black	Difference	White	Black	Difference
All[a]	36.3	32.6	3.7	31.1	26.2	4.9
< $10,000[b]	35.8	32.7	3.1	27.3	25.2	2.1
$10,000–$14,999[b]	37.4	33.5	3.9	30.3	28.1	2.2
$15,000–$24,999[b]	37.8	36.3	1.5	32.4	31.3	1.1
≥ $25,000[b]	38.5	36.5	2.0	33.9	32.6	1.3

[a]Figures are for 1989–1991.

[b]Figures are for 1979–1989.

Source: National Center for Health Statistics.

of race/ethnicity and how these communal and societal patterns of socioeconomic and racial/ethnic stratification affect the socioeconomic and racial/ethnic status of individuals and their health. Finally, we conclude with an assessment of what we know and need to know about how to reduce socioeconomic and racial/ethnic disparities in health and hence to improve population health.

Several themes pervade our discussion. First, there are multiple indicators of socioeconomic position and hence multiple indices of socioeconomic disparities in health, and these are best comprehended in a multivariate, causal, and life course framework. Second, socioeconomic and racial/ethnic disparities in health, and the reasons for and means of reducing them, are inextricably related but also distinctive. This also can best be comprehended in a multivariate causal framework. Third, it is important to understand the pathways or mechanisms linking socioeconomic and racial/ethnic status to health. What is most striking and important here is to recognize that socioeconomic and racial/ethnic status shape and operate through a very broad range of pathways or mechanisms, including almost all known major psychosocial and behavioral risk factors for health. Thus socioeconomic and racial/ethnic status are, in the terms of Link and Phelan (1995), the "fundamental causes" of corresponding socioeconomic and racial/ethnic disparities in risk factors and hence health and consequently also the fundamental levers for reducing these health disparities. Finally, existing evidence strongly suggests that the nature of the socioeconomic and racial/ethnic stratification of individuals can be changed in ways beneficial to health and, coincidentally, to a broad range of other indicators of individual and societal well-being.

THE NATURE OF SOCIOECONOMIC AND RACIAL/ETHNIC DISPARITIES AND THEIR RELATION TO HEALTH

We take the size, persistence, and even increase of socioeconomic and racial/ethnic disparities as given. Here we seek to clarify the nature of socioeconomic and racial/ethnic status and their relations to each other and to health.

A Multivariate, Causal, and Life Course Framework

Socioeconomic status (SES) refers to individuals' position in a system of social stratification that differentially allocates the major resources enabling people to achieve health or other desired goals. These resources centrally include education, occupation, income, and assets or wealth, which are related to each other and to health in a causal framework first elucidated by Blau and Duncan (1967) and shown in its simplest form in Figure 3.1. This model suggests that over the life course, individuals first acquire varying levels and types of education, which in turn help them to enter various types of occupations, which then yield income, which finally enables them to accumulate assets or wealth. Each subsequent variable in this causal chain is generally most affected by the immediately prior variable, with potential residual effects of earlier variables. This model is simple because it omits potential feedback loops other than from assets or wealth to income (e.g., a person's occupation may facilitate further educational attainment) and fails to incorporate variations in each of these indicators that will occur over the life course (e.g., progressions or regressions in terms of occupation or income).

Although this causal framework has been used routinely in the study of socioeconomic attainment, it has seldom been explicitly applied to the study of socioeconomic disparities. It is important, however, that it be utilized more explicitly in future research on the relation of socioeconomic status to health and especially in thinking about how socioeconomic disparities in health have been or could be reduced. The framework helps, for example, to understand why income is perhaps the strongest and most robust predictor of health (McDonough et al., 1997; Lantz et al., 1998), because to some degree the impacts of all other variables are mediated through it. Also, some health outcomes are more strongly affected by certain socioeconomic indicators than others (education, for example, more strongly affects health behaviors, patterns of which form early in life, and the diseases or health indicators affected most by them). Overall, in the United States, education and income have proved most predictive of health, with occupation often adding little additional explanatory power and assets or wealth somewhat more. More research is needed, however,

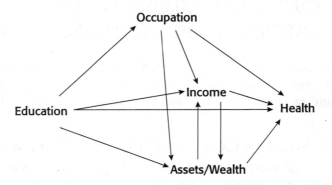

Figure 3.1. Simple Intragenerational Causal Model Relating Major Indicators of Socioeconomic Position to Each Other and to Health.

to estimate explicitly the relative effects on health of these different indicators of socioeconomic position and how much the total effect of any given variable is spuriously produced by temporally antecedent confounding variables, mediated via temporally subsequent intervening variables, or acts more directly on health (see Sorlie, Backlund, and Keller, 1995; Lantz et al., 2001; and Robert and House, 2000a, 2000b).

From the point of view of reducing health disparities, we need to have such an analysis of the variance in health explained by different socioeconomic factors in order to understand or predict the health effects of planned or unplanned change in each indicator. Further, by adding other variables to Figure 3.1, we can extend our understanding of how disparities in health across these indicators of socioeconomic position may be generated by antecedent factors or mediated via subsequent factors. Several such elaborations are important in thinking about reducing other socioeconomic and racial disparities in health.

First, socioeconomic position (SEP) has to be thought of as an intergenerational as well as intragenerational phenomenon. Thus parental socioeconomic position may importantly shape childhood well-being and hence educational and later adult socioeconomic attainment and health, as shown in Figure 3.2. The work of Barker (e.g., Barker and Osmond, 1986) and others (Kaplan and Salonen, 1990; Elo and Preston, 1992; Blane et al., 1996; Kuh and Ben-Shlomo, 1997) has indicated that childhood socioeconomic position and experiences can have long-term effects on adult health. This is sometimes interpreted to mean that childhood socioeconomic position is a more important determinant of health than adult socioeconomic position. However, Figure 3.2 suggests that most such effects are likely to be channeled through and reinforced by later socioeconomic attainment, and the unique impact of childhood SEP or its sequelae must be evaluated net of later socioeconomic or other experiences. When this is done, the unique effects of childhood SEP on adult health are often found to be small or even nonexistent relative to the effects of later adult socioeconomic attainment and experiences (e.g., Lynch et al., 1994).[1] Thus although the impact of socioeconomic position on childhood health and well-being is a very important problem in its own right, it cannot and should not be viewed as a major explanation of adult socioeconomic or racial/ethnic disparities in health or hence as the major, preferred, or necessary route for reducing such adult disparities.

However, Figure 3.2 is also highly simplified, neglecting the changing socioeconomic position of the families of many children. Thus the socioeconomic position of a child often changes from preschool to elementary school to secondary school and onward through adulthood. Socioeconomic advantage and disadvantage may be viewed as ebbing and flowing or cascading over a person's life course. Although recent socioeconomic position is usually the best

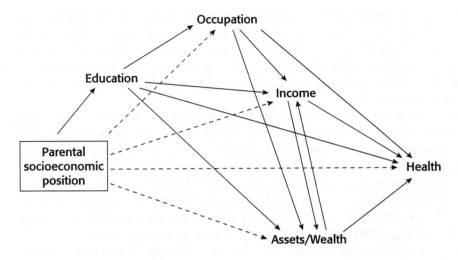

Figure 3.2. Simple Intergenerational Extension of the Model in Figure 3.1.

predictor of future outcomes, sustained socioeconomic deprivation over time is likely to be even more damaging (Wolfson et al., 1993, Lynch, Kaplan, and Salonen, 1997), and uncertainty or variability in socioeconomic position may be deleterious even to those of generally solid middle- or higher-level SEP (McDonough et al., 1997). Thus knowledge of the full life course of socioeconomic position is ideally desirable for understanding socioeconomic disparities in health and a target for efforts to alleviate such disparities.

Finally, Figures 3.1 and 3.2 must be further elaborated, as in Figure 3.3, to take account of the impact of more ascribed and relatively fixed social statuses—most notably for our purposes, race/ethnicity, but also age and gender. Figure 3.3 reveals two simple but very important truths about racial/ethnic disparities in health. First, racial/ethnic status is a major determinant of every indicator of socioeconomic position, even net of all prior variables in the model. For example, not only are African Americans disadvantaged in terms of level of education, but even given the same education, they are disadvantaged occupationally and in terms of income and still disadvantaged in income even within the same educational and occupational levels (Featherman and Hauser, 1978). Most egregiously, their assets/wealth lag far behind other Americans of equivalent income, occupation, and education (Oliver and Shapiro, 1995; Conley, 1999). Not surprisingly, then, a great deal of racial/ethnic disparity in health is explainable in terms of the socioeconomic disadvantages associated with membership in the most historically disadvantaged racial/ethnic groups (Williams and Collins, 1995).

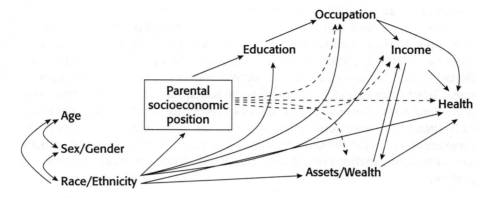

Figure 3.3. Extension of the Model in Figure 3.2, Incorporating Race/Ethnicity, Sex/Gender, and Age.

Note: For clarity of presentation, no arrows are drawn from "Age" and "Sex/Gender" to subsequent variables, but these would and should be exactly parallel to those for "Race/Ethnicity."

However, the second important truth of Figure 3.3 is that race/ethnicity has effects on health that are independent of socioeconomic differences between racial/ethnic groups (Williams and Collins, 1995; Williams et al., 1997). For example, African Americans generally exhibit poorer health outcomes even when compared to whites with statistically equivalent levels of socioeconomic position (see Table 3.1). Thus race carries its own burdens for health beyond those associated with socioeconomic disadvantage. We can properly estimate and understand how race/ethnicity and socioeconomic position combine to affect health only within a multivariate framework such as Figure 3.3. Further, such a framework can also reveal that race/ethnicity sometimes has salutary effects on health that may compensate in part for the deleterious effects of socioeconomic disadvantages. For example, African Americans exhibit better levels of mental health, and Latinos better levels of infant and child health, than would be expected based on their socioeconomic position. The next major section of this chapter focuses on elucidating the pathways or mechanisms through which both socioeconomic position and race/ethnicity affect health, for better as well as for worse.

Due to constraints of space and the desire for clarity, Figure 3.3 fails to represent other important issues for understanding and reducing socioeconomic disparities in health. First is the issue of reciprocal or reverse causality, especially between socioeconomic position and health. Ours and others' discussions of reducing socioeconomic and racial/ethnic disparities in health are predicated on the assumption that by far the predominant causal flow is from socioeconomic position and race/ethnicity to health rather than vice versa. This assumption is self-evident for a fixed attribute such as race/ethnicity and is generally borne out in empirical research on socioeconomic position, for example, by introducing baseline controls on health into the framework of Figure 3.1 (see Robert and House, 2000b), though clearly health events or shocks can and do affect subsequent labor force participation and income (often more in the short term than in the long term). Second, time and space prevent us from fully and systematically attending to variations by age, sex, race/ethnicity, and other factors in the presence of size of the causal paths/effects in Figure 3.1, though we will on occasion note such variations (see Robert and House, 2000b, for more discussion of such issues).

Shape of the Relationship Between SES and Health

Before turning more explicitly to how we may explain and reduce socioeconomic and racial/ethnic disparities in health, it is important to clarify our understanding of the shape of the relationship between socioeconomic position and health. An intriguing finding of some research on socioeconomic inequalities in health is that it is not simply that those who are in the lowest socioeconomic groups have worse health than those in higher socioeconomic groups. Rather, a relationship between socioeconomic position and health has been observed across the socioeconomic hierarchy, with even those in relatively high socioeconomic groups having better health than those just below them in the socioeconomic hierarchy (Adler et al., 1994; Marmot et al., 1991). Perhaps the most important implication of this finding is that it is not just the material, psychological, and social conditions associated with severe deprivation or poverty (such as lack of access to safe housing, healthy food, and adequate medical care) that explain socioeconomic inequalities in health among those already at relatively high levels of socioeconomic position.

Despite some evidence for gradient effects of socioeconomic position on health, it is also important to note the many studies indicating that the relationship of socioeconomic position, especially as indexed by income, to health is monotonic but not a linear gradient. Although increasingly higher levels of socioeconomic position may be associated with increasingly better levels of health, there are also substantially diminishing returns of higher socioeconomic position to health. For example, studies have found diminishing and even nonexistent relationships between income and mortality (Wolfson et al., 1993; Backlund, Sorlie, and Johnson, 1996; Chapman and Hariharan, 1996; McDonough et al., 1997) or morbidity (House et al., 1990, 1994; Mirowsky and Hu, 1996) at higher levels of income (e.g., above the median). This trend partially reflects a health "ceiling effect" caused by the fact that people in the upper socioeconomic strata maintain overall good health until quite late in life, leaving little opportunity for improvement in health among these groups throughout much of adulthood (House et al., 1994). Thus it is most important to understand what accounts for socioeconomic inequalities in health across the broad lower range (e.g., lower 40–60%) of socioeconomic position, rather than focusing mainly or only on factors that might explain this relationship across the gradient or at higher levels.

PATHWAYS LINKING INDIVIDUAL SOCIOECONOMIC AND RACIAL/ETHNIC STATUS TO HEALTH
Pathways from SES to Health

We have increased understanding of how and why socioeconomic status has such strong pervasive and even increasing impacts on health. Several aspects of this deserve emphasis. First, access to and utilization of medical care play only a limited role in explaining the impact of socioeconomic factors on health, although research is needed to reassess the size of the role played by medical care. Second, there is no single or small set of factors, psychosocial or physiological, that provides the pathways linking socioeconomic position to health. Rather, what makes socioeconomic position such a powerful determinant of health is that it shapes people's experience of, and exposure to, virtually all psychosocial and environmental risk factors for health—past, present, and future— and these in turn operate through a very broad range of physiological mechanisms to influence the incidence and course of virtually all major causes of disease and health. Thus in the end, socioeconomic position itself is a fundamental cause (Link and Phelan, 1995) of levels of individual and population health and a fundamental lever for improving health in American society.

The Limited but Insufficiently Understood Role of Medical Care. Several types of evidence point to the limited role of medical care in understanding how and why socioeconomic position affects health. First, there is evidence that modern preventive and therapeutic medical care can account for only a minor fraction of the dramatic improvements in individual and population health over the last 250 years (McKeown, 1979, 1988; McKinlay and McKinlay, 1977). Even analysts admiring of the impact of medical science on health, for example, estimate that only about five years of the 30-year increase in life expectancy in the United States in the twentieth century has been due to preventive or therapeutic medical care (Bunker, Frazier, and Mosteller, 1994). The remainder is attributable primarily to increasing socioeconomic development and associated gains in nutrition, public health and sanitation, and living conditions. Second, improvements in access to medical care occasioned by the introduction of national health insurance or service plans have, quite unexpectedly, done little or nothing to reduce socioeconomic differences in health. The rediscovery of the importance of socioeconomic disparities in health as a major public health problem was probably stimulated most by the publication in England in 1980 of the Report of the Working Group on Inequalities in Health, better known as the Black Report after the chair of the working group, Sir Douglas Black, then chief scientist of the U.K. Department of Health and subsequently president of the Royal College of Physicians. The report showed that occupational class differences in health were greater than differences by gender, race, or regional background and, most distressingly, had actually increased between 1949–1953 and 1970–1972 over the first quarter-century of existence of the British National Health Service. Nor did things improve between the early 1970s and 1980s (Marmot, Kogevinas, and Elston, 1987). During the 1980s and early 1990s, the British experience was replicated in other developed countries including Canada, where the introduction of national health insurance in the early 1970s had little effect on socioeconomic differences in health (Wilkins, Adams, and Brancker,, 1989). Finally, adjustments for gross access to and utilization of medical care have contributed little or nothing to explaining socioeconomic and racial/ethnic differences in health in our and other data.

However, we believe that the role of medical care in socioeconomic and racial/ethnic health differences deserves renewed examination and research. First, compared to whites, racial/ethnic minorities have lower levels of access to medical care in the United States (Blendon et al., 1989; Trevino et al., 1991). Second, higher incidence rates for racial/ethnic minorities do not fully account for the higher death rates (Schwartz et al., 1990). Later initial diagnosis of disease, comorbidity, delays in medical treatment, and disparities in the quality of care also play a role. There is growing evidence of large racial/ethnic differences in the quality of medical care. Many studies have found racial/ethnic differences in the receipt of therapeutic procedures for a broad range of conditions even after adjustment for insurance status and severity of disease (e.g., Wenneker and Epstein, 1989; Harris, Andrews, and Elixhauser, 1997). These disparities exist even in contexts where differences in economic status and insurance coverage are minimized, for example, the Veterans Administration Health System (e.g., Whittle et al., 1993) and the Medicare program (e.g., McBean and Gornick, 1994). Recent studies document that these differences in medical treatment adversely affect the health of minority group members (Peterson et al., 1997; Hannan et al., 1999). Moreover, medical care appears to play a modest role in accounting for racial differences in mortality (Woolhandler et al., 1985; Schwartz et al., 1990), and other evidence suggests that medical care has a greater impact on the health status of vulnerable racial and low-SES groups than on their more advantaged counterparts (Williams, 1990). More generally, behind declining socioeconomic and racial/ethnic disparities in gross levels of access to and utilization of medical care may lie persisting differences in access to more continuous care from a concerned and responsive provider, associated differences in access to and utilization of important standards of preventive care (e.g., blood pressure, prostate, and colorectal screening; Pap smears and mammograms; and professional advice on health behaviors), and differences in the timeliness and appropriateness of access to state-of-the-art standards of therapeutic care. Thus socioeconomic and racial/ethnic disparities in standards and appropriateness of medical care merit increased attention in research and policy.

Psychosocial and Environmental Risk Factors. As evidence grew of the more limited impact of medical care in explaining socioeconomic and racial/ethnic disparities in health, research increasingly established a growing and even predominant role of behavioral and psychosocial risk factors in the etiology and course of human health and disease. First, and still most compelling, was the evidence of the adverse effects of cigarette smoking on mortality and morbidity, especially adult lung cancer and heart disease (e.g., Surgeon General's Advisory Committee, 1964). This was followed by increasing evidence of the health risks of other behaviors, including immoderate levels of eating (and hence weight) and of alcohol consumption, lack of exercise, and dietary composition, e.g., fat and fiber (Lalonde, 1975; Berkman and Breslow, 1983, U.S. Department of Health and Human Services, 1990). Evidence has also accumulated on the deleterious health effects of chronic and acute stress in work and life (Theorell, 1982), hostility and depression (Scheier and Bridges, 1995), lack of social relationships and supports (House, Landis, and Umberson, 1988), and lack of control, efficacy, or mastery (Rodin, 1986), with the impact of lack of social relationships, for example, on all-cause mortality being not incomparable to that of cigarette smoking (House, Landis, and Umberson, 1988). Notably, these psychosocial factors all tend to affect a broad range of health outcomes, rather than being focused on a single outcome.

Socioeconomic Status and Psychosocial and Environmental Risk Factors. One factor (e.g., smoking) or a small set of factors (e.g., health behaviors) is sometimes seen as crucial in explaining and alleviating problems of premature morbidity and mortality more generally (e.g., U.S. Department of Health and Human Services, 1990; McGinnis and Forge, 1993) and socioeconomic and racial/ethnic disparities in health in particular (Mechanic, 1989; Satel, 1996). However, increasing evidence suggests that there are few or no analogues in our current problems of public health to the necessary and sufficient microbial causes of many infectious diseases, nor are there any comparable "magic bullets" for treating, preventing, or eradicating them. Rather, the current causes of morbidity and mortality, especially from major chronic diseases, are broadly multifactorial, with no one or few decisive, but the accumulation of many being as debilitating or deadly as a virulent infectious agent (Kunitz, 1987). For example, all major health behaviors combined (i.e., cigarette smoking, immoderate weight and drinking, and lack of physical activity) appear able to explain only 10–20%, at most, of socioeconomic differences in mortality (Lantz et al., 1998). Rather, what is most striking and important about socioeconomic (and, to a lesser degree, racial/ethnic) status is the degree to which it shapes exposure to, and perhaps also the impact of, a wide range of psychosocial and environmental risk factors for health. Our data (House et al., 1992, 1994) and those of others (e.g., Marmot et al., 1991; Lynch et al., 1996) show that lower-SES individuals have a higher prevalence of almost all major psychosocial risk factors for health. That is, they manifest higher levels of risky health behaviors such as smoking, lack of exercise, immoderate eating and drinking, and high-fat–low-fiber diets. They also experience more chronic and acute stress due to, for example, their more vulnerable economic status and the higher rates of ill health and death among friends and relatives. They generally report lower levels of social relationships and supports and of personal efficacy or control, along with *higher* levels of hostility and depression.

Figures 3.4 and 3.5 show, for national samples of the U.S. population, the distribution and range of these psychosocial risk factors by education and income. The prevalence of each psychosocial risk factor is always highest among those with the lowest level of education and income, with rate ratios (of the lowest- to the highest-SES groups) ranging from 1.1 to 3.8 and averaging 2.0 (see Lantz et al., 1998, for parallel data on health behaviors).

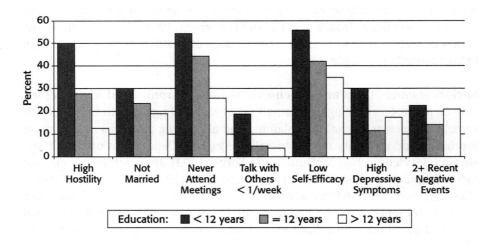

Figure 3.4. Psychosocial Risk Factors by Education for Persons Aged Forty-Five to Sixty-Four in the United States.

Source: House and Williams, 1995.

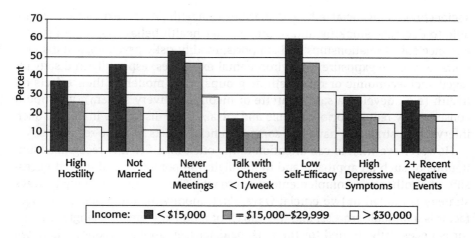

Figure 3.5. Psychosocial Risk Factors by Income for Persons Aged Forty-Five to Sixty-Four in the United States.

Source: House and Williams, 1995.

Persons of lower socioeconomic status in adulthood are also more likely to live and work in physical-chemical-biological environments that are hazardous to health. Further, they are more likely to have grown up in lower-socioeconomic environments, which may have residual adverse effects on health in adulthood that research is just beginning to examine (e.g., Power et al., 1990). At this point we are only beginning to explore the causal pathways and complexities that link socioeconomic position to exposure to behavioral, psychosocial, and environmental risk factors and in turn link these risk factors to health outcomes. Our own analyses and those of others find that although any single behavioral, psychosocial, or environmental risk factor, or small set thereof, can account for only a small fraction of the association between SES and health, a set of 10 to 20 such risk factors can account for 50–100% of the association between a given SES indicator and health outcome. Marmot et al.(1991) and Lynch et al.(1996) have reported that adjusting for 10 to 20 such risk factors reduces the predictive association of SES with mortality by 50–100%. We get similar results for the cross-sectional relationship between education or income and functional status (House et al., 1994).

Potentials and Limits of Understanding and Intervening in Pathways. Better understanding of the pathways and mechanisms linking socioeconomic and racial/ethnic status to health is often and appropriately seen as crucial to reducing socioeconomic and racial/ethnic disparities in health. Once an intervening variable or mechanism is understood, efforts can be made to reduce this variable or mechanism or to weaken its impact on health, hence reducing the socioeconomic or racial/ethnic disparities in health. To the extent that we are able to decrease smoking and improve other health behaviors, lessen stress, enhance social relationships and supports, modify risky psychological dispositions, or reduce exposure to environmental exposures, especially in disadvantaged socioeconomic or racial/ethnic groups, or to moderate their effects on health (e.g., develop a safe cigarette or nicotine delivery system), we should consequently reduce socioeconomic and racial/ethnic disparities in health. Such intervention strategies have had some beneficial effects in these regards.

However, we wish to call attention to the often insufficiently recognized limitations of such an approach and to highlight the potential, and indeed necessity, of another and complementary approach. The potential of the pathways strategy is limited in two crucial ways. First, modifying any psychosocial risk factor is a difficult process, and the impact of modifying one or a single risk factor is necessarily limited for the reasons discussed above. Second, where we have had substantial success in reducing a behavioral or psychosocial risk factor (e.g., smoking), this success is often greatest among the more advantaged due to the persistence or even accentuation (e.g., targeting of disadvantaged groups for cigarette advertising) of the causal forces giving rise to the risk factor in less advantaged groups. Thus as overall levels of smoking have decreased in the United States, socioeconomic differences in smoking have increased. Finally, it is important to recognize that the mechanisms that currently link socioeconomic status to health are not the same ones that did so in the past or will in the future. Prior socioeconomic differences undoubtedly had more to do with differences in exposure to infectious agents and access to medical care than is currently the case. Indeed, many of the currently most important diseases and risk factors—such as coronary heart disease and its risk factors of smoking, lack of exercise, and high-fat diet—were at one time more characteristic of upper socioeconomic strata, but have become more incident and prevalent in lower socioeconomic strata as these diseases and risk factors have become more deleterious to health. A similar trend has characterized AIDS, which emerged first as a disease among higher socioeconomic strata but has rapidly become more prevalent in disadvantaged socioeconomic and racial/ethnic groups. Thus whatever the major diseases (or risk factors for them) are in future years, they too are likely to be importantly determined by socioeconomic status (Link and Phelan, 1995).

In sum, as Link and Phelan (1995) have cogently argued, we need to think increasingly of disparities in socioeconomic position as the "fundamental cause" of socioeconomic disparities in health. Hence, ameliorating these socioeconomic disparities themselves may be the best strategy for reducing disparities in health. A parallel, but not identical, argument can be made regarding racial/ethnic disparities, to which we now turn, before returning to evidence that socioeconomic improvement and policy are a major form of health improvement and policy in our and other societies, arguably the most important and essential one for reducing socioeconomic disparities in health.

Understanding Racial/Ethnic Differences in Health

Race/Ethnicity and Health. National mortality data reveal that African Americans (or blacks) have an overall death rate that is more than 1.5 times higher than that of whites (National Center for Health Statistics, 1998). The magnitude of the racial difference in death rates varies by the specific cause of death, but a pattern of elevated death rates for blacks compared to whites exists for almost all the leading causes of death in the United States. In contrast, all other racial/ethnic groups have an overall death rate that is lower than that of whites. However, there is considerable variability for subgroups of these populations and for specific health conditions. All nonblack minorities have considerably lower rates than whites for the two leading causes of death (heart disease and cancer) but higher rates for some conditions. Hispanics have higher mortality rates than non-Hispanic whites for tuberculosis, septicemia, HIV/AIDS, chronic liver disease and cirrhosis, diabetes, and homicide (Sorlie et al., 1993; Vega and Amaro, 1994). Subgroups of the Asian and Pacific Islander population also have elevated mortality rates for some health conditions (Lin-Fu, 1993). For example, the Native Hawaiian population has the highest death rate due to heart disease of any racial group in the United States (Chen, 1993). Similarly, American Indians who receive care from the Indian Health Service (60% of that population) have age-adjusted mortality rates higher than the national average for tuberculosis, alcoholism, diabetes, accidents, homicides, suicides, and pneumonia and influenza (National Center for Health Statistics, 1993).

What Is Race? Early studies of racial variations in health viewed race as primarily reflecting biological homogeneity and racial differences in health as largely genetically determined. This view predated modern scientific theories of genetics and carefully executed genetic studies. In contrast, scientific evidence suggests that our current racial categories are more alike than different in terms of biological characteristics and genetics (Lewontin, 1972; Gould, 1977; Latter, 1980). All human beings are identical for about 75% of known genetic factors, with about 95% of human genetic variation existing *within* racial groups (Lewontin, 1982). Thus there is more genetic variation within races than between them, and racial categories do not capture biological distinctiveness. Race is thus more of a social than a biological category, and racial classification schemes have been influenced by larger social and political considerations (Cooper and David, 1986; Williams, 2001).

Race and SES. Although not useful as biological markers, current racial/ethnic categories capture an important part of the inequality and injustice in American society (See and Wilson, 1988). There are important power and status differences between groups. For example, in 1995 the poverty rate for Asians was almost twice that of whites, while the rate for blacks and Hispanics was more than three times that of non-Hispanic whites (National Center for Health Statistics, 1998). Data on poverty tell only a part of the story of economic vulnerability. In addition to persons who actually fall below the government's poverty threshold, a large number of persons are only slightly above this level. Many of these persons are at a high risk of becoming poor. The combination of the poor and near-poor (annual income above the poverty threshold but less than twice the poverty level) categories reveals that one in every three persons in the United States falls into this economically vulnerable category—26% of whites, 33% of Asians, 54% of blacks, and 62% of Hispanics (National Center for Health Statistics, 1998). Although there is a strong relationship between race and SES, they are not equivalent. For example, the rate of poverty is three times higher for blacks than for whites, but two-thirds of blacks are not poor, and two-thirds of all poor Americans are white.

Race, SES, and Health. Research reveals that SES differences between races account for much of the racial differences in health. Adjusting racial (black-white) disparities in health for SES sometimes eliminates, but always substantially reduces, these differences (Krieger et al., 1993; Williams and Collins, 1995; Lillie-Blanton et al., 1996). However, race often has an effect on health independent of SES: within levels of SES, blacks still have worse health status than whites.

Table 3.1 illustrates these issues with life expectancy data. At age 45, white males have a life expectancy that is almost five years more than black males (National Center for Health Statistics, 1990). Similarly, the life expectancy at age 45 for white females is 3.7 years longer than that of similarly aged black women. However, there is considerable socioeconomic variation in life expectancy within both racial groups (National Center for Health Statistics, 1998). When we consider the distribution of life expectancy by race and income, two important trends emerge. First, for both racial groups, income is strongly linked to health status. Consistently, persons of lower levels of income report lower life expectancy than their more economically favored peers. Black men in the highest-income group live 7.4 years longer than those in the lowest-income group. The comparable numbers for whites was 6.6 years. Thus the SES difference within each racial group is larger than the racial difference across groups. A similar pattern is evident for women, although the SES differences are smaller. At age 45, black women in the highest-income group have a life expectancy that is 3.8 years longer than those in the lowest-income group. Among whites, the SES difference is 2.7 years. Moreover, for men and women of both racial groups, increasing levels of income are associated with longer life expectancy. The power of SES in shaping racial differences in health is clearly evident by comparing the highest-SES blacks with the lowest-SES whites, especially among males. High-income black males have a life expectancy that is 5.3 years longer than low-income white males. Thus the disproportionate concentration of African Americans at lower SES levels is a major factor behind the overall racial differences in health.

The second pattern that clearly emerges in these data is that race is more than socioeconomic status. Consistently, there is an independent effect of race even when SES is controlled. At every level of income, for both men and women, African Americans have lower levels of life expectancy than whites. In these data, the differences are greater at the two lower levels of income than the two higher economic status categories. However, for some indicators of health status such as infant mortality, the racial gap becomes larger as SES increases (National Center for Health Statistics, 1998).

Role of Racism or Discrimination. The construct of racism can structure and inform our understanding of racial inequalities in health (Cooper et al., 1981; Krieger et al., 1993; Hummer, 1996; La Veist, 1996; Williams, 1997, 2001). The term *racism* refers to an ideology of inferiority that is used to justify the differential treatment of members of racial outgroups by both individuals and societal institutions, usually accompanied by negative attitudes and beliefs toward these groups. Racism has been a central organizing principle within American society and has played a key role in shaping major social institutions and policies (Omi and Winant, 1986; Quadagno, 1994). Historically, ideologies about racial groups were translated into policies and societal arrangements that have limited the opportunities and social mobility of stigmatized groups. The strong association between race/ethnicity and SES in the United States reflects the successful implementation of social policies that were designed to limit societal resources and rewards to socially marginalized groups.

There have been important positive changes in the racial attitudes of whites toward blacks in recent decades and broad current support for the *principle* of equality in most societal institutions (Schuman et al., 1997). At the same time, there is considerably less support for policies that would actually implement equal access to education, housing, jobs, and so forth (Schuman et al., 1997). Moreover, national data on stereotypes reveal that whites view blacks, Hispanics, and Asians more negatively than themselves, with blacks viewed more negatively than all other groups and Hispanics twice as negatively as Asians (Davis and Smith, 1990). Such a high level of acceptance of negative stereotypes of minority groups is an ominous harbinger of widespread societal discrimination. Psychological research indicates that the endorsement of negative racial stereotypes leads to discrimination against minority groups (Devine, 1995; Hilton and von Hippel, 1996). Moreover, well-learned stereotypes are resistant to disconfirmation (Stangnor and McMillan, 1992), and their activation is an automatic process, with individuals spontaneously becoming aware of relevant stereotypes after encountering someone to whom the stereotypes are applicable (Devine, 1989; Hilton and von Hippel, 1996).

Research reveals that considerable racial/ethnic discrimination persists in the United States in domains that affect socioeconomic mobility, such as housing and employment (Kirschenman and Neckerman, 1991; Neckerman and Kirschenman, 1991; Fix and Struyk, 1993). Thus the advent of civil rights legislation and changes in the racial attitudes of whites have not been sufficient to eradicate discrimination, and there has been remarkable stability over time on multiple dimensions of racial inequality (Clinton, 1998). For example, the median income of African Americans was 59 cents for every dollar earned by whites in 1996—identical to what it was in 1978.

Racism affects disparities in health in multiple ways. First, racism restricts and truncates socioeconomic attainment. The consequent racial differences in SES and poorer health reflect, in part, the impact of economic discrimination produced by large-scale societal structures. Residential segregation has been a primary mechanism by which racial inequality has been created and reinforced. Racial segregation has determined access to educational and employment opportunities that has importantly led to truncated socioeconomic mobility for blacks and American Indians (Jaynes and Williams, 1987; Massey and Denton, 1993). Residence in segregated neighborhoods can lead to exposure to environmental toxins, poor-quality housing, and other pathogenic living conditions, including inadequate access to a broad range of services provided by municipal authorities (Collins and Williams, 1999). These conditions importantly account for the large racial difference in homicide. The combination of concentrated poverty, male joblessness, and residential instability leads to high rates of single-parent households, and these factors together account for variation in the levels of violent crime (Sampson and Wilson, 1995). Importantly, the association between these factors and violent crime for whites was virtually identical in magnitude with the association for African Americans. Several studies have found a positive association between both adult and infant mortality and residence in segregated areas. One recent study has documented elevated mortality rates for both blacks and whites in cities high on two indices of segregation compared to cities with lower levels of segregation (Collins and Williams, 1999). This pattern suggests that beyond some threshold of segregation, the adverse conditions linked to highly segregated cities may negatively affect the health of all persons who reside there.

Moreover, because of racism, SES indicators are not commensurate across racial groups, which makes it difficult to truly adjust racial differences in health for SES (Kaufman, Cooper, and McGee, 1997). There are racial differences in the quality of education, income returns for a given level of education or occupational status, wealth or assets associated with a given level of income, the purchasing power of income, the stability of employment, and the health risks associated with occupational status (Williams and Collins, 1995; Kaufman, Cooper, and McGee, 1997).

Racial differences are especially marked for wealth. Eller (1994) shows that while white households have a median net worth of $44,408, the median net worth is $4,604 for black households and $5,345 for Hispanic ones. Moreover, racial/ethnic differences in wealth are evident at all levels of income and are greatest at the lowest income level. For persons in the lowest quintile of income in the United States, the net worth of whites is 10,000 times higher than that of blacks ($10,257 versus $1).

As noted earlier, systematic discrimination can also affect the quantity and quality of services received, including medical care. Recent research has focused on the potential health consequences of subjective experiences of discrimination. Racism in the larger society can also lead to systematic differences in exposure to personal experiences of discrimination. These experiences of discrimination may be an important part of subjectively experienced stress that can adversely affect health. A growing body of evidence indicates that self-reported measures of discrimination are adversely related to physical and mental health in a broad range of racial/ethnic minority populations (Amaro, Russo, and Johnson, 1987; Salgado de Snyder, 1987; Krieger, 1990; Dion, Dion, and Pak, 1992; Jackson et al., 1996; Krieger and Sidney, 1996; Kessler, Mickelson, and Williams, 1999; Noh et al., 1999). Two recent studies suggest that exposure to discrimination plays a role in explaining observed racial differences in self-reported measures of health (Williams et al., 1997; Ren, Amick, and Williams, 1999).

A small body of research suggests that the prevalence of negative stereotypes and cultural images of stigmatized groups can adversely affect health status. First, the widespread societal stigma of inferiority can create specific anxieties, expectations, and reactions that can affect health indirectly by having an adverse impact on socioeconomic performance and mobility (Fischer et al., 1996; Steele, 1997). There may also be more direct health effects. Researchers have long identified that one response of minority populations would be to accept the dominant society's ideology of their inferiority as accurate. A few studies have operationalized the extent to which African Americans internalize or endorse these negative cultural images. These studies have found that internalized racism is positively related to psychological distress, depressive symptoms, substance use, and chronic physical health problems (Taylor and Jackson, 1990; Taylor, Henderson, and Jackson, 1991; Williams and Chung, forthcoming).

SOCIOECONOMIC AND RACIAL/ETHNIC CHARACTERISTICS OF SOCIAL SYSTEMS AS DETERMINANTS OF INDIVIDUAL AND POPULATION HEALTH

Individuals occupy particular socioeconomic positions and racial/ethnic status within broader systems of socioeconomic and racial/ethnic stratification at the level of communities, metropolitan areas, regions, nations, and even the world. Research and theory increasingly suggest the importance in at least two ways of these broader stratification systems for individual and population health. First, the nature of socioeconomic and racial/ethnic stratification at these more macrosocial levels is a major determinant of the nature and meaning of the socioeconomic and racial/ethnic status occupied by individuals. For example, the level of economic growth and development in communities, metropolitan areas, regions, nations, and the world and the relative equality or inequality in the distribution of the fruits of economic growth and development shape the absolute and relative levels of income of individuals. In particular, living in an area with lower levels of average income or higher levels of income inequality will increase the likelihood of individuals having low income levels. Similarly, as discussed in the preceding section, higher levels of racial/ethnic segregation are likely to adversely affect the socioeconomic position and other life chances of members of disadvantaged racial/ethnic groups. Second, the socioeconomic and racial/ethnic composition of areas may have effects on individual health that are not mediated through individual socioeconomic and racial/ethnic status. Such effects may be additive or interactive, as shown in Figure 3.6. The socioeconomic and racial/ethnic characteristics of areas may affect individuals' (and hence population) health independently of individuals' personal socioeconomic and racial/ethnic characteristics, presumably by shaping the nature of the social and physical environment in the area in terms of variables specified in Figure 3.6 or other unspecified features of the environment that can affect individual health. The area-level socioeconomic, racial/ethnic, and environmental characteristics may also interact with and potentiate or buffer the impact of individual socioeconomic and racial/ethnic status on health. For example, living in a poor area may increase the impact of individual income on health because personal resources become even more consequential in the relative absence of benign environmental influences and, conversely, living in a better-off area may soften the impact of personal economic deprivation.

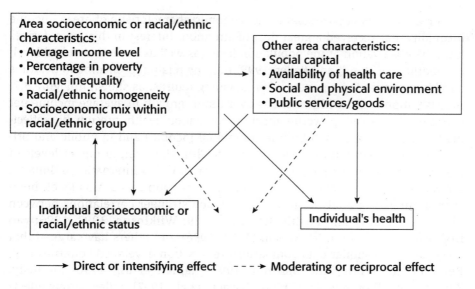

Figure 3.6. Pathways for Effects of Area Socioeconomic and Racial/Ethnic Characteristics on Health.

Contextual Effects: Real but Limited

Effects of area characteristics on individuals are usually referred to as context effects (e.g., Hauser, 1970, 1974). Evidence of aggregate or ecological correlation between the socioeconomic and racial/ethnic characteristics of areas and the population health parameters of the areas (e.g., mortality rates) are suggestive of context effects, but do not demonstrate them because they fail to control for the characteristics of individuals, which, as shown in Figure 3.6, may either select people into areas or be shaped by the characteristics of the area. A small number of studies exist that test the effects of area socioeconomic and racial/ethnic characteristics net of individual-level characteristics. As in other areas of research (e.g., Jencks and Mayer, 1990), the general finding is that there are significant effects of context, but that a far greater portion of the variance in individual health outcomes is explained by the socioeconomic and racial/ethnic characteristics of individuals (see Robert, 1999, and Robert and House, 2000b, for reviews of the socioeconomic literature; and Collins and Williams, 1999, for a review of the racial/ethnic literature). However, because social contexts also exert effects on individual characteristics, they remain a potential target for interventions to promote health.

In recent years, a particular socioeconomic characteristic of areas, income inequality, has received a great deal of attention. Interest in this topic derives from the observation at the population level (as well as at the individual level; e.g., Sorlie, Backlund, and Keller, 1995) that the relation of income to health is curvilinear, reflecting a pattern of diminishing returns, as shown in Figure 3.7. Across nations (and within nations over time), growth in average income per capita has had a very powerful effect on population health, presumably reflecting the associated growth both in individual incomes and in public and private social infrastructures productive of health. However, at higher levels of per capita income (e.g., about $5,000 per person, 1991 international dollars), the relationship becomes much weaker. Across countries at this level, however, a number of analyses have found much stronger correlations between income inequality and health (Rodgers, 1979; Wilkinson, 1992, 1996; van Doorslaer et al., 1997). Wilkinson (1992, 1996) and others have argued that these data, and similar data comparing areas within developed countries (e.g, Ben-Shlomo, White, and Marmot, 1996; Kaplan et al., 1996; Kennedy, Kawachi, and Prothrow-Stith, 1996; Kawachi et al., 1997), reflect strong effects of income inequality per se, operating through variables such as social capital, cohesion, and trust in the population. A large body of conceptual and

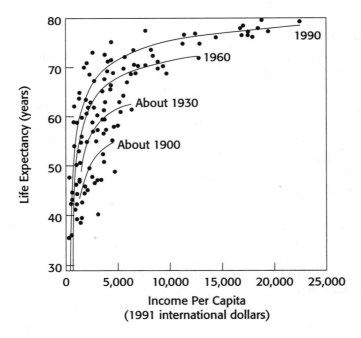

Figure 3.7. Life Expectancy and Income Per Capita for Selected Countries and Periods.

Source: World Bank, 1993.

empirical analyses suggests, on the contrary, that income inequality has its effects primarily via the underlying high level of individuals with relatively low income that necessarily characterizes areas with more unequal incomes, at least given the average levels of income in these populations (Gravelle, 1998; Deaton, 1999; Mellor and Milyo, 1999). Some evidence exists in methodologically sound studies for contextual effects of income inequality, but these are equally or more plausibly interpretable as reflecting a lower investment in public goods, especially for the disadvantaged, in areas or political units characterized by greater income inquality (Robert and House, 2000a; Lynch et al., 2000). Again, these data still suggest that interventions that affect income inequality (or correlates of it) can be a potential means of improving individual or population health, if only or mainly by improving the incomes of more disadvantaged individuals.

In sum, the socioeconomic and, especially, racial/ethnic (due to the powerful deleterious effects of segregation on African Americans discussed at the end of the previous section) characteristics of areas are important components of understanding socioeconomic and racial/ethnic disparities. Hence they must also be important in policies aimed at alleviating such disparities.

IMPROVING POPULATION HEALTH AND REDUCING SOCIOECONOMIC AND RACIAL/ETHNIC DISPARITIES THROUGH PLANNED SOCIAL POLICY AND UNPLANNED SOCIAL CHANGE

What has been said thus far provides powerful evidence of how social and behavioral science knowledge can contribute to societal and governmental objectives of improving population health and reducing socioeconomic and racial/ethnic disparities in health. It is these socioeconomic and racial/ethnic disparities in health that we believe largely explain why the United States has levels of population health significantly below those of peer nations such as Canada, Japan, or Sweden, and no better than those of many less developed countries (see Figure 3.8), despite national expenditures on health care and health research that far exceed those of any other nation. Indeed, disadvantaged portions of the U.S. population have levels of health no better than those of some of the least developed nations in the world (McCord and Freeman, 1990).

The main message we want to deliver is that socioeconomic policy and practice and racial/ethnic policy and practice are the most significant levers for reducing socioeconomic and racial/ethnic disparities and hence improving overall population health in our society, more important even than health care policy.

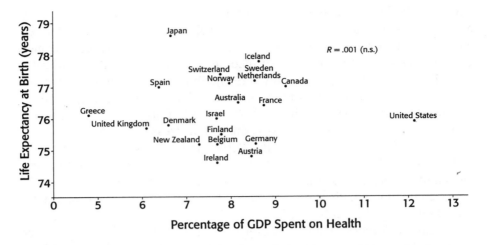

Figure 3.8. Life Expectancy at Birth, Expressed as a Percentage of Gross Domestic Product Spent on Health, 1990 (for Selected OECD Countries).

Interventions in Pathways or Mechanisms: Promise and Problems

One of the major reasons for understanding the pathways or mechanisms linking a health outcome to its more distal causes such as socioeconomic and racial/ethnic status is the promise that we may be able to intervene in the pathways or mechanisms, even if we cannot alter the more distal causes and thus eliminate or mitigate the deleterious effects of the distal cause. Preventive and therapeutic pharmacological interventions via "magic bullets" epitomize this strategy for preventing disease and promoting health. Even if we cannot eradicate the bacteria, viruses, or toxins that cause infectious diseases, we can reduce or eliminate their deleterious effects via vaccination or prophylaxis. Even where we may only partially understand, much less be able to intervene in, the ultimate causes of disease, as in hypertension, we can mitigate or eliminate its deleterious effects by acting on better-understood intervening mechanisms.

This paradigm of disease prevention and health promotion has great appeal, based on the dramatic instances of its success just alluded to. However, it remains generally more effective and efficient to approach disease promotion from a broader population or public health standpoint where feasible. This has been and may continue to be particularly true for socioeconomic and racial/ethnic disparities in health, for reasons discussed earlier. Returning to the case of cigarette smoking, efforts to understand or intervene in the physiological pathway through which it operates have not yet been successful, and extensive efforts at behavioral and pharmacological interventions to stop smoking behavior at the level of individuals have been only modestly successful. Nevertheless, in the United States at least, we have made major progress in reducing levels of cigarette consumption, due in large part to broader population-wide interventions via pricing, labeling, regulation of pro- and anti-smoking advertising, and increasingly severe restrictions on where and when persons may smoke, all contributing to an increasingly strong set of social norms against smoking. Further, and paradoxically, the success of efforts to reduce smoking may have contributed, as noted above, to the perplexing pattern from which we began—overall improvements in population health but widening socioeconomic and racial/ethnic disparities in health. This is because persons of higher socioeconomic position, especially education, have been much more likely to stop or not start smoking, thus creating a growing inverse association between socioeconomic position and smoking (Moore, Williams, and Quails, 1996).

We believe that efforts to intervene on many other psychosocial pathways linking socioeconomic and racial/ethnic status to health are likely to confront similar problems and potentially exacerbate rather than alleviate socioeconomic and racial/ethnic differences in health, unless they very carefully take account of the ways in which these pathways and mechanisms may operate differentially across socioeconomic or racial/ethnic groups. This would be true for plausibly promising interventions such as modifying other health behaviors (eating, drinking, exercise); stress management and reduction; enhancing social relationships and supports and social capital; or modifying psychological dispositions such as anger or hostility and control or efficacy. This is primarily because such interventions generally presume that the intervening risk factor can be modified largely by individual choice and effort and hence does not alter the strong forces in our systems of socioeconomic and racial/ethnic stratification that produce differences in the first place. These forces include (1) differential access or exposure to opportunities for desirable health behaviors (e.g., areas populated by disadvantaged socioeconomic and racial/ethnic minorities tend to be long on convenience and liquor stores selling cigarettes and junk food and short on supermarkets or groceries selling fresh fruits and vegetables or on safe and supportive venues and facilities for physical activity); (2) the increased risks in disadvantaged socioeconomic groups and areas of stressful events at work or home or of disruptions of social relationships, networks, and support by illness and death; (3) greater exposure to experiences generative of discrimination, hostility, or inefficacy; and (4) heightened exposure to social, and to physical, chemical, and biological environmental hazards. In addition, as noted above, the tendency is for new health problems (e.g., AIDS) and risk factors to arise, which may operate via quite different mechanisms and pathways and yet become rapidly stratified by socioeconomic and racial/ethnic status.

Nevertheless, there are opportunities for intervening in pathways and mechanisms that offer promise of reducing socioeconomic and racial/ethnic disparities and hence improving overall population health. These must involve, however, sensitivity to the specific sources of risk and also of resilience in disadvantaged socioeconomic and racial/ethnic groups and areas. Let us consider two examples—medical care and sources of resilience and health promotion in disadvantaged racial/ethnic groups.

Medical Care. What we know and do not know about the role of medical care in producing and alleviating socioeconomic and racial/ethnic disparities in health is illustrative. As already noted, there can be no question that wider availability of effective therapeutic and preventive medical care has improved population health, though to a more limited degree than is often presumed. However, Preston and Haines (1991) argued that improvements in medical care may also have exacerbated socioeconomic and racial/ethnic disparities in health to the extent that differential access to care has become more consequential for health. As we have seen, the implementation of national health services or insurance has failed to reduce socioeconomic and racial/ethnic disparities in health to the degree we had hoped or expected, if at all. Growing evidence suggests, however, that gross equalization of access or utilization fails to equalize access to maximally appropriate and effective care.

Addressing three kinds of issues offers the promise of reducing socioeconomic and racial/ethnic disparities in the quality and appropriateness of care and hence in health. The first is to recognize that differentials in the ways the medical care system deals with different groups can lead to problems in the delivery of care. If disadvantaged socioeconomic and racial/ethnic groups do not have access to the same type and quality of providers and the same kind of relationships and communication with them as more advantaged persons, the result is likely to be their receiving less regular, preventive, and appropriate care. Second, the focus of the medical care system on different types of care differentially affects the health of different groups. Disadvantaged groups may benefit more from improvements in basic primary and preventive care; advantaged groups, from secondary and tertiary care. Thus relatively poor societies (e.g., China, Costa Rica, Sri Lanka, Kerala state in India) have achieved "good health at low cost" by focusing their limited resources on ensuring equal access to basic primary and preventive care (Halsted, Walsh, and Warren, 1985). Finally, as discussed above, even secondary and tertiary care appears to be distributed inequitably by racial/ethnic groups and probably also by socioeconomic status. This may explain why the United States generally lags behind other developed nations in population life expectancy but surpasses all in life expectancy at age 80, where a high-technology system supports a relatively elite set of survivors in the population.

Finally, we must also give more attention in medical care to identifying the ways in which the lives of individuals are constrained by broader social, economic, and political forces. Some evidence suggests that the effectiveness of behavioral interventions varies by the degree that they attend to social situations in which individuals are embedded. Syme's study of 244 hypertensive patients (1987) clearly illustrates how addressing underlying social and economic conditions appears to enhance the management of hypertension and improve the effectiveness of antihypertensive therapy. The patients in this study were matched on age, race, gender, and blood pressure history and randomly assigned to one of three groups. The first group received routine hypertensive care from a physician. In addition to routine hypertensive care, the second group also attended 12 weekly clinic meetings providing health education with regard to hypertension by a health educator and nurse practitioner. In addition to routine hypertensive care, the third group was visited by community health workers who had been recruited from the immediate community and provided with one month of training to address the diverse social and medical needs of persons with hypertension. These outreach lay workers provided information on hypertension but also discussed family difficulties, financial strain, and employment opportunities and, as appropriate, provided support, advice, referral, and direct assistance.

After seven months of follow-up, patients in the third group were more likely to have their blood pressure controlled than patients in the other two groups. In addition, those in the third group knew twice as much about blood pressure and were more compliant with taking their hypertensive medication than patients in the other two groups, and the good compliers in the third group were twice as successful at controlling their blood pressure as good compliers in the health education intervention group. Thus even the effectiveness of the pharmacological treatment appeared to be enhanced in the group that also addressed the underlying stressful conditions of these hypertensive persons.

A study by Buescher and colleagues (1987) further illustrates how addressing underlying economic and social issues can improve the impact of medical care. This study compared the effectiveness of two approaches to delivering prenatal care in a population of predominantly black low-SES women in Guilford County, North Carolina. One group received prenatal care at the county health department. The other group received prenatal care from private practice physicians. Women who received care from the community-based physicians were twice as likely to have a low-birthweight baby, compared to those visiting the health department. The health department's prenatal care program attempted to comprehensively address the medical and social needs of the pregnant mothers. Prenatal care was provided by nurse practitioners instead of physicians. Time was devoted during prenatal care visits to counseling the women about nutrition and other aspects of personal care. As appropriate, referrals were made to the Women, Infants and Children Program, which provides nutritional supplements to poor women. These referrals, as well as missed clinic appointments, were followed up aggressively. James (1993) argues that the positive cultural features of this program may have been very important. It appears that the county health department's program offered low-income women an extended network of social support, capable of meeting their needs in much the same way that older, more knowledgeable women have traditionally guided and supported young inexperienced mothers (James, 1993).

Adaptive Attributes of Disadvantaged Groups. One of the major paradoxes in U.S. population health is that African Americans and Latinos are not as disadvantaged on some aspects of health as their socioeconomic positions would lead us to expect. Thus, although African Americans tend to have higher levels of ill health than whites for most indicators of physical health and are also disadvantaged compared to whites on indicators of subjective well-being such as life satisfaction and happiness (Hughes and Thomas, 1998), they have comparable or better health status than whites for other indicators of mental health. Community-based studies using measures of psychological distress show an inconsistent pattern of black–white differences. Some studies show that blacks have higher rates of distress compared to whites, while other studies show higher rates of psychological distress for whites compared to blacks (Dohrenwend and Dohrenwend, 1969; Neighbors, 1984; Vega and Rumbaut, 1991; Williams and Harris-Reid, 1999). However, when rates of psychiatric illness are considered, African Americans have comparable or lower rates of mental illness than whites. In the Epidemiologic Catchment Area Study (ECA), the largest study of psychiatric disorders ever conducted in the United States, there were very few differences between blacks and whites in the rates of both current and lifetime psychiatric disorders. Anxiety disorders, especially phobias, stand out as one area in which blacks had considerably higher rates than Caucasians. In the National Comorbidity Study, blacks do not have higher rates of disorder than whites for any of the major classes of disorders (Kessler et al., 1994). Instead, lower rates of disorders for blacks than whites are especially pronounced for the affective disorders (depression) and the substance abuse disorders (alcohol and drug abuse).

These findings emphasize the need for renewed attention to identify the cultural strengths and health-enhancing resources within the black community. Two social institutions—the family and the church—stand out as crucial for the black population. Strong family ties and an extended family system are important resources that may reduce some of the negative effects of stress on the health of black Americans. At the same time, a recognition of the strengths of black families should not be used to romanticize them as if they were a panacea for a broad range of adverse living conditions. While these networks of mutual aid and support do facilitate survival, they are also likely to provide both stress and support. Moreover, it is likely that cutbacks in government-provided social services in recent years have increased the burdens and demands on the support services provided by the black family. The black American church has been the most important social institution in the black community. These churches have historically been centers of spiritual, social, and political life. Black churches may promote mental health by providing a broad range of social and human services to the African-American community, serving as a conduit to the formal mental health system, providing a base for friendship networks, and facilitating collective catharsis and stress reduction through religious rituals and participation (Williams, 1998).

A second paradox is evident for Mexican Americans. In spite of high rates of poverty and comparatively low levels of access to medical care, Mexican Americans tend to have similar or better levels of health than the white population. Moreover, across a broad range of health status indicators, foreign-born Hispanics have a better health profile than their counterparts born in the United States. This pattern may reflect the impact of migration. Rates of infant mortality, low birthweight, cancer, high blood pressure, adolescent pregnancy, and psychiatric disorders increase with length of stay in the United States for Hispanics (Vega and Amaro, 1994). It is likely that increasing length of stay and greater acculturation of the Hispanic and Asian populations will lead to worsening health. Early studies of acculturation found that rates of heart disease among Japanese increased progressively as they moved from Japan to Hawaii to the U.S. mainland (Marmot and Syme, 1976). As groups migrate from one culture to another, immigrants often adopt the diet and behavior patterns of the new culture. Several behaviors that adversely affect health status appear to increase with acculturation. These include decreased fiber consumption, decreased breast feeding, increased use of cigarettes and alcohol—especially in young women—driving under the influence of alcohol, and use of illicit drugs (Vega and Amaro, 1994). However, the association between acculturation, length of stay in the United States, and the prevalence of disease may be complex. Migration studies of the Chinese and Japanese show that the rates of some cancers, such as prostate and colon, increase when these populations migrate to the United States, while the rates of other cancers, such as liver and cervical, decline (Jenkins and Kagawa-Singer, 1994). Research is needed to identify the extent to which there are specific aspects of culture that promote health and the strategies that may be utilized to facilitate their maintenance over time.

Social and Economic Change and Policy as Major Determinants of Health

For all the reasons discussed to this point, we believe the reduction of socioeconomic and racial/ethnic disparities in health depends most on social changes and public policies that reduce disparities in socioeconomic and racial/ethnic status or, more exactly, ensure that all citizens live under conditions that protect against disease and promote health. We would emphasize that we do not believe that there is evidence that inequality or hierarchy per se produces large social disparities in health, though it may always be a residual difference in any situation of inequality. This is because socioeconomic and other forces of advantage have diminishing returns to health. Thus, the issue is not reducing or eliminating inequality, but reducing or eliminating the relatively severe social and economic deprivations that still characterize the broad lower range (e.g., lower 25–50%) of the U.S. population in terms of socioeconomic and/or racial/ethnic status. The history of our own and other countries suggests that the poor (and truly disadvantaged) need not always be with us, and that as their conditions of life improve so does their health and hence also overall population health.

Improvements in the status of the socioeconomically or racially/ethnically disadvantaged can be made through the provision of either private or public goods or a combination thereof. That is, we can ensure their access to education, income, and other resources that allow them to obtain in the private market housing, health care, and good living and working conditions productive of health. Alternatively, we can provide many of these as public goods. Different societies at different times have chosen different mixes, but all have converged on a mix of these strategies. How good is the evidence that they work to reduce health disparities and promote population health? It is both better and worse than we might expect or like.

Macrosocial Change and Health. Not to be ignored is the evidence of history that improvements in the educational, occupational, and income levels of populations have produced massive improvements in population health that in turn improve the human capital necessary for further socioeconomic advancement (see Figure 3.7). This has included reductions in health disparities by socioeconomic position, gender, and race/ethnicity. Not surprisingly, educational and economic development are major priorities of less developed societies and also of the developed countries.

Social Welfare and Health. Similarly, evidence from the more developed countries strongly suggests that ensuring that the fruits of development are broadly distributed, especially to the broad lower range of the population, assists in promotion of health. The rise of Sweden and then Japan to the highest levels of population health in the world and the clearly reduced socioeconomic disparities in the case of Sweden, must be significantly attributed to their emphasis on ensuring good conditions of life for all, albeit via different mixes of social policy and provision of private and public goods.

More Focused Social Policies. One would like to have clearer evidence, however, that specific policies that improve the social and economic status of disadvantaged groups also improve their health. Unfortunately, we have not always evaluated the effects of such policies, and rarely their health impacts, and this remains an agenda for future research. However, limited and developing evidence is at least consistent with our thesis.

At least one study from the evaluation of the negative income tax experiments of the early 1970s shows positive effects on maternal and child health. In a study of expanded income support, Kehrer and Wolin (1979) found that the birth weight of infants born to mothers in the experimental income group was higher than that of those born to mothers in the control group although neither group experienced any experimental manipulation of health services. Improved nutrition, probably a result of the income manipulation, appeared to have been the key intervening factor. Evaluation of the long-term effects of early childhood interventions, such as the Perry preschool study, also suggests long-term effects of socioeconomic factors (median income and rates of home ownership) as well as on other behavior and beliefs (e.g., staying in school, avoiding delinquency and crime, achieving better jobs) that should promote health.

Major Exogenous Income Policies. An ideal test of our thesis would be the examination of social policies that have markedly improved the economic status of all or some of the disadvantaged population. In the United States, two stand out. One is Social Security, which has provided an income support program for the elder portion of the population that has, over time, lifted or kept most of them out of poverty. We (Arno and House, 2003) have undertaken to see if one can find evidence that Social Security has also improved the health of the elderly. We have sought to do so by examining the mortality experience of different adult age groups in the population over the course of the twentieth century. We hypothesized that the two largest exogenous income improvements from Social Security occurred first at its inception in the late 1930s and second when it was indexed to inflation in the late 1960s and early 1970s. Hence we expected that one should see discontinuous improvements in the health of the elderly, but not in other age groups, after these two periods. Our initial results, shown in Figure 3.9, seem to us consistent with this. We recognize that there may be other compelling explanations of these two discontinuities, but we do not believe that others have or would have predicted both of them ex ante or that other explanations can explain both as well or as parsimoniously ex post. Further, these trends are consistent with the evidence that socioeconomic differences in health are markedly reduced among the elderly as compared to working-age adults (House et al., 1990, 1994). The other major income support program in our country has been the earned income tax credit, but we know of no research on its effects and would certainly see such research as a high priority for the future.

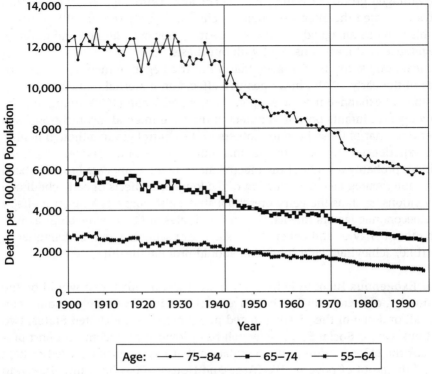

Figure 3.9. Total Mortality, United States, 1900–1995.

Source: National Center for Health Statistics.

Investment in Public Goods and Infrastructure. Limited data also indicate that efforts to improve the public good and infrastructure of communities improve the health of their residents. Some research suggests that policy changes to improve neighborhoods can importantly enhance health. Dalgard and Tambs (1997) provide findings from a ten-year follow-up study of residents in five neighborhood types in Norway. This study found that residents in a poorly functioning neighborhood that had experienced dramatic changes in its social environment over time reported improved mental health ten years later. The improvements in the neighborhoods included a new public school, a playground extension, establishment of a sports arena and park, the organization of activities for adolescents by the sports association of the municipality, establishment of a shopping center with restaurants and a cinema, and a subway line extension into the neighborhood. This effect was not explained by selective migration. Similarly, an intervention in England for a poorly functioning neighborhood also had dramatic effects (Halpern, 1995). Over a two-year period, this intervention refurbished housing, with a special emphasis on making it safe and sheltered from strangers. Changes included improved traffic regulations, improved lighting and strengthening of windows, enclosure of gardens for apartments, closure of alleyways, and landscaping. In this project, residents were involved in the planning process. A one-year follow-up study, conducted after the intervention had been in place, documented that the changes in the physical environment were associated with changes in the social environment and mental health as well. That is, the contact between neighbors had increased, and neighbors reported more trust in each other. Levels of optimism and belief in the future had increased, and residents felt a stronger identification with their neighborhood. In addition, levels of anxiety and depression were significantly reduced among residents. This study reveals that improvement in the quality of life in a neighborhood can increase both the quality of social interaction or cohesion and health.

The Case of Racial/Ethnic Disparities. Racial/ethnic disparities in health should clearly be reduced by policies that reduce absolute and relative socioeconomic deprivation. However, they also need special approaches, obviously not aimed at changing race/ethnicity per se, but rather at changing the way race/ethnicity and associated racial/ethnic status are socially defined and constructed. Again, available evidence suggests there are reduced racial/ethnic disparities in health. Mullings (1989) has suggested that the civil rights movement, for example, had important positive effects on black health. By reducing occupational and educational segregation, it improved the SES of at least a segment of the black population and also influenced public policy to make health care accessible to larger numbers of people. Consistent with this hypothesis, one study found that between 1968 and 1978, blacks experienced a larger decline in mortality rates (on both a percentage and absolute basis) than whites (Cooper et al., 1981).

CONCLUSION

We hope this chapter has produced an appreciation that socioeconomic and racial/ethnic disparities in health are the product of a broad and complex system of social stratification that will continue to structure the experience of and exposure to virtually all behavioral and psychosocial risk factors to health, hence producing large, persistent, and even increasing socioeconomic and racial/ethnic disparities in health. These health disparities largely explain why the United States increasingly lags behind other developed and even less developed nations in levels of population health, with the most disadvantaged portions of our population characterized by levels of population health comparable to some of the least developed nations in the world.

Socioeconomic and racial/ethnic disadvantages affect almost all forms of disease; almost all behavioral, psychosocial, and environmental risk factors producing these diseases; and also access to the most appropriate and effective forms of medical care. These effects are persistent over time. Thus as the major public health problems of society and the risk factors producing them change, they still will be more incident and prevalent among lower socioeconomic classes. Thus, intervening in or changing one or a few major risk factors for health (including inadequate medical care) can have only a limited effect on socioeconomic and racial/ethnic disparities in health, though this effect is clearly enhanced if interventions or changes are attentive to the broader social forces that produce these disparities.

The greatest past accomplishments and future potential for reducing socioeconomic and racial/ethnic disparities in health and improving overall population health involve improving socioeconomic status and reducing invidious racial/ethnic distinctions themselves, especially among the more disadvantaged portions of the population. Thus economic growth and development and progress toward greater racial/ethnic equality have had and can have dramatic effects on individual and population health, especially if these changes impact the more disadvantaged socioeconomic and racial/ethnic groups in our society.

Note

1. Link and Phelan (forthcoming) have similarly shown that although cognitive ability contributes to socioeconomic attainment, its effects on health are mediated entirely through such attainments, and it in no way can explain away or make spurious the considerable impact of adult SEP on health.

References

Adler, N.E., et al. "Socioeconomic Inequalities in Health: No Easy Solution." *Journal of the American Medical Association,* 1993, *269,* 3140–3145.

Adler, N. E., et al. "Socioeconomic Status and Health: The Challenge of the Gradient." *American Psychologist,* 1994, *49*(1), 15–24.

Amaro, H., Russo, N. F., and Johnson, J. "Family and Work Predictors of Psychological Well-Being Among Hispanic Women Professionals." *Psychology* of *Women Quarterly,* 1987, *11,* 505–521.

Arno, P., and House, J. S. "Can Socioeconomic Policy Improve Population Health and Reduce Social Disparities in Health? The Case of Social Security." Unpublished manuscript, 2003.

Backlund, E., Sorlie, P. D., and Johnson, N. J. "The Shape of the Relationship Between Income and Mortality in the United States: Evidence from the National Longitudinal Mortality Study." *Annals of Epidemiology,* 1996, *6,* 12–20.

Barker, D.J.P., and Osmond, C. "Infant Mortality, Childhood Nutrition and Ischaemic Heart Disease in England and Wales." *Lancet,* 1986, *1,* 1077–1081.

Ben-Shlomo, Y., White, I. R, and Marmot, M. G. "Does the Variation in the Socio-Economic Characteristics of an Area Affect Mortality?" *British Medical Journal,* 1996, *312,* 1013–1014.

Berkman, L. F., and Breslow, L. *Health and Ways of Living.* New York: Oxford University Press, 1983.

Blane, D., et al. "Association of Cardiovascular Disease Risk Factors with Socioeconomic Position During Childhood and During Adulthood." *British Medical Journal,* 1996, *313,* 1431–1438.

Blau, P., and Duncan, O. D. *The American Occupational Structure.* New York: Wiley, 1967.

Blendon, R., et al. "Access to Medical Care for Black and White Americans." *Journal of the American Medical Association,* 1989, *261,* 278–281.

Buescher, P. A., et al. "Source of Prenatal Care and Infant Birth Weight: The Case of a North Carolina County." *American Journal of Obstetrics and Gynecology,* 1987, *53,* 204–210.

Bunker, J. P., Frazier, H. S., and Mosteller, F. "Improving Health: Measuring Effects of Medical Care." *Milbank Quarterly,* 1994, *72,* 225–258.

Chapman, K. S., and Hariharan, G. "Do Poor People Have a Stronger Relationship Between Income and Mortality Than the Rich? Implications of Panel Data for Health Analysis." *Journal of Risk and Uncertainty,* 1996, *12,* 51–63.

Chen, M. S. "A 1993 Status Report on the Health Status of Asian Pacific Islander Americans: Comparisons with *Healthy People 2000* Objectives." *Asian American and Pacific Islander Journal of Health,* 1993, *1,* 37–55.

Clinton, W. J. *Economic Report of the President.* Washington, D.C.: U.S. Government Printing Office, 1998.

Collins, C. A., and Williams, D. R. "Segregation and Mortality: The Deadly Effects of Racism?" *Sociological Forum,* 1999, *14,* 495–523.

Conley, D. *Being Black, Living in the Red: Race, Wealth, and Social Policy in America.* Berkeley: University of California Press, 1999.

Cooper, R. S., and David, R. "The Biological Concept of Race and Its Application to Public Health and Epidemiology." *Journal of Health and Politics, Policy and Law,* 1986, *11,* 97–116.

Cooper, R. S., et al. "Racism, Society, and Disease: An Exploration of the Social and Biological Mechanisms of Differential Mortality." *International Journal of Health Services,* 1981, *11,* 389–414.

Dalgard, O. S., and Tambs, K. "Urban Environment and Mental Health: A Longitudinal Study." *British Journal of Psychiatry,* 1997, *171,* 530–536.

Davis, J. A., and Smith, T. W. *General Social Surveys, 1972–1990.* Chicago: National Opinion Research Center, 1990.

Deaton, A. *Inequalities in Income and Inequalities in Health.* Working Paper no. 7141. Washington, D.C.: National Bureau of Economic Research, 1999.

Devine, P. G. "Stereotypes and Prejudice: Their Automatic and Controlled Components." *Journal of Personality and Social Psychology,* 1989, *56,* 5–18.

Devine, P. G. "Prejudice and Out-Group Perception." In A. Tesser (ed.), *Advanced Social Psychology.* New York: McGraw-Hill, 1995.

Dion, K. L., Dion, K. K., and Pak, A.W.P. "Personality-Based Hardiness as a Buffer for Discrimination-Related Stress in Members of Toronto's Chinese Community." *Canadian Journal of Behavioral Science,* 1992, *24,* 517–536.

Dohrenwend, B. P., and Dohrenwend, B. S. *Social Status and Psychological Disorder: A Casual Inquiry.* New York: Wiley, 1969.

Eller, T. J. *Household Wealth and Asset Ownership, 1991.* Current Population Reports, no. P70-34. Washington, D.C.: U.S. Bureau of the Census, 1994.

Elo, I. T., and Preston, S. H. "Effects of Early-Life Conditions on Adult Mortality: A Review." *Population Index,* 1992, *58,* 186–212.

Evans, R. G., Barer, M. L., and Marmor, T. R. *Why Are Some People Healthy and Others Not? The Determinants of Health of Populations.* Hawthorne, N.Y.: Aldine de Gruyter, 1994.

Featherman, D. L, and Hauser, R. M. *Opportunity and Change.* San Diego, Calif.: Academic Press, 1978.

Fischer, C. S., et al. *Inequality by Design: Cracking the Bell Curve Myth.* Princeton, N.J.: Princeton University Press, 1996.

Fix, M., and Struyk, R. J. *Clear and Convincing Evidence: Measurement of Discrimination in America.* Washington, D.C.: Urban Institute Press, 1993.

Gould, S. J. "Why We Should Not Name Human Races: A Biological View." In S. J. Gould (ed.), *Ever Since Darwin.* New York: Norton, 1977.

Gravelle, H. "How Much of the Relation Between Population Mortality and Unequal Distribution of Income Is a Statistical Artifact?" *British Medical Journal,* 1998, *316,* 382–385.

Halpern, D. *Mental Health and the Built Environment: More Than Bricks and Mortar?* Bristol, Pa.: Taylor & Francis, 1995.

Halsted, S. B., Walsh, J. A., and Warren, K. S. *Good Health at Low Cost.* Proceedings of a Conference at the Bellagio Conference Center, Bellagio, Italy, Apr. 29–May 3, 1985. New York: Rockefeller Foundation, 1985.

Hannan, E. L., et al. "Access to Coronary Artery Bypass Surgery by Race/Ethnicity and Gender Among Patients Who Are Appropriate for Surgery." *Medical Care,* 1999, *37,* 68–77.

Harris, D. R, Andrews, R., and Elixhauser, A. "Racial and Gender Differences in Use of Procedures for Black and White Hospitalized Adults." *Ethnicity and Disease,* 1997, *7,* 91–105.

Hauser, R. M. "Context and Convex: A Cautionary Tale." *American Journal of Sociology,* 1970, *75,* 645–664.

Hauser, R. "Contextual Analysis Revisited." *Sociological Methods and Research,* 1974, *3,* 365–375.

Hilton, J. L., and von Hippel, W. "Stereotypes." *Annual Review of Psychology,* 1996, *47,* 237–271.

House, J. S., Landis, K., and Umberson, D. "Social Relationships and Health." *Science,* 1988, *241,* 540–545.

House, J. S., and Williams, D. R. "Psychosocial Pathways Linking SES and CVD." In National Institutes of Health, National Heart, Lung, and Blood Institute's Report of the Conference on Socioeconomic Status and Cardiovascular Health and Disease, November 6–7, 1995.

House, J. S., et al. "Age, Socioeconomic Status, and Health." *Milbank Quarterly,* 1990, *68,* 383–411.

House, J. S., et al. "Social Stratification, Age, and Health." In K. W. Schaie, D. Blazer, and J. S. House (eds.), *Aging, Health Behaviors, and Health Outcomes.* Mahwah, N.J.: Erlbaum, 1992.

House, J. S., et al. "The Social Stratification of Aging and Health." *Journal of Health and Social Behavior,* 1994, *35,* 213–234.

Hughes, M., and Thomas, M. E. "The Continuing Significance of Race Revisited: A Study of Race, Class, and Quality of Life in America, 1972 to 1996." *American Sociological Review,* 1998, *63,* 785–795.

Hummer, R. A. "Black-White Differences in Health and Mortality: A Review of a Conceptual Model." *Sociological Quarterly,* 1996, *37,* 105–125.

Jackson, J. S., et al. "Racism and the Physical and Mental Health Status of African Americans: A Thirteen-Year National Panel Study." *Ethnicity and Disease,* 1996, *6,* 132–147.

James, S. A. "Racial and Ethnic Differences in Infant Mortality and Low Birth Weight: A Psychosocial Critique." *Annals of Epidemiology,* 1993, *3,* 131–136.

Jaynes, G. D., and Williams, R. M. *A Common Destiny: Blacks and American Society.* Washington, D.C.: National Academy Press, 1987.

Jencks, C., and Mayer, S. E. "The Social Consequences of Growing Up in a Poor Neighborhood." In L. E. Lynn Jr. and M.G.H. McGeary (eds.), *Inner-City Poverty in the United States.* Washington, D.C.: National Academy Press, 1990.

Jenkins, C.N.H., and Kagawa-Singer, M. "Cancer." In N.W.S. Zane, D. T. Takeuchi, and K.N.J. Young (eds.), *Confronting Critical Health Issues of Asian and Pacific Islander Americans.* Thousand Oaks, Calif.: Sage, 1994.

Kaplan, G. A., and Salonen, J. T. "Socioeconomic Conditions in Childhood and Ischaemic Heart Disease During Middle Age." *British Medical Journal,* 1990, *301,* 1121–1123.

Kaplan, G. A., et al. "Inequality in Income and Mortality in the United States: Analysis of Mortality and Potential Pathways." *British Medical Journal,* 1996, *312,* 999–1003.

Kaufman, J. S., Cooper, R. S., and McGee, D. L. "Socioeconomic Status and Health in Blacks and Whites: The Problem of Residual Confounding and the Resiliency of Race." *Epidemiology,* 1997, *8,* 621–628.

Kawachi, I., et al. "Social Capital, Income Inequality, and Mortality." *American Journal of Public Health,* 1997, *87,* 1491–1498.

Kehrer, B. H., and Wolin, C. M. "Impact of Income Maintenance on Low Birth Weight: Evidence from the Gary Experiment." *Journal of Human Resources,* 1979, *14,* 434–462.

Kennedy, B. P., Kawachi, I., and Prothrow-Stith, D. "Income Distribution and Mortality: Cross-Sectional Ecological Study of the Robin Hood Index in the United States." *British Medical Journal,* 1996, *312,* 1004–1007.

Kessler, R. C., Mickelson, K. D., and Williams, D. R. "The Prevalence, Distribution, and Mental Health Correlates of Perceived Discrimination in the United States." *Journal of Health and Social Behavior,* 1999, *40,* 208–230.

Kessler, R. C., et al. "Lifetime and 12-Month Prevalence of DSM-III-R Psychiatric Disorders in the United States." *Archives of General Psychiatry,* 1994, *51,* 8–19.

Kirschenman, J., and Neckerman, K. M. "We'd Love to Hire Them, but . . . : The Meaning of Race for Employers." In C. Jenkins and P. E. Peterson (eds.), *The Urban Underclass.* Washington, D.C.: Brookings Institution, 1991.

Krieger, N. "Racial and Gender Discrimination: Risk Factors for High Blood Pressure?" *Social Science and Medicine,* 1990, *30,* 1273–1281.

Krieger, N., and Sidney, S. "Racial Discrimination and Blood Pressure: The CARDIA Study of Young Black and White Adults." *American Journal of Public Health,* 1996, *86,* 1370–1378.

Krieger, N., et al. "Racism, Sexism, and Social Class. Implications for Studies of Health, Disease, and Well-Being." *American Journal of Preventive Medicine,* 1993, *9*(6 suppl.), 82–122.

Kuh, D., and Ben-Shlomo, Y. *A Lifecourse Approach to Chronic Disease Epidemiology.* Oxford: Oxford University Press, 1997.

Kunitz, S. J. "Explanations and Ideologies of Mortality Patterns." *Population and Development Review,* 1987, *13,* 379–408.

Lalonde, M. *A New Perspective in the Health of Canadians.* Ottawa: Information Canada, 1975.

Lantz, P. M, et al. "Socioeconomic Factors, Health Behaviors, and Mortality." *Journal of the American Medical Association,* 1998, *279,* 1703–1708.

Lantz, P. M., et al. "Socioeconomic Disparities in Health Change in a Longitudinal Study of U.S. Adults: The Role of Health Risk Behaviors." *Social Science and Medicine,* 2001, *53*(1), 29–40.

Latter, B.D.H. "Genetic Differences Within and Between Populations of the Major Human Subgroups." *American Naturalist,* 1980, *116,* 220–237.

La Veist, T. A. "Why We Should Continue to Study Race but Do a Better Job: An Essay on Race, Racism, and Health." *Ethnicity and Disease,* 1996, *6,* 21–29.

Lewontin, R. C. "The Apportionment of Human Diversity." In T. Dobzhansky, M. K. Hecht, and W. C. Steere (eds.), *Evolutionary Biology,* Vol. 6. Upper Saddle River, N.J.: Appleton-Century-Crofts, 1972.

Lewontin, R. C. *Human Diversity.* New York: Scientific American Books, 1982.

Lillie-Blanton, M., et al. "Racial Differences in Health: Not Just Black and White, but Shades of Gray." *Annual Review of Public Health,* 1996, *17,* 411–448.

Lin-Fu, J. S. "Asian and Pacific Islander Americans: An Overview of Demographic Characteristics and Health Care Issues." *Asian and Pacific Islander Journal of Health,* 1993, *1,* 20–36.

Link, B. G. and Phelan, J. "Social Conditions as Fundamental Causes of Disease." *Journal of Health and Social Behavior,* 1995 (special issue), 80–94.

Link, B. G., and Phelan, J. (forthcoming).

Lynch, J. W., Kaplan, G. A., and Salonen, J. T. "Why Do Poor People Behave Poorly? Variation in Adult Health Behaviors and Psychosocial Characteristics by Stages of the Socioeconomic Lifecourse." *Social Science and Medicine,* 1997, *44,* 809–819.

Lynch, J. W., et al. "Childhood and Adult Socioeconomic Status as Predictors of Mortality in Finland." *Lancet,* 1994, *343,* 524–527.

Lynch, J. W., et al. "Do Cardiovascular Risk Factors Explain the Relation Between Socioeconomic Status, Risk of All-Cause Mortality, Cardiovascular Mortality, and Acute Myocardial Infarction?" *American Journal of Epidemiology,* 1996, *144,* 934–942.

Lynch, J. W., et al. "Income Inequality and Health: Importance to Health of Individual Income, Psychosocial Environment or Material Conditions." *British Medical Journal,* 2000, *320,* 1200–1204.

Marmot, M. G., Kogevinas, M., and Elston, M. A. "Social/Economic Status and Disease." *Annual Review of Public Health,* 1987, *8,* 111–135.

Marmot, M. G., and Syme, S. L. "Acculturation and Coronary Heart Disease in Japanese-Americans." *American Journal of Epidemiology,* 1976, *104,* 225–247.

Marmot, M. G., et al. "Health Inequalities Among British Civil Servants: The Whitehall II Study." *Lancet,* 1991, *337,* 1387–1393.

Massey, D. S., and Denton, N. A. *American Apartheid. Segregation and the Making of the Underclass.* Cambridge, Mass.: Harvard University Press, 1993.

McBean, A. M., and Gornick, M. "Differences by Race in the Rates of Procedures Performed in Hospitals for Medicare Beneficiaries." *Health Care Financing Review,* 1994, *15*(4), 77–90.

McCord, C., and Freeman, H. P. "Excess Mortality in Harlem." *New England Journal of Medicine,* 1990, *322,* 173–177.

McDonough, P., et al. "Income Dynamics and Adult Mortality in the United States, 1972 through 1989." *American Journal of Public Health,* 1997, *87,* 1476–1483.

McGinnis, M. J., and Forge, W. H. "Actual Causes of Death in the United States." *Journal of the American Medical Association,* 1993, *270,* 207–221.

McKeown, T. J. *The Role of Medicine: Dream, Mirage, or Nemesis.* Princeton, N.J.: Princeton University Press, 1979.

McKeown, T. J. *The Origins of Human Disease.* Malden, Mass.: Blackwell, 1988.

McKinlay, J. B., and McKinlay, S. J. "The Questionable Contribution of Medical Measures to the Decline of Mortality in the United States in the Twentieth Century." *Milbank Memorial Fund Quarterly,* 1977, *55,* 405–428.

Mechanic, D. "Socioeconomic Status and Health: An Explanation of Underlying Processes." In J. P. Bunker, D. S. Gomby, and B. H. Kehrer (eds.), *Pathways to Health: The Role of Social Factors.* Menlo Park, Calif.: Henry J. Kaiser Family Foundation, 1989.

Mellor, J., and Milyo, J. *Income Inequality and Individual Health: Evidence from the Current Population Survey.* Robert Wood Johnson Health Policy Scholars Working Paper no. 8. Boston: Boston University School of Management, 1999.

Mirowsky, J., and Hu, P. N. "Physical Impairment and the Diminishing Effects of Income." *Social Forces,* 1996, *74,* 1073–1096.

Moore, D. J., Williams, J. D., and Quails, W. J. "Target Marketing of Tobacco and Alcohol-Related Products to Ethnic Minority Groups in the United States." *Ethnicity and Disease,* 1996, *6,* 83–98.

Mullings, L. "Inequality and African-American Health Status: Policies and Prospects." In W. A. Van Horne and T. V. Tonnesen (eds.), *Race: Twentieth Century Dilemmas, Twenty-First Century Prognoses.* Madison: Institute on Race and Ethnicity, University of Wisconsin, 1989.

National Center for Health Statistics. *Mortality Detail Files, 1990:* Vol. 7. ICPSR Study no. 07632. Ann Arbor, Mich.: Inter-University Consortium for Political and Social Research, 1990.

National Center for Health Statistics. *Trends in Indian Health, 1993.* Rockville, Md.: U.S. Department of Health and Human Services, 1993.

National Center for Health Statistics. *Health, United States: Socioeconomic Status and Health Chartbook.* Hyattsville, Md.: U.S. Department of Health and Human Services, 1998.

Neckerman, K. M., and Kirschenman, J. "Hiring Strategies, Racial Bias, and Inner-City Workers." *Social Problems,* 1991, *38,* 433–447.

Neighbors, H. W. "The Distribution of Psychiatric Morbidity in Black Americans." *Community Mental Health Journal,* 1984, *20,* 169–181.

Noh, S., et al. "Discrimination and Emotional Well-Being: Perceived Racial Discrimination, Depression, and Coping: A Study of Southeast Asian Refugees in Canada." *Journal of Health and Social Behavior,* 1999, *40,* 193–207.

Oliver, M. L., and Shapiro, T. M. *Black Wealth/White Wealth: A New Perspective on Racial Inequality.* New York: Routledge, 1995.

Omi, M., and Winant, H. *Racial Formation in the United States: From the 1960s to the 1980s.* New York: Routledge, 1986.

Pappas, G., et al. "The Increasing Disparity in Mortality Between Socioeconomic Groups in the United States, 1960 and 1986." *New England Journal of Medicine,* 1993, *329,* 103–109.

Peterson, E. D., et al. "Racial Variation in the Use of Coronary Revascularization Procedures: Are the Differences Real? Do They Matter?" *New England Journal of Medicine,* 1997, *336,* 480–486.

Power, C., et al. "Health in Childhood and Social Inequalities in Young Adults." *Journal of the Royal Statistical Society,* 1990, *153,* 17–28.

Preston, S. H., and Haines, M. R. *Fatal Years.* Princeton, N.J.: Princeton University Press, 1991.

Quadagno, J. *The Color of Welfare: How Racism Undermined the War on Poverty.* New York: Oxford University Press, 1994.

Ren, X. S., Amick, B., and Williams, D. R. "Racial/Ethnic Disparities in Health: The Interplay Between Discrimination and Socioeconomic Status." *Ethnicity and Disease,* 1999, *9,* 151–165.

Robert, S. A. "Socioeconomic Position and Health: The Independent Contribution of Community Context." *Annual Review of Sociology,* 1999, *25,* 489–516.

Robert, S. A., and House, J. S. "Socioeconomic Inequalities in Health: An Enduring Sociological Problem." In C. Bird, P. Conrad, and A. Fremont (eds.), *Handbook of Medical Sociology.* Upper Saddle River, N.J.: Prentice Hall, 2000a.

Robert, S. A., and House, J. S. "Socioeconomic Inequalities in Health: Integrating Individual-, Community-, and Societal-Level Theory and Research." In G. L. Albrecht, R. Fitzpatrick, and S. C. Scrimshaw (eds.), *Handbook of Social Studies in Health and Medicine.* London: Sage, 2000b.

Rodgers, G. B. "Income and Inequality as Determinants of Mortality: An International Cross-Section Analysis." *Population Studies,* 1979, *33,* 343–351.

Rodin, J. "Aging and Health: Effects of the Sense of Control." *Science,* 1986, *237,* 143–149.

Salgado de Snyder, V. N. "Factors Associated with Acculturative Stress and Depressive Symptomatology Among Married Mexican Immigrant Women." *Psychology of Women Quarterly,* 1987, *11,* 475–488.

Sampson, R. J., and Wilson, W. J. "Toward a Theory of Race, Crime, and Urban Inequality." In J. Hagan and R. D. Peterson (eds.), *Crime and Inequality.* Stanford, Calif.: Stanford University Press, 1995.

Satel, S. "The Politicization of Public Health." *Wall Street Journal,* Dec. 12, 1996, p. 12.

Scheier, M. F., and Bridges, M. W. "Person Variables and Health: Personality Predispositions and Acute Psychological States as Shared Determinants for Disease." *Psychosomatic Medicine,* 1995, *57,* 255–268.

Schuman, H., et al. *Racial Attitudes in America: Trends and Interpretations.* Cambridge, Mass.: Harvard University Press, 1997.

Schwartz, E., et al. "Black/White Comparison of Deaths Preventable by Medical Intervention: United States and the District of Columbia, 1980–1986." *International Journal of Epidemiology*, 1990, *19*, 591–598.

See, K. O., and Wilson, W. J. "Race and Ethnicity." In N. J. Smelser (ed.), *Handbook of Sociology*. Thousand Oaks, Calif.: Sage, 1988.

Sorlie, P. D., et al. "Mortality by Hispanic Status in the United States." *Journal of the American Medical Association*, 1993, *270*, 2464–2468.

Sorlie, P. D., Backlund, E., and Keller, J. B. "U.S. Mortality by Economic, Demographic, and Social Characteristics: The National Longitudinal Mortality Study." *American Journal of Public Health*, 1995, *85*, 949–956.

Stangnor, C., and McMillan, D. "Memory for Expectancy-Congruent and Expectancy-Incongruent Information: A Review of the Social and Social Development Literatures." *Psychological Bulletin*, 1992, *111*, 42–61.

Steele, C. M. "A Threat in the Air: How Stereotypes Shape Intellectual Identity and Performance." *American Psychologist*, 1997, *52*, 613–629.

Surgeon General's Advisory Committee on Smoking and Health. *Smoking and Health*. Washington, D.C.: U.S. Public Health Service, 1964.

Syme, S. L. "Drug Treatment of Mild Hypertension: Social and Psychological Considerations." *Annals of the New York Academy of Science*, 1987, *304*, 99–106.

Taylor, J., Henderson, D., and Jackson, B. B. "A Holistic Model for Understanding and Predicting Depression in African American Women." *Journal of Community Psychology*, 1991, *19*, 306–320.

Taylor, J., and Jackson, B. B. "Factors Affecting Alcohol Consumption in Black Women, Part 2." *International Journal of Addictions*, 1990, *25*, 1415–1427.

Theorell, T. G. "Review of Research on Life Events and Cardiovascular Illness." *Advances in Cardiology*, 1982, *29*, 140–147.

Trevino, F. M., et al. "Health Insurance Coverage and Utilization of Health Services by Mexican Americans, Mainland Puerto Ricans, and Cuban Americans." *Journal of the American Medical Association*, 1991, *265*, 2233–2237.

U.S. Department of Health and Human Services. *Healthy People 2000: National Health Promotion and Disease Prevention Objectives*. DHHS Publication no. 91-50212. Rockville, Md.: U.S. Department of Health and Human Services, 1990.

U.S. Department of Health and Human Services. *Healthy People 2010: Objectives: Draft for Public Comment*. 1999. [http://web.health.gov/healthypeople/2010Draft/object.htm].

van Doorslaer, E., et al. "Income-Related Inequalities in Health: Some International Comparisons." *Journal of Health Economics*, 1997, *16*, 93–112.

Varmus, H. E. Statement Before the House and Senate Appropriations Subcommittees on Labor, Health and Human Services, and Education, Feb. 23–24, 1999. [http://www.nih.gov/welcome/director/022299.htm].

Vega, W. A., and Amaro, H. "Latino Outlook: Good Health, Uncertain Prognosis." *Annual Review of Public Health*, 1994, *15*, 39–67.

Vega, W. A., and Rumbaut, R. G. "Ethnic Minorities and Mental Health." *Annual Review of Sociology,* 1991, *17,* 351–383.

Wenneker, M. B., and Epstein, A. M. "Racial Inequalities in the Use of Procedures for Patients with Ischemic Heart Disease in Massachusetts." *Journal of the American Medical Association,* 1989, *261,* 253–257.

Whittle, J., et al. "Racial Differences in the Use of Invasive Cardiovascular Procedures in the Department of Veterans Affairs." *New England Journal of Medicine,* 1993, *329,* 621–626.

Wilkins, R., Adams, O. and Brancker, A. "Changes in Mortality by Income in Urban Canada from 1971 to 1986." *Health Reports,* 1989, *1,* 137–174.

Wilkinson, R. G. "Income Distribution and Life Expectancy." *British Medical Journal,* 1992, *301,* 165–168.

Wilkinson, R. G. *Unhealthy Societies: The Afflictions of Inequality.* New York: Routledge, 1996.

Williams, D. R. "Socioeconomic Differentials in Health: A Review and Redirection." *Social Psychology Quarterly,* 1990, *53,* 81–99.

Williams, D. R. "Race and Health: Basic Questions, Emerging Directions." *Annals of Epidemiology,* 1997, *7,* 322–333.

Williams, D. R. "African-American Health: The Role of the Social Environment." *Journal of Urban Health: Bulletin of the New York Academy of Medicine,* 1998, *75,* 304–321.

Williams, D. R. "Racial Variations in Adult Health Status: Patterns, Paradoxes and Prospects." In N. J. Smelser, W. J. Wilson, and F. Mitchell (eds.), *America Becoming: Racial Trends and Their Consequences,* Vol. 2. Washington, D.C.: National Academy Press, 2001.

Williams, D. R., and Chung, A.-M. "Racism and Health." In R. Gibson and J. S. Jackson (eds.), *Health in Black America.* Thousand Oaks, Calif.: Sage, forthcoming.

Williams, D. R., and Collins, C. "U.S. Socioeconomic and Racial Differences in Health." *Annual Review of Sociology,* 1995, *21,* 349–386.

Williams, D. R., and Harris-Reid, M. "Race and Mental Health: Emerging Patterns and Promising Approaches." In A. V. Horwitz and T. L. Scheid (eds.), *A Handbook for the Study of Mental Health: Social Contexts, Theories, and Systems.* New York: Cambridge University Press, 1999.

Williams, D. R., et al. "Racial Differences in Physical and Mental Health: Socioeconomic Status, Stress, and Discrimination." *Journal of Health Psychology,* 1997, *2,* 335–351.

Wolfson, M., et al. "Career Earnings and Death: A Longitudinal Analysis of Older Canadian Men." *Journal of Gerontology,* 1993, *48,* 167–179.

Woolhandler, S., et al. "Medical Care and Mortality: Racial Differences in Preventable Deaths." *International Journal of Health Services,* 1985, *15,* 1–11.

World Bank. *World Development Report.* Washington, D.C.: World Bank, 1993.

CHAPTER FOUR

Gender, Health, and Equity

The Intersections

Piroska Östlin
Asha George
Gita Sen

A s a fundamental basis for grouping people, gender is a social stratifier that both influences and is influenced by multiple forms of discrimination. The resulting inequalities in health between women and men have not only stimulated medical and social science research during the last decade but also become one of the major public health concerns in policy debates in many countries. Research aimed at a deeper understanding of the social and biological determinants of gender inequalities in health and how such inequalities reflect and sustain social discrimination is an important prerequisite to enabling policy makers to address the health gap between women and men more effectively.

The purpose of this chapter is to illustrate the ways in which gender influences health inequalities. A more detailed discussion is found in our forthcoming review of the subject (G. Sen et al. 2002). This chapter is divided into three parts. In the first part, we describe what we mean by gender and how it informs a health equity perspective. In the second part, we focus on gender influences in four key areas of health: (1) mortality and longevity in general and maternal mortality in particular, (2) morbidity, (3) health care, and (4) medical research. The final section draws on selected examples of policies from both developing and developed countries that have a strong bearing on gender inequalities in health.

CONCEPTUAL INTERSECTIONS: GENDER, HEALTH, AND EQUITY

The terms *sex* and *gender* are often used synonymously, but in gender research the two concepts have fundamentally different meanings. Sex refers to the biologically recognized differences between men and women—chromosomes, internal and external sex organs, hormonal makeup and secondary sex characteristics. In contrast, the concept of *gender* "is related to how we are perceived and expected to think and act as women and men because of the way society is organized, not because of our biological differences" (World Health Organization, 1998a). In this way, what is considered "appropriate" female and male behavior can vary across cultures.

However, gender is much more than the socialized relations between individuals. It is a key form of social stratification, which also determines unequal access to resources, biased public representation, and discriminatory institutional policies. Gender is distinct from but *interactive* with other social features like social class or race/ethnicity. All these social factors combine to determine power relations in society that lead not only to inequalities *between* women and men, but also to inequalities *within* different groups of women and different groups of men.

Lastly, although gender and sex are conceptually distinct, in practice, variations of interaction between the two exist. Biological differences between the sexes may be in part socially determined, while social differences arising from gender relations may also have a biological element (Hammarström et al., 2001; Krieger and Zierler, 1995).

There are systematic gender differences in income, resources, and benefits. These include, for example, the division of labor both within the household and outside of it, levels of education or medical care received, and liberties that different members of society are permitted to enjoy (A. Sen, 1992a). Gender equity, including equity in health, is contingent on fairness in the distribution of resources, benefits, and responsibilities between women and men. This idea of equity envisions health as being located within the larger realm of societal well-being and within overarching social and political contexts.

The gender, health, and inequity interface can initially be broken down into two conceptually distinct dimensions: (1) biologically specific health needs of men and women that are not fairly accommodated and (2) inequalities in health and health care arising from unfair gender relations and not from biological differences between the sexes.

The failure to recognize the biologically specific health needs of women and men is most obviously related, but not limited to, the reproductive system. Perhaps the clearest and most appalling expression of this type of gender inequity is the persistence of extremely high rates of maternal death in childbirth in many developing countries despite the widespread public health know how to prevent such catastrophes (Figure 4.1 and further discussion below).

Despite the need to recognize and address such differences, care must be taken to note that such specific needs do not lead to "naturally" different social roles or fewer social opportunities for women or men. Another example of this type of gender and health inequity is the tendency to interpret women's biological reproductive capacity as a basis to justify exclusive responsibility for reproduction to women. Instead, occupational regulations should protect both male and female reproductive health from exposure to toxic chemicals and radiation, and employment policies should support both male and female parenting.

Once these specific needs are addressed fairly, all other differences in health between women and men must be hypothesized as being caused by unequal social relations of gender. For example, although both females and males have similar biological risks for trachoma infection, males at all ages have a lower prevalence of the disease (West et al. 1991a, 1991b). This reflects not only the higher exposure of females through their domestic roles as caregivers to young children who carry the infection, but also a gender bias in access to trachoma treatment favoring males (Congdon et al., 1993; Lane and Inhorn, 1987).

Gendered patterns of employment also underlie differentials in occupational health. Women are also disproportionately hired in export factories notorious for their lack of occupational health standards and labor policies that respect their needs. At the same time, rigid gender roles are also dangerous to men's

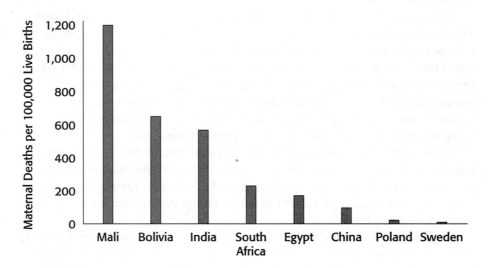

Figure 4.1. Maternal Mortality Ratios in Selected Countries, 1990.

Source: United Nations Development Programme, 1999.

health. The pervasive expectation of men as the family breadwinner forces many poor men to take jobs that expose them to excessive health risks. If they are unable to meet expectations, they may also resort to health-damaging behaviors such as alcohol abuse and smoking (Sabo and Gordon 1993). Hence gender roles and the extent to which health care provision is skewed along gender lines underlie male–female differences in health outcomes (Okojie, 1994; Doyal, 1995).

Women are also disproportionately affected by harmful traditional practices, such as female genital mutilation, which causes health problems and suffering in millions of girls and women (Santow, 1995; Craft, 1997a; World Health Organization, 1997). Although female genital mutilation has recently attracted much public attention, it is only one part of the larger problem of violence against women implicitly and explicitly sanctioned by gender discrimination (Heise et al., 1994). Another disturbing form of social discrimination against women is the health and economic destitution of female-headed households and widows in many developing countries (Chen and Drèze, 1995).

EVIDENCE OF GENDER INEQUALITY IN HEALTH
Mortality

Globally, the observed higher rates of male mortality are assumed to be based in biological fact. Women's survival advantage at all ages has been demonstrated in a wide range of countries (Waldron, 1983; Hemström, 1998). The degree of gender difference in life expectancy, however, varies across the age spectrum and across time periods (Hemström, 1998). In an 11 country study, Hemström identified a range in the mortality rate ratio of men to women from a low of 1.25 at either end of the age spectrum to a high of 2.4 in the early adult years (Figure 4.2). As demonstrated in Sweden, the pattern of excess male mortality has varied considerably over the last 50 years (Figure 4.3). The variations across age, time, and place suggest that social factors have a significant influence on the biological difference in survival between the sexes.

Where social discrimination against women is less pervasive, women tend to increase their life expectancy beyond that of men (Waldron, 1983). In countries where women's mortality rate is higher or equal to that of men, differential female deprivation of extraordinary proportions exists (A. Sen, 1992a). Extremes in the range of gaps in life expectancy at birth between males and females are expressed as ratios in Table 4.1. At the low end are countries such as Nepal and India where women's survival advantage is suppressed, and at the other extreme are former socialist countries where men's survival has decreased even more than women's. In 1994, Russian women could expect to live 13.5 years longer than men, a gender gap in life expectancy that had widened significantly since 1989.

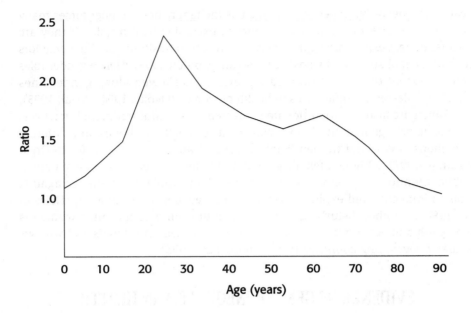

Figure 4.2. Average Lifetime Pattern of Male-to-Female Mortality Rate Ratios.

Source: Adapted from Hemström, 1998.

Note: Figure is based on data from Ecuador, Egypt, Finland, Hungary, Israel, Japan, the Netherlands, Portugal, Sri Lanka, Sweden, and the United States. There are two observations for each country (three for Sweden), the first for a year in the 1970s and the second for a year in the 1990s (or the most recent year available). For Sweden, data for 1945 are also used.

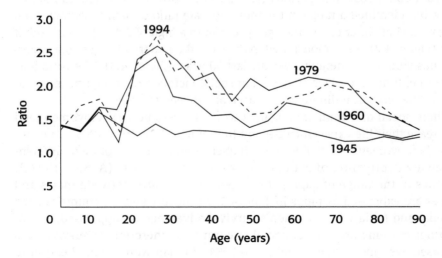

Figure 4.3. Male-to-Female Mortality Rate Ratio in Sweden, Selected Years, 1945–1994.

Source: Adapted from Hemström, 1998.

Table 4.1. Ratio of Female to Male Life Expectancy at Birth in Selected Countries, 1997.

Country	Ratio
Maldives	0.96
Nepal	0.99
Bangladesh	1.00
India	1.01
Afghanistan	1.02
Belarus	1.16
Estonia	1.17
Lithuania	1.17
Latvia	1.19
Russia	1.23

Source: United Nations Development Programme, 1999.

In comparing survival between sexes, one has to be careful not to confuse equality with equity. Amartya Sen argues that a "shortfall" from the optimal value each sex could ideally achieve would be more useful in measuring gender differences in survival (A. Sen, 1992a). A shortfall measure controls for biological differences between men and women and reveals the extent of social discrimination faced by both men and women across different countries. Such an approach raises the important issue of how an optimal value of life expectancy for each sex is agreed upon.

In some countries where female survival is inferior or equal to that of males, sex ratios at birth provide another indication of gender inequity. Under normal circumstances, the male to female ratio at birth is expected to be 1.05 (105 males for every 100 females). In a number of countries, such as China, South Korea, and India, attention has been drawn to sex ratios that are significantly higher than the expected ratio of 1.05. These countries are facing a phenomenon of "missing" girls and women, reflecting differential treatment of women and men, and particularly of girls vis-à-vis boys (A. Sen, 1992b; Das Gupta, 1998). In China, gender discrimination against females before birth is particularly worrisome: 116.3 males (instead of an expected 105) were born for every 100 females in 1994 (State Statistical Bureau, 1995). This unusually high ratio arises from sex-selective abortions, informal adoption of girl babies and concealment or nonregistration of female birth, and female infanticide—reflecting both China's one child per family policy and the culturally rooted preference for sons (Dalsimer and Nisonoff, 1997.

Within countries, average differentials in survival between men and women may mask significant variation across specific causes of death. For example, despite greater overall survival probabilities, women in China (and perhaps in many other countries of South and Southeast Asia) have markedly higher death rates from suicide than men, contradicting the pervasive global trend of greater suicide mortality among males (World Health Organization, 2000).

Gender also interacts with occupational class and race to differentially influence survival. Between 1987 and 1991 British male life expectancy at birth in the upper two occupational classes was 75 years while for the lower two classes it was 70 years. For women, life expectancy at birth was considerably longer, and the differences between the occupational classes were narrower (80 years in the upper two occupational classes and 77 years in the lower occupational classes (Hattersley, 1997). In the United States in 1996, mean life expectancy for white women was 6 years longer than for black women, and white men lived an average of 8 years longer than black men (U.S. Department of Health and Human Services, 1993).

A third example suggests differences in male–female survival gaps according to level of wealth (Figure 4.4). Within a given country, as expected, nonpoor (rich) adult men have a significantly higher probability of dying between the ages of 15 and 59 years than do nonpoor (rich) women. Among the poor, beyond the markedly higher probability of deaths, we also observe that the female advantage in survival has virtually disappeared: from minimal female survival advantage in India and South Africa; to equal survival chances in Egypt, Niger, and Nicaragua; to a situation in which poor women have inferior survival in Sri Lanka, China, Poland, and the Czech Republic.

Although poor women and men in developing countries suffer primarily and disproportionately from infectious diseases, malnutrition, and lack of quality primary health care services, persistently high rates of maternal mortality in the developing world are symptomatic of more profound global gender inequities (see Figure 4.1). Of the 585,000 annual deaths among young women in pregnancy or childbirth, 99% occur in developing countries (World Health Organization, 1998c). In Africa the risk of dying is 1 in 16 pregnancies compared with 1 in 65 in Asia and 1 in 1400 in Europe (World Health Organization, 1998c). For the most part, maternal deaths are entirely preventable, yet remain unchecked due to lack of emergency health services for the poor and to historical neglect of women's broader reproductive health needs in developing countries. Such societal discrimination has restricted women's health issues to a narrow focus on the control of their fertility rather than on their rights to societal well being.

The social and economic costs of maternal mortality are enormous not only for the women themselves but also for their children's survival and well-being, their households, and society as a whole. When a mother dies or is disabled, household income for children's food, education, and health care is reduced. In

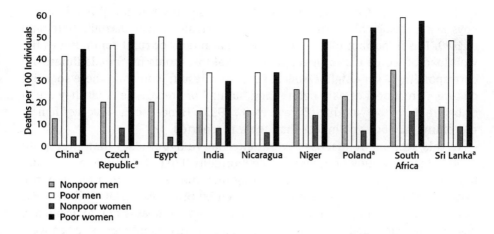

Figure 4.4. Probability of Dying Between the Ages of Fifteen and Fifty-Nine, by Poverty Status and Sex, in Selected Countries, c. 1990.

Source: World Health Organization, 1999b.

[a]Country in which poor women have higher mortality rates than men.

such circumstances, daughters are at particular risk in societies in which sons are more valued than girls. For example, in Bangladesh one study found that a mother's death sharply increased the chances that surviving children, predominantly girls, up to the age of 10 years would die within 2 years (World Health Organization, 1998b).

Morbidity

Because death is frequently preceded by illness, we might expect that those with higher mortality rates would similarly suffer from higher rates of morbidity. In other words, we might expect men, who are more likely to die prematurely, to be more affected by illness. Paradoxically, most research on gender differences in health shows higher rates of illness among women. Studies on morbidity, which are almost exclusively conducted in developed countries, indicate that women, more than men, perceive their health as worse and suffer greater disability. Thus, women's potential for greater longevity rarely results in them feeling healthier than men during their lifetimes. Furthermore, excess female morbidity can be observed in all socioeconomic groups, as illustrated in the Anglo-Swedish study (Diderichsen and others, 2001).

Although literature on morbidity in developing countries is scarce, several community surveys conducted in developing countries show similar patterns of higher female morbidity across the life cycle. A number of studies indicate that women are more likely than men to report feelings of anxiety and depression

(Paltiel, 1987). In China, a remarkably high disability rate for girls relative to boys under the age of 4 years is reflected in a female to male disability rate ratio of 1.89. It is important to note, however, that in poor or rural communities the workload of women is so heavy that societal thresholds for female illness are correspondingly very high (Okojie, 1994). As a result, women in these societies endure a great deal of pain before they "admit" or "recognize" that they are ill or before they stop working (Zurayk et al., 1993). Hence, actual levels of female morbidity may be even higher than what is reported.

In this section we discuss several alternative hypotheses that attempt to explain the patterning of excess female morbidity. First, the weaker association between mortality and morbidity among men may suggest that many of the excess deaths among men are not preceded by prolonged related illness. For example, deaths from external causes such as violent deaths due to accidents, suicide, homicide, and war, and perhaps some deaths from heart attack as well, often occur without a preceding period of illness (Hemström, 1998). Correspondingly, women's greater longevity in and of itself could be a cause of their higher rates of recorded morbidity. Longer life spans increase both biological and social risks associated with common disabling conditions among elderly women such as rheumatoid arthritis, osteoporosis, and Alzheimer's disease (World Health Organization, 1998a; Verbrugge, 1985). Even when controlling for differential life span, however, research has also found consistently poorer self-reported health for women in developing countries (Rahman et al., 1994).

Second, it has been hypothesized that women's reproductive ill health may account for their greater morbidity. In many parts of the world, pregnancy-related complications account for between 25% and 33% of all deaths of women of reproductive age and 18% of the global burden of disease for women of this age group (World Health Organization, 1996). The true range of morbidity actually suffered is hard to quantify, however, and is potentially much larger than what is currently measured. Many argue that maternal mortality figures only represent the tip of the iceberg—for every maternal death, there are over 100 acute morbidity episodes (Koblinsky et al., 1993).

Although women are more likely to suffer health problems connected to their reproductive functions, one should not conflate all women's health issues with reproduction. This is especially important given the historical antecedents of attributing many female health problems, including mental disorders, to gynecological dysfunction—so-called "globus hystericus" (Johannisson, 1995; Laqueur, 1994). A Dutch study has shown that 60% of women's health problems were unrelated to reproductive morbidity (Gijsbers van Wijk et al., 1995). Furthermore, women who do not report reproductive health problems still report worse health than men (Popay et al., 1993).

Third, cultural norms governing gender roles may determine the likelihood of reporting illness and therefore affect the apparent degree of morbidity differentials between the sexes. Some have interpreted excess female morbidity in developed countries as a sign that women may be more observant and more conscious of their bodies and consequently find it easier to report health problems and/or seek medical care. The traditional masculine ideal of remaining impervious to infirmities, on the other hand, may also contribute to gender differences in self-reported illness. Men may underreport morbidity, in keeping with their perceived gender roles (Sabo and Gordon, 1993). Thus it is hypothesized that women exaggerate real morbidity while men underreport it. The few studies in developed countries that compare reporting of morbidity with clinical examination, however, fail to support this hypothesis (Gijsbers van Wijk et al., 1995; Stenberg and Wall, 1995).

An important corollary to mortality studies that document greater female longevity is the assessment of female morbidity, as longevity does not seem to translate into greater health and well-being during women's lives. The multidimensionality of morbidity makes gender equity assessments in this area a thorny issue. None of the aforementioned hypotheses provides a wholly convincing explanation of higher female morbidity relative to men. From an equity perspective, this argues against a reliance on single measures of mortality or morbidity when comparing the ill health of women and men. Rather, on a case by case basis, the social and biological antecedents of specific gender inequalities in health must be assessed in order to make an equity judgment.

Health Care

Gender inequities are endemic in health care systems globally. In part, this reflects a lack of gender analysis in the planning and provision of health care systems. It also reflects more general gender inequalities in society that impact on the equitable utilization or consumption of health care. Here we describe some manifestations of these inequities in the planning, provision, and utilization of health care.

In many health care systems there is often insufficient attention to the differential needs of men and women in planning health services. As a result, health services for women often focus on only reproductive functions. The widespread priority of maternal child health has focused primarily on children to the relative neglect of the mothers. Important women's health issues, unrelated to their reproductive role, tend to be shortchanged (Paolissio and Leslie, 1995; Vlassoff, 1994). In Tanzania, the gender bias in adolescent health policies has led to a disproportionate focus on female reproductive health to the virtual exclusion of policies addressing both male adolescents and young women with nonreproductive health needs (Nantulya and others, 2001).

Gender inequality may also be manifest in the ways men and women are treated by the health care system. Mounting evidence suggests that male and female health providers may be gender biased in their perception of patient preferences and problems (Pittman and Hartigan, 1996). Patient–physician differences in age, class, sex, race, or ethnicity are found to accentuate gender bias in quality of care. Studies from rural communities in West Africa (Prevention of Maternal Mortality Network, 1992) and from Chile (Vera, 1993) have shown that women are not always treated with respect by health providers. In many societies women complain about lack of privacy, confidentiality, and information about treatment options (Vlassoff, 1994). Underpaid, overworked, and gender-insensitive health care workers will be unlikely to communicate with, examine, and prescribe appropriately for women (or men). Not surprisingly, women in some cultures prefer traditional providers (healers), who take the time to listen and explain ailments in easily understood terms. Given that many women are reluctant to be examined by male doctors, the lack of female medical personnel—itself a reflection of gender bias in educational opportunity—is an important barrier to utilization for many women (Zaidi, 1996).

Studies in the Netherlands, Sweden, and the United States highlight gender inequalities in the provision of certain technologies or treatment services for the same disease. Women with heart disease are less likely than men to receive coronary bypass surgery, and women are less likely to receive organ transplants such as kidney transplants (Kutner and Brogan, 1990; Held et al., 1988). In the case of lung cancer, it has been found that women are less likely than men to have cytological tests of sputum ordered by their doctors (Wells and Feinstein, 1988).

A wide variety of sociodemographic factors such as employment status and age interact with gender relations to generate inequalities in accessing health care (Puentes-Markides, 1992). Although health care services may be available, girls and women may be unable to access them due to discrimination within the household, granting preferential allocation of resources to male needs. Girls are likely to receive less expensive and more home-based care than boys (Lane and Inhorn, 1987) and also more likely to suffer from outright neglect of their health needs than boys (Chen et al., 1981; Das Gupta, 1987; Ahmed et al., 2000). In general, vulnerable sections of society, such as poor, illiterate, or less educated rural women, may not even be aware of their legal rights to adequate health care (Gijsbers van Wijk et al., 1996).

Clinical Research

Medical research and clinical trials for new drugs have been heavily criticized during the last decade for their general lack of a gender perspective (Freedman and Maine, 1993). Health problems that specifically or predominantly affect women have received less attention and funding than research on health problems mainly prevalent among men. The lack of research is obvious in areas concerning menstruation and nonlethal chronic diseases that affect women disproportionately, such as rheumatism, fibromyalgia, and chronic fatigue syndrome (Doyal, 1995). The only exception to this trend is contraceptive research, which has historically neglected male methods and focused on controlling fertility rather than on enhancing women's contraceptive and reproductive options.

In the field of occupational health and safety, women are overlooked in toxicological studies. Even when women are considered, their biological specificity is seldom noted. For example, the effects of occupational exposures on lactating women have received little study despite research results indicating the adverse health effects of their exposure to certain chemicals (Messing et al., 1993). This is a particularly important issue for women, as their greater level of body fat means that they store more fat-soluble toxic material even when exposed to the same levels as men (Sims and Butter, 2002).

An even more serious problem has been the exclusion of female subjects from study populations for medical and drug research. One rationale for excluding female subjects from research is that the menstrual cycle introduces a potentially confounding variable. Additional grounds for omitting women of childbearing age is the fear that experimental treatments or drugs may affect their fertility. Experimental use of treatment might, moreover, expose fetuses to unknown risk. Despite such concerns, the consequences for women of interpreting research results based on studies of male models and without convincing evidence of their applicability to women, continue to be harmful to women (Hammarström et al., 2001). Accumulating evidence shows that technology for diagnoses, treatment of diseases, and rehabilitation programs are not adapted to the specific characteristics and needs of women in general, let alone to women in various socioeconomic circumstances or cultural backgrounds.

Encouragingly, emerging research on gender differences in cardiovascular epidemiology has revealed the serious shortcomings of applying "male-based" diagnostic techniques and treatments to female patients (Gijsbers van Wijk et al., 1996). In part, this stems from increased recognition that symptoms of heart attack differ significantly between men and women (Loring and Powell, 1988). Of particular concern is recent evidence that life-threatening delays in diagnosis (via EKG) of women may occur because of lack of awareness of the unique nature of female symptomatology (Lerner and Kannel, 1986; Green and Raffin, 1993; Heston and Lewis, 1992).

There is an obvious need for further research to improve health care professionals' perception of, and response to, gender-specific needs and preferences. Greater gender sensitivity will minimize the risk of attitudinal biases in diagnostic and treatment decisions and help improve health outcomes. Formal medical education and training can be an excellent forum for sensitization to avoid gender bias by providers. Accordingly medical textbooks should reduce the stereotypic representation of the sexes (Mendelsohn et al., 1994). Apart from educational measures, funding guidelines, review boards, and the engagement of women's advocacy groups in research and policy also provide important institutional incentives for change.

POLICIES FOR ADDRESSING GENDER INEQUITIES

The recognition by policy makers that something can be done about gender inequalities in health has long been obscured by the strong biological and individualistic orientation of medical research. Analysis of socioeconomic, cultural, and environmental influences has consequently been overshadowed by genetic and biomedical models. The resulting view that the determinants of gender inequalities in health are mainly of genetic and biological origin has led policy makers and practitioners to pay insufficient attention to which of these inequalities are genuinely unchangeable and fixed and which are in fact quite amenable to change (Hammarström et al., 2001).

Today there is a growing recognition that the most powerful determinants of health for both women and men are to be found in social, economic, and cultural circumstances. These include, among other things, economic growth, income distribution, sanitation, housing, nutrition, consumption, work environment, employment, social and family structures, education, community influences, and individual behaviors (Blane et al., 1996). All of these circumstances differentially affect women and men due to the positions they occupy in society, the different roles they perform, and the variety of social and cultural expectations and constraints placed on them.

Health promotion, disease prevention, and rehabilitation have until now been recognized as largely the responsibility of those working in the health sector. Health, however, does not arise from actions solely by the health sector, but as the result of all public policies and how they individually, or in interaction with each other, promote or damage health. A narrow focus on the health sector alone obscures the socially constructed gender roles and expectations that may exacerbate health inequalities.

The multisectoral responsibility for creating sustainable health has recently been recognized by the World Health Organization policy document *Health 21: The Health for All Policy for the WHO European Region—21 Targets for the 21st Century* (1999a). The document emphasizes solidarity, equity, and gender sensitivity. It notes that "decision-makers in all sectors should take into consideration the benefits to be gained from investing for health in their particular sector and orient policies and actions accordingly." Furthermore, "Member States should have established mechanisms for health impact assessment and [ensure] that all sectors become accountable for the effects of their policies and actions on health." Accordingly, an evaluation of the health impacts of various policies on women or men occupying different positions in the social hierarchy is desirable.

In the following section we give examples of strategies that are important from a gender health equity perspective, ranging from macro to micro public policy levels. These strategies include interventions aimed at promoting gender equity in society in general and in health in particular by (1) ensuring a supportive macroeconomic and sectoral policy framework, (2) promoting gender equity in access to essential goods and services, and (3) reducing gender bias in communities and empowering women.

Gender and Macroeconomic Policies

Policies at the structural level include macroeconomic and social policies spanning sectors such as labor market, trade, environment, and more general efforts to improve women's status. Such major structural policies are seldom introduced for the specific purpose of filtering the health status of the population, but they all have great potential to reduce or exacerbate gender inequality, including inequalities in health (Whitehead, 1995).

Developing Countries. The dramatic declines in mortality observed in developing countries during the last 50 years are due in part to advances in public health measures and in part to policies at the macroeconomic level. The most important policies leading to improved life expectancy are those aimed at poverty reduction and increased spending on public health measures (Anand, 1996). Supportive macroeconomic and sectoral policies that increased income and educational levels allowed greater proportions of the population to obtain the prerequisites for good health—food, housing, clean water, and employment opportunities. Investments in schooling, particularly for girls, and policies that increased women's political and economic power have contributed to significant health improvements for women and for whole populations.

In Mauritius, the fertility rate of the population declined dramatically from 6.2 in 1963 to 3.2 in 1972. The rapid success is attributed to advances in girls' education, supportive policies that improved access to health and family planning services, and pension schemes providing for improved social security for all (Lutz et al., 1994). A striking feature of this change in Mauritius, as is also true for similar changes in Sri Lanka and the state of Kerala in India, is that it occurred in the absence of significant economic growth. Per capita income in Mauritius, for example, not only was relatively low but also actually fell during its period of rapid fertility decline in the 1960s before accelerating significantly during the subsequent decades. The ability of governments to retain and even strengthen supportive policies toward sectors such as health, education, and social security in an environment promoting gender equality made these advances possible (G. Sen, 1992).

Equity-oriented policies in a social context in which women had traditional matrilineal rights to property and girls were valued as much as boys have resulted in laudable health gains in Kerala, India. Although state policies in Kerala during the twentieth century were not particularly focused on reducing gender inequalities, because the social and cultural environment was not strongly biased against women, it was possible for women to benefit from improvements in health care provision and to achieve high levels of literacy. Not surprisingly,

Kerala is the only state in India where the population's sex ratio has been favorable to women throughout the twentieth century and is not plagued by the problem of "missing women."

Unfortunately there are many examples, particularly in the last two decades, of macroeconomic policies that have brought about increased gender inequalities in living conditions and health by worsening the position of women in absolute and/or relative terms. Many developing countries have, for example, introduced structural adjustment policies aimed at halting inflation, gaining economic efficiency, improving the balance of payments, promoting sustainable growth by switching resources to production of tradable goods and services, and allowing liberalization of imports. When, as in many cases, these policies have been implemented without adequate or effective safeguards for the social sectors, they have resulted in severe cuts in public expenditure on health, education, and other social programs. Privatization of many services including health care; tolerance of higher unemployment rates; promotion of more flexible and informal labor markets; removal of subsidies for food and other basic goods; and increased prices for drugs, foods, and health and educational services have been important parts of structural adjustment policy packages.

The impact of cuts in public expenditure tends to fall most heavily on the most disadvantaged sections of the population and especially on girls and women who have to shoulder the heaviest burden of poverty (Stewart, 1992; Whiteford, 1993). Econometric proof of causal associations between macroeconomic policies and health outcomes is quite challenging to obtain because of the complex web of associations inherent in such broad social and economic changes. The reallocation and cuts in public resources can, however, clearly lead to serious failures of access to health care, worsening of service delivery, and greater gender inequality as existing gender biases within communities and households interact with shrinking resource availability. A few examples below serve to illustrate the multidimensional impact of some macroeconomic policies on gender inequalities in developing countries.

Increased food prices and removal of food subsidies are major elements of adjustment programs at the macro level. These measures, together with declining earnings, translate into a steep fall in real household incomes and have a strong gender-differentiated impact on poor households (Stewart, 1992). Available evidence indicates that decreases in household incomes result in significant malnutrition in girls and women—especially pregnant and lactating women. Many countries, including Brazil, Barbados, and Jamaica, have reported increases in the proportion of low-birth-weight babies during periods of structural adjustment (Dias et al., 1986).

Price reform has also involved the introduction of user charges for health and educational services. In Nigeria, enrollment was reduced by one-third when fees for primary and secondary schools were introduced, while in Sri Lanka several schools were shut down. The introduction of user charges for health care in

Ghana was associated with lower attendance at clinics (Stewart, 1992). Similar results were also found in Zambia. Cuts in public expenditure on health, drugs and educational services hit women harder than men. When these services are in short supply or increase costs for households, girls more often than boys are taken out of schools and deprived of health services such as immunizations (McPake, 1993). Under the pressure of increased male unemployment and rising inflation, mothers are often forced to leave home in order to earn incomes. Girls are then withdrawn from school to care for younger siblings.

Evidence is just beginning to emerge from Southeast Asian countries on the health implications of the budget cuts and inflation following the late 1990s financial crisis. In Asia, International Monetary Fund–supported policies of budget deficit management without effective safeguards for social sector expenditures are, in part, blamed for the crisis. Relief organizations and nongovernmental organizations working at the community level report increasing incidences of hunger, school drop-outs, homelessness, and street children. Based on past experience it would not be farfetched to anticipate rising gender inequalities from these macro policies. Few countries in the South have been able to protect the social sectors adequately in the face of structural adjustment programs. More recently however, there have been calls for ensuring adequate resources for the social sectors through such measures as the 20–20 compact (the proposition that both governments and international aid donors should allocate 20% of their resources to social sectors) and taxes on financial transactions.

Industrialized Countries. In industrialized countries where evidence suggests that the magnitude of income differences is strongly linked to population health status (Wilkinson, 1996), policies at the structural level aimed at reducing poverty and social disadvantage are just as important from a public health perspective as in developing countries. The strong association between more inequitable income distribution and lower life expectancy suggests that economic policies that increase income inequalities can therefore be characterized as "unhealthy."

Examples of "healthy" economic policies, on the other hand, aim at compensating those who for different reasons (e.g., unemployment, early retirement, parental leave) experience loss of income (Dahlgren, 1997). High rates of universal family benefits are usually found to be linked to low rates of infant mortality (Wennemo, 1993). It is likely that "healthy" economic policies influence not only the overall health profile of a population but also the health status of the most disadvantaged sections of the populations, such as single parents, early retirees, and people with very low incomes, many of whom are women.

Sweden, for example, has focused on full employment by developing a parent-worker model through extensive public child care provision and family-friendly employment policies. With gender equity already a national goal, this full employment policy has led to increased job opportunities for women in the public sector. Expanded provision of social services not only directly enabled more women to find employment but also indirectly enabled other women to pursue careers in other sectors. A cohort study by Vågerö and Lahelma (1998) has followed up and compared the mortality of women who took advantage of these employment policies with that of women who did not. The findings show significantly greater decreases in mortality among those employed. Positive health selection could not alone account for this mortality differential. Other than improving the health of employed women, the provision of social services in Sweden has also mitigated the negative effects of poverty for more disadvantaged women. As a result, poor Swedish women are no more likely than women who are not poor to report fair or poor health.

Promoting Gender Equity in Access to Essential Goods and Services

Many developing countries continue to suffer from weak or deteriorating health services, infrastructures, and unaffordable services, a situation that disproportionately affects women. The inadequacy and lack of affordability of health services are compounded by physical and psychological barriers to care. At the national level, there have been some attempts to tackle the cost and affordability barriers to health services for women. For example, both South Africa and Sri Lanka provide free maternal and infant health services. Flat fee structures that cover not only regular antenatal and postnatal care but also delivery care, including complications, may be one way to ensure that cost barriers do not prevent families from bringing women in for such services, especially during obstetric emergencies (World Health Organization, 1998b). When health insurance schemes are introduced, care should be taken to ensure that poor women are adequately covered (Carrin and Politi, 1997).

Even such services as are available or affordable to the poor in general may still be out of the reach for girls and women. In some settings, this is a matter of distance or transport access, which may make it impossible for girls or women to visit health centers, particularly where gender taboos limit women's mobility. Upgrading local (village-level) health centers, setting up systems for reliable emergency transport, and making it possible for women and their attendants to stay near a health facility can help to bridge this gap (World Health Organization, 1998b). Such measures have yielded good results in countries such as Cuba, Sri Lanka, Uganda, and, in the Matlab project, in Bangladesh.

Poor quality in patient-provider interactions can also make women unwilling to use health services. There is now substantial evidence showing that improving the quality of care in reproductive health services can significantly increase women's willingness to use such services (Jain et al., 1992). This requires, among other measures, improvement in the attitudes of providers toward women clients through effective training and gender sensitization.

Particularly nefarious are the health systems that exacerbate health inequalities through lack of gender sensitivity. All too often health policy makers tend to view women primarily as "reproducers" and narrowly focus their attention on women in the reproductive ages. In 1994, the International Conference on Population and Development attempted to correct this bias by including actions to meet the health needs of girls, adolescents, and older women.

Perhaps the most comprehensive attempt to design a more holistic policy has been the Comprehensive Program for Women's Health Care, which was created in Brazil in 1983. This program includes a range of reproductive and sexual health services, as well as occupational and mental health services. It includes not only women in the reproductive ages but also postmenopausal women and preadolescents, and it emphasizes that women need access to both preventive and curative care as well as information about their bodies and health (Garcia-Moreno and Claro, 1994).

Another positive example of an integrated and gender-sensitive health policy is the "Health for Women, Women for Health" policy enunciated by the Ministry of Health in Colombia in 1992, which explicitly aims to reduce gender inequalities through a comprehensive approach. Its five programs include the promotion of self-help, reproductive health and sexuality, violence prevention and care for victims of violence, mental health, and occupational health. The policy document states explicitly that a "woman has the right to treatment and care from the health services as a whole being, with specific needs—according to her age, activity, social class, race, and place of origin, and not to be treated exclusively as a biological reproducer. She has the right to respectful and dignified treatment by health workers of her body, her fears, and her needs for intimacy and privacy" (Colombia Ministry of Health, 1992).

Thus, quality of care and attention to women's health needs throughout the life cycle are critical components in the health system—and as essential to ensuring utilization as physical access and affordability.

Reducing Gender Bias at the Community Level and Empowering Women

Promoting gender equality and equity also requires tackling gender biases in communities and households through community education, empowering women, and training boys and men to reduce gender biases by promoting gender-sensitive behavior and reducing violence. The International Conference on Population and Development initiated a broad-based policy discussion on this subject. There are also many examples from both developed and developing countries of person-based strategies aimed at strengthening individuals in disadvantaged positions (Whitehead, 1995). From a gender equity perspective, such strategies have focused mainly on strengthening women to better respond to, and control determinants of, health in the physical or social environment.

The most effective interventions have been those with an *empowerment* focus. They aim to help disadvantaged women to gain their rights, improve their access to essential facilities and services, address perceived deficiencies in their knowledge, acquire personal or social skills, and thereby improve their health (for more discussion of empowerment strategies, see Batliwala, 1994; G. Sen and Batliwala, 2000; Whitehead, 1995; Hashemi and Schuler, 1996).

Empowerment initiatives aim at encouraging both sexes to challenge gender stereotypes. One of these projects, described by Craft (1997b), is The Girl Child Project (see also International Planned Parenthood Federation, 1995), established by the Family Planning Association of Pakistan. The project raises awareness among young girls and their families about unfair and unnecessary discrimination against girls and thereby promotes the status and the value of the girl child. For example, according to the girls involved, the project made them aware that unequal food allocation in the family is wrong. In fact, just a few years ago, Pakistan was one of the countries where the female life expectancy was inferior to male life expectancy. By 1997, this situation had reversed (World Health Organization, 1998c), indicating a positive trend toward the greater gender equity in longevity.

In Bangladesh, one of the initiatives (BRAC) integrated into a poverty alleviation project focused on the empowerment of poor rural women by provision of women's microcredit and female education. Gender equity in health was improved considerably via increased economic independence and improved social status relative to men in both public and personal spheres (Bhuiya and Ansary, 1998). Positive changes were also reported in food allocation and educational attainment that led to decreasing male bias in a society where preference for sons is deeply rooted. The BRAC initiative, designed to increase gender equity, has also successfully contributed to the sharp decline in the socioeconomic gap in child mortality but has not significantly altered the gender gap in child mortality.

CONCLUSION

This chapter has explored the ways in which gender acts as an important determinant of health inequalities and inequity in both high- and low-income countries. The analysis of mortality, morbidity, health care, and clinical health research suggests that gender biases are important and pervasive stratifiers of health outcomes for women and men. These outcomes not only arise from sociocultural beliefs and behaviors but may be sustained and accentuated by policies that are insensitive to the multiple manifestations of gender bias.

The chapter has also provided a range of examples of more gender-sensitive approaches to policy at the macro, sectoral, community, and individual levels.

As stated at the outset, gender equity in health depends on fairness in the distribution of health-promoting resources, benefits, and responsibilities between girls and boys and women and men. It also requires policy assurance that men and women will be treated equally where they share common needs, as well as recognition that where their needs are different, these differences will be addressed in an equitable manner. The chapter illustrates that when policies are framed in this manner, they can go a fair way toward closing the health gaps between women and men.

References

Ahmed, S. M., and others. "Gender, Socioeconomic Development and Health-Seeking Behavior in Bangladesh." *Social Science and Medicine*, 2000, *51*, 361–372.

Anand, S. "Global Health Equity: Some Issues." Paper presented at the Workshop on Global Health Equity, Harvard Center for Population and Development Studies, Sept. 20, 1996.

Batliwala, S. "The Meaning of Women's Empowerment: New Concepts from Action." In G. Sen, A. Germain, and L. C. Chen (eds.), *Population Policies Reconsidered: Health, Empowerment, and Rights*. Cambridge, Mass.: Harvard University Press, 1994.

Bhuiya, A., and Ansary, S. "Status of Health and Health Equity in Bangladesh." Report prepared for the Global Health Equity Initiative (GHEI) meeting in Dhaka, Bangladesh, Dec. 11–17, 1998.

Blane, D., Brunner, E., and Wilkinson, R. G. (eds.). *Health and Social Organization: Toward a Health Policy for the 21st Century*. London: Routledge, 1996.

Carrin, G., and Politi, C. *Poverty and Health: An Overview of Basic Linkages and Public Policy Measures*. Geneva: Task Force on Health Economics, World Health Organization, 1997.

Chen, L.C., Huq, E., and D'Souza, S. "Sex Bias in the Family Allocation of Food and Health Care in Rural Bangladesh." *Population and Development Review*, 1981, *7*, 147–183.

Chen, M., and Drèze, J. "Widowhood and Well-Being in Rural North India." In M. Das Gupta, L. C. Chen, and T. N. Krishnan (eds.), *Women's Health in India: Risk and Vulnerability*. Delhi: Oxford University Press, 1995.

Colombia Ministry of Health. *Salud para las mujeres, mujeres para la salud* [Health for Women, Women for Health]. Bogotá: Colombia Ministry of Health, 1992.

Congdon, N., and others. "Exposure to Children and Risk of Active Trachoma in Tanzanian Women." *American Journal of Epidemiology*, 1993, *137*, 366–372.

Craft, N. "Life Span: Conception to Adolescence." *British Medical Journal*, 1997a, *315*, 1227–1230.

Craft, N. "Women's Health Is a Global Issue." *British Medical Journal*, 1997b, *315*, 1154–1157.

Dahlgren, G. "Strategies for Reducing Social Inequalities in Health: Visions and Reality." In E. Ollila, M. Koivusalo, and T. Partonen (eds.), *Equity in Health Through Public Policy.* Helsinki, Finland: STAKES, 1997.

Dalsimer, M., and Nisonoff, L. "Abuses Against Women and Girls Under the One-Child Family Plan of the People's Republic of China." In N. Visvanathan and others (eds.), *The Women, Gender and Development Reader.* London: Zed Books, 1997.

Das Gupta, M. "Selective Discrimination Against Female Children in Rural Punjab, India." *Population and Development Review,* 1987, *13,* 77–100.

Das Gupta, M. *"Missing Girls" in China, South Korea and India: Causes and Policy Implications.* Working Paper no. 98-03. Cambridge, Mass.: Harvard Center for Population and Development Studies, Harvard School of Public Health, 1998.

Dias, L. R., Camarano, R., and Lechtig, A. "Drought, Recession, and Prevalence of Low-Birthweight Babies in Poor Urban Populations of Northeastern Brazil." Letter to the editor. *Journal of Tropical Pediatrics,* 1986.

Diderichsen, F., Whitehead, M., Burström, Åberg, M, and Östlin, P. "Sweden and Britain: The Impact of Policy Context on Inequities in Health." In T, Evans, M. Whitehead, F. Diderichsen, A. Bhuiya, M. Wirth (eds.), *Challenging Inequities in Health: From Ethics to Action.* Oxford: Oxford University Press, 2001.

Doyal, L. *What Makes Women Sick? Gender and the Political Economy of Health.* London: Macmillan, 1995.

Freedman, L., and Maine, D. "Women's Mortality: A Legacy of Neglect." In M. Koblinsky, J. Timyan, and J. Gay (eds.), *The Health of Women: A Global Perspective.* Boulder, Colo.: Westview Press, 1993.

Garcia-Moreno, C., and Claro, A. "Challenges from the Women's Health Movement: Women's Rights Versus Population Control." In G. Sen, A. Germain, and L. C. Chen (eds.), *Population Policies Reconsidered: Health, Empowerment, and Rights.* Cambridge, Mass.: Harvard University Press, 1994.

Gijsbers van Wijk, C. M., van Vliet, K. P., and Kolk, A. M. "Gender Perspectives and Quality of Care: Toward Appropriate and Adequate Health Care for Women." *Social Science and Medicine,* 1996, *43,* 707–720.

Gijsbers van Wijk, C. M., and others. "Male and Female Health Problems in General Practice: The Differential Impact of Social Position and Social Roles." *Social Science and Medicine* 1995, *40,* 597–611.

Green, L. A., and Raffin, M. T. "Differences in Management of Suspected Myocardial Infarction in Men and Women." *Journal of Family Practice,* 1993, *36,* 389–393.

Hammarström, A., Härenstam, A., and Östlin, P. 2001. "Gender and Health: Concepts and Explanatory Models." In P. Östlin P. and others (eds.), *Gender Inequalities in Health: A Swedish Perspective.* Cambridge, Mass.: Harvard School of Public Health, 2001.

Hashemi, S. M., and Schuler, S. R. "Rural Credit Programs and Women's Empowerment in Bangladesh." *World Development,* 1996, *24,* 635–653.

Hattersley, L. "Expectation of Life by Social Class." In F. Drever and M. Whitehead (eds.), *Health Inequalities*. London: Stationery Office, 1997.

Heise, L., Pitanguy, J., and Germain, A. *Violence Against Women: The Hidden Health Burden*. Washington, D.C.: World Bank, 1994.

Held, P. J., and others. "Access to Kidney Transplantation: Has the United States Eliminated Income and Racial Differences?" *Archives of Internal Medicine*, 1988, *148*, 2594–2600.

Hemström, Ö. "Male Susceptibility and Female Emancipation: Studies on the Gender Difference in Mortality." Doctoral thesis, University of Stockholm, 1998.

Heston, T. F., and Lewis, L. M. "Gender Bias in the Evaluation and Management of Acute Nontraumatic Chest Pain." *Family Practice Research Journal*, 1992, *12*, 383–389.

Jain, A. K., Bruce, J., and Kumar, S. "Quality of Services, Program Efforts, and Fertility Reduction." In J. F. Phillips and J. A. Ross (eds.), *Family Planning Programs and Fertility*. Oxford: Clarendon Press, 1992.

Johannisson, K. *Den mörka kontinenten: Kvinnan, medicinen och fin-de-siècle* [*The Dark Continent: Woman, Medicine, and Fin-de-Siécle*]. Stockholm: Norstedt, 1995.

Koblinsky, M., Campbell, O., and Harlow, S. "Mother and More: A Broader Perspective on Women's Health." In M. Koblinsky, J. Timyan, and J. Gay (eds.), *The Health of Women: A Global Perspective*. Boulder, Colo.: Westview Press, 1993.

Krieger, N., and Zierler, S. "Accounting for the Health of Women." *Current Issues in Public Health*, 1995, *1*, 251–256.

Kutner, N. G., and Brogan, D. "Sex Stereotypes and Health Care: The Case of Treatment for Kidney Failure." *Sex Roles*, 1990, *24*, 279.

Lane, S. D., and Inhorn, M. "The 'Hierarchy of Resort' Examined: Status and Class Differentials as Determinants of Therapy for Eye Disease in the Egyptian Delta." *Urban Anthropology*, 1987, *16*, 151–182.

Laqueur, T. *Making Sex*. Cambridge, Mass.: Harvard University Press, 1994.

Lerner, D. J., and Kannel, W. B. "Patterns of Coronary Heart Disease Morbidity and Mortality in the Sexes: A 26-Year Follow-Up of the Framingham Population." *American Heart Journal*, 1986, *111*, 383–390.

Loring, M., and Powell, B. "Gender, Race, and DSM-III: A Study of the Objectivity of Psychiatric Diagnostic Behavior." *Journal of Health and Social Behavior*, 1988, *29*, 1–22.

Lutz, W., and others. *Population-Development-Environment: Understanding Their Interactions in Mauritius*. Berlin: Springer-Verlag, 1994.

McPake, B. "User Charges for Health Services in Developing Countries: A Review of the Economic Literature." *Social Science and Medicine*, 1993, *36*, 1397–1405.

Mendelsohn, K. D., and others. "Sex and Gender Bias in Anatomy and Physical Diagnosis Text Illustrations." *Journal of the American Medical Association*, 1994, *272*, 1267–1270.

Messing, K., Dumais, L., and Romito, P. "Prostitutes and Chimney Sweeps Both Have Problems: Toward Full Integration of Both Sexes in the Study of Occupational Health." *Social Science and Medicine,* 1993, *36,* 47–55.

Nantulya, V.M., Semakafu, A. M., Muli-Musiime, F., Massawe, A., and Munyetti, L. "Tanzania: Gaining Insights into Adolescent Lives and Livelihoods". In T, Evans, M. Whitehead, F. Diderichsen, A. Bhuiya, M. Wirth (eds.), *Challenging Inequities in Health: From Ethics to Action.* Oxford: Oxford University Press, 2001.

Okojie, C.E.E. "Gender Inequalities of Health in the Third World." *Social Science and Medicine,* 1994, *39,* 1237–1247.

Paltiel, F. "Women and Mental Health: A Post-Nairobi Perspective." *World Health Statistics Quarterly,* 1987, *40,* 233–266.

Paolissio, M., and Leslie, J. "Meeting the Changing Needs of Women in Developing Countries." *Social Science and Medicine,* 1995, *40,* 55–65.

Pittman, P., and Hartigan, P. "Gender Inequity: An Issue for Quality Assessment Researchers and Managers." *Health Care for Women International,* 1996, *17,* 469–486.

Popay, J., Bartley, M., and Owen, C. "Gender Inequalities in Health: Social Position, Affective Disorders, and Minor Physical Morbidity." *Social Science and Medicine,* 1993, *36,* 21–32.

Prevention of Maternal Mortality Network. "Barriers to Treatment of Obstetric Emergencies in Rural Communities of West Africa." *Studies in Family Planning,* 1992, *23,* 279–291.

Puentes-Markides, C. "Women and Access to Health Care." *Social Science and Medicine,* 1992, *35,* 619–626.

Rahman, O., and others. "Gender Differences in Adult Health: An International Comparison." *Gerontological Society of America,* 1994, *34,* 463–469.

Sabo, D., and Gordon, G. *Men's Health and Illness: Gender, Power and the Body.* London: Sage, 1993.

Santow, G. "Social Roles and Physical Health: The Case of Female Disadvantage in Poor Countries." *Social Science and Medicine,* 1995, *40,* 147–161.

Sen, A. K. *Inequality Reexamined.* Cambridge, Mass.: Harvard University Press, 1992a.

Sen, A. K. "Missing Women: Social Inequality Outweighs Women's Survival Advantage in Asia and North Africa." *British Medical Journal,* 1992b, *304,* 587–588.

Sen, G. "Social Needs and Public Accountability: The Case of Kerala." In M. Wuyts and others (eds.), *Development Policy and Public Action.* Oxford: Oxford University Press, 1992.

Sen, G., and Batliwala, S. "Empowering Women for Reproductive Rights." In H. Presser and G. Sen (eds.), *Women's Empowerment and Reproductive Rights: Moving Beyond Cairo.* Oxford: Oxford University Press, 2000.

Sen, G., George, A., and Östlin, P. "Engendering Health Equity: A Review of Research and Policy." In G. Sen, A. George, and P. Östlin (eds.), *Engendering International Health: The Challenge of Equity.* Cambridge, Mass.: MIT Press, 2002.

Sims, J., and Butter, M. "Health and Environment: Moving Beyond Conventional Paradigms". In G. Sen, A. George, and P. Östlin (eds.), *Engendering International Health: The Challenge of Equity.* Cambridge, Mass.: MIT Press, 2002.

State Statistical Bureau. *Social Statistical Information of China.* Beijing: State Statistical Publishing House, 1995.

Stenberg, B., and Wall, S. "Why Do Women Report 'Sick Building Symptoms' More Often Than Men?" *Social Science and Medicine,* 1995, *40,* 491–502.

Stewart, F. "Can Adjustment Programs Incorporate the Interests of Women?" In H. Asfhar and C. Dennis (eds.), *Women and Adjustment Policies in the Third World.* London: Macmillan, 1992.

United Nations Development Programme. *Human Development Report.* New York: Oxford University Press, 1999.

U.S. Department of Health and Human Services. *Health in the United States, 1992.* Hyattsville, Md.: U.S. Department of Health and Human Services, 1993.

Vågerö, D., and Lahelma, E. "Women, Work, and Mortality: An Analysis of Female Labor Participation." In K. Orth-Gomér, M. A. Chesney, and N. K. Wenger (eds.), *Women, Stress, and Heart Disease.* Mahwah, N.J.: Erlbaum, 1998.

Vera, H. "The Client's View of High-Quality Care in Santiago, Chile." *Studies in Family Planning,* 1993, *24*(1): 40-49.

Verbrugge, L. M. "Gender and Health: An Update on Hypotheses and Evidence." *Journal of Health and Social Behavior,* 1985, *26,* 156–182.

Vlassoff, C. "Gender Inequalities in Health in the Third World: Uncharted Ground." *Social Science and Medicine,* 1994, *39,* 1249–1259.

Waldron, I. "Sex Differences in Human Mortality: The Role of Genetic Factors." *Social Science and Medicine,* 1983, *17,* 321–333.

Wells, C. K., and Feinstein, A. R. "Detection Bias in Diagnostic Pursuit of Lung Cancer." *American Journal of Epidemiology,* 1988, *128,* 1016–1026.

Wennemo, I. "Infant Mortality, Public Policy, and Inequality: A Comparison of 18 Industrialized Countries." *Sociology of Health and Illness,* 1993, *15,* 429–446.

West, S. K., and others. "Epidemiology of Ocular Chlamydial Infection in a Trachoma-Hyperendemic Area." *Journal of Infectious Diseases,* 1991a, *163,* 752–756.

West, S. K., and others. "The Epidemiology of Trachoma in Central Tanzania." *International Journal of Epidemiology,* 1991b, *20,* 1088–1092.

Whiteford, L. "Child and Maternal Health and International Economic Policies." *Social Science and Medicine,* 1993, *37,* 1391–1400.

Whitehead, M. "Tackling Inequalities: A Review of Policy Initiatives." In M. Benzeval, K. Judge, and M. Whitehead (eds.), *Tackling Inequalities in Health. An Agenda for Action.* London: King's Fund, 1995.

Wilkinson, R. G. *Unhealthy Societies. The Afflictions of Inequality.* London: Routledge, 1996.

World Health Organization. *Safe Motherhood Progress Report, 1993–1995.* Geneva: World Health Organization, 1996.

World Health Organization. *Female Genital Mutilation: A Joint WHO/UNICEF/UNFPA Statement.* Geneva: World Health Organization, 1997.

World Health Organization. *Gender and Health: Technical Paper.* Geneva: World Health Organization, 1998a.

World Health Organization. *Report of the Technical Consultation on Safe Motherhood* [held in Sri Lanka, Oct. 19–23, 1997]. Geneva: World Health Organization, 1998b.

World Health Organization. *World Health Report, 1998: Life in the 21st Century— A Vision for All.* Geneva: World Health Organization, 1998c.

World Health Organization. *Health 21: The Health for All Policy for the WHO European Region—21 Targets for the 21st Century.* Copenhagen: World Health Organization Regional Office for Europe, 1999a.

World Health Organization. *World Health Report, 1999.* Geneva: World Health Organization, 1999b.

World Health Organization. *World Health Report, 2000.* Geneva: World Health Organization, 2000.

Zaidi, A. S. "Gender Perspectives and Quality of Care in Underdeveloped Countries: Disease, Gender, and Contextuality." *Social Science and Medicine,* 1996, *43,* 721–730.

Zurayk, H., and others. "Concepts and Measures of Reproductive Morbidity." *Health Transition Review,* 1993, *3,* 17–40.

CHAPTER FIVE

Getting a Grip on the Global Economy

*Health Outcomes and the Decoding
of Development Discourse*

John Gershman
Alec Irwin
Aaron Shakow

*I sometimes wonder whether there is any way
of making poverty terribly infectious. If that were to happen,
its general elimination would be, I am certain, remarkably rapid.*
—Amartya Sen

Poverty, inequality, and patterns of economic change directly and indirectly shape health policy and health outcomes. This chapter investigates the issues at stake on the economic side of these relationships, in order to understand how economic forces and institutions affect health in vulnerable communities. Although the precise relationship between poverty and ill health has been debated in industrial North America and Europe since the early eighteenth century, this chapter takes the causal link between poverty and unfavorable health outcomes as a given.[1] Our purpose is to examine institutions, policy measures, and development strategies that exacerbate poverty, thereby rendering the poor more vulnerable to ill health.[2]

Our examination of selected concepts, institutions, and historical trends will be helpful in understanding how the health of poor communities is affected by processes such as privatization, trade liberalization, and deregulation, as well as by actors such as transnational corporations (TNCs), international financial institutions, and non-governmental institutions. We explore historical factors, including the legacy of colonialism and sociopolitical dynamics within countries. At the same time, we question the accuracy and appropriateness of the indicators usually used to evaluate economic progress and calculate the benefits of globalization.

Since the end of the Second World War, economic development, conflated with economic growth, has often been heralded as the necessary and sufficient solution to poverty. Critical tools are necessary for assessing this claim and the ideological assumptions on which it rests. Today, while some critics question long-dominant economic paradigms (see, for example, Stiglitz, 2002), *growth* remains for many economists and noneconomists a word charged with almost magical power. We aim to challenge the belief that ensuring strong economic growth is the primary requirement for combating poverty and inequality and thereby improving health status.

Recently, international development organizations have begun to acknowledge that growth must follow particular patterns if it is to benefit the poor. This realization itself, however, raises new problems. If the pattern of growth is important, what kind of pattern is required? Will beneficial patterns emerge naturally, through the action of intrinsic market mechanisms, or will they have to be created by sustained political effort? Who would stand to gain from such effort, and whose interests might be threatened? How do our assumptions about the benefits of economic growth square with the economic history of the past several decades? What effects are processes of economic globalization likely to have on poverty and inequality in the years ahead? This chapter provides a framework for exploring such questions critically.

Economic growth is not irrelevant to struggles against poverty. Yet we argue that growth, as such, is an insufficient objective; alternative ways of evaluating development are required. Our claim is that concrete effects on the health and well-being of the poor provide criteria for analyzing and judging the value of development efforts.

We begin by examining some basic concepts associated with poverty, health, and development in order to arrive at a clearer sense of the scope and nature of poverty. We then examine the history of poverty and development in the post–World War II era, focusing on such crucial episodes as the "debt crisis" of the 1980s and the subsequent period of "structural adjustment." We explore the implications of the new relationships emerging at this time between poor countries and the international financial institutions that took the lead in responding to a global financial crisis. Finally, we survey selected aspects of the current international economic landscape, seeking to discern traits that will be especially pertinent to ongoing debates on economic policy, poverty, growth, and health.

POVERTY AND THE PANACEA OF GROWTH

To deplore the magnitude of human suffering caused by poverty is a familiar ritual for public figures. Moreover, in recent years, a consensus has emerged among many economists, political leaders, and businesspeople about the most effective way to combat this scourge. They argue that poverty can be significantly reduced only through the long-term benefits of sustained economic growth. Inequalities within and between countries, including egregious disparities in health outcomes, will diminish as more countries enter and become competitive in the market-driven global economy. Therefore, all who are committed to fighting poverty, narrowing inequality, and improving global health must make growth, economic globalization, and modernization their priorities.

However, as we try to bring the relations between poverty, inequality, economic growth, and health into focus, this conventional wisdom seems problematic. It may be, in part, because the exact meanings of the key terms remain elusive. What do sweeping terms like *poverty* and *global inequality* actually refer to? First, some quantitative measures:

- An estimated 2.8 billion people today survive on the equivalent of under $2 a day, 1.2 billion on less than $1 a day.[3] Well over a billion people (about a fifth of the world's population) lack access to safe water. Every day, some 840 million people go hungry (United Nations Development Programme [UNDP], 1997).

- At the end of 2002, fifteen million people in southern Africa faced the threat of imminent starvation. Yet while international media tended to portray the famine as an abrupt catastrophe, in reality the disaster perpetuated a long-standing pattern. Through the 1990s, millions of people in southern Africa suffered severe malnourishment. In 1991, the chronic malnutrition (stunting) rate of children aged six months to five years in Zambia, for example, already stood at 39 percent. By 2002, the rate had reached 55 percent (Patel and Delwiche, 2002). Since 1990, immunization rates for children in sub-Saharan Africa have dropped below 50 percent (UNDP, 2002).

- The number of poor people worldwide between 1970 and 1985 increased by 17 percent—even as total global production rose by 40 percent. Two hundred million people saw their income fall during the period 1965–1980; during 1980–1993, this fate befell more than a *billion* people (UNDP, 1996). Between 1990 and 2000, as U.S. stock markets soared to unprecedented heights, fifty-two countries, including twenty in sub-Saharan Africa, experienced not growth but shrinkage of their national economies (UNDP, 2000).

- According to the United Nations Development Programme, a girl born in Japan in 2002 may have a 50 percent chance of living to see the twenty-second century. A child born in Afghanistan at the same moment has a one-in-four chance of dying before reaching age five. Every day, more than thirty thousand children worldwide, the vast majority in developing regions, die of preventable diseases (UNDP, 2002).

- The deadliest infectious diseases, including HIV/AIDS, tuberculosis, and malaria, are overwhelmingly concentrated in the world's poorer regions. Poverty raises people's risk of exposure to infections and constrains their ability to obtain treatment when they fall ill. At the end of 2002, of forty-two million men, women, and children estimated to be infected with HIV/AIDS worldwide, 95 percent lived in developing countries. In sub-Saharan Africa, only 1 percent of people in acute need of AIDS treatment with antiretroviral medicines (ARVs) could obtain access to ARV therapy (International HIV Treatment Access Coalition, 2002).

- In 1960, the poorest 20 percent of the world's people received only 2.3 percent of global income. By 1991, their share had shrunk to 1.4 percent. At the end of the 1990s, the poorest 20 percent of people in the world were receiving only 1.1 percent of global income (UNDP, 1997). The economic boom of the 1990s propelled inequalities in global wealth and income to new levels. As that decade closed, according to the UNDP, the world's 225 richest individuals enjoyed a combined wealth of over $1 trillion, equal to the annual income of the poorest 47 percent of the world's population (2.5 billion people). The three richest people on the planet possessed assets that exceeded the combined gross domestic product (GDP) of the forty-eight least developed countries. Meanwhile, in about one hundred countries, incomes at the end of this period of vaunted economic growth were lower in real terms than they had been a decade or more earlier. In seventy countries with a combined population of a billion people, consumption at the end of the recent boom was lower than it had been twenty-five years before (UNDP, 1998).

  What do such figures and descriptions reveal? First, they remind us that *poverty kills.* The World Health Organization (WHO) underscores that poverty signifies brutal suffering and premature death for those in its grasp. Poverty is the "main reason why babies are not vaccinated, clean water and sanitation not provided, and curative drugs and other treatments [remain] unavailable." Around the world, poverty is the chief cause "of reduced life expectancy, of handicap and disability, and of starvation" (WHO, 1995). Furthermore, it is a major contributor to mental illness, stress, suicide, family disintegration, and substance abuse (Desjarlais and others, 1995).

These figures reveal, too, that *poverty and inequality are worsening* today in many parts of the world, despite decades of efforts to stimulate economic growth and despite strong economic figures in countries like the United States during the 1990s. Even in regions where robust economic performance sustained itself for years or decades, the anticipated benefits of growth have failed to materialize for many people.

Finally, implicit in these quantitative indicators are issues of *power*. In distributing wealth, economic structures both assign and respond to power. Within these structures, certain interests are privileged over others, and resources are distributed for the benefit of some groups and at other groups' expense. Decisions of a political nature determine, for example, whether a poor nation's limited resources will be used to construct local health clinics or to purchase new weapons for the military. The political dimension emerges again when poor countries slash funding for social services in order to make payments on staggering foreign debts—and again when U.S. health corporations reap record profits while increasing numbers of American citizens find themselves unable to afford basic health insurance. The relationship between health and the economy cannot be separated from questions of power—who wields it, how, and to what ends.

Many discussions of poverty rely on numerical measures and cast poverty itself as a quantitative phenomenon. People are categorized as poor if their income falls below a certain numerical threshold, calculated as a function of their country's economic indicators—the poverty line. Conservative estimates based on such calculations show poverty to be a condition that characterizes the lives of over one billion people—well more than three times the total population of the United States (UNDP, 1997).

The quantitative character of poverty statistics implies objectivity where objectivity may not exist. For example, the income level at which a poverty line is set can be quite arbitrary; thresholds vary widely from one part of the world to another, and their configuration inevitably reflects political interests. Poverty is a value-laden concept with a heavy historical subtext; even its measurement is fraught with moral and ideological difficulties. Small wonder that economists remain deeply divided on the questions of how best to define poverty and calculate its effects. Clearly, we need quantitative information to help us grasp specific aspects of poverty. Yet a sound analysis strives to connect numerical data with social and political dimensions of poor people's experience that numbers may not adequately capture.

Our understanding of poverty must pay attention not only to the lack of basic economic resources (including money and food) but also to how material deprivation leads to poor health and to the lack of social resources, including access to education and health care. Over the years, many theorists have emphasized the inadequacy of trying to grasp poverty simply by means of income statistics. Some scholars have tried to examine the causes and consequences of poverty and well-being by using a variety of alternative frameworks based, for example, on concepts of social exclusion and human capabilities (Sen, 1993). Nobel laureate in economics Amartya Sen has argued that poverty and wealth must be conceived in relation to "human capabilities": people's capacity to pursue a diverse range of desirable activities, meet their self-defined goals, and lead the sorts of lives they consider valuable. For Sen, human beings must be seen not merely as "recipients of income," but as "people attempting to live satisfactory lives" (Sen, 1995, p. 17; see also Sen, 1992, ch. 6–7).[4] Tables of income statistics fail to capture the "texture" of people's lives and aspirations and at the same time mask distinctions fundamental for those confronting the lived reality of poverty. For example, poverty definitions based on household incomes say nothing about uneven income distribution within a household, which leads to an "invisible" poverty affecting mostly women and children. Likewise, most quantitative measures cannot "account for the 'double jeopardy' experienced by minority groups in which poverty is created by or exacerbated by discrimination, overt or covert" (Spencer, 1996, p. 4).

The analyses developed by economists like Sen suggest that eliminating poverty would require not just increasing GDP but also changing the distribution of economic output, economic resources, and social services so as to nurture human capacities more equitably. Such changes in distribution will demand a shift in political power in favor of the poor. The need to modify the balance of political power in order to combat poverty is not apparent if one thinks that simply raising per capita GDP or lifting a society's standard of living in broad terms will eliminate poverty. But making a bigger aggregate pie does not guarantee that disadvantaged communities or individuals will receive more adequate portions. Addressing global hunger exemplifies these difficulties and underscores the need to consider not just the existence of resources in a society but the mechanisms that distribute those resources. Merely increasing food production and containing population growth cannot eliminate hunger (Nikiforuk, 1993; Giblin, 1992). Historical studies of famine demonstrate that ending hunger requires addressing entrenched forms of structural inequality, transforming the political and economic conditions that prevent millions from having *access* to food or from owning their own land to grow it (Sen, 1985; Lappe, 1978).

In trying to arrive at a more accurate understanding of poverty, theorists have developed statistical tools such as the United Nations Development Programme's Human Development Index (HDI).[5] The HDI goes beyond traditional definitions of poverty by including variables such as life expectancy and educational attainment that reflect the satisfaction of a range of basic human needs, rather than simply income or consumption figures. These more sophisticated analytical frameworks also focus attention on issues of political power—for example, the extent of grassroots organizing in poor communities—and on questions about the role of public policy in poverty reduction.

Since the 1940s and the emergence of development economics as a distinct field, producing expert knowledge about poverty has been a profitable enterprise. Prominent institutions such as the World Bank owe much of their perceived importance to their role in addressing world poverty. Indeed, "attacking poverty" is now one of the World Bank's central stated policy objectives (World Bank, 2000). The vital question, of course, is whether the World Bank's policies and programs and those of similar institutions actually contribute to helping substantial numbers of people escape the disempowerment and multiple forms of vulnerability poverty imposes.

GROWTH AS A MIRACLE DRUG

The solution to poverty routinely proffered by leading economic analysts in the world's most powerful nations over the past half-century is disarmingly simple: *development,* defined primarily in terms of *economic growth.*[6] The consensus concerning these notions among influential thinkers—even those whose political, social, and philosophical views are otherwise sharply opposed—has been little short of miraculous. At the root of this consensus lies the belief that growth and development are virtually interchangeable. This tendency takes hold not only in the minds of analysts and policymakers but also among the general public. The belief that economic growth automatically translates into greater prosperity and a better life for all persists even when this assumption is contradicted by experience in a country like the United States, where relatively robust economic growth through the 1990s went hand in hand with a palpable erosion of the quality of life for many citizens.[7]

Poverty and Inequality

The nature and effects of poverty are closely associated with income inequality, itself often closely related to other social disparities. The conventional measure of income inequality is the *Gini coefficient.* The coefficient is a number between zero and one, where zero represents perfect income equality (all people have equal incomes) and one represents perfect inequality (all income is received by one person).

Explaining disparities in wealth and income requires examining factors like geography, gender, race, and ethnicity. For example, an estimated 70 percent of people living in absolute poverty today are women, while in the Americas indigenous communities suffer disproportionately (Buvinic, Gwin, and Bates, 1996; Çagatay, Elson, and Grown, 1995; Sparr, 1994).

The concept of *vulnerability* (or *insecurity*), as distinguished from the concept of poverty, helps us analyze the exposure of particular social groups to external risks, shocks, and stresses, and assess their capacity to respond to these challenges. Subsistence farmers who diversify their crop selection, for example, may be poor without being vulnerable. If, by contrast, they enter the market by selling high-risk export crops, their income may rise, but their vulnerability may also increase. As with vulnerability to economic fluctuation, vulnerability to disease both reflects the severity of poverty and contributes to its perpetuation. Examining vulnerability can highlight structural and institutional factors that are important in understanding the effects on poverty and inequality of different health policies and of particular patterns of growth.

Some recent analyses of poverty focus on the concept of social exclusion, the "process through which individuals or groups are wholly or partially excluded from full participation in the society in which they live" (de Haan and Maxwell, 1998, p. 2).[8] Social exclusion further expands the measurement and analysis of poverty.

Analysts' decisions about which economic and social indicators to use carry important consequences. Specific indicators can clarify some dynamics and processes while obscuring others. We need to pay close attention to the indicators different sources select in evaluating the claims made for or against particular development policies.

Stimulating and maintaining economic growth is widely understood as the primary objective of national and international economic policy and as the surest way to reduce poverty in local communities and around the world. Growth is desirable because it enables the community to consume more private goods and services, and it contributes to the provision of a greater quantity of social goods and services (health, education, and so on) (*HarperCollins,* 1991).

Indeed, many analysts view growth as the key indicator of a country's economic success. Conventionally, growth is measured by the annual percentage change in a given country's real (inflation-corrected) gross domestic product (GDP). Gross domestic product is similar to but distinct from gross national product (GNP). GDP measures the value of all goods and services produced within a country, regardless of the nationality of the producers. In contrast, GNP is the value of the total output of goods and services generated by a country's citizens, whether they reside in that country or abroad. Thus, for example, GNP does not include the value of goods and services produced by foreign workers living on a country's soil.[9]

Wealthy countries consider an annual GDP growth rate of between 3 and 4 percent to be healthy. Under optimal conditions, poorer economies should be showing a more rapid rate of expansion, on the order of 5 to 7 percent annually. Economic policies are considered successful if they contribute to GDP growth and often judged unsuccessful if they diminish GDP growth rates, regardless of what other goods they may provide. In this view, economic growth benefits all segments of the population, even the poorest, to whom increased wealth will gradually "trickle down" in a variety of forms.

This model involves significant problems. GDP growth figures provide a convenient scorecard on which to base judgments about a country's economic health. However, the tendency to focus exclusively on growth figures subtly shifts our perspective from growth as a means of enhancing human lives to economic growth as an end in itself. Meanwhile, trends in the United States and other regions during the 1990s confirmed that strong economic growth can occur simultaneously with significant increases in the level of inequality. The "long-term" future in which the gains of growth will seep down to reach the poor continues to be deferred. The World Bank's own data from almost two decades of structural adjustment programs (SAPs) imposed on developing countries suggest that growth-oriented SAPs worsen inequality in many cases (World Bank, 1995a, 1995b; 1996; Ravallion, 1997).

Furthermore, critiques from the environmental movement challenge the notion of unlimited growth and endless productive expansion as the normative framework for our thinking about the world economy. Since the 1970s, many economists and natural scientists have underscored the material constraints on economic expansion. Policies that push growth at all costs can lead to the depletion of nonrenewable resources and cause serious environmental degradation (Meadows and others, 1972). Such concerns have led to efforts to formulate a "sustainable" world development program, as well as to calls for a more equitable redistribution of resources between rich and poor countries. "Sustainable development," however, remains unproven as an effective tenet of economic policy. Moreover, proponents of sustainable development, on the one hand, and advocates of short-term action to reduce poor people's suffering, on the other, may at times find themselves opposed on particular political issues, requiring difficult forms of negotiation as they attempt to reconcile their agendas.

Per capita GDP can be an important predictor of health and life quality in a country. A very strong relationship appears to exist between per capita GDP and certain crucial health indicators, such as life expectancy and infant mortality. However, GDP per capita, as an average indicator, tells us nothing about the distribution of wealth or income, that is, whether the benefits of growth are shared widely among the population or are restricted to a narrow elite (see, for example, Halstead and Cobb, 1996). Growth must be consciously crafted and shaped for a pro-poor impact. "In too many countries, growth has failed to reduce poverty, either because growth has been slow or stagnant *or because its quality and structure have been insufficiently pro-poor*" (UNDP, 1997, p. 71; emphasis added).

Growth *can* benefit the poor. Yet there is no *guarantee* that growth in GDP per capita will translate into improvements in income for the poorest and most vulnerable groups in society. Still less automatic "are the links between economic growth and reduction in other aspects of human poverty—such as illiteracy, a short lifespan, ill health, lack of personal security" (UNDP, 1997, p. 72). UNDP researchers have correctly stressed that "distribution, government policies and public provision" decisively affect the translation of a given level of consumption and growth into effective poverty reduction.

Unfortunately, GDP growth today remains the most commonly used indicator of progress toward the reduction of poverty and of the overall economic health of a society. For decades, this theory has been used inappropriately to legitimate growth-oriented economic policies in the United States and elsewhere. Understanding where and why growth fails to fulfill the promises made about its beneficial effects involves attention not only to GDP but to the *pattern* of growth as it expresses itself in human experience at various economic levels. This pattern influences and is influenced by social conditions and government policies, including commitment to health as a fundamental political imperative. Significant factors influencing the way growth circulates through the complex structures of a society include initial asset distributions (land, human capital, natural resources, and the like), the redistributive nature of government programs, and the extent to which growth is more labor- or capital-intensive.[10] Therefore, to discern patterns and their consequences correctly, we must consider equality (or inequality) of asset ownership, the success or failure of government services in reaching the poor, and measures of the extent to which growth is labor-intensive, since labor power is typically the poor's most significant asset.

HISTORICAL PERSPECTIVES ON GROWTH: THE "GOLDEN AGE" AND BEYOND

If economic growth is actually a relatively unreliable indicator of improvement in life quality for poor people, how did growth become so widely accepted as the royal road to reducing poverty? A brief review of the history of development economics will help explain how an uncritical ideology of growth came to occupy a dominant position in contemporary economic theory and political discourse.

Development Discourse in the Golden Age

Early writing on development economics as a field of its own coincided with the post–World War II era and the identification of the majority of the world as "underdeveloped."[11] The fundamental assumption linking the ideologically heterogeneous writings produced in this early phase of development was a version of the "rising tide" principle. Following the classical economists, most development economists viewed the accumulation of physical capital (if it embodied technical progress) as leading quasi-automatically to a reduction in poverty.[12] As technical progress and the accumulation of physical capital generated an expansion of economic activity, economic growth would ipso facto create greater wealth, which would eventually be distributed through market interactions to all segments of the population. As this process unfolded, "developing" nations would pass through socioeconomic and demographic transitions, some of which might be painful in the short term but would eventually yield greater wealth and higher quality of life for all.

During the period of rapid expansion of the world economy between 1945 and the mid-1970s (referred to broadly as the "Golden Age"), industrialized economies grew at almost 5 percent annually, nearly double the industrialized countries' long-term historical rate. The Golden Age brought prosperity to many citizens of established industrial powers and increased wealth dramatically, even in certain parts of the world where economic modernization was more recent.

Three key international institutions emerged during the Golden Age and have continued to play a pivotal role in the world economy: the International Monetary Fund (IMF), the World Bank, and the General Agreement on Tariffs and Trade (GATT), this last of which gave birth to the World Trade Organization (WTO) in 1994.[13] The original mission of the IMF, conceived in the aftermath of the Great Depression, was to constitute a permanent international body capable of coordinated action to prevent or contain economic crises like those that marked the 1930s. The IMF strove to eliminate trade restrictions and the destructive economic policies, such as competitive currency devaluations, that had paralyzed investment and trade in the 1930s (see International Monetary Fund, 2002). Maintaining a clear, fair exchange rate structure, the IMF would facilitate the conversion of currencies and smooth the way for orderly international commerce. The World Bank's first purpose was to aid in the reconstruction of economies devastated by the Second World War, primarily those of Western European countries and Japan. Rapidly, however, the World Bank began providing development loans to poor countries (George and Sabelli, 1994). The GATT was an integrated set of trade agreements aimed at the reduction of tariffs and other barriers to trade. Signed in 1947 by twenty-three countries, the GATT, originally intended as an interim arrangement, sustained itself through several decades as an effective instrument for trade liberalization in manufactured goods.

The overarching objective associated with the IMF, the World Bank, and the GATT was to shape and then maintain a system that encourages free trade at the international level, combined with restrictions on capital mobility and a domestic social contract sufficient to maintain relative peace between labor and capital (Helleiner, 1994). The purpose of the reconstructed global economy was to nurture growth in the underdeveloped world while protecting the interests of the dominant capitalist powers.

The relation of economic development to social equality or inequality concerned some development economists. They assumed that growth in low-income countries would necessarily be inequitable at first and that economic disparities would probably have to increase initially while the process of growth was launched and gathered momentum.[14] Calling this model into question, most recent research suggests that greater initial *equality,* not inequality, is beneficial for growth itself. Initial equality also enhances the degree to which GDP growth enables poverty reduction (UNDF, 1997). These findings demonstrate the extent to which government policies—as opposed to some "natural" process of economic development or an intrinsic law of market forces—play a key role in shaping the interaction of growth, poverty, and inequality.

The 1978 Alma Ata declaration promised "Health for All by the Year 2000" as a reward for pressing forward with development.[15] By 1978, however, the Golden Age of (relative) prosperity for both rich and poor countries was over. The oil crisis of 1973 is often seen as symbolically marking the conclusion of the era of rapid expansion and economic optimism.[16] Since then, the GDP growth rates for the twenty-nine wealthy countries that constitute the Organization for Economic Cooperation and Development (OECD) and the rates for the world as a whole have been nearly halved.[17]

Three decisive developments marked the conclusion of the Golden Age: the decline in growth rates in the OECD countries and "stagflation" (high levels of both inflation and unemployment) in the United States in the 1970s; the election of rhetorically antistatist governments in Great Britain (Thatcher), the United States (Reagan), and Germany (Kohl); and in the early 1980s, the debt crisis.[18] The debt crisis and its aftermath reshaped the global economic landscape and redefined relationships between developing countries and the major international financial institutions. The lasting effects of the crisis have played an important role in configuring the power dynamics of the new era of globalization and economic restructuring.

Crisis and Adjustment

The *debt crisis* refers to the panic generated in international financial and political circles from the mid-1970s to the mid-1980s, when a substantial number of heavily indebted Third World nations appeared unable to continue making payments on their debts to commercial banks in wealthy countries. Fears arose that the looming default of debtor countries, toppling the banks, might produce a collapse of the global financial system. This collapse was averted by the energetic intervention of wealthy countries, acting through the World Bank and the IMF. These institutions took center stage in the resolution (or perhaps more accurately, the effective displacement) of the crisis. "Solving" the debt crisis involved imposing structural adjustment programs on the economies of debtor countries, thus allowing them to "return to growth" and, most important, to continue making interest payments on their foreign loans.[19]

Before exploring the consequences of structural adjustment schemes and in particular their effects on health outcomes among the poor, a brief consideration of the historical roots of the debt crisis will refute the all-too-common assumption among some economists and politicians that the crisis was primarily the result of mismanagement and corruption in poorer countries. The economic problems of heavily indebted poor countries reached crisis proportions under the combined impact of three principal factors:

- *Changes in the international economy.* The oil price increases spurred by OPEC in and after 1973 created new pressures for foreign exchange among oil-importing countries worldwide. Interest rates skyrocketed after 1979 with the shift in monetary policy by the U.S. Federal Reserve, increasing the cost of developing countries' loans. As these pressures combined with the recession and declining commodity prices of the early 1980s, developing countries were squeezed by higher debt payments, smaller markets for their exports, and reduced inflows of foreign loans.

- *Expanded bank lending.* The enormous revenues generated by OPEC countries required a mechanism to circulate the capital. The OPEC monies joined a larger, growing supply of dollars not deposited in U.S. banks but held by financial institutions in other parts of the world. This capital was available to fund foreign investment. Third World governments, in need of foreign exchange to promote industrialization in the face of declining demand in the developed countries, were prime clients for these so-called petrodollars.[20]

- *Development strategies in crisis.* Many poorer countries had pursued development strategies that relied heavily on state intervention in the economy to promote industrialization through mechanisms like state-owned corporations, subsidies to urban consumers, and restrictions on foreign trade and investment. These strategies had led to significant growth and industrialization in some parts of the Third World. Yet where industries never became internationally competitive, countries were unable to earn foreign exchange by exporting their goods overseas. The combination of three factors—small domestic markets for industrial goods, increased foreign exchange demands for oil and petroleum-related imports, and increasing pressure from the poor and middle classes for greater redistribution of the benefits of economic growth—led, in the 1970s, to challenges to these political regimes. Governments responded primarily through increased borrowing from abroad.

Worldwide, initial responses to the debt crisis were based on the then-prevalent belief that the crisis was merely a short-term problem of liquidity (see, for example, Cline, 1983). Yet it soon became clear that the damaged economies were not rebounding, nor was foreign capital flowing back into developing countries. The World Bank and IMF, pushed by their most powerful shareholders—the United States, Britain, and Germany—intervened more dramatically to address the crisis. A consensus emerged among policymakers in the development institutions and their backer governments: what was required was a radical restructuring of Third World economies.

The policy objectives of this restructuring were linked to ideological changes among leading rich-country governments and among some Third World, particularly Latin American, technocrats and elites. Their prescription for poorer countries, as previously noted, became known as structural adjustment or more broadly as neoliberalism (see Williamson, 1990, 1996; see also Chapter Fourteen of this volume).

Neoliberal thinkers believe that the state plays too great a role in the economy, inhibiting markets and firms from operating in a manner that would raise overall welfare.[21] Misguided state intervention that prevented markets from acting efficiently explained why countries were and remained poor. Even when market mechanisms failed, neoliberal economists opposed government intervention because the direct and indirect costs of governmental action would almost inevitably outweigh its benefits. The state's legitimate role in the economy was limited to protecting property rights, enforcing contracts, and (in some cases) investing in human capital (see Bauer, 1972, 1981, 1984; Toye 1993).

The Mechanics of Adjustment

The debt crisis required an explanation, and neoliberal economics provided one: excessive state intervention had bred uncompetitive, inefficient industries sheltered behind protectionist walls, and state interference had distorted markets and prices. The answer was an "adjustment" of poor countries' fundamental economic structures and strategies.

The first step in treating the ailing debtor economy was stabilization, in order to reduce inflation and even out the country's balance of payments. Such goals could, in theory, be achieved by reducing demand for goods and services in the economy (for example, by cutting government spending or lowering wages). These methods focused on a quick reduction in effective demand. The free market's own self-regulating mechanisms would come into play, subsequent to stabilization providing the cure for previous distortions, understood to have been largely the result of state interference.

The structural adjustment prescription was (and is) usually seen as embracing three interrelated aims and processes (Woodward, 1992):

- To reduce the role of the state relative to the market in the economy

- To enhance economic efficiency by allowing prices to be determined by market forces, such as exchange rates, interest rates, and real wages

- To integrate the national economy into the world economy by lifting barriers to trade and investment.[22]

Did structural adjustment address the debt crisis and its consequences? Clearly, adjustment worked very well to manage one dimension of the crisis: ensuring repayment of debts to lending institutions in wealthy countries.[23] But SAPs did little to reduce debts, cut poverty, or enable robust economic growth in the majority of countries where such programs have been implemented (see Schoepf, Schoepf, and Millen, 2000).

Although the debt crisis is now often discussed in the past tense, its destructive effects persist in many regions. Poor countries' debt problems continue to exact a cruel toll in deteriorating life quality, massive physical and psychological suffering, and squandered human potential, as urgently needed social investment in health, nutrition, education, and basic social services becomes subordinate to debt service. The food crisis unfolding in southern Africa in 2002 provided a cruel illustration (see Pettifor, 2002). Two decades after the debt crisis began, halting steps toward debt reduction for the poorest, most heavily indebted countries began to be seen.[24] Yet progress has been agonizingly slow. The Heavily Indebted Poor Countries (HIPC) Initiative, launched in 1996, aimed to reduce the debt burdens of the forty-one poorest heavily indebted countries (thirty-three in Africa, four in Asia, and four in Latin America.[25] The HIPC program has brought some significant successes; evidence shows that debt reduction has enabled some countries to increase their levels of investment in health, education, and other vital social sectors (Greenhill and Blackmore, 2002). Yet debt relief under the HIPC plan has thus far failed to address the full dimensions of the crisis. Critics argue that IMF-imposed conditions make it difficult for countries to progress through the program and that even when countries successfully complete the initiative, many continue to face unsustainable debt burdens (Clark, Vanderslice, and Joyner, 2002).

The Many Faces of Structural Adjustment

The structural adjustment paradigm rapidly encountered criticism from relatively early on, both outside and within development institutions. In 1987, analysts associated with UNICEF published the first major critique of adjustment, titled *Adjustment with a Human Face* (Cornia, Jolly, and Stewart, 1987). UNICEF's analysis focused on how the poor, in particular women and children, bear a disproportionate share of the costs of adjustment. The study stressed the need to incorporate compensatory programs for those negatively affected by economic change (Gibbon, 1992). *Adjustment with a Human Face* inaugurated a series of efforts to weigh the gains and losses of the SAP model, an undertaking that continues to the present day (See Chossudovsky, 1997; Danaher, 1994; Global Exchange, 2001; Stiglitz, 2002).

Isolating the specific impact of structural adjustment programs on poverty is difficult. One way of approaching the issue is to bracket temporarily some of our own critical questions and grant the general premise that encouraging economic growth is one important component of a realistic poverty reduction program. We can then consider how adjustment affects growth.

Public investment is a key determinant of growth. Virtually all studies agree that a correlation exists between structural adjustment and declining public investment (see, for example, Conway, 1994). This is important because investment priorities are directly related to future growth. Public investment funds social infrastructure and other needs that are unlikely to be adequately addressed by the private sector: for example, sanitation, drinking water, schools, and health clinics. Clearly, not all public investment is inherently and necessarily beneficial. Governments have bankrolled notorious development disasters like large dams that have uprooted communities and wrought environmental havoc (see Schoepf, Schoepf, and Millen, 2000). Yet adequate, properly managed public investment is vital to a society's long-term viability and to the well-being of its citizens, particularly the poor.

Unsurprisingly, IMF programs are associated with a significant decline in public investment (Bird, 1996; Edwards, 1989; Khan, 1990; Killick, Malik, and Manuel, 1992; Conway, 1994). If an IMF program aims to strengthen the balance of payments in the short term by reducing aggregate demand relative to supply, then the brunt of the change will fall on domestic expenditure, of which public investment is a significant component. It is politically easier for a government facing pressure to reduce spending to cut back on building new roads or new sanitation systems—or to reduce maintenance on existing facilities—than to cut other types of direct consumption expenditures. Falling public investment undermines the prospects for future growth. This produces a destructive contradiction, since finding ways to increase their rate of economic growth is a major reason countries seek IMF assistance in the first place (see Bird, 1996).

The World Bank (1990b) itself notes that "when structural adjustment issues came to the fore, little attention was paid to the effects on the poor" (p. 103). The injury to the poor has come in two main forms: lower incomes and declining access to quality social services. Poverty increased in both absolute and relative terms over the 1980s in Africa, Latin America, and the Caribbean.

The distributional impact of adjustment within a country depends significantly on the extent of initial equality of asset ownership. In rural areas, for example, if land ownership is highly concentrated, the benefits of adjustment will flow to the landed elite (Lele, 1990; Bourguignon and Morrisson, 1992). Adjustment has its most significant effect through its impact on employment, which is almost "invariably negative in the short run" (Killick, 1995b, p. 314). Under "stabilization" programs in Latin America, observers have noted a "strong and consistent pattern of reduction of labor share in income" (Pastor, 1987), which continued through 1990s (see Economic Commission, 1997).

Growth rebounded in Latin America in the late 1990s, yet neither its level nor its pattern was sufficient to alter severe inequalities or reduce the number of poor. The Inter-American Development Bank (1997) concedes, in a gross understatement, that "the relatively well-off groups of Latin American society appear to have benefited from the recovery of the 1990s somewhat more than the poorest classes" (p. 18).[26] In Africa, home to twenty-five of the thirty-two countries classified by the World Bank as severely indebted low-income countries, the situation is even bleaker.[27]

In sum, the poor often suffered in the period of economic crisis immediately prior to the adjustment program and suffered even more severely as adjustment proceeded and access to publicly funded social services dwindled. However, some countries, such as Costa Rica and Malaysia, were able to successfully combine adjustment with committing higher shares of government expenditure to the social sectors. This more positive outcome was largely a function of political factors. In some cases, policymakers committed themselves to poverty alleviation, whether for reasons of conviction or to purchase political stability. In some countries, groups of poor people organized to voice demands and effectively advance their interests (Mehrotra and Jolly, 1987; Watkins, 1998; Ribe and others, 1990; World Bank, 1990a; Shapiro and Taylor, 1990).

A number of reviews describing the economic situation in Latin America in the 1980s suggest that the distribution of the costs of adjustment was not determined by immutable laws of economics. Rather, the distribution was significantly shaped by the equality or inequality of asset distribution, the extent and strength of social safety nets prior to the crisis, the nature of the political regime (democratic or authoritarian), and the relative political power exercised by unions, business, and other groups (Birdsall and Londoño, 1997; Inter-American Development Bank, 1997; Killick, 1995a, 1995b; Londoño and Székely, 1997; Lustig, 1995; Pastor, 1987; Taylor, 1993; Vivian, 1995). The existence of these differences suggests that the negative effects of adjustment on the poor were not inevitable. Political forces influence the extent to which the costs of adjustment were borne disproportionately by the disadvantaged. Simply striving to improve the internal mechanisms of an adjustment program is insufficient. Moreover, focusing on technical minutiae may distract attention from the broader political and economic structures that decisively configure growth, poverty, and inequality—and thus policy strategies' impact on health.

The 1990s and Beyond: A New Poverty Agenda

The debates over the costs of adjustment and the decadelong decline of many economies in Africa and Latin America in the 1980s pushed poverty back onto the international agenda. In its 1990 *World Development Report,* the World Bank announced a shift toward "poverty reduction" as its overarching objective and described a three-pronged strategy to attain this goal: labor-intensive growth, investing in the poor via the development of human capital (mainly in health and education), and the promotion of safety nets and targeted social programs. The regional development banks quickly followed the World Bank's lead in presenting their own poverty reduction agendas.

Several general trends distinguished the 1990s climate from the earlier era of "defensive modernization," during which the Bank had sought to "give people a stake, however minimal, in the system" (Ayres, 1983, p. 226) primarily to undercut demands for more radical types of political change. In the World Bank's new stance on poverty, still evolving in the early 2000s, more attention is given to direct targeting of resources to the poor and underserved, as opposed to a belief that growth will automatically trickle down to benefit the poor (Gershman and Fox, 1996; Lipton and Maxwell, 1992). The Bank focuses on providing public goods that benefit poor people, rather than emphasizing, for example, agricultural development per se, since elite groups often captured the credit and other input subsidies provided under earlier integrated rural development programs. Bank analysts are therefore now expected to examine the composition of public spending with an eye toward the effects of social spending on the poor. Analysts now ask, for example, whether health spending targets the poor or the urban elite and if resources for education fund primary schools in poor regions or college education for the urban middle class. The Poverty Reduction Strategy approach, officially adopted at the 1999 annual meetings of the World Bank and the IMF, further advanced this agenda, with an emphasis on national "ownership" of programs and broad-based civil society participation in setting antipoverty agendas (see World Bank, 2003).

Despite these positive developments, the World Bank's approach continued to exhibit significant problems through the 1990s. A 1996 World Bank report called *Taking Action for Poverty Reduction in Sub-Saharan Africa* found that in reality few projects provided for adequate monitoring and evaluation of their effects on the poor communities. *Taking Action*'s review of ninety-six investment and adjustment projects approved by the World Bank in fiscal 1992–1994 found that less than a third included pro-poor components (World Bank, 1996). The World Bank clearly has some way to go in developing approaches to policy lending that genuinely reduce poverty by promoting equitable patterns of growth.

The Bank's 1990s poverty agenda involved increased recognition of the importance of investing in human capital (health and education), based on the principle that efficient and equitable delivery of social services (particularly primary education and basic health care) can actually contribute to economic growth as well as to promoting equity (Birdsall and James, 1990; Angell and Graham, 1995). In this new framework, World Bank policies affect the health of the poor in at least three dimensions: via economic policies shaped by the Bank's structural and sectoral adjustment loans, through lending targeted specifically to the health sector, and by means of the Bank's role in promoting particular kinds of health care policies, represented most clearly in the publication of *Investing in Health,* the Bank's highly influential 1993 World Development Report.[28] The appearance of this study marked, according to Buse and Gwin (1998), "a shift in leadership on international health from the World Health Organization to the World Bank" (p. 666).

In the *Investing in Health* era, the Bank increased its lending and research output to the health sector as part of its antipoverty agenda. World Bank lending in the population, health, and nutrition sectors increased in absolute terms from an annual average of $103 million in the 1981–1984 period to $1.3 billion in the fiscal 1991–1994 period and $1.8 billion in fiscal years 1995–1997. Health advocates applauded *Investing in Health* for its emphasis on primary care but criticized its promotion of market-oriented health care systems (including managed care), its reluctance to identify the weaknesses of such systems, and its emphasis on cost recovery.

The World Bank's policy dialogue with borrowing countries has at least as great an impact on health policy as specific World Bank–sponsored projects. In the 1980s, Bank-approved adjustment programs focused on cutting government expenditures while giving little attention to the impact that such cuts would have on the poor. In the 1990s, the Bank's policy recommendations, outlined in *Investing in Health,* included shifting public health expenditures from tertiary to primary care; developing more targeted interventions, such as micronutrient programs and early childhood interventions; decentralization; and the use of "cost recovery" mechanisms like user fees.

The World Bank has played an important role in the debate over shifting health policy from public to private financing. In 1987, *Financing Health Services in Developing Countries: An Agenda for Reform* directly challenged the idea of free, universally available health care: "The . . . common approach to health care in developing countries has been to treat it as a right of citizenry and to attempt to provide free services for everyone. This approach does not usually work. It prevents the government health system from collecting revenues that many patients are both able and willing to pay." In line with this stance, typical components of adjustment programs have been reductions in government spending and the introduction of user fees for social services such as health care. The World Bank has recognized that health measures such as the control of communicable diseases and public health education are basic public goods that will likely be undersupplied by the market. Yet despite this recognition of the market's failure to guarantee health care, the Bank still promotes market-driven policies such as cost recovery.

A key component of the World Bank's 1990s antipoverty agenda was the targeting of social services and safety nets, using two distinct but related approaches.[29] One was expenditure shifting within social service programs like health and education to services most likely to be used by the poor. This meant, for example, shifting the education budget away from university education to primary schools and moving health care funds from urban hospitals toward rural primary care. The second type of targeting consisted in developing specific programs for the poor, either through reform of an existing general subsidy or the adoption of a new program.

A number of problems confront programs that shift from universal provision to "targeted" benefits. One is the increased administrative cost associated with a targeted program; another is the impact of reduced political support for targeted programs. The political argument around targeting is the more important consideration. Universal programs tend to have greater popular support (see Ahmad, 1993).

Our survey of poverty reduction efforts in the 1990s and at the dawn of the new millennium shows a mixture of positive intentions and inconclusive, sometimes negative results. At a minimum, enormous challenges remain. Amid the current global instability, gaps and uncertainties have emerged in what was the conventional wisdom of the 1980s and 1990s. These provide some new (albeit modest) opportunities to bring new questions, issues, and voices into the development debate.

Redistribution and Politics: Restoring the Missing Links

Several analysts have argued that adding safety nets and social funds long after economic adjustment has begun does not make a new antipoverty agenda. Without a sustained effort to redistribute economic resources among the members of society, antipoverty interventions will be piecemeal, fragile, and often ineffectual (Lipton, 1985). The missing link in both the World Bank's changing poverty agenda and in UNICEF's *Adjustment with a Human Face* (Cornia, Jolly, and Stewart, 1987) is redistribution on grounds of both social justice and economic efficiency. Economist Michael Lipton (1996) suggests that the "constriction of the ability of the poor to operate in the marketplace may help explain why the unprecedented decline in world poverty from 1945–80 appears to have stopped and not to have resumed, though growth has. . . . Though set up as caricature enemies, redistributive and market reforms need each other if they are to accelerate growth or help the poor" (p. 73).[30] Birdsall and Londoño (1997) note that while the new World Bank poverty agenda has belatedly identified social spending as a key element of a pro-poor growth agenda, "World Bank and other development economists have neglected . . . a second key determinant of poverty reduction and aggregate growth: the distribution of assets," including both physical assets and human capital. "More concern earlier with the causes and the consequences of income inequality would have called greater attention to a fundamental constraint on poverty reduction: the poor's lack of access to the assets necessary for increased productivity and income" (p. 36).

While it is simplistic to assign all blame for the negative effects of structural adjustment programs and their successors to the international financial institutions, it is equally apparent that the concrete operations and policy analyses of institutions like the World Bank need to support pro-poor patterns of growth and development instead of allowing the health of various markets routinely to take unquestioned priority over the health and lives of poor people.

Past and Present

Our survey of some major episodes in recent economic history—in particular the debt crisis and its aftermath—yields important lessons. The first are flaws in theories that argued that strong growth, at least in its initial phases, requires (and will probably exacerbate) socioeconomic inequalities. Second, reviewing the history of structural adjustment programs shows that the disproportionately destructive effects of these programs on poor communities were not inevitable but were often the result of political choices. The World Bank itself, recognizing grave flaws in its earlier approach, has more recently articulated an antipoverty framework that represents a theoretical step forward from previous policies, though a considerable gap still separates theory from practice. However, even in theory, the Bank's modified strategies leave much to be desired in terms of their capacity to protect the health of the poor. To prevent the poor from bearing a disproportionate share of the social costs of economic restructuring, current discussions of market reform and growth must reintroduce the theme of redistribution as the "missing link.

Perhaps most important, the economic principles many of us tend to regard as self-evident and in some sense "natural" are the products of a specific history. Neither the notion of a free market nor the thesis that economic growth will sooner or later benefit all members of a society is natural. But pointing out the historical roots of these notions does not mean we think they are irrelevant to current realities. On the contrary, these historically embedded ideas continue to shape the present and, surely, will exert a powerful influence on our collective future.

We now consider the economic "new world order" emerging under the impact of a relatively broad consensus whose watchwords include *globalization, free markets,* and *competitiveness.* We examine some of the main architectural features of the global economy with an eye to their implications for the health of the poor.

GLOBALIZATION AND THE NOT SO NEW WORLD ORDER

Although global economic patterns have been developing since at least the sixteenth century, the concept of "globalization" is now increasingly deployed in the United States and Europe both as a description and an explanation of contemporary social phenomena. In the United States, for example, the debate about globalization fuses with discussions of job loss and of the growth in trade and trade agreements (such as the North American Free Trade Agreement). Worries over imports from developing countries as well as "runaway" firms seeking tax and pollution havens abroad have coincided with growing domestic inequality and falling real wages since the late 1970s, generating a new level of public concern about globalization and its consequences.

This concern is not unreasonable, although it would be a serious mistake to blame trade per se for America's social ills. Many of these problems have their roots in an economy that gives primacy to the goal of economic growth over the assurance that workers and ordinary citizens can meet their basic human needs, policies that enable and even encourage corporations to abandon local communities to go where the largest profit can be made, tax structures favorable to corporations, the lack of social policies such as job retraining to protect laid-off workers, and the promotion of labor-displacing technologies. In the early 2000s, the United States, despite its wealth and its status as the largest economy in the world, has poverty rates and inequalities of both wealth and income that are among the highest of all established market economies (see United for a Fair Economy, 2002). Not coincidentally, the United States also exhibits egregious disparities in basic health indicators such as life expectancy and infant mortality rates, and approximately 43 million Americans are unprotected by health insurance of any kind—including 24.1 percent of those with annual household incomes of under $25,000 (Sklar, Mykyta, and Wefald, 2001, p. 122).

We cannot analyze the intricacies of the global economy here, but we can touch on a few crucial aspects of global capitalism: the growth of "free" trade, the role of transnational corporations, and expanding and accelerated capital flows mingling with the impacts of privatization. These trends are endorsed as the route to success and, eventually, an improved life for all in the new world economy. The idolatry of growth has broadened to include globalization as a companion deity.

Trade, Free and Otherwise

A cornerstone of the emerging global economic order is understood to be free trade: the unhindered movement of capital, goods, and services in an increasingly open worldwide marketplace. Yet "free" trade and the global triumph of market freedom are not without ambiguities. Though theoretically at liberty to roam the globe, most trade today remains concentrated among the rich OECD countries, above all the member states of the European Union, the United States, and Japan. Moreover, a significant amount of "trade" (estimates range from 30 to 40 percent) actually consists of transactions within the same transnational firm.[31]

It is difficult to determine whether expansion in world trade has benefited developing countries because the differential impact of trade on wealthy and poorer countries reflects, in part, differences in what the respective traders bring to the market. While most wealthy countries export manufactured goods and services, many developing countries rely most heavily on the export of primary commodities like unprocessed agricultural products, minerals, oil, wood, or fish. A higher proportion of exports composed of manufactured goods is associated with higher growth. Developing countries in which manufactured exports made up at least 50 percent of total exports grew four times as fast as countries that were predominately commodity exporters. Today, developing countries as a group account for about 25 percent of world exports in manufactured goods, compared to 5 percent in the early 1970s. However, three-quarters of this growth in manufacturing for export is accounted for by East Asia. Although primary commodities are of diminishing significance in world trade flows, some countries remain heavily dependent on them (see Overseas Development Institute, 1995; Coote and Lequesne, 1996).

The growth in world trade and investment has generated a search for new ways to govern "free" economic exchange. It may seem contradictory to suggest that increasing free trade requires increased regulation. Yet this paradox is at the heart of the contemporary global economy. "Free trade" actually involves a particular way of *managing* trade. It is a misrepresentation to say that free trade demands only deregulation. "Free" trade and "free" markets require extensive sets of regulations: recognition of patents, copyrights, and other intellectual property rights; the ability to enforce contracts; and so forth. Given the importance of TNCs in world trade, it is moreover not surprising that so-called free trade agreements include numerous provisions reflecting the interests of corporations concerned, above all, to maximize their own profitability. Harvard economist Robert Lawrence (1996) notes that such agreements are "motivated by the desire to facilitate international investment and the operations of multinational firms as much as to promote trade" (p. 17).

Freedom is a sacred term in American society. "Free markets" and "free trade" strike us intuitively as desirable things: a free market has to be better than the alternative, and open, unfettered trade must be the optimal condition for flourishing economic activity. Speeches endorsing the new global economic order almost invariably connect the promised advantages of globalization with the idea of greater freedom.

In implementing the North American Free Trade Agreement (NAFTA) in 1988, U.S., Canadian, and Mexican officials underscored their "long-term goal . . . to remove barriers to trade worldwide." NAFTA, claimed those who drafted it, sought to "reinforce free-market reforms" and "stimulate cross-border economic activity" among the partner countries (Epping, 1995, pp. 82–83). This aim sounds legitimate. But this variety of "freedom" refers to markets maintained by complex international legislation and commercial agreements and substantially dominated by the demands of transnational corporations. Under these circumstances, freedom can describe only partially the nature of economic activity. More precisely, *freedom* becomes a code word for a particular way of managing market interactions.

Our intuitive idea that a free market would be one in which firms and individuals engaged in fair, open exchange with no outside interference (above all from states) does not correspond to the realities of international trade or to the way in which wealthy countries have developed and prospered historically. Free trade requires a complex network of legislation and framing agreements (for instance, to govern the enforcement of patents and copyrights). Moreover, trade itself and individual firms involved in it benefit substantially from "state interference" in the form of publicly funded infrastructure projects (such as transportation and communications networks) and government financing of costly research and development programs. The development of the American computer industry from the 1950s onward represents one of the most spectacular examples of this pattern, more the rule than the exception among modern high-tech industries (Chomsky, 1996).

These considerations are important for evaluating current economic policy recommendations from supporters of "free market reforms." Through institutions such as the World Trade Organization and the IMF, wealthy countries are today urging poorer countries to adopt free market principles, opening their economies to unconstrained foreign investment and foreign competition. In theory, the laws of the open market will push people and firms in the newly opened economies to seek their "comparative advantage." People, firms, and countries would focus their productive efforts on the raw materials, goods, or services they can generate most cheaply. They will use these products to trade for items that cannot be produced locally in an efficient manner. In this way, market forces will lead the developing economy to be more streamlined and rational.

Convincing as the free market theory may appear, it does *not* reflect the pattern by which wealthy countries' industries developed and were able to achieve power and preeminence. Countries such as the United States and Japan made substantial and systematic use of protectionist or anti–free market devices (high import tariffs and other barriers to free trade) during the periods in which their fledgling industries were beginning to mature but still remained vulnerable to foreign competition. The pattern of free market rhetoric combined with restrictive protectionist practices continued in the American case through the Reagan era of the 1980s and has flourished anew since 2001 with the Bush administration's domestic agricultural subsidies and tariffs on imported steel.

The role of transnational corporations in promoting free trade agreements reflects their growing power within the global economy as a whole. Governments' role in providing tax breaks and other incentives to TNCs (such as bans on union organizing or strikes) illustrates how the logic of competitiveness, or of "creating a good investment climate" to promote growth, may work against the well-being of workers and citizens. Rising global investment coupled with declining health indicators demands reexamination of the prevalent assumption that increased levels of corporate investment in developing countries' economies will naturally bring improvements in life quality to these countries' disadvantaged and vulnerable citizens.

Finance Capital and Globalization

While many of the contemporary debates on globalization focus on free trade agreements like NAFTA and on the growth of foreign direct investment by TNCs, the most dramatic globalization of economic activity has been in the movement of finance capital. Traders shift currency, bonds, and stocks via digital networks twenty-four hours a day. At first glance, the activities of high-rolling international financial speculators seem unrelated to the struggles of poor people who lack adequate food, shelter, and health care. Yet as far apart as their respective worlds may seem, international traders exert an increasingly direct influence over the lives of the poor. Indeed, the increasing vulnerability of poor communities to shocks and fluctuations emanating from the world of global finance is a key trait of the global economy.

The speed, ubiquity, and sheer volume of international financial transactions in portfolio investments (stocks and bonds) have exploded in the past thirty years. This accelerates the impact of the contagious panics intrinsic to deregulated capital markets. Investors can easily move billions of dollars in or out of countries, thereby undermining the stability of national economies and placing entire governments at the mercy of individuals in quest of short-term profits (Kindleberger, 2000). Poor-country governments operating in such an uncertain economic environment therefore have an increasingly difficult time making the kinds of long-term budgetary commitments necessary for real improvements in health and welfare.

Portfolio investment in the so-called emerging markets of the developing world increased significantly in the early 1990s. The volatility of that investment has been implicated in a series of recent economic crises: in Mexico and Latin America in 1994–1995 and again in 1998, in Asia in 1997–1998, and in Russia in 1998.[32] The historically unprecedented growth of stock markets in developing countries in the past twenty years has been shaped by external financial liberalization (sometimes as part of sectoral or structural adjustment programs) and inflows of portfolio capital (sometimes linked to the privatization of public enterprises).

In contrast to the image of growing democratization of corporate capitalism, control over capital is in some respects becoming increasingly centralized (Harmes, 1998; Koppes, 1999). This means that decisions about where capital will flow are often determined by people far from the places where the consequences of these choices will be felt most acutely. This tendency complicates the challenge of shaping capital investment to obtain pro-poor patterns of growth.

In recent years, the IMF has been preparing to amend its charter to adopt a liberalization of capital controls. This is a radical departure from the original Bretton Woods vision of promoting free trade while restricting the mobility of capital. There is a real need for a fundamental debate over the international financial regime that has emerged since the 1970s. A number of proposals have been advanced, including Nobel laureate James Tobin's idea for a tax on currency transactions (see Ul Haq, Kaul, and Grunberg, 1996). In any event, as political scientist Robert Wade (1998b) suggests, "We should keep at the forefront of discussion the . . . abundance of historical evidence that free international capital markets are prone to excesses that inflict huge social costs" (p. 23; see also Bhagwati, 1998; Rodrik, 1998; Stiglitz, 1998; Wade, 1998a).

People's lives have been directly and brutally affected by the transformations associated with development strategies founded on the unreflective pursuit of economic globalization and the unrestricted electronic mobility of capital. The manipulation of money has consequences for the health and indeed the very survival of vulnerable individuals, families, and communities. Responsible economic analysis must systematically interrelate quantitative data and the "laws" of the market with the level of human experience where international capital movements translate into hunger, sickness, and despair.

CONCLUSION: CHALLENGING THE IDOLATRY OF GROWTH

This chapter has explored the conceptual tools and historical background for an investigation of relations between global economic patterns and the health of poor people, critiquing the presuppositions that underlie today's conventional wisdom on relations among poverty, inequality, economic growth, and globalization. The notion of economic development, understood as equivalent to strong growth in annual per capita GDP, is often construed today as the necessary and sufficient solution to the problem of poverty. This belief forms a part of that fund of commonsense knowledge that, in the words of Princeton economist Paul Krugman, "has a profound influence on actual policies in the real world" (1996, p. 732).[33] Our survey of the recent history of development economics suggested that the influence of this particular idea on "actual policies in the real world" has been pronounced, durable, and in many instances destructive. We saw, on the one hand, that economic policies intended to stimulate growth often fail to do so and, on the other, that even where GDP growth is strong, there is no guarantee that improvement in broad economic indicators will translate into improvements in the health and well-being of poor people. Growth per se does not automatically make poor people's lives better, and policies legitimated by the perceived need to generate growth at all costs have often made the living conditions of poor and middle-income people demonstrably worse.

Economic growth can bring important benefits for the poor. Yet to assume that growth will automatically generate such benefits neglects the dimension of political responsibility inseparable from meaningful discussions of poverty, inequality, and economic reform. We can all understand the seduction of simple theories and quick-fix solutions that would take responsibility and initiative out of our hands and assign them to some providential, invisible force. However, the pattern of growth that shapes (and that can destroy) real human lives is to a considerable extent the fruit of political choices, which are not magical but quite mundane.

At the most basic level, to emphasize a political dimension to the relationship between economic growth and the health of the poor is to argue for engaging our human responsibility and creativity. The relations between growth and health are not simply programmed by inflexible economic laws over which we have no influence, although, clearly, structural factors set limits to what can be achieved by individual initiative. This is why we argue for coordinated action that takes the health of the poor as its fundamental compass point and its concrete measure of success.

Our claim is not that growth in and of itself is bad or unnecessary. For many poor countries and communities, expansion in economic activity and GDP may be a key component of programs for improving health and life quality. However, if growth is to benefit poor communities, the health and wellbeing of poor people cannot be dealt with only as an afterthought, through palliative measures framed in terms of poverty alleviation, the prevention of social unrest, or the repair of social safety nets. Rather, the goals of ending poverty and decreasing inequality must be integrated and prioritized within the institutional policy mechanisms that promote growth and distribute its benefits. Stated another way, the challenge is to make improved health for poor people a central goal and a binding criterion in the planning, execution, and evaluation of economic and social policy on the local, national, and international levels.

Debates over poverty rates, foreign debt as a percentage of GDP, structural adjustment packages, and cost recovery mechanisms are of course highly technical discussions of economic matters; yet the problems they raise are also political and moral. If the poor and their advocates are to be more than passive bystanders in the drama of economic transformation, we have a responsibility to examine the implicit assumptions that guide patterns of change and to learn about the concrete effects of these patterns on human lives.

Notes

1. For detailed explorations of the relationship of poverty, inequality, and health, see Berkman and Kawachi (2000); Evans and others (2001); Kawachi and Kennedy (2002); Kawachi, Kennedy, and Wilkinson (1999); and World Bank (2000).

2. For a comprehensive examination of these problems, see Fort and Mercer (2004).

3. These figures (World Bank, 2001) are calculated in terms of purchasing power parity (PPP). Purchasing power parity is defined as the number of units of a country's currency required to buy the same amounts of goods and services in the domestic market as $1 would buy in the United States. Converting incomes to purchasing power parity corrects for problems caused by calculating incomes in U.S. dollars by using exchange rates. In order that the relative PPP of, say, India and Pakistan should not be affected by the prices prevailing in the United States, over-all GDP per person is calculated at "regional prices," representative of, for example, South Asia or East Asia. Afterward, the regions are linked statistically to enable global comparisons of the GDP per person and of its components, such as private consumption per person. This is very important for attempts to compare average GDP per person between countries. It may not make much sense to do so between, say, India and the United States because the average U.S. national's "bundle" of goods and services is so different from the average Indian's bundle. But between two countries in the same region, such as India and Pakistan, such differences should be much less, and comparisons accordingly make more sense. All such comparisons should nonetheless be taken as approximations.

4. For related issues, see Rodgers (1995). The concept of capabilities was an inspiration for the Human Poverty Index used in the UNDP's 1997 *Human Development Report* (see Sen, 1997, p. 201, n. 136). The roots of this approach are ideologically heterogeneous. For example, Adam Smith, in *The Wealth of Nations*, wrote of the importance of "appearing in public without shame." Income-based poverty measures may also miss elements of household dynamics of poverty (particularly on generational and gender lines), with significant implications for health outcomes. For another classic article, see Seers (1972).

5. See also the Human Poverty Index (HPI), introduced in the UNDP's *Human Development Report 1997*.

6. For discussions of the concept of development, see Sachs (1992) and Sen (2002), as well as the various issues of the *Human Development Report* published by the United Nations Development Programme.

7. During the 1990s, for example, almost all the benefits of economic growth in the United States went to the richest 5 percent of U.S. households. The next 15 percent fared moderately well, while the bottom 80 percent barely remained in place. This may be one reason that more people are working longer hours than at any other time in modern history, a fact that contributes to the erosion of both family and community life (see Mishel, Bernstein, and Schmitt, 1999).

8. This definition is from the European Foundation for the Improvement of Living and Working Conditions; see de Haan, Maxwell, and Wilkinson (1998) for application of the concept to health.

9. For countries that rely on migrant labor, for example, income from workers' remittances can be significant. Similarly, countries that have a high level of foreign-owned companies as their production base can see substantial funds depart in remitted profits.

10. Labor or capital intensity is a measure of the extent to which production uses greater amounts of human labor or capital per unit of production. Sometimes people think it is a contrast between agriculture and industry, but in fact both can be either: agriculture can be labor-intensive (generally, small-scale family farming) or capital-intensive (plantations); industry can be labor-intensive (generally, garment factories) or capital-intensive (high-tech auto plants).

11. For discussion from an economic perspective, see Lipton and Ravallion (1995). See Escobar (1995) for a postmodern reading.

12. *Physical capital* consists of buildings, machinery, and other structures and materials that are intended for some productive use. The term is used in contrast to *human capital,* which includes skills, education, or health; *social capital,* such as networks of trust that facilitate cooperation and collective action; and *environmental capital,* such as land, water, forests, or air.

13. The GATT operated from 1948 onward as an agreement among nation-states committed to reducing tariff (and later nontariff) barriers to trade. Reductions were to take effect as the result of agreements reached in rounds of negotiations, typically named for the locations where that particular round began. In the case of the decisive Uruguay Round, negotiations began in 1986 in Punta del Este, Uruguay, and the agreements were signed in April 1994 in Marrakesh, Morocco. By the late 1980s, the GATT framework, which focused primarily on manufactured goods, could not address the concerns of corporations and states interested in promoting freer trade in agricultural products and services (among other items). The agreement to form the World Trade Organization was a key product of the GATT's final round.

14. The general idea was that poor countries had low average income and low-income inequality in the rural, agricultural sector of the economy while displaying higher average income and at the same time higher income inequality in the urban industrial sector. During modernization, the distribution of income would first become more unequal as people migrated from the countryside to the city. The need for investment, and savings to fund investment, would also exacerbate inequality, as there would have to be a concentration of wealth to enable savings and investment to occur. As industrialization continued however, income inequality would eventually decline. This dominant view thus posited a trade-off between growth and inequality in the early stages of development.

15. Several international meetings initiated during this period, including Alma Ata, were held to respond to, and ultimately diffuse, demands for fundamental social

transformation. Declarations resulting from these meetings tended to appropriate the language of the more radical movements ("health for all," "primary health care") but ignored radicals' call to address inequalities in power and wealth.

16. In reality, the causes of the economic decline were more complex. They appear to have had (and to continue to have) more to do with the dismantling of the Bretton Woods system and the reckless liberalization of financial dealings begun in the early 1970s than with any real effects of the oil crisis itself.

17. Formed in 1961, the OECD is a group of the world's twenty-nine wealthiest nations dedicated to building strong economies in member countries and expanding free trade. OECD countries account for more than two-thirds of the world's production of goods and services but represent a much smaller portion of the world's population.

18. The antistatist, free market rhetoric of these administrations was significantly at odds with their actual practice in certain areas of economic policy, which tended in many cases to reinforce protectionism. In a review of the 1980s, Shafiqul Islam (1990) describes the Reagan administration as having presided over a significant swing toward protectionism in United States trade policy.

19. *Structural adjustment* is the formal IMF term to describe the programs the fund designs for Third World debtors. Others call them *austerity programs* (George, 1990).

20. For good discussions of the supply side of the debt crisis, see Lissakers (1990) and Devlin (1989). For an accessible introduction to the political economy of the crisis, see George (1992).

21. John Toye (1993), among others, has noted how the neoclassical public choice school of political economics, also known as the New Political Economy (NPE), has imported many "vulgar" Marxist arguments regarding the role of the state in capitalist economies. Neoclassical economics has discarded some of the more interesting insights of classical economists like Adam Smith, who saw the importance of embedding markets within a sociopolitical framework of laws and regulations and who also stressed cultural norms of solidarity ("fellow-feeling").

22. One emphasis of adjustment programs is to increase the "flexibility of labor" by deregulating labor markets. Typically, this means reducing minimum wages, shifting from industrial to enterprise-level collective bargaining, and making it easier for firms to hire workers on a temporary or subcontractual basis (see Oxfam, 1994; World Bank, 1995a).

23. In 1997, the net long-term private flows rose to $256 billion (see World Bank, 1998).

24. Until the Heavily Indebted Poor Country Initiative (to be discussed shortly), creditor governments had agreed in a series of negotiations to various terms for debt reduction for the severely indebted low-income countries. The latest of these was called the Naples Terms, which provided for a two-thirds reduction in present-value terms of certain categories of official debt.

25. The independent Jubilee Research Institute tracks the ongoing results of the HIPC initiative; see http://www.jubileeplus.org/hipc/tracking_hipc.htm.

26. In the late 1990s, the Inter-American Development Bank (1997, pp. 40–41) contended that 150 million Latin Americans were poor.

27. During the 1990s, sub-Saharan Africa received less than 1 percent of global private capital flows and so remained largely dependent on financial flows from wealthy-country governments and the international financial institutions. From 1990 to 1993, Africa transferred more than $13.4 billion annually to its external creditors, more than it spent on health and education combined (see Oxfam, 1995).

28. *Investing in Health* acknowledges the economic roots of ill-health and states that improvements in health are likely to result primarily from advances in nonhealth sectors. The study calls for increased family income, admits that the market is not perfect in shaping health care systems, and acknowledges that structural adjustment programs were "indiscriminate" in their impact on health services. *Investing* encourages increased health spending, focuses on violence against women as a major health problem, advocates essential drug programs, and argues that smoking cessation is integral to the achievement of health goals. The endorsement of essential drug programs and the antismoking position are especially striking in light of the Bank's history of enforcing substantive measures to preserve the tobacco and pharmaceutical industries' liberal access to Third World markets.

29. The issue of targeting emerged in part because of the recognition that the benefits of some universal social programs (like general food subsidies) were received disproportionately by the nonpoor.

30. Land reform, understood as redistribution of land rights to the rural poor, can play a major role in poverty reduction if combined with other policies like agricultural extension and credit. The benefits include generally greater farm output and a greater capacity among the rural poor to raise their voice in debates over economic and social policies. The key seems to be redistributive policies that enhance productivity.

31. Roughly equal shares of world trade are accounted for by transnational corporations trading with their own affiliates, by TNC corporate trade with nonaffiliates, and by trade among domestic firms. The expansion of TNCs has been a major source of the proliferation of trade. The rise of processing and assembly operations under the aegis of TNCs spurred trade growth in the 1990s while at the same time highlighting transactions among and within TNCs as a significant portion of global commerce. See Brenner and others (2000).

32. The Mexican and Asian crises had different roots. In Mexico, it was government bonds (public debt) that was at issue, while in Asia it was a private debt crisis (private corporations owed foreign banks money or owed domestic banks debts denominated in foreign currencies).

33. Krugman argues that "Washington consensus" policies bear a striking resemblance to the conventional wisdom before the Great Depression.

References

Ahmad, E. "Protecting the Vulnerable: Social Security and Public Policy." In M. Lipton and J. van der Gaag (eds.), *Including the Poor*. Washington, D.C.: World Bank, 1993.

Angell, A., and Graham, C. "Social Sector Reform and the Adjustment Process." Paper presented at the meeting of the Latin American Studies Association, Washington, D.C., Sept. 28–30, 1995.

Ayres, R. L. *Banking on the Poor*. Washington, D.C.: Overseas Development Council, 1983.

Bauer, P. T. *Dissent on Development*. London: Weidenfeld & Nicolson, 1972.

Bauer, P. T. *Equality, the Third World, and Economic Delusion*. London: Methuen, 1981.

Bauer, P. T. *Reality and Rhetoric: Studies in the Economics of Development*. London: Weidenfeld & Nicolson, 1984.

Berkman, L. F., and Kawachi, I. *Social Epidemiology*. New York: Oxford University Press, 2000.

Bhagwati, J. "The Capital Myth." *Foreign Affairs*, 1998, *73*(3), 7–12.

Bird, G. "Borrowing from the IMF: The Policy Implications of Recent Empirical Research." *World Development*, 1996, *24*, 1753-1760.

Birdsall, N., and James. E. *Efficiency and Equity in Social Spending: How and Why Governments Misbehave*. Working Paper no. 274. Washington, D.C.: World Bank, 1990.

Birdsall, N., and Londoño, J. L. "Assets Inequality Matters: An Assessment of the World Bank's Approach to Poverty Reduction." *American Economic Review Papers and Proceedings*, 1997, *87*(2), 32–37.

Bourguignon, F., and Morrisson, C. *Adjustment and Equity in Developing Countries: A New Approach*. Paris: Organization for Economic Cooperation and Development, 1992.

Brenner, J., and others. "Neoliberal Trade and Investment and the Health of *Maquiladora* Workers on the U.S.-Mexico Border." In J. Kim and others (eds.), *Dying for Growth: Global Inequality and the Health of the Poor*. Monroe, Maine: Common Courage, 2000.

Buse, K., and Gwin, C. "The World Bank and Global Cooperation in Health: The Case of Bangladesh." *Lancet*, 1998, *351*(9103), 665–669.

Buvinic, M., Gwin, C., and Bates, L. M. *Investing in Women: Progress and Prospects for the World Bank*. Washington, D.C.: Overseas Development Council, 1996.

Çagatay, N., Elson, D., and Grown, C. (eds.). "Gender, Adjustment, and Macroeconomics" [special issue]. *World Development*, 1995.

Chomsky, N. *Powers and Prospects: Reflections on Human Nature and the Social Order*. Boston: South End Press, 1996.

Chossudovsky, M. *The Globalisation of Poverty: Impacts of IMF and World Bank Reforms.* London: Zed Books, 1997.

Clark, M., Vanderslice, M., and Joyner, K. *Determined to Fail: The Heavily Indebted Poor Country Initiative.* Washington, D.C.: Jubilee USA Network, 2002.

Cline, W. (ed.). *Trade Policy in the 1980s.* Washington, D.C.: Institute for International Economics, 1983.

Conway, P. "IMF Lending Programs: Participation and Impact." *Journal of Development Economics,* 1994, *45,* 365-391.

Coote, B., and Lequesne, C. *The Trade Trap: Poverty and the Global Commodity Markets.* Oxford: Oxfam, 1996.

Cornia, G. A., Jolly, R., and Stewart, F. *Adjustment with a Human Face: Protecting the Vulnerable and Promoting Growth.* Oxford: Oxford University Press, 1987.

Danaher, K. (ed.). *50 Years Is Enough: The Case Against the World Bank and the International Monetary Fund.* Boston: South End Press, 1994.

de Haan, A., and Maxwell, S. "Poverty and Social Exclusion in North and South." *IDS Bulletin,* 1998, *29*(1), 1-9.

de Haan, A., Maxwell, S., and Wilkinson, R. G. "What Health Tells Us About Society." *IDS Bulletin,* 1998, *29*(1).

Desjarlais, R., and others (eds.). *World Mental Health: Problems and Priorities in Low-Income Countries.* New York: Oxford University Press, 1995.

Devlin, R. *Debt and Crisis in Latin America: The Supply Side of the Story.* Princeton, N.J.: Princeton University Press, 1989.

Economic Commission for Latin America and the Caribbean. *La Brecha de la Equidad: Latin America, the Caribbean, and the Social Summit.* Santiago, Chile: U.N. Economic Commission on Latin America, 1997.

Edwards, S. *The IMF and Developing Countries: A Critical Analysis.* Washington, D.C.: Holland, 1989.

Epping, R. C. *A Beginner's Guide to the World Economy: Seventy-Seven Basic Economic Concepts That Will Change the Way You See the World.* New York: Vintage, 1995.

Escobar, A., *Encountering Development: The Making and Unmaking of the Third World.* Princeton, N.J.: Princeton University Press, 1995.

Evans, T., and others (eds.). *Challenging Inequities in Health: From Ethics to Action.* New York: Oxford University Press, 2001.

Fort, M., and Mercer, M. A. (eds.). *Globalization and Health.* Boston: South End Press, forthcoming, 2004.

George, S. *A Fate Worse Than Debt.* New York: Grove Weidenfeld, 1990.

George, S. *The Debt Boomerang: How Third World Debt Harms Us All.* Boulder, Colo.: Westview Press, 1992.

George, S., and Sabelli, F. *Faith and Credit: The World Bank's Secular Empire.* Boulder, Colo.: Westview Press, 1994.

Gershman, J., and Fox, J. "Taking on Poverty Targeting." *Bankcheck Quarterly*, May 1996, *14*.

Gibbon, P. "The World Bank and African Poverty, 1973–91." *Journal of Modern African Studies*, 1992, *30*, 193–220.

Giblin, J. L. *The Politics of Environmental Control in Northeastern Tanzania.* Philadelphia: University of Pennsylvania Press, 1992.

Global Exchange. *How the International Monetary Fund and the World Bank Undermine Democracy and Erode Human Rights: Five Case Studies.* San Francisco: Global Exchange, 2001.

Greenhill, R., and Blackmore, S. *Relief Works: African Proposals for Debt Cancellation and Why Debt Relief Works.* London: Jubilee Research/New Economics Foundation, 2002.

Halstead, T., and Cobb, C. "The Need for New Measurements of Progress." In J. Mander and E. Goldsmith (eds.), *The Case Against the Global Economy.* San Francisco: Sierra Club Books, 1996.

Harmes, A. "Institutional Investors and the Reproduction of Neoliberalism." *Review of International Political Economy*, 1998, *5*, 92–121.

HarperCollins Economic Directory. New York: HarperCollins, 1991.

Helleiner, E. *States and the Reemergence of Global Finance: From Bretton Woods to the 1990s.* Ithaca, N.Y.: Cornell University Press, 1994.

Inter-American Development Bank. *Economic and Social Progress in Latin America: Latin America After a Decade of Reforms.* Washington, D.C.: Inter-American Development Bank, 1997.

International HIV Treatment Access Coalition. *A Commitment to Action for Expanded Access to HIV/AIDS Treatment.* Geneva: World Health Organization, 2002.

International Monetary Fund, External Relations Department. "What Is the International Monetary Fund?" 2002. [http://www.imf.org/external/pubs/ft/exrp/what.htm].

Islam, S. "America and the World." *Foreign Affairs*, 1990, *69*, 172–182.

Kawachi, I., and Kennedy, B. P. *The Health of Nations: Why Inequality Is Harmful for Your Health.* New York: New Press, 2002.

Kawachi, I., Kennedy, B. P., and Wilkinson, R. G. *Income Inequality and Health.* New York: New Press, 1999.

Khan, M. S. *The Macroeconomic Effects of Fund-Supported Adjustment Programs.* IMF Staff Papers, no. 37. Washington, D.C.: International Monetary Fund, 1990.

Killick, T. (ed.). *IMF Programs in Developing Countries: Design and Impact.* New York: Routledge, 1995a.

Killick, T. "Structural Adjustment and Poverty Alleviation: An Interpretive Survey." *Development and Change*, 1995b, *26*, 305–331.

Killick, T., Malik, M., and Manuel, M. "What Can We Know About the Effects of IMF Programmes?" *World Economy*, 1992, *15*, 575–597.

Kindleberger, C. P. *Manias, Panic, and Crashes: A History of Financial Crises.* (4th ed.) New York: Wiley, 2000.

Koppes, R. H. "Corporate Governance in the New Millennium: Concentrated Ownership Swells Activist Influence." *Directorship,* 1999, *25*(2), 4–5.

Krugman, P. "Cycles of Conventional Wisdom on Economic Development." *International Affairs,* 1996, *71,* 717–732.

Lappe, F. M. *Food First: Beyond the Myth of Scarcity.* Boston: Houghton Mifflin, 1978.

Lawrence, R. *Regionalism, Multilateralism, and Deeper Integration.* Washington, D.C.: Brookings Institution, 1996.

Lele, U. *Structural Adjustment, Agricultural Development, and the Poor: Some Lessons from the Malawian Experience.* Washington, D.C.: World Bank, 1990.

Lipton, M. *Land Assets and Rural Poverty.* Working Paper no. 744. Washington, D.C.: World Bank, 1985.

Lipton, M. "Comment on 'Research on Poverty and Development Twenty Years After *Redistribution with Growth,*' by Pranab Bardahn." In M. Bruno and B. Pleskovic (eds.), *Annual World Bank Conference on Development Economics, 1995.* Washington, D.C.: World Bank, 1996.

Lipton, M., and Maxwell, S. *The New Poverty Agenda: An Overview.* Discussion Paper no. 306. Brighton, England: Institute for Development Studies, University of Sussex, 1992.

Lipton, M., and Ravallion, M. "Poverty and Policy." In H. Chenery and T. N. Srinivasan (eds.), *Handbook of Development Economics.* (3rd ed.) New York: North-Holland, 1995.

Lissakers, K. *Banks, Borrowers, and the Establishment: A Revisionist Account of the International Debt Crisis.* New York: Basic Books, 1990.

Londoño, J. L., and Székely, M. *Distributional Surprises After a Decade of Reform: Latin America in Nineties.* Working Paper no. 352. Washington, D.C.: Inter-American Development Bank, 1997.

Lustig, N. (ed.). *Coping with Austerity: Poverty and Inequality in Latin America.* Washington, D.C.: Brookings Institution, 1995.

Meadows, D. H., and others. *Limits to Growth: A Report for the Club of Rome's Project on the Predicament of Mankind.* New York: Universe Books, 1972.

Mehrotra, S., and Jolly, R. (eds.). *Development with a Human Face: Experiences in Social Achievement and Growth.* Oxford: Clarendon Press, 1987.

Mishel, L., Bernstein, J., and Schmitt, J. *The State of Working America, 1998–99.* Ithaca, N.Y.: Cornell University Press, 1999.

Nikiforuk, A. *The Fourth Horseman: A Short History of Epidemics, Plagues, Famine, and Other Scourges.* New York: Evans, 1993.

Overseas Development Institute. *Commodity Markets: Options for Developing Countries.* Briefing Paper no. 5. London: Overseas Development Institute, 1995.

Oxfam. *Structural Adjustment and Inequality in Latin America: How IMF and World Bank Policies Have Failed the Poor.* Oxford: Oxfam, 1994.

Oxfam. *The Oxfam Poverty Report.* Oxford: Oxfam, 1995.

Pastor, M. "The Effects of IMF Programs in the Third World: Debates and Evidence from Latin America." *World Development,* 1987, *15,* 249–262.

Patel, R., and Delwiche, A. "The Profits of Famine: Southern Africa's Long Decade of Hunger." *Food First Backgrounder,* 2002, 8(4). [http://www.foodfirst.org/pubs/backgrdrs/2002/f02v8n4.html].

Pettifor, A. "Debt Is Still the Lynchpin: The Case of Malawi." Jubilee Research, July 2002. [http://www.jubileeplus.org/opinion/debt040702.htm].

Ravallion, M. *Can High-Inequality Developing Countries Escape Absolute Poverty?* Poverty Research Working Paper no. 1775. Washington, D.C.: World Bank, 1997.

Ribe, H., and others. *How Adjustment Programs Can Help the Poor: The World Bank's Experience.* Washington, D.C.: World Bank, 1990.

Rodgers, G. (ed.). *The Poverty Agenda and the ILO: Issues for Research and Action.* Geneva: International Labour Organization, 1995.

Rodrik, D. "Why Do More Open Economies Have Bigger Governments?" *Journal of Political Economy,* 1998, *106,* 997–1032.

Sachs, W. (ed.). *The Development Dictionary: A Guide to Knowledge as Power.* London: Zed Books, 1992.

Schoepf, B. G., Schoepf, C., and Millen, J. V. "Theoretical Therapies, Remote Remedies: SAPs and the Political Ecology and Poverty and Health in Africa." In J. Kim and others (eds.), *Dying for Growth: Global Inequality and the Health of the Poor.* Monroe, Maine: Common Courage, 2000.

Seers, D. "What Are We Trying to Measure?" In N. Baster (ed.), *Measuring Development.* London: Cass, 1972.

Sen, A. K. *Commodities and Capabilities.* New York: North-Holland, 1985

Sen, A. K. *Inequality Reexamined.* Cambridge, Mass.: Harvard University Press, 1992.

Sen, A. K. "Capability and Well-Being." In M. Nussbaum and A. K. Sen (eds.), *The Quality of Life.* New York: Oxford University Press, 1993.

Sen, A. K. "The Political Economy of Targeting." In D. van de Walle and K. Nead (eds.), *Public Spending and the Poor: Theory and Evidence.* Baltimore: Johns Hopkins University Press, 1995.

Sen, A. K. *On Economic Inequality.* Oxford: Clarendon Press, 1997.

Sen, A. K. "The Concept of Development." In H. Chenery and T. N. Srinivasan (eds.), *Handbook of Development Economics.* (4th ed.) New York: North Holland, 2002.

Shapiro, H., and Taylor, L. "The State and Industrial Strategy." *World Development,* 1990, *18,* 861–878.

Sklar, H., Mykyta, L., and Wefald, S. *Raise the Floor: Wages and Policies That Work for All of Us.* New York: Ms. Foundation for Women, 2001.

Sparr, P. (ed.). *Mortgaging Women's Lives: Feminist Critiques of Structural Adjustment.* London: Zed Books, 1994.

Spencer, N. *Poverty and Child Health.* Oxford: Radcliffe Medical Press, 1996.

Stiglitz, J. "More Instruments and Broader Goals: Moving Toward the Post-Washington Consensus." WIDER Annual Lecture, Helsinki, Finland, Jan. 7, 1998.

Stiglitz, J. *Globalization and Its Discontents.* New York: Norton, 2002.

Taylor, L. (ed.). *The Rocky Road to Reform: Adjustment, Income Distribution, and Growth in the Developing World.* Cambridge, Mass.: MIT Press, 1993.

Toye, J. *Dilemmas of Development: Reflections on the Counter-Revolution in Development Economics.* (2nd ed.) Oxford: Blackwell, 1993.

Ul Haq, M., Kaul, I., and Grunberg, I. (eds.). *The Tobin Tax: Coping with Financial Vulnerability.* Oxford: Oxford University Press, 1996.

United for a Fair Economy. "Wealth Inequality Charts." 2002. [http://www.ufenet.org/research/wealth_charts.html].

United Nations Development Programme. *Human Development Report 1996.* New York: Oxford University Press, 1996.

United Nations Development Programme. *Human Development Report 1997.* New York: Oxford University Press, 1997.

United Nations Development Programme. *Human Development Report 1998.* New York: Oxford University Press, 1998.

United Nations Development Programme. *Human Development Report 2002.* New York: Oxford University Press, 2002.

Vivian, J. (ed.). *Adjustment and Social Sector Restructuring.* London: Cass, 1995.

Wade, R. "The Asian Debt-and-Development Crisis of 1997–?: Causes and Consequences." *World Development,* 1998a, *26,* 1535–1554.

Wade, R. "From Miracle to Meltdown: Vulnerabilities, Moral Hazard, Panic, and Debt Deflation in the Asian Crisis." Working Paper prepared for the Russell Sage Foundation, June 1, 1998b.

Watkins, K. *Economic Growth with Equity: Lessons from East Asia.* Oxford: Oxfam, 1998.

Williamson, J. *Latin American Adjustment: How Much Has Happened?* Washington, D.C.: Institute for International Economics, 1990.

Williamson, J. "Lowest Common Denominator or Neoliberal Manifesto? The Polemics of the Washington Consensus." In R. M. Auty and J. Toye (eds.), *Challenging the Orthodoxies.* New York: St. Martin's Press, 1996.

Woodward, D. *Debt, Adjustment, and Poverty in Developing Countries.* London: Pinter/Save the Children, 1992.

World Bank. *Financing Health Services in Developing Countries: An Agenda for Reform.* Washington, D.C.: World Bank, 1987.

World Bank. *Zimbabwe: Issues in the Financing of Health Services.* Washington, D.C.: World Bank, 1990a.

World Bank. *World Development Report 1990*. Washington, D.C.: World Bank, 1990b.

World Bank. *World Development Report 1993: Investing in Health*. Washington, D.C.: World Bank, 1993.

World Bank. *Global Economic Prospects and the Developing Countries*. Washington, D.C.: World Bank, 1995a.

World Bank. *World Development Report 1995*. Washington, D.C.: 1995b.

World Bank. *Taking Action for Poverty Reduction in Sub-Saharan Africa*. Washington, D.C.: World Bank, 1996.

World Bank. *Global Development Finance*. Washington, D.C.: World Bank, 1998.

World Bank. *World Development Report 2000/01: Attacking Poverty*. Washington, D.C.: World Bank, 2000.

World Bank. "Income Poverty: The Latest Global Numbers." 2001. [http://www.worldbank.org/poverty/data/trends/income.htm].

World Bank. "Overview of Poverty Reduction Strategies." 2003. [http://www.worldbank.org/poverty/strategies/overview.htm].

World Health Organization. *World Health Report*. Geneva: World Health Organization, 1995.

CHAPTER SIX

The Political Context of Social Inequalities and Health

Vicente Navarro
Leiyu Shi

This analysis reflects on the importance of political parties, and the policies they implement when in government, in determining the level of equalities/inequalities in a society, the extent of the welfare state (including the level of health care coverage by the state), the employment/unemployment rate, and the level of population health. The study looks at the impact of the major political traditions in the advanced OECD countries during the golden years of capitalism (1945–1980)—social democratic, Christian democratic, liberal, and ex-fascist—in four areas: (1) the main determinants of income inequalities; (2) levels of public expenditures and health care benefits coverage; (3) public support of services to families; and (4) the level of population health as measured by infant mortality. The results indicate that political traditions more committed to redistributive policies (both economic and social) and full-employment policies, such as the social democratic parties, were generally more successful in improving the health of populations. The erroneous assumption of a conflict between social equity and economic efficiency is also discussed. The study aims at filling a void in the growing health and social inequalities literature, which rarely touches on the importance of political forces in influencing inequalities.

THE IMPORTANCE OF POLITICS

A very important development in the social science and health literature over the last ten years has been a focus on how social inequalities are affecting the health of populations (see Kawachi, Wilkinson, and Kennedy, 1999,(1) for an extensive review of the literature in this area and Navarro, 1998a,(2) for a description of how these types of studies have not always been so "popular"). In this growing area of research, however, a subject rarely studied is the impact on social inequalities and health of political forces (such as political movements and parties) and the public policies they follow when in government. Indeed, a review of the latest literature on the relationship between social inequalities and health shows the dearth of references that either include or focus on political variables and their impact on health (Kawachi, Wilkinson, and Kennedy, 1999). This lack of attention to the importance of political variables also appears in the growing field of research on comparative international studies of health status. The state of Kerala in India, for example, has been widely studied, showing the relationship between its impressive reduction of inequalities in the last 40 years and improvements in the health status of its population. With very few exceptions (Navarro, 1993; Cereseto and Waitzkin, 1986), however, these reductions in social inequalities and improvements in health have rarely been traced to the public policies carried out by the state's governing party, the Indian Communist Party, which has governed in Kerala for the longest period during those 40 years.

Similarly, we have seen several studies that refer admiringly to the developments occurring in the northeastern regions of Italy in the last 40 years, with active popular participation in the governance of these regions paralleling active policies of reducing social inequalities and discouraging hierarchical relations. These studies are silent, however, on a critical element: all those regions were governed by the Italian Communist Party, which was to a large degree responsible for such policies. (An example here is the otherwise excellent book by Richard Wilkinson, 1996.)

Some studies have included political variables to explain variations in health status, tracing the variations to different political configurations. Cereseto and Waitzkin (1986) have analyzed the health status and quality of life in capitalist countries and in countries they define as socialist. And Navarro (1993) has analyzed changes in the health status of populations during the 20th century, comparing the performance of countries at similar levels of development under different political regimes. But these are exceptions. For the most part, the abundant literature on health status and health inequalities does not include many studies on the importance of political variants in shaping social inequalities and population health.

Our chapter aims at correcting this deficit. Its objective is to show the importance of political parties, and the policies they implement when in government, in determining the level of equalities or inequalities in a society and in explaining the level of health of its population. We also analyze the mechanisms by which these political influences take place and their social and health consequences in advanced countries of the Organization for Economic Cooperation and Development (OECD). Data for this study are largely from OECD Health Data Set 98 (1998b), an interactive database comprising systematically collated data on key aspects of the health care systems of the 29 OECD member countries within their general demographic, economic, and social contexts. Also used are data on political, economic, and social variables derived from the Comparative Welfare State Data Set assembled by Evelyn Huber, Charles Ragin, and John D. Stephens (1998); data on household income and wage differentials are extracted from the OECD Data Set 1997 (1998a) and the U.S. Bureau of Labor Statistics.

THE MAJOR POLITICAL REGIMES IN DEVELOPED CAPITALIST COUNTRIES

To show the importance of political forces in explaining social phenomena, including the level of inequalities and the health and well-being of populations, we have grouped the major developed capitalist countries according to the dominant type of political force that governed them during the time when their welfare states were established (from the end of World War II to the 1980s): social democratic, Christian democratic (or conservative parties within the Christian tradition), liberal, and fascist (the typology is adapted from Huber and Stephens, 1998; see also Navarro, 1999). The assignment of a country to a particular political tradition is based on the political orientation of parties that governed either alone or as the major partner in a coalition for the greatest proportion of the time between 1945 and 1980. This period (1945–1980) was selected because, for most OECD countries, these were the years when welfare states were established and fully developed. It was in these expansive years, the golden years of capitalism, that the major characteristics of welfare states were shaped.

The Social Democratic Tradition

In the first group—the social democracies—we include those countries (Sweden, Finland, Norway, Denmark, and Austria) that have been governed by social democratic parties (either alone or as the major party in a coalition) for the majority of years during the period 1945–1980. As Table 6.1 shows, the social democratic parties governed for an average of 23.5 years in these countries during that period. In this group of countries, the labor movements and their socialist parties have been very strong, while the capitalist classes and the political parties they have chosen to represent their interests have been weak and usually fragmented (see Huber and Stephens, 1998, for an explanation of this situation). Table 6.1 also shows how these countries have been characterized by high union density (percentage of the working population enrolled in unions), high social security expenditures (as percentage of GDP), high taxation (as percentage of GDP), and high public employment in health services, education, and welfare (as percentage of the working-age population). They have the most extensive welfare states. (For an expansion of the description of the political economy of these countries, see Navarro, 1999.)

Table 6.2 shows that (on average) the social democratic countries also had the largest public expenditures in health care during the period 1960–1990, followed by the Christian democratic countries. The liberal countries and the ex-fascist countries had, in general, the lowest public expenditures on health in that same period. And the data in Table 6.3 show that (on average) the social democratic countries covered almost the entire population with a public medical care program; this coverage was lower (on average) in Christian democratic countries and even lower in liberal countries. The coverage in the ex-fascist countries, although low (during the fascist dictatorships, the lowest in all countries studied in this article), increased significantly during the democratic periods to a high level, primarily because of the social democratic governance during these periods.

The social democratic parties governing these countries were also characterized by their implementation of (a) full-employment policies, which explains their low unemployment (the lowest in these OECD countries during the period 1945–1980; see Table 6.4), and (b) universalistic social policies, aimed at covering the whole population. Table 6.3 shows, for example, how health care benefits coverage includes the entire population.

Such policies have used the social services of the welfare state (health, education, and family supportive services such as child care and domiciliary services) as a means of creating employment and facilitating the integration of women into the labor force—which explains the high rate of female employment in these countries (see Table 6.1). The social democratic countries have had a very large percentage of the adult population working in the labor market, a consequence of the high rate of women's participation in the labor force, in particular in the social services of the welfare state. The exception here is Austria, where a Catholic tradition emphasizing the family (rather than the state) as the primary provider of services to children and the elderly has kept women out of the labor force. This also accounts for the very low percentages— 4 percent—of the working-age population in Austria employed in the social services of the welfare state, compared with 20 percent in Sweden, 18 percent in Denmark, and 15 percent in Norway. There is a clear relationship between the size of these sectors and the percentage of women in the labor force. This explains why the percentage of the working-age population employed in the social services of the welfare state and the percentage of women who are working are lower in Christian democratic countries (6.2 percent and 46 percent, respectively), and much lower in ex-fascist countries (2.6 percent and 26 percent), than in social democratic countries (13.2 percent and 65.2 percent). It is also the social democratic countries that have smaller inequalities in household income (Table 6.5), larger supportive services for families (such as child care services and domiciliary services for the elderly and disabled), and lower poverty rates for the overall population and for children (Table 6.5).

Why do the social democratic countries have the lowest household income inequalities? To answer this question, we need to understand the primary reasons for income inequalities in a country: (a) the percentage of national income that goes to capital versus labor, (b) the wage disparities within labor, and (c) the redistributive effect of state interventions—that is, changes in disposable income of households and individuals as a result of adding transfers from the state and subtracting income paid in taxes and fees to the state. The social democratic countries have (a) the lowest percentage of national income derived from capital and the highest derived from labor; profits derived from ownership of capital have historically tended to be the lowest among the countries under study (Table 6.6); (b) the lowest wage disparities within the labor force (Table 6.6); and (c) the highest redistributive effect of the state (Table 6.1).

, It is important to note that although mean wage differentials in social democratic countries (2.24 in 1990) were lower than those in Christian democratic countries (2.56 in 1990), they were not much different (Table 6.6). The mean household income inequalities in social democratic countries (2.79 in 1990–91), however, were much lower than those in Christian democratic countries (3.14) as a result of the much more favorable treatment of capital and lower redistributive effect of the state in the Christian democratic countries (Table 6.5).

We should also mention that while income derived from capital was lower in social democratic countries than in Christian democratic countries (Table 6.6), the rate of investment, measured by gross fixed capital formation as percentage of GDP (Table 6.6), and economic growth (Table 6.4) were higher than in the Christian democratic and liberal countries. Only during the years 1989–1995 was the rate of economic growth of the social democratic countries lower, on average, than that of the Christian democratic and liberal countries. These empirical data question the assumption made by the Christian democratic and liberal parties that public policies favoring income derived from capital and high-income groups are required to stimulate investment and economic growth. Tables 6.4 and 6.6 show otherwise. Rather than inequalities being a

Table 6.1. Political Characteristics, Policy Outcomes, and the Welfare State, Late 1970s.

	Years of Social Democratic Government, 1946–1980[a]	Years of Christian Democratic Government, 1946–1980[a]	Union Density[b]	Social Pact[c]	Social Security Expenditures[d]	Total Taxes[e]	Public Employment in Health, Education, and Welfare[f]	Redistributive Effect of the State[g]	Women's Participation[h]
Social Democratic Political Economies									
Sweden	30	0	82	4	31	56	20	53	74
Norway	28	1	59	4	20	53	15	40	62
Denmark	25	0	70	3	26	52	18	39	71
Finland	14	0	73	3	17	36	9	35	70
Austria	20	15	66	4	21	46	4	—	49
Mean	23.5	3.2	70	3.6	23.2	48.8	13.2	41.8	65.2
Christian Democratic Political Economies									
Belgium	14	19	72	3	21	43	7	47	47
Netherlands	8	22	38	4	27	53	4	41	35
Germany	11	16	40	3	23	45	5	38	51
France	3	4	28	1	25	45	9	35	54
Italy	3	30	51	2	20	33	5	29	39
Switzerland	9	10	35	3	13	33	7	19	54
Mean	7.8	16.7	43.9	3.0	21.6	41.8	6.2	34.8	46

	Years of Social Democratic Government, 1946–1980[a]	Years of Christian Democratic Government, 1946–1980[a]	Union Density[b]	Social Pact[c]	Social Security Expenditures[d]	Total Taxes[e]	Public Employment in Health, Education, and Welfare[f]	Redistributive Effect of the State[g]	Women's Participation[h]
Liberal Anglo-Saxon Political Economies									
Canada	0	0	31	1	13	36	4	25	57
Ireland	3	0	68	3	19	39	—	34	36
Great Britain	16	0	48	2	17	40	8	36	58
United States	0	0	25	1	12	31	5	26	60
Mean	4.7	0.0	43.0	1.8	15.2	36.5	5.7	30.3	52.8
Conservative or Fascist Dictatorships									
Spain	0	3	0	0	9	18	3	5	28
Greece	0	2	0	0	6	16	2	18	24
Portugal	2	3	0	0	8	15	3	16	26
Mean	0.7	2.6	0	0	7.7	16.3	2.6	16.3	26

Sources: Huber and Stephens, 1998; for conservative dictatorship countries, our own elaboration.
[a]Years in cabinet, scored 1 per year, less for coalition (Huber and Stephens, 1998).
[b]Union density as a percentage of the labor force.
[c]Scale of 1 to 4 used to measure social pact (Huber and Stephens, 1998).
[d]Social security as a percentage of GDP.
[e]Total taxes as a percentage of GDP.
[f]Public employment in health, education, and welfare as a percentage of the working-age population.
[g]Percentage reduction of income inequality affected by direct taxes and transfer payments.
[h]Percentage of working-age women in the labor force.

Table 6.2. Public Expenditures on Health, 1960–1990, as a Percentage of GDP.

	1960	1970	1980	1990
Social Democratic Political Economies				
Austria	3.0	3.4	5.3	5.3
Sweden	3.2	6.1	8.7	7.9
Denmark	3.2	5.2	7.7	7.1
Norway	2.3	4.1	5.9	6.5
Finland	2.1	4.2	5.1	6.5
Mean	2.8	4.6	6.5	6.7
Christian Democratic Political Economies				
Belgium	2.3	5.0	5.5	6.9
Germany	3.2	4.6	7.0	6.7
Netherlands	1.3	5.0	5.9	6.1
France	2.4	4.3	6.0	6.6
Italy	3.0	4.5	5.6	6.3
Switzerland	1.9	3.1	4.6	5.7
Mean	2.4	4.4	5.8	6.4
Liberal Anglo-Saxon Political Economies				
United Kingdom	3.3	3.9	5.0	5.1
Ireland	2.9	4.3	7.1	4.9
United States	1.3	2.7	3.9	5.1
Canada	2.3	5.0	5.5	6.9
Mean	2.4	3.9	5.3	5.5
Former Fascist Dictatorships				
Spain	—	2.4	4.4	5.7
Portugal	—	—	—	—
Greece	—	—	3.1	3.5
Mean	—	2.4	3.8	4.6

Source: Organization for Economic Cooperation and Development, 1998b.

Table 6.3. Total Public Medical Care Coverage, 1960–1996, as a Percentage of Total Population.

	1960	1970	1980	1990	1996
Social Democratic Political Economies					
Austria	78.0	91.0	99.0	99.0	99.0
Sweden	100.0	100.0	100.0	100.0	100.0
Denmark	95.0	100.0	100.0	100.0	100.0
Norway	100.0	100.0	100.0	100.0	100.0
Finland	55.0	100.0	100.0	100.0	100.0
Mean	85.6	98.2	99.8	99.8	99.8
Christian Democratic Political Economies					
Belgium	58.0	97.8	99.0	97.3	99.0
Germany	85.0	88.0	91.0	92.2	92.2
Netherlands	71.0	86.0	74.6	70.7	72.0
France	76.3	95.7	99.3	99.5	99.5
Italy	87.0	93.0	100.0	100.0	100.0
Switzerland	74.0	89.0	96.5	99.5	100.0
Mean	75.0	91.6	93.4	93.2	93.8
Liberal Anglo-Saxon Political Economies					
United Kingdom	100.0	100.0	100.0	100.0	100.0
Ireland	85.0	85.0	100.0	100.0	100.0
United States	20.0	40.0	42.0	44.0	45.0
Canada	71.0	100.0	100.0	100.0	100.0
Mean	69.0	81.3	85.5	86.0	86.3
Former Fascist Dictatorships					
Spain	54		61	99	99.8	99.8
Portugal	18		40	100	100	100
Greece	30		55	100	100	100
Mean	34		52	99.7	99.9	99.9

Source: Organization for Economic Cooperation and Development, 1998b.

Table 6.4. Economic Growth and Unemployment (percent change during the period indicated).

	Economic Growth				Unemployment					
	1960–1973	1974–1979	1979–1989	1989–1995	1960–1973	1974–1979	1980–1988	1990	1993	1995
Social Democratic Political Economies										
Sweden	3.4	1.5	1.8	-0.1	1.9	1.9	2.5	1.6	8.2	7.7
Norway	3.5	4.3	2.3	2.9	1.0	1.8	2.5	5.2	6.0	4.9
Denmark	3.6	1.6	1.8	1.6	1.4	6.0	8.1	8.3	10.7	7.0
Finland	4.5	1.8	3.2	-1.1	2.0	4.6	53	3.6	17.9	17.1
Austria	4.3	3.0	2.0	1.3	1.7	1.6	3.3	3.2	4.2	3.8
Mean	3.9	2.4	2.2	0.9	1.6	3.2	4.3	4.4	9.4	8.1
Christian Democratic Political Economies										
Belgium	4.4	2.1	1.8	1.3	2.2	5.7	11.5	8.8	12.0	12.9
Netherlands	3.6	1.9	1.1	1.8	1.3	5.0	10.0	7.5	6.7	7.1
Germany	3.7	2.5	1.7	1.3	0.8	3.4	6.7	6.2	7.9	8.1
France	4.3	2.3	1.6	0.8	2.0	4.6	9.0	9.1	11.7	11.5
Italy	4.6	3.2	2.4	1.1	5.3	6.3	9.1	10.5	10.6	12.0
Switzerland	3.0	-0.1	1.7	-0.5	0.0	0.4	0.6	0.5	3.8	3.3
Mean	3.9	2.0	1.7	1.0	1.9	4.2	7.8	7.1	8.7	9.2
Liberal Anglo-Saxon Political Economies										
Canada	3.6	2.9	1.8	-1.0	5.0	7.2	9.5	8.1	12.0	9.5
Ireland	3.7	3.3	2.7	5.8	5.2	7.6	14.2	13.7	15.6	12.1
Great Britain	2.6	1.5	2.2	0.7	1.9	4.2	9.9	5.4	10.2	8.6
United States	2.6	1.4	1.5	0.9	5.0	7.0	7.8	5.6	6.8	5.5
Mean	3.1	2.3	2.1	1.6	4.3	6.5	10.3	8.2	11.0	8.9

Source: Huber and Stephens, 1998, tabs. 2 and 3.

Table 6.5. Household Income and Poverty.

	Household Income Inequality Relative to National Median Incomes (ratio of 90th to 10th percentile, 1990–1991)	Poverty Rate (percentage of population)	
		Total	Children
Social Democratic Political Economies			
Sweden	2.78	6.7	3.0
Denmark	2.86	7.5	5.1
Norway	2.80	6.6	4.9
Finland	2.75	6.2	2.7
Mean	2.79	6.75	3.92
Christian Democratic Political Economies			
France	3.48	7.5	7.4
Germany	3.21	7.6	8.6
Belgium	2.79	5.5	4.4
Netherlands	3.05	6.7	8.3
Italy	3.14	6.5	10.5
Mean	3.14	6.7	7.84
Liberal Anglo-Saxon Political Economies			
United States	5.78	19.1	24.9
Canada	3.90	11.7	15.3
United Kingdom	4.67	14.6	18.5
Ireland	4.18	11.1	13.8
Mean	4.63	14.25	18.1
Former Fascist Dictatorships			
Spain	4.4	10.4	12.8

Sources: Mishel, Bernstein, and Schmitt, 1999; Smeeding, 1997.

requirement for growth (as classical economics maintains), the reduction of such inequalities has been a precondition for economic efficiency and economic growth (Navarro, 1998b, expands on this point). These social democratic countries have also been the countries with the lowest infant mortality rates (Table 6.7) during the period 1960–1996.

It is not our purpose here to analyze the pathways by which reduction of income inequalities affects infant mortality rates. But our data show that the political forces that have been more successful in reducing income inequalities, such as the social democratic parties, have also been more successful in reducing infant mortality rates. The policies in the social democratic countries resulted from the strength of the labor movements, which, in alliance with other sectors and classes (rural farmers in Northern Europe and the middle class in Austria), have been the major force behind the reduction of inequalities and, consequently, the declines in infant mortality rates. It is important to stress that even in countries, such as Italy, that have not been governed by social democratic forces, those regions of the country that have been governed by parties following social democratic policies of reducing inequalities and creating employment, such as the former Italian Communist Party (today the Left Democratic Party), have had lesser inequalities and better mortality indicators than other regions. The regions of northern Italy—Tuscany and Piedmont, for example—mentioned in Richard Wilkinson's book *Unhealthy Societies* (1996) were governed by Communist parties following social democratic policies. Explaining the reduction of mortality rates in these countries (or regions) in terms of specific interventions such as higher population participation in civil and political societies or other types of interventions is insufficient. Rather, mortality reductions result from a larger set of related interventions guided by a political party or parties (socialist, social democratic, communist, labor, or whatever name is used to define these labor-oriented social democratic parties) that generate and reproduce a culture of solidarity and opportunity. Attempts to disaggregate these collective responses into their different components ignore the Hegelian dictum that the totality is more than the sum of its parts. These data seem to allow the conclusion, therefore, that to reduce income inequalities and infant mortality, it is advisable to support labor-based social democratic parties.

The Christian Democratic Tradition

In this group we include countries that from 1945 to 1980 were governed for long periods by conservative parties based in the Christian tradition—parties that define themselves as Christian democratic and those that, while not defining themselves in this way, consider themselves based in the Christian tradition. These countries (Belgium, the Netherlands, Germany, France, Italy, and Switzerland) form the least homogeneous group of all the countries considered here—a consequence of Christian democratic parties sometimes having to govern in coalition with other parties, including social democrats (as in Belgium, Germany, and the Netherlands). But despite the party alliances and coalitions in these countries, the conservative parties of Christian tradition were either the dominant forces in the coalitions or were the parties governing for greater lengths of time in the 1945–1980 period (Table 6.1), and this is what explains their common characteristics.

First, the Christian democratic countries rely primarily on the family for the provision of social services to the elderly, the disabled, and children. Families in these societies have been burdened with caring work that in the social democracies is the responsibility of the state and in the liberal countries the responsibility of the market. This extra burden on the family in Christian democratic countries explains the very low rate of women's participation in the labor force (Table 6.1): only 46 percent of women participate in the labor market, compared with 65.2 percent in social democratic and 52.8 percent in liberal countries. Only the former fascist countries (Spain, Greece, and Portugal) have a lower percentage of women in the labor force (26 percent). In the Christian democratic countries, class inequalities have been compounded by large gender inequalities, including gender inequalities in health. Spain's government commission on inequalities in health (the Spanish equivalent of the U.K. Black Commission) found, for example, that in the 30- to 50-year age group, women have twice as many stress-related conditions as men (Navarro and Benach, 1996). In fact, women in this group suffer more stress-related conditions than any other group in Spain. Table 6.8 shows, for example, the number of hours that women work at home in Spain and Italy, versus those in Denmark, Sweden, and the United States. Women in southern European countries work much longer hours than those in northern Europe.

The second characteristic shared by the Christian democratic countries is the heavy reliance of families' standard of living on the salary and pension of the male breadwinner, considered the head of the family. This explains the enormous importance given by the labor movements of these countries to both maintaining and expanding wages and expanding social transfers (in particular, pensions) as a way of assuring families' standard of living. Thus these countries have large social transfers and underdeveloped social services. As Table 6.1 shows, the average level of social expenditures in the Christian democratic countries (21.6 percent of GDP) was lower than that in the social democratic countries (23.2 percent of GDP), although much higher than that in the liberal countries (15.2 percent of GDP). The same table also shows that only 6.2 percent of the working-age population was employed in services in the Christian democratic countries, compared with 13.2 percent in the social democracies. And the Christian democratic countries have lower public expenditures on health (Table 6.2) and a lower degree of health benefits coverage than the social democratic countries, although higher than in the liberal countries.

Table 6.6. Total Profits, Wage Inequalities, and Gross Fixed Capital Formation, 1960–1989.

	Operative Surplus and Profits from Unincorporated Businesses (percent of national income)[a]			Wage Inequality (ratio of highest to lowest earners)[b]		Gross Fixed Capital Formation (percent of GDP)		
	1960–1973	1974–1979	1980–1989	1980	1990	1960–1973	1974–1979	1980–1989
Social Democratic Political Economies								
Sweden	21	15	17	2.04	2.21	23	21	19
Norway	27	20	27	2.06	—	28	33	25
Denmark	30	24	24	2.14	2.18	24	22	17
Finland	32	24	22	2.46	2.34	25	27	24
Austria	30	23	24	—	—	27	26	24
Mean	28.1	21.4	22.8	2.17	2.24	25.6	25.9	21.8
Christian Democratic Political Economies								
Belgium	34	25	29	—	2.07	22	22	18
Netherlands	32	25	29	—	2.59	24	21	20
Germany	30	23	23	2.69	2.32	25	21	21
France	32	25	24	3.24	3.06	24	24	20
Italy	41	28	40	2.94	2.80	25	24	21
Switzerland	31	38	23	—	—	28	23	25
Mean	33.3	27	28	2.95	2.56	24.4	22.4	20.8

	Operative Surplus and Profits from Unincorporated Businesses (percent of national income)[a]			Wage Inequality (ratio of highest to lowest earners)[b]		Gross Fixed Capital Formation (percent of GDP)		
	1960–1973	1974–1979	1980–1989	1980	1990	1960–1973	1974–1979	1980–1989
Liberal Anglo-Saxon Political Economies								
Canada	26	25	26	4.01	4.20	22	24	21
Ireland	31	30	33	—	—	20	26	20
Great Britain	21	24	20	2.79	3.37	18	19	17
United States	25	32	21	3.65	4.43	18	19	17
Mean	25.7	27.8	25	3.48	4.00	19.4	21.9	18.8

Source: Huber and Stephens, 1998, tab. 4.

[a]Operative surplus reflects corporate profits, including those of state enterprises; profits from unincorporated business include the earnings of self-employed persons.

[b]Ratio of earnings of the 90th percentile of workers to those of the 10th percentile of workers.

Table 6.7. Infant Mortality, 1960–1996.

	Deaths per 1,000 Live Births				
	1960	1970	1980	1990	1996
Social Democratic Political Economies					
Austria	37.5	25.9	14.3	7.8	5.1
Sweden	16.6	11.0	6.9	6.0	4.0
Denmark	21.5	14.2	8.4	7.5	5.2
Norway	18.9	12.7	8.1	7.0	4.0
Finland	21.0	13.2	7.6	5.6	4.0
Mean	23.1	15.4	9.1	6.8	4.5
Christian Democratic Political Economies					
Belgium	31.2	21.1	12.1	8.0	6.0
Germany	33.8	23.6	12.6	7.0	5.0
Netherlands	17.9	12.7	8.6	7.1	5.2
France	27.4	18.2	10.0	7.3	4.9
Italy	43.9	29.6	14.6	8.2	5.8
Switzerland	21.1	15.1	9.1	6.8	4.7
Mean	29.2	20.1	11.2	7.4	5.3
Liberal Anglo-Saxon Political Economies					
United Kingdom	22.5	18.5	12.1	7.9	6.1
Ireland	29.3	19.5	11.1	8.2	5.5
United States	26.0	20.0	12.6	9.2	7.8
Canada	27.3	18.8	10.4	6.8	6.0
Mean	26.3	19.2	11.6	8.0	6.4
Former Fascist Dictatorships					
Spain	43.7	26.3	12.3	7.6	5.0
Portugal	77.5	55.1	24.3	11.0	6.9
Greece	40.1	29.6	17.9	9.7	7.3
Mean	53.8	37.0	18.2	9.4	6.4

Source: Organization for Economic Cooperation and Development, 1998b.

Table 6.8. The Overburdening of Families and Women.

	Percentage of Elders Living with Children	Percentage of Adolescents Living with Parents	Weekly Hours of Household Work Done by Women
Northern European Countries			
Denmark	4	8	24.6
Norway	11	—	31.6
Sweden	5	—	34.2
Southern European Countries			
Italy	39	81	45.4
Spain	37	63	45.8
Other Countries			
United States	15	28	31.9
Great Britain	16	35	30.0
Japan	65	—	33.0

Source: Adapted from Esping-Andersen, 1999, tab. 4.3.

The relatively large social expenditures in the Christian democratic countries have required relatively large fiscal revenues (41.8 percent of GDP), lower than in the social democratic countries (48.8 percent of GDP) but much higher than in the liberal countries (36.5 percent of GDP).

The labor movement in the Christian democratic countries has been weaker than that in the social democratic countries, which explains the following situations. First, income derived from capital represented a much larger percentage of the national accounts than in the social democratic countries (Table 6.6). Second, unemployment was higher than in the social democratic countries for most of the years 1960–1995 (Table 6.4). Third, wage disparities were larger than in the social democratic countries (Table 6.6). And fourth, the redistributive effect of the state was lower than in the social democratic countries (Table 6.1). Poverty in general and among children was also greater in Christian democratic than in social democratic countries. These are the causes of the greater household income inequalities (Table 6.5) and higher infant mortality (Table 6.7) in the Christian democratic countries.

Former Fascist Dictatorships in
Southern European Countries (1945–1975)

In this group of countries (Spain, Greece, and Portugal), fascist regimes governed for the entire 1945–1980 period or for most of that time. These were class dictatorships against the working and popular classes. There has been interest recently in defining such regimes as *caudillistas,* regimes based on the personal power of a *caudillo* or clan, rejecting their class character. However, an analysis of the nature of the state in these three countries during that period, of its repressive nature and its social and fiscal policies, reveals its class character. Fascism was a class response by the land-based oligarchies and other sectors of capital, including financial capital, to the threat posed by the growing power of the working class, expressed through democratic institutions—which those dictatorships disrupted. The class character of the fascist regimes was clearly evident in (a) the highly repressive nature of the states, a repression directed primarily at the working class; (b) the most regressive fiscal policies in existence in Europe at that time; and (c) the underdeveloped welfare states. In Spain in 1960, for example, public expenditures on health and education amounted to only 60 percent of the spending on the armed police forces (United Nations Development Programme, 1992). And in 1980, social expenditures in Spain (9 percent of GDP) were much lower than those in the Christian democratic countries (21.6 percent of GDP). During the fascist periods, the public medical care expenditures and the level of public medical care coverage were the lowest among the countries under study. And the percentage of the working population employed in service (2.6 percent) was much lower than in the Christian democratic (6.2 percent) and social democratic (13.2 percent) countries.

It was in the former fascist countries that labor was weakest. While much has been done since the democracies have been established (primarily by social democratic parties) to correct the underdevelopment of the welfare states and to reduce the large income inequalities, these countries still have the greatest income inequalities in the European Union. This results from the very large percentage represented by capital in the national accounts, the very large wage disparities, and the small redistributive effect of the state. These countries were heavily influenced by Catholic teachings that relied on women for the care of family members. They did not have supportive services for families, and poverty among children was very high. They also had high infant mortality rates during the 1945–1980 period, when they were governed by fascist regimes for the longest times. In all these countries, during the democratic periods, income inequalities have been reduced, the welfare state expanded, women's participation in the labor force expanded, and infant mortality reduced.

The Liberal Countries

This group (the United States, Canada, Ireland, and Great Britain) consists of the Anglo-Saxon countries where labor has been particularly weak and the capitalist class particularly strong. With the partial exception of Great Britain, social democratic parties have never governed at the national level (the United States and Canada) or, if they have, have done so for only short periods. These countries have been governed for the most part by parties clearly committed to a full expression of market forces, with as little interference from the state as possible. Some readers may be surprised that we have included Great Britain in this group, since the Labour Party governed for as long as 14 years in the period 1960–1980. We have done so—following the Huber and Stephens (1998) typology—because Great Britain has more similarity with this group of countries than with the Christian democratic or social democratic countries. The British welfare state, for example, is not fully universal or comprehensive—with the exception of the National Health Service (which Churchill called the jewel in the British crown)—and has a relatively low level of social expenditures. Canada also has a universal national health program. Both countries, however, share with the other liberal countries the residual and assistential nature of the welfare state. Benefits are provided based on proven financial need (means-tested programs) rather than on citizenship alone (as in social democracies) or on workers' rights (as in the Christian democracies). The liberal countries also have, after the ex-fascist countries, the lowest public expenditures on health care (Table 6.2) and (with the exception of Britain and Canada) the lowest coverage by public medical care.

In all these liberal countries, social transfers by the welfare state are supplemented by benefits acquired through the labor market through collective bargaining, with public social expenditures concentrated on the needy (need being defined by political-administrative criteria). Welfare functions are assigned to the private sector, with the state covering only the minimum. Wages tend to be low, requiring involvement of all family members in the labor force; this explains the large percentage of employed women in the liberal countries (with the exception of Ireland, whose Catholic tradition emphasizes a reliance on the family and which thus has a lower percentage of women in the labor force). The integration of women into the labor force in the liberal countries is facilitated by an extensive, privatized personal and social services sector, the size of which is made possible by very low wages and low social protection—characteristics responsible for the marked social polarization in these societies.

In the liberal countries, the market reigns supreme. Capital has the strongest influence, labor the weakest. Inequalities are largest in these countries. Income derived from capital is the largest, wage disparities the most accentuated, and the state the least redistributive (only the fascist states were less redistributive). Tables 6.5 and 6.7 show how the liberal countries have the largest income differentials and the lowest rates of improvement in infant mortality rates. This group includes the country (of those included in the study) with the highest infant mortality—the United States (Table 6.7).

CONCLUSION

The empirical information provided in this study allows several conclusions. First, political variables such as the political party in government (either alone or as a majority partner in a coalition) for longer periods of time are important in influencing a country's level of income inequalities and social inequalities and its health indicators such as infant mortality. Second, these political forces represent the interests of classes and other social forces with different interests in redistributive policies. Third, the labor movements and the social democratic parties that have governed as a majority for long periods since World War II have generally been the most committed to redistributive policies, contributing to better health indicators such as lower infant mortality rates. Fourth, and conversely, in countries with weaker labor movements and social democratic parties and stronger capitalist classes, such as the liberal Anglo-Saxon countries, there has been a weaker commitment to redistributive policies and worse health indicators. Finally, the Christian democratic parties (or conservative parties rooted in the Christian tradition) have made a compromise, with redistributive policies that are weaker than those in the social democracies but stronger than those in the liberal countries. The Christian democratic parties have emphasized the key role of the family rather than the state (as in the social democratic tradition) or the market (as in the liberal tradition) in the care of children and the elderly, overburdening families (especially women) with these tasks.

Our conclusions need to be qualified, of course. This is an introductory study. We hope it will stimulate some much needed research on the relationship between political forces and health. For instance, it would be interesting to use the typology presented here to analyze countries that, for specific periods, do not seem to fit the type; such atypicality calls for an expansion of the study to better explore its causes. Also, further study is required on the possible impact of a "dose-response" effect of the length of time a particular party was in power—that is, a possibly more direct causal relationship between time in government, either alone or in coalition, and reduction of inequalities and improvements in health. Also requiring further study are "mixed cases" in which the balance of forces within government may have had different effects on redistributive policies. Belgium and the Netherlands, for example, with conservative governments of the Christian tradition during most of the period 1945–1980, still have had large social democratic parties. This explains, in part, their different redistributive intensity within the conservative and Christian democratic tradition compared with other countries in the same group. Comparative policy studies, such as the one reported here, also need to be complemented by more traditional and equally informative case studies analyzing experiences and making evaluations country by country. These further areas of investigation could overcome some of the limitations of the present study, which cannot be resolved at this aggregate multicountry level.

We believe, however, that this study offers more than just pointers on the road to understanding the complex and highly sensitive (and extremely relevant) work on the relationship between politics, policy, and health. None other than Rudolph Virchow, one of the founders of public health, wrote that politics is "public health in the most profound sense" (Taylor and Rieger, 1985, p. 547).

The empirical information provided here already suggests we can conclude that, for those wishing to optimize the health of populations by reducing social and income inequalities, it seems advisable to support political forces such as the labor movements and social democratic parties, which have traditionally supported larger, more successful redistributive policies than have the Christian democratic or liberal parties.

References

Cereseto, S., and Waitzkin, H. "Capitalism, Socialism, and the Physical Quality of Life." *International Journal of Health Services,* 1986, *16,* 643–658.

Esping-Andersen, G. *The Social Foundations of Post-Industrial Economies.* Oxford: Oxford University Press, 1999.

Huber, E., and Stephens, J. D. "Internationalization and the Social Democratic Model: Crisis and Future Prospects." *Comparative Political Studies,* 1998, *13,* 353–397.

Huber, E., Ragin, C., and Stephens, J. D. "Comparative Welfare State Data Set." 1998. [http://www.unc.edu ~ jcsteph].

Kawachi, I, Wilkinson, R. G., and Kennedy, B. P. (eds.). *Income Distribution and Health: A Reader.* New York: New Press, 1999.

Mishel, L., Bernstein, L., and Schmitt, J. "International Comparisons." In *State of Working America, 1998–1999.* Ithaca, N.Y.: Cornell University Press, 1999.

Navarro, V. "Has Socialism Failed? Health Indicators Under Capitalism and Socialism." *Science and Society,* 1993, *57*(1), 6–30.

Navarro, V. "A Historical Review (1965–1997) of Studies on Class, Health, and Quality of Life: A Personal Account." *International Journal of Health Services,* 1998a, *28,* 389–406.

Navarro, V. "Neoliberalism, 'Globalization,' Unemployment, Inequalities, and the Welfare State." *International Journal of Health Services,* 1998b, *28,* 607–682.

Navarro, V. "The Political Economy of the Welfare State in Developed Capitalist Countries." *International Journal of Health Services,* 1999, *29,* 1–50.

Navarro, V., and Benach, J. *Health Inequalities in Spain.* Madrid: Ministry of Health and Consumer Affairs, 1996.

Organization for Economic Cooperation and Development. *OECD Data Set 1997: Main Economic Indicators: Historical Statistics, 1960–1997.* Paris: Organization for Economic Cooperation and Development, 1998a.

Organization for Economic Cooperation and Development. *OECD Health Data Set 98.* Paris: Organization for Economic Cooperation and Development, 1998b.

Smeeding, T. M. *Financial Poverty in Developed Countries: The Evidence from the Luxembourg Income Study.* Working Paper no. 155. New York: United Nations, 1997.

Taylor, R., and Rieger, A. "Medicine as Social Science: Rudolph Virchow on the Typhus Epidemic in Upper Silesia." International Journal of Health Services, 1985, *15,* 547–559.

United Nations Development Programme. *Historical Series.* New York: United Nations, 1992.

Wilkinson, R. G. *Unhealthy Societies: The Afflictions of Inequality.* London: Routledge, 1996.

CHAPTER SEVEN

Income Inequality and Mortality

Importance to Health of Individual Income, Psychosocial Environment, or Material Conditions

John W. Lynch
George Davey Smith
George A. Kaplan
James S. House

S tudies on the health effects of income inequality have generated great interest The evidence on this association between countries is mixed (see Wilkinson, 1992; Judge, 1995; Judge, Mulligan, and Benzeval, 1998; Lynch and Kaplan, 1997), but income inequality and health have been linked within the United States (Kaplan and others, 1996; Kennedy, Kawachi, and Prothrow-Stith, 1996; Kennedy and others, 1998; Lynch and others, 1998; Daly and others, 1998; Waitzman and Smith, 1998; Soobader and Le Clere, 1999), Britain (Stainstreet, Scot-Samuel, and Bellis, 1999), and Brazil (Szwarcwald and others, 1999). Questions remain over how to interpret these findings and the mechanisms involved. We discuss three interpretations of the association between income inequality and health: the individual income interpretation, the psychosocial environment interpretation, and the neo-material interpretation.

The idea for this chapter arose from a meeting of invited participants who discussed the effects of income inequality on health in June 1998 at the University of Michigan School of Public Health. The meeting was sponsored by the University of Michigan Initiative on Inequalities in Health; the Survey Research Center at the University of Michigan; the Health Institute at the New England Medical Center; the Canadian Institute for Advanced Research Population Health Program, and the Population Health Program at the University of Texas at Houston, Health Sciences Center.

Funding: James S. House was supported by a health investigator award from the Robert Wood Johnson Foundation. The other authors received no funding for this research.

We reviewed the literature through traditional and electronic means and supplemented this with correlational analyses of gross domestic product and life expectancy and of income inequality and mortality trends based on data from the World Bank (1997), the World Health Organization (1999) and two British sources (Goodman and Webb, 1994; Charlton and Murphy, 1994).

THE INDIVIDUAL INCOME INTERPRETATION

According to the individual income interpretation, aggregate-level associations between income inequality and health reflect only the individual-level association between income and health. The curvilinear relation between income and health at the individual level (Backlund, Sorlie, and Johnson, 1996; Ecob and Davey Smith, 1999) is a sufficient condition to produce health differences between populations with the same average income but different distributions of income (Lynch and Kaplan, 1997; Gravelle, 1998). This interpretation assumes that determinants of population health are completely specified as attributes of independent individuals and that health effects at the population level are merely sums of individual effects (Koopman and Lynch, 1999; Diez-Roux, 1998). In contrast, research on income inequality recognizes that there may also be important contextual determinants of health. To understand these potential multilevel effects, analyses are needed that use measures of income distribution and individual income to examine health differences across individuals and aggregated units.

In examinations of health differences among individuals, contextual health effects of income distribution have remained after adjustment for individual income in most studies (Daly and others, 1998; Kennedy and others, 1998; Waitzman and Smith, 1998; Soobader and Le Clere, 1999)—but not all (Fiscella and Franks, 1997). Not surprisingly, these studies found that individual income was more strongly related to individual differences in health than to income distribution. Only one study has examined the role of individual income and income distribution on health differences among aggregated units: Wolfson and colleagues (1999) used a simulation technique to explore the contribution of individual income to aggregate health differences. They showed that the individual mechanism explained only a modest proportion of the observed aggregate variation in mortality at the level of U.S. states.

Though empirical tests of this hypothesis indicate that the association between income and health at the individual level is important in understanding differences in health between individuals, they also indicate that individual income may be less important in understanding variation in health across aggregated units. Policies on wages, investments, and taxes help determine the extent of unequal income distribution across the population, and this distribution then influences individual incomes. The statistical adjustment for individual income reveals an important pathway linking aggregate income inequality and individual health—but it may also encourage underestimation of the overall population effects of unequal income distribution.

THE PSYCHOSOCIAL ENVIRONMENT INTERPRETATION

The psychosocial environment interpretation proposes that psychosocial factors are paramount in understanding the health effects of income inequality. Wilkinson (1996) has argued that income inequality affects health through perceptions of place in the social hierarchy based on relative position according to income. Such perceptions produce negative emotions such as shame and distrust that are translated "inside" the body into poorer health via psycho-neuro-endocrine mechanisms and stress induced behaviours such as smoking. Simultaneously, perceptions of relative position and the negative emotions they foster are translated "outside" the individual into antisocial behaviour, reduced civic participation, and less social capital and cohesion within the community. In this way, perceptions of social rank—indexed by relative income—have negative biological consequences for individuals and negative social consequences for how individuals interact. Perceptions of relative income thus link individual and social pathology.

Wilkinson's demonstration (1997) that absolute income was unrelated ($r = 0.08$) to health among developed countries has been important in staking a claim for this psychosocial theory of health inequalities. Figures 7.1 and 7.2 show the association between gross domestic product per person and life expectancy for 155 countries and for the 33 countries where gross domestic product was greater than $10,000—the cut-off used by Wilkinson. Our results, however, include data for all the countries above $10,000, not a selection of some countries in the Organisation for Economic Cooperation and Development as used by Wilkinson. The correlation between life expectancy and gross domestic product per person in the complete sample is $r = 0.51$ ($p = .003$). Thus the association between absolute income and life expectancy among wealthier countries depends on which countries are included.

For 15 developed countries with comparable income inequality data, Lynch and colleagues (2000) showed that indicators of social capital, such as trust and belonging to and volunteering for community organisations, were all much more strongly related to gross domestic product per person than to income inequality. Diener, Diener, and Diener (1995) showed that absolute income was a better predictor of subjective wellbeing than relative income, and concluded that "exposure in natural settings to others who are better off will not automatically influence one's moods in a negative way" (p. 856). In other analyses, social

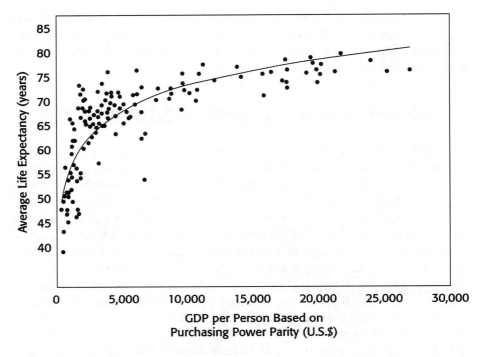

Figure 7.1. Gross Domestic Product per Person and Life Expectancy in 155 Countries, c. 1993.

World Bank, 1997; World Health Organization, 1999.

capital measured as trust and organisational membership mediated the cross-sectional association between income inequality and mortality in U.S. states (Kawachi and others, 1997). However, this association is difficult to interpret given that time series analyses of data from the same source show little decline in levels of trust, fairness, and helpfulness from the mid-1960s to 1994 (Smith, 1997). The psychosocial hypothesis would lead to the expectation that these indicators of social capital should have deteriorated during this period of unprecedented increases in income inequality. In sum then, a broader consideration of relevant research raises questions about the evidence used to exclude absolute income and material conditions, and about the evidence in favour of a mainly psychosocial interpretation of health inequalities.

We do not deny negative psychosocial consequences of income inequality, but we argue that interpretation of links between income inequality and health must begin with the structural causes of inequalities, and not just focus on perceptions of that inequality (Davey Smith, 1996; Davey Smith and Egger, 1996; Lynch and others, 2000; Muntaner and Lynch, 1999; Muntaner, Lynch, and

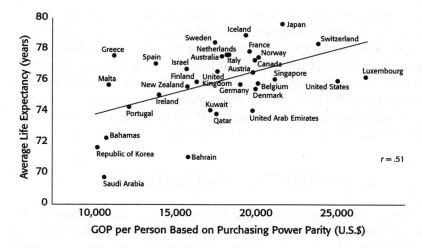

Figure 7.2. Gross Domestic Product per Person in All Thirty-Three Countries with Per Capita GDP Greater Than $10,000.

World Bank, 1997; World Health Organization, 1999.

Oates, 1999; Newman, 1999). In this regard, the psychosocial interpretation raises several areas of concern.

Firstly, it conflates the structural sources with the subjective consequences of inequality and reinforces the impression that the impact of psychosocial factors on health can be understood without reference to the material conditions that structure day to day experience (Lynch, 2000). The structural, political-economic processes that generate inequality exist before their effects are experienced at the individual level.

Secondly, it underplays the ambiguous health consequences of tightknit social networks and greater social cohesion. Strong social networks can be coercive and can be sources of strain as well as support in relationships. In some contexts, network ties function to enhance health; in others they can be detrimental (S. Kunitz, unpublished data).

Thirdly, a shallow definition of social cohesion or capital as informal social relations limits its potential relevance for public health (Lynch and others, 2000). In health research, social cohesion and capital have been discussed as horizontal social relations, ignoring the crucial role that vertical, institutional social relations (political, economic, legal) play in structuring the environments in which informal relations play out (Woolcock, 1998; Szreter, 1999; Lynch and others, 2000).

Finally, the psychosocial interpretation encourages understanding of psychosocial health effects in a vacuum. Although clearly not intended by its proponents, a decontextualised psychosocial approach can be appropriated for regressive political agendas, leading to claims that we lack the social cohesion of the past; that problems of poor and minority communities are really a result of deficits of strong social networks; and that local communities must solve their own problems. There has been little discussion of the possibility that focusing on what materially and politically disenfranchised communities can do for themselves may be akin to victim blaming at the community level that reinforces low expectations for structural change (Wainwright, 1996).

THE NEO-MATERIAL INTERPRETATION

The neo-material interpretation says that health inequalities result from the differential accumulation of exposures and experiences that have their sources in the material world. Under a neo-material interpretation, the effect of income inequality on health reflects a combination of negative exposures and lack of resources held by individuals, along with systematic underinvestment across a wide range of human, physical, health, and social infrastructure (Davey Smith, 1996; Kaplan and others, 1996; Lynch and Kaplan, 1997; Lynch and others, 1998). An unequal income distribution is one result of historical, cultural, and political-economic processes. These processes influence the private resources available to individuals and shape the nature of public infrastructure—education, health services, transportation, environmental controls, availability of food, quality of housing, occupational health regulations—that form the "neo-material" matrix of contemporary life. In the United States, higher income inequality is significantly associated with many aspects of infrastructure—unemployment, health insurance, social welfare, work disability, educational and medical expenditure, and even library books per capita (Kaplan and others, 1996).

Thus income inequality per se is but one manifestation of a cluster of neo-material conditions that affect population health. This implies that an aggregate relation between income inequality and health is not necessary—associations are contingent on the level and distribution of other aspects of social resources. If income inequality is less linked to investments in health related public infrastructure, the aggregate level association between income inequality and health may break down. In fact, recent evidence from Canada supports this view (Ross and others, 2000). This is in contrast to the psychosocial hypothesis, which implies a universal association.

Perceptions of relative position will always be present, regardless of the actual living conditions for those at the bottom of the social hierarchy. Evidence from animal studies on the role of social hierarchy itself in generating health differences has been used to support this aspect of the psychosocial hypothesis (Wilkinson,

1996). Health effects of social hierarchy in animals are, however, contingent on relations between social position and material living conditions such as availability of food, water, and space. Robert Sapolsky, an eminent primate researcher, has recently proclaimed that "it seems virtually meaningless to think about the physiological correlates of rank outside the context of a number of other modifiers—the sort of society in which the rank occurs" (1999, p. 39).

A Metaphor

To appreciate how neo-material conditions can influence health, it may be useful to consider the metaphor of airline travel. Differences in neo-material conditions between first and economy class may produce health inequalities after a long flight. First class passengers get, among other advantages such as better food and service, more space and a wider, more comfortable seat that reclines into a bed. First class passengers arrive refreshed and rested, while many in economy arrive feeling a bit rough. Under a psychosocial interpretation, these health inequalities are due to negative emotions engendered by perceptions of relative disadvantage. Under a neo-material interpretation, people in economy have worse health because they sat in a cramped space and an uncomfortable seat, and they were not able to sleep. The fact that they can see the bigger seats as they walk off the plane is not the cause of their poorer health. Under a psychosocial interpretation, these health inequalities would be reduced by abolishing first class, or perhaps by mass psychotherapy to alter perceptions of relative disadvantage. From the neo-material viewpoint, health inequalities can be reduced by upgrading conditions in economy class. Of course, this simplistic metaphor assumes that conditions in first class and economy class are independent—in the real world, improvements in economy are often resisted by those able to travel first class.

Examples from India and Britain

Cross nationally, higher levels of social expenditures—markers of neo-material conditions—are associated with greater life expectancy, lower maternal mortality, and a smaller proportion of low birthweight babies (Gough and Thomas, 1994). Thus, strategic social investment may be important in determining health differences between countries. Interpretation of health differences between and within countries should be based on a historical view of social conditions and policies. Consider, for example, the widely discussed favourable health situation in Kerala state, India (World Bank, 1996). Despite low individual income the infant mortality, maternal mortality, childhood mortality, and overall mortality in Kerala are better than in other Indian states and approach levels in richer, industrialised countries. Greater redistributive actions of the Kerala government over recent decades have been viewed as the phenomenon underlying this. It is also the case, however, that the social and cultural basis for these favourable health outcomes can be traced to over a century of social activities that have promoted greater gender equality, education, and general public investment in human resources (Kabir and Krishnan, 1996).

In Britain, income inequality increased greatly from the mid-1970s to the 1990s, but mortality in middle age and at older ages declined dramatically. Correlations between income inequality and mortality range from $r = -.76$ for men aged 55–64 to $r = -.86$ for women aged 45–54 (Figure 7.3). Understanding the rapid decline in mortality in middle age against a background of escalating income inequality in Britain may require consideration of earlier social investments. Expansion of the welfare state, educational opportunities, and introduction of the National Health Service had positive influences in early life for those cohorts in which mortality is currently declining, and social circumstances in early life can have important long term effects on later risk of death (Davey Smith and others, 1997, 1998). Such findings encourage a view that health in adulthood is the outcome of socially patterned processes acting across the entire life course (Lynch, Kaplan, and Salonen, 1997). This perspective would lead to attention being paid to how income inequality—and the broader social processes which income inequality indexes—influences health across the life course of successive cohorts. In several countries, the burden of increased income inequality has fallen disproportionately on poor households containing young children, and this may lead to poor health outcomes in the future (Lynch and Kaplan, 2000; Lynch, Kaplan, and Salonen, 1997; Davey Smith and others, 1997, 1998).

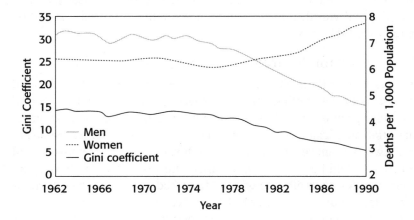

Figure 7.3. Income Inequality and Mortality in Men and Women Aged 45–54 in Britain, 1962–1990.

Lynch and Kaplan, 2000; Lynch, Kaplan, and Salonen, 1997; Davey Smith and others, 1997, 1998; Goodman and Webb, 1994; Charlton and Murphy, 1994.

CONCLUSIONS

A combination of the individual income and neo-material interpretations is a better fit to the available evidence on income inequality and health, is more comprehensive, and has greater potential to inform interventions that advance public health and reduce inequalities. The psychosocial environment interpretation focuses attention on aspects of personal psychological functioning such as trust, respect, and support. It is hard to understand how this emphasis on psychological functioning and informal interpersonal relations would serve as a basis for a public policy agenda to reduce health inequalities. The neo-material interpretation is an explicit recognition that the political and economic processes that generate income inequality influence individual resources and also have an impact on public resources such as schooling, health care, social welfare, and working conditions. It is strategic investments in neo-material conditions via more equitable distribution of public and private resources that are likely to have the most impact on reducing health inequalities and improving public health in both rich and poor countries in the 21st century.

References

Backlund, E., Sorlie, P. D., and Johnson, N. J. "The Shape of the Relationship Between Income and Mortality in the United States: Evidence from the National Longitudinal Mortality Study." *Annals of Epidemiology,* 1996, *6,* 1–9.

Charlton, J., and Murphy, M. *The Health of Adult Britain, 1841–1994.* London: Stationery Office, 1994.

Daly, M., and others. "Macro-to-Micro Linkages in the Inequality-Mortality Relationship." *Milbank Quarterly,* 1998, *76,* 315–339.

Davey Smith, G. "Income Inequality and Mortality. Why Are They Related? Income Inequality Goes Hand in Hand with Underinvestment in Human Resources." *British Medical Journal,* 1996, *312,* 987–988.

Davey Smith, G., and Egger, M. "Commentary: Understanding It All—Health, Meta-Theories, and Mortality Trends." *British Medical Journal,* 1996, *313,* 1584–1585.

Davey Smith, G., and others. "Lifetime Socioeconomic Position and Mortality: Prospective Observational Study." *British Medical Journal,* 1997, *314,* 547–552.

Davey Smith, G., and others. "Adverse Socioeconomic Circumstances in Childhood and Mortality: Prospective Observational Study." *British Medical Journal,* 1998, *316,* 1631–1635.

Diener, E., Diener, M., and Diener, C. "Factors Predicting the Subjective Well-Being of Nations." *Journal of Personality and Social Psychology,* 1995, *69,* 851–864.

Diez-Roux, A. V. "Bringing Context Back into Epidemiology: Variables and Fallacies in Multilevel Analysis." *American Journal of Public Health,* 1998, *88,* 216–222.

Ecob, R., and Davey Smith, G. "Income and Health: What Is the Nature of the Relationship?" *Social Science and Medicine*, 1999, *48*, 693–705.

Fiscella, K., and Franks, P. "Poverty or Income Inequality as Predictor of Mortality: Longitudinal Cohort Study." *British Medical Journal*, 1997, *314*, 1724–1727.

Goodman, A., and Webb, S. *For Richer, for Poorer: The Changing Distribution of Income in the UK*. London: Institute for Fiscal Studies, 1994.

Gough, I., and Thomas, T. "Why Do Levels of Human Welfare Vary Among Nations?" *International Journal of Health Services*, 1994, *24*, 715–748.

Gravelle, H. "How Much of the Relation Between Population Mortality and Unequal Distribution of Income Is a Statistical Artefact?" *British Medical Journal*, 1998, *316*, 382–385.

Judge, K. "Income Distribution and Life Expectancy. A Critical Appraisal." *British Medical Journal*, 1995, *311*, 1282–1285.

Judge, K., Mulligan, J., and Benzeval, M. "Income Inequality and Population Health." *Social Science and Medicine*, 1998, *46*, 567–579.

Kabir, M., and Krishnan, T. N. "Social Intermediation and Health Change: Lessons from Kerala." In M. Das Gupta, L. C. Chen, and T. N. Krishnan (eds.), *Health, Poverty and Development in India*. Delhi: Oxford University Press, 1996.

Kaplan, G. A., and others. "Inequality in Income and Mortality in the United States: Analysis of Mortality and Potential Pathways." *British Medical Journal*, 1996, *312*, 999–1003.

Kawachi, I., and others. "Social Capital, Income Inequality, and Mortality." *American Journal of Public Health*, 1997, *87*, 1491–1499.

Kennedy, B. P., Kawachi, I., and Prothrow-Stith, D. "Income Distribution and Mortality: Cross-Sectional Ecological Study of the Robin Hood Index in the United States." *British Medical Journal*, 1996, *312*, 1004–1007.

Kennedy, B. P., and others. "Income Distribution, Socioeconomic Status, and Self-Rated Health in the United States: Multilevel Analysis." *British Medical Journal*, 1998, *317*, 917–921.

Koopman, J. S., and Lynch, J. W. "Individual Causal Models and Population Systems Models in Epidemiology." *American Journal of Public Health*, 1999, *89*, 1170–1175.

Lynch, J. W. "Income Inequality and Health: Expanding the Debate." *Social Science and Medicine*, 2000, *51*, 1001–1005.

Lynch, J. W., and Kaplan, G. A. "Understanding How Inequality in the Distribution of Income Affects Health." *Journal of Health Psychology*, 1997, *2*, 97–314.

Lynch, J. W., and Kaplan, G. A. "Socioeconomic Position." In L. F. Berkman and I. Kawachi (eds.), *Social Epidemiology*. New York: Oxford University Press, 2000.

Lynch, J. W., Kaplan, G. A., and Salonen, J. T. "Why Do Poor People Behave Poorly? Variations in Adult Health Behaviour and Psychosocial Characteristics, by Stage of the Socio-Economic Lifecourse." *Social Science and Medicine*, 1997, *44*, 809–820.

Lynch, J. W., and others. "Income Inequality and Mortality in Metropolitan Areas of the United States." *American Journal of Public Health*, 1998, *88*, 1074–1080.

Lynch, J. W., and others. "Social Capital—Is It a Good Investment Strategy for Public Health?" *Journal of Epidemiology and Community Health*, 2000, *54*, 404–408.

Muntaner, C., and Lynch, J. W. "Income Inequality and Social Cohesion Versus Class Relations: A Critique of Wilkinson's Neo-Durkheimian Research Program." *International Journal of Health Services*, 1999, *29*, 59–81.

Muntaner, C., Lynch, J. W., and Oates, G. "The Social Class Determinants of Income Inequality and Social Cohesion." *International Journal of Health Services*, 1999, *29*, 699–732.

Newman, K. S. *No Shame in My Game: The Working Poor in the Inner City.* New York: Knopf, 1999.

Ross, N. A., and others. "Relation Between Income Inequality and Mortality in Canada and in the United States: Cross-Sectional Assessment Using Census Data and Vital Statistics." *British Medical Journal*, 2000, *320*, 898–902.

Sapolsky, R. M. "Hormonal Correlates of Personality and Social Contexts: From Non-Human to Human Primates." In C. Panter-Brick and C. M. Worthman (eds.), *Hormones, Health and Behavior.* New York: Cambridge University Press, 1999.

Smith, T. "Factors Relating to Misanthropy in Contemporary American Society." *Social Science Research*, 1997, *26*, 170–196.

Soobader, M.-J., and Le Clere, F. B. "Aggregation and the Measurement of Income Inequality: Effects on Morbidity." *Social Science and Medicine*, 1999, *48*, 733–744.

Stainstreet, D., Scot-Samuel, A., and Bellis, M. A. "Income Inequality and Mortality in England." *Journal of Public Health Medicine*, 1999, *21*, 205–207.

Szreter, S. "A New Political Economy for New Labour: The Importance of Social Capital." *Renewal*, 1999, *7*, 30–44.

Szwarcwald, C. L., and others. "Income Inequality and Homicide Rates in Rio de Janeiro, Brazil." *American Journal of Public Health*, 1999, *89*, 845–880.

Wainwright, D. "The Political Transformation of the Health Inequalities Debate." *Critical Social Policy*, 1996, *49*, 67–82.

Waitzman, N. J., and Smith, K. R. "Separate but Lethal: The Effects of Economic Segregation on Mortality in Metropolitan America." *Milbank Quarterly*, 1998, *76*, 341–373.

Wilkinson, R. G. "Income Distribution and Life Expectancy." *British Medical Journal*, 1992, *304*, 165–168.

Wilkinson, R. G. *Unhealthy Societies: The Afflictions of Inequality.* New York: Routledge, 1996.

Wilkinson, R. G. "Socio-Economic Determinants of Health: Health Inequalities— Relative or Absolute Material Standards?" *British Medical Journal*, 1997, *314*, 591–595.

Wolfson, M., and others. "The Relation Between Income Inequality and Mortality Is Not a Statistical Artefact." *British Medical Journal*, 1999, *319*, 953–957.

Woolcock, M. "Social Capital and Economic Development: Toward a Theoretical Synthesis and Policy Framework." *Theory and Society.* 1998, *27*, 151–208.

World Bank. *Improving Women's Health in India.* Washington, D.C.: World Bank, 1996.

World Bank. *World Bank Development Indicators.* CD-ROM. Washington D.C.: World Bank, 1997.

World Health Organization. "WHO Statistical Database." 1999. [http://www3.who.int/whosis/menu.cfm].

CHAPTER EIGHT

Zoning, Equity, and Public Health

Juliana A. Maantay

Many public health concerns are location specific and location dependent. It behooves us to consider the role of zoning as the primary planning tool that governs what goes where. Most major U.S. cities; many suburban, exurban, and even rural areas of the United States; and many other countries use zoning as their primary means of land use planning (Haar and Wolf, 1989).[1] Zoning is used to designate certain areas as "appropriate" for certain uses (separated into broad categories such as residential, commercial, institutional, and industrial), as well as to determine "appropriate" densities, building bulk, lot coverage, and a host of other factors. Zoning can also be employed to restrict or prohibit certain land uses in certain areas.

Zoning therefore determines the allowable uses to which land may be put. The uses to which land may be put, in turn, influence what environmental and human health impacts may result from the activities allowed to take place on the land. The determination of zoning, then, can have substantial ramifications for public health matters. In fact, the idea of zoning and much of the seminal public health legislation came of age at approximately the same time in many American and European cities (Platt, 1991).

The modern disciplines of public health and urban planning developed from the same roots in the late 19th century, with similar objectives, strategies, and standards. Although the fields of planning and public health diverged during the intervening century, in both theoretical focus and practical applications, it may now be timely to consider the shared roots and experiences of the two fields and return to a state of collaborative effort and awareness of each other's work. Planners need to take into account the potential public health impacts of their planning actions, and public health professionals can benefit from understanding the implications and importance of land use planning decisions in public health issues.

This chapter is based on an analysis of past and present conditions in New York City's industrial areas, as well as specific case-study industrial communities within the city (Maantay, 2000). I examined, for the four-decade period 1961 through 1998,[2] the location of the city's industrial zones[3] and where industrial zones had been increased or decreased in size.[4] I then compared these rezoned areas in terms of the proximate population's characteristics and changes over time (Adams, 1992; U.S. Bureau of the Census, 1980, 1990)[5] and examined the public policies relevant to the rezonings.[6] One goal of the study was to determine whether public policies pertaining to zoning and land use planning are inherently (if inadvertently) discriminatory regarding the disproportionate distribution of potentially noxious land uses in poorer communities and communities of color.

New York City was the nation's first municipality to adopt a comprehensive zoning ordinance, and its experiences should be relevant to many other major cities as well as other places where zoning is used.

NOXIOUS LAND USES AND ZONING

In its most basic form, zoning separates land areas into broad categories of land use—for example, residential, commercial, and industrial—with the assumption that separation of land uses promotes the public health and welfare of the population. In New York City, as in many other cities developed during 19th-century industrialization and before the advent of inexpensive public transportation, industrial neighborhoods typically contain or are adjacent to large residential populations.

Industrial areas generally carry a higher environmental burden than do purely residential neighborhoods in terms of pollution impacts and risks (Miller and de Roo, 1996). Some of these burdens include adverse air quality, noise, traffic safety, congestion, and vibrations from heavy truck traffic; use and storage of hazardous materials; emission of hazardous and toxic substances, which enter the air, soil, and water; illegal dumping of hazardous materials; proliferation of waste handling facilities; and poor enforcement of environmental regulations and inadequate response to environmental complaints. These burdens all contribute to the undesirable and unhealthy living conditions in industrial areas.

In recent years, industrial processes have been accompanied or supplanted by noxious waste-related facilities in New York City's manufacturing zones, and this situation threatens to worsen with the 2001 closing of Staten Island's Freshkills Landfill, the city's last remaining landfill. Because city residents generate approximately 13,000 tons per day of municipal solid waste, alternative management plans will undoubtedly include many additional waste transfer stations and potentially thousands of additional truck trips per day on city roads (Office of the Bronx Borough President, 1997).

Yet only certain areas are zoned to accommodate the predicted increase in waste-related facilities as well as to continue to host the existing ones. Waste-related facilities can legally be located only in manufacturing (M) zones; this requirement negates the city's attempt to achieve equitable distribution of noxious waste facilities, since M zones are not distributed evenly around the city (see Figure 8.1; New York City Department of City Planning, 1991).[7]

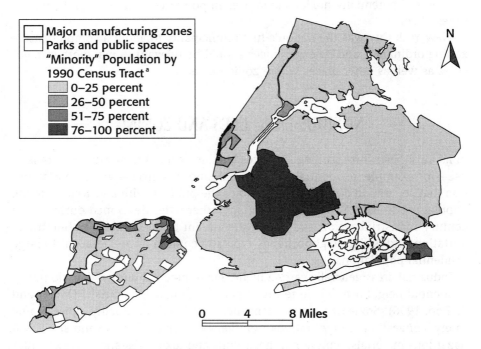

Figure 8.1. Major Manufacturing Zones and Percentage Minority Population, New York City, 1990.

Sources: Based on data from New York City Department of City Planning (1993a, 1993b) and U.S. Bureau of the Census (1990).

[a]In 1990, New York City's population was approximately 56 percent "minority."

In addition to the uneven distribution of M zones, there is the ongoing issue of zoning changes. Since the last major overhaul of the New York City zoning ordinance in 1961, there have been thousands of individual zoning map changes, many affecting M zones. These changes have enlarged M zones in some areas and decreased them in others. There have also been changes within the category "M zone" so that some zones have been changed from one type of M zone to another, with different uses permitted and restricted. In some industrial areas, M zones have not been changed at all (Maantay, 2000).

These zoning changes have ramifications for the distribution and concentration of noxious waste facilities, and therefore for health impacts on the nearby populations. How is policy made on changing zones from one type to another, and what are the potential impacts of these policies? What are the characteristics of the populations most affected by these zoning changes?

NOXIOUS LAND USES AND PUBLIC HEALTH

We would not be concerned about people living in or near industrial areas if these areas were not potentially noxious and harmful to human health. There are numerous reported cases of noxious land uses and of nearby communities' being affected by abnormally high rates of cancer and other debilitating, chronic, life-threatening, or rare diseases (Novotny, 1998).[8] These cases include such places as Triana, Alabama, which was dubbed the "unhealthiest town in America" by *National Wildlife* magazine owing to high levels of serious illness, possibly caused by DDT contamination from a nearby chemical plant (Haggerty, 1996); "Cancer Alley," a string of towns along the petrochemical refining corridor in Louisiana (Wright, Bryant, and Bullard, 1996; Costner and Thornton, 1989); Sunnyside, Arizona, where rare cancers and immune system disorders in the community may be a result of pollution caused by nearby aircraft industries (Nienaber-Clarke and Gerlak, 1998); and West Dallas, Texas, a community that has a lead smelter and several toxic waste dumps among its land uses and whose population suffers from high levels of cancer, heart disease, liver damage, and blood disorders (Robinson, 1996).

In a more urban context, the industrial area of Hunts Point–Mott Haven in the South Bronx section of New York City has one of the nation's highest rates of childhood asthma hospitalization—nearly 150% higher than that of New York City overall, and 1,000% higher than the rest of New York State (Nossiter, 1995; New York City Department of Health, 1999). Hunts Point is also home to a disproportionately high number of New York City's waste-handling facilities, including the largest wastewater sludge pelletization plant in the Northeast and, until it was forced to close in 1997, the region's largest medical waste incinerator (Maantay, 1996).

Definitive links have not been established between these land uses, the environmental burdens they impose on the nearby communities, and the health impacts borne by the communities. Although conventional wisdom and intuitive logic would suggest that there is a correlation between the high rates of respiratory illness and high levels of air pollution, there has been little research demonstrating such a correlation.

Unfortunately, it is difficult to prove a cause-and-effect relationship between noxious land uses and adverse health impacts. One reason is that there is a lack of scientific consensus on health-based standards for toxic substances. Clear data do not exist regarding the effects of exposures to many toxic substances. There are also difficulties in assessing impacts from substances that have not yet been tested, especially considering that, on average, 1500 new chemicals are introduced each year (Head, 1995). The effects of distance on toxicity are not well documented, either: "Little is known about the relationship between distance from a pollution source, such as a hazardous waste site, and actual health risks. . . . Accurate estimation of human exposures to hazardous air pollutants across all levels of geographic aggregation is constrained by the paucity of suitable monitoring methods, relevant ambient measures, and validated models for predicting exposures to populations of interest" (Perlin and others, 1995, pp. 70, 71).

Another factor is the difficulty in assessing cumulative and synergistic impacts of various chemicals emitted together or in close proximity. Exposure and risk from each toxic substance is evaluated separately, because there are different thresholds and measurement techniques for each. However, chemicals can combine to create synergistic impacts that are more deadly than the impacts of individual substances, and this is not taken into account in traditional risk assessments.

There are also uncertainties in assessing the impacts of substances emitted through different media pathways, such as air, water, and soil, and whether exposure to humans occurs through ingestion, inhalation, or dermal contact. There are significant uncertainties when we try to model exposures and outcomes, since the relationship between emissions and exposures is poorly understood. The correlation between exposure dose (ambient levels), body dose (amount inhaled or ingested), and target dose (amount reaching a sensitive organ) is affected by many variables that may not be well understood and may be difficult to model (Regeski, 1993).

Even for many substances for which there are standards, the thresholds are set for harm to the average individual, not the most vulnerable members of the community, such as young children, the elderly, pregnant women, or persons with compromised immune systems (Commoner, 1989). In many poorer communities and communities of color, it is precisely the preponderance of such individuals that makes the community so disproportionately burdened.

A mundane but very real drawback in impact assessment is the lack of reliable measurements of actual emissions. Since most regulated polluters are responsible for reporting their own toxic emissions, these measurements are notoriously inaccurate, and of course they do not take into account the emissions of the many nearby unregulated polluters (Hearne, 1996; Maantay and others, 1997).

Some of the problems involved in correlating public health impacts and the environmental effects of noxious land uses are summarized by Head (1995, p. 48):

> Current criteria for potential causal relationships are based on complicated assumptions and assessments of available data, because, as explained the absolute cause-and-effect relationship is often difficult to establish. Hence, scientists may seek data associations that suggest a correlation as the basis for inferring a causal relationship. It is interesting to note that this absolute relationship of causality may have been less of a factor when combating past public health epidemics than in current efforts related to investigating and responding to environmentally induced diseases. In those past epidemics, unequivocal cause and effect was not necessarily determined prior to action being taken to mitigate the disease (e.g., malaria).

Additionally, in many cases where an association between noxious land uses and adverse health impacts was suspected, a formal health study of the affected community was never conducted. For instance, in Texarkana, Arkansas, several federal agencies (such as the Environmental Protection Agency, the Agency for Toxic Substances and Disease Registry, and the Department of the Interior) issued reports admitting that there were severe health risks to the people living near a former wood-treatment facility. Although people were suffering from rare cancers and otherwise unexplained diseases, no public health survey was undertaken (Oliver, 1996). In most of these cases, the public health linkages remain inconclusive in terms of strict scientific proof.

With noxious land uses and environmental burdens, exposures are uncertain and risks cannot be definitively determined; therefore, health outcomes are hypothetical. The question is, should this lack of absolute certainty prevent public health action on behalf of the populations most likely to be affected by noxious land uses and zoning decisions about industrial districts?

WHY DO WE HAVE ZONING?

Zoning began as an attempt to control land use in order to protect the health, lives, safety, morals, properties, and welfare of the population within an existing constitutional framework of the state's police powers. These police powers are upheld by the courts only when such powers pass tests of reasonableness and when they are clearly related to the general interest of the community as a whole (Freund, 1904; Bassett, 1936; Plotkin, 1987). Zoning case law varies widely in how "the general interest" is interpreted. "The myth begins with the assumption that there is an objective reference for the concept of what is best" (Mandelker, 1971, p. 14). The goals of public protection have been interpreted according to the policymakers' standards and the values of the day, and they have changed and increased over time. In general, zoning ordinances do not specify a definition of public welfare. Each government is free to determine the limits to public welfare and exactly who constitutes the public that is being protected.

Zoning separates land uses from each other, as adjacency and mixture of disparate uses were seen as detrimental. In addition to zoning's public health purpose, early planning documents overtly stated that the reason for zoning was to protect private property, and "private property" was generally understood to refer to the "better" residential and commercial properties (Makielski, 1966).

It can also be said that the purpose of zoning is to prevent change, or at least to seriously retard change, so as to make real estate investment a more predictable and less risky endeavor and therefore more profitable in the long run. Encouragement of stability in the real estate industry was seen by policymakers to be beneficial to the general public (Perin, 1977; Weaver and Babcock, 1979).

Other zoning experts have argued that zoning is not a control but a "thermometer" that measures the amount of economic heat on a property: as the heat goes up, zoning responds by changing. In other words, zoning is the result of economic and real estate market conditions and trends, rather than the result of a well-considered comprehensive plan, as is considered proper planning practice. According to some observers, real estate speculation and profit seeking are actually driving the American planning process (Bryant, 1968; Siegan, 1972).

Babcock, in his 1966 book *The Zoning Game,* speculated on the purposes of zoning: "These [purposes] may vary from a fear of 'Negro infiltration' to a vague identification of zoning with 'good government.' To most real estate brokers, and to some land economists, lawyers, and judges, zoning is a means of maximizing the value of property. . . . I suppose what really disturbs me is that because zoning is the most universal of the legal tools for shaping the character of the municipality, any unwise use of the process has a far greater impact upon our national character than does the abuse of a less widely employed device" (pp. 116, 124).

THE NATION'S FIRST COMPREHENSIVE
ZONING ORDINANCE: NEW YORK CITY

New York City has a long history of legislating land use for public health purposes. As early as 1664, only a few decades after the first permanent European settlement in this area, New York City had adopted land use laws designed for the protection of public health, such as the prohibition of tanneries and tallow makers in the densely settled parts of the city. City officials believed these activities were noxious and potentially injurious to human life and, perhaps more important, injurious to property and property values. Other acts throughout the 17th and 18th centuries further restricted noxious land uses, for example, by prohibiting distilleries and slaughterhouses in heavily populated areas of the city. Comprehensive building codes, tenement house laws, and sanitary and public health regulations of the 19th century helped make both laypeople and government officials more receptive to the promulgation of universally restrictive land use controls and environmental regulations in the 20th century (Citizens' Association of New York, [1866] 1970; De Forest and Veiller, 1903; Ford, 1936; Lubove, 1962; Plunz, 1983).

In 1916, New York City was the first municipality in the nation to adopt a comprehensive zoning ordinance. Other cities had instituted laws that could be considered protozoning ordinances, including restrictions on building height in Boston and the prohibition of certain land uses, such as brick kilns, within the city limits of Los Angeles (Haar and Wolf, 1989). But New York City was the first to create a zoning ordinance that regulated land use, building height, bulk, and density for every property within the city.

The main impetus for the 1916 Zoning Resolution was the desire to protect property values for certain types of landowners, thus protecting public welfare, since real estate values were seen as critical to the success of the whole city's economy. The push for zoning in New York City was spearheaded by a strange coalition of groups. The Fifth Avenue Association was a group of owners of exclusive shops catering to the wealthy; its members feared what the encroachment of manufacturing lofts and the immigrant workforce might do to the value of their properties and to their profits from retail trade. They wanted zoning to protect them by giving them an exclusive zone closed to industry.

Another group of zoning advocates consisted of property owners in the Wall Street area, who feared reductions in property values and rent profits owing to the loss of light and air from adjacent overbuilt skyscrapers. The huge bulk and resultant seven-acre shadow of the Equitable Building, constructed in 1913 at 120 Broadway, had made property owners in the area aware of the financial impacts that a lack of land use controls could have on their properties. And then there were the good-government types, public health advocates, and reformers who wanted zoning for the same reasons they had wanted tenement building codes, sanitary infrastructure investment, and worker safety laws: to improve the lives of everyday people (Toll, 1969; Willis, 1993).

The 1916 Zoning Resolution divided the city into commercial zones, residential zones, and unrestricted zones where nearly any land use could go (Committee on City Planning, 1913; Board of Estimate and Apportionment, 1916). Since New York City's existing industrial areas usually included residential enclaves or contiguous residential areas, these unrestricted zones had significant residential populations. These populations gained little protection from the new zoning resolution compared with the people in the officially designated residential zones, which were the city's more exclusive and affluent neighborhoods.

New York City revamped its entire zoning apparatus in 1961, creating three broad use categories—residential (R), commercial (C), and manufacturing (M)—and eliminating the unrestricted category implemented in 1916 (*Plan for Re-Zoning*, 1950; New York City Department of City Planning, 1961). This approach required a determination of existing predominant land use for each part of the city so that planners could assign the most appropriate of the three zones to each area. This was especially difficult in the old unrestricted zones that had permitted residential uses to exist side by side with industry. Residential, commercial, and industrial uses were supposed to be in separate zones, and the planners anticipated that the nonconforming uses would in time disappear; however, in many neighborhoods both industry and residential uses remained (*Zoning New York City*, 1958; New York City Department of City Planning, 1969). The result is that most industrial zones in New York still have rather large residential communities within or surrounding them.

A BRIEF HISTORY OF INDUSTRIAL NEIGHBORHOODS IN NEW YORK CITY

There are 58 major industrially zoned districts in New York City (New York City Department of City Planning, 1993a). According to the 1990 census, approximately 22% of New York City population lives in census tracts that are within these M zones (Maantay, 2000). Many of these industrial districts have existed since the 19th century, when New York City was the nation's most important port (Albion, 1939) and most of the city's industrial areas are on the waterfront (Buttenwieser, 1987). Because of historic settlement patterns, many industrial districts developed with worker housing within walking distance (Blackmar, 1989). Therefore, most industrial districts were essentially mixed-use areas, combining manufacturing activities with residential uses.

By the second half of the 20th century, new industrial enterprises were choosing not to locate in central cities, owing to changes in manufacturing technology, transportation, and demographics (New York City Department of City Planning, 1993b; Hoover and Vernon, 1959; Castells and Hall, 1994). New York City, like many U.S. cities, was entering a period of deindustrialization. This process was exacerbated by the decline of the city's port activities as a result of containerization and relocation of the port to New Jersey. New York City has lost hundreds of thousands of manufacturing and port-related jobs since the 1960s (O'Neill and Moss, 1991).

Industrial areas and their nearby residential communities were profoundly affected by this decline of industry and job loss. Historically, the populations of these communities had been predominantly working-class and employed by local industries. As industry left the city in the 1960s and 1970s, these areas became the repositories of noxious waste–related uses without the benefit of viable industries' providing jobs for local residents. At the same time, other planning policies and private sector decisions intensified the deleterious impacts to industrial areas. Large-scale public housing projects, urban renewal areas, and highway projects were often located in or near industrial areas, furthering the downward spiral of neglect and decline. Considerable private disinvestment usually accompanied these planning efforts, to the further detriment of these communities (Fitch, 1993; Caro, 1974).

As manufacturing activities diminished in industrial areas, both private and public waste-related facilities proliferated.[9] The substitution of waste facilities— private solid waste transfer stations, marine transfer stations, wastewater treatment plants, combined sewer overflow outfalls, sludge treatment facilities, recycled materials handling facilities, junkyards, auto salvage yards, scrap metal and construction debris processing facilities, and medical waste disposal plants— for viable manufacturing furthers the impression that these communities are being disproportionately "dumped on." The fact that the neighborhoods most affected by waste facilities are poorer and with a higher percentage of minority people[10] and immigrants than the city average means that the health burden of the city's waste problem falls on this already more vulnerable population.

EQUITY ISSUES IN ZONING

Ironically, zoning, which was intended to protect the public health, safety, and welfare, has often proved to be exclusionary, offering differential protection to different segments of the public. Indeed, as many see it, the original purpose of zoning in this country was to promote exclusion. Some early zoning ordinances, such as San Francisco's 1885 prohibition against laundries in residential areas, were blatant attempts to prevent Chinese people from living in White neighborhoods (Shenkel, 1972). One of the main purposes of New York City's 1916 Zoning Resolution was to keep the factory worker rabble away from the wealthy ladies shopping on Fifth Avenue by creating an exclusive zone for the "better" commercial and residential uses.

For the most part, the courts have upheld municipalities' right to craft their own zoning ordinances in the way that serves their community best and to define the public welfare for their own jurisdictions as they see fit; however, several important legal battles have been won by groups claiming racial and economic discrimination resulting from exclusionary zoning ordinances. The best-known instance was the landmark 1974 New Jersey State Supreme Court case *Southern Burlington County NAACP* v *Township of Mount Laurel, N.J.* The town's zoning and other land use regulations had made it physically and economically impossible to provide low- and moderate-income housing in the municipality, thereby excluding low- and moderate-income people from living within the confines of the town (Haar and Wolf, 1989).

In the 1960s and 1970s, it was widely acknowledged by zoning experts that many zoning ordinances are discriminatory: by requiring minimum lot sizes and house sizes, specifying allowable housing types and construction materials, and even specifying minimum dollar values, such ordinances keep out lower-income people and maintain community homogeneity (Elias, 1974; Lauber, 1974; National Committee Against Discrimination, 1974; Williams and Norman, 1974; Perin, 1977). In many cases, the effort to keep out lower-income people was directed at minorities, primarily African Americans, as opposed to poor White people (Branfman, Cohen, and Trubek, 1974).

Thus, zoning has limited the choices of certain groups as to where they can live, often relegating poor and discriminated-against people to the least desirable locations. In addition, rezoning an area where such people already live to permit heavier industrial uses or noxious nonmanufacturing uses can further degrade the area and have adverse impacts on the people who live there.

REZONING INDUSTRIAL AREAS

New York City has rezoned a substantial portion of its industrial land since 1961, mainly from manufacturing uses to other uses.[11] There were 409 zoning changes affecting industrial districts from 1961 through 1998, and for every two changes from nonmanufacturing uses to manufacturing uses, there were about three changes in the opposite direction. The city was rezoning *from* M zones much more than it was rezoning *to* M zones.

Approximately 20% of the total changes to industrial zones can be classified as large (affecting four to ten square blocks) or very large (more than ten square blocks). Of these 82 changes, 60 resulted in major decreases to M zones and 22 resulted in major increases to M zones, again indicating that the city was more interested in promoting new uses for zones previously designated M zones than in increasing the number of M zones overall. The Bronx, the city's least affluent borough, had the largest number of major increases and the fewest major decreases to M zones. Manhattan, the city's most affluent borough, had the fewest major increases and the largest number of major decreases to M zones.

The inventory and mapping of the rezoning activities indicated that there was not only a disparity between the number of actions resulting in M zone decreases and the number resulting in increases, but also a disparity in where and when these changes occurred. Some boroughs had experienced few or no major increases in M zones since the late 1960s, while others had undergone relatively few M zone decreases (Maantay, 2000).

RACE, CLASS, AND HOME OWNERSHIP IN INDUSTRIAL ZONES AND REZONED NEIGHBORHOODS

Nearly one quarter of New Yorkers live in census tracts within major M zones.[12] What are the characteristics of these people? In each decade between 1961 and 1998, major M zones in New York City generally had a higher percentage of minority populations than borough or city averages, except in Manhattan, where the percentage of minorities living within M zones has dropped each decade in relation to borough averages. M zones also generally contain people with lower than average incomes and rates of home ownership.

In general, the city was rezoning to increase M zones in areas with higher than average minority populations, lower than average incomes, and lower than average rates of home ownership. Conversely, the city was rezoning to decrease M zones in areas with lower than average minority populations, higher than average incomes, and higher than average rates of home ownership. Years after rezoning, the affected areas were often even more divergent from city, borough, and M-zone averages with regard to income, percentage minority population, and home ownership rates.

A detailed analysis of land use maps from 1956 through 1990 revealed that in industrial areas where M zones were increased or recategorized as "heavier" industrial zones, industrial uses had increased in concentration in the years after the rezoning. Conversely, in industrial areas where M zones were decreased or recategorized as "lighter" industrial zones, industrial uses had decreased in the years after the rezoning.

PLANNING FOR ZONING CHANGES

The zoning change applications and other documents state the ostensible planning rationales for proposing areas for rezoning. For instance, "marginal" or "deteriorated" residential neighborhoods were considered more appropriate for rezoning to industrial use than "stable" communities that have been "maintained." Sometimes "market forces" or "market pressures" were cited as reasons for decreasing M zones, along with evidence that the proposed zoning change reflected conformance with existing (if illegal) conditions.[13] Thus, a zoning change can contribute to neighborhood transformation in either of two ways: it provides the mechanism to facilitate or jump-start the change, or it legitimizes the change that is already under way, encouraging the trend to continue.

THE ZONING PROCESS AND THE PUBLIC

New York City has developed an elaborate and extensive procedure to enable public participation in certain planning activities, and these participation opportunities are theoretically available to all residents and all communities equally. However, there are great disparities in how successful various communities are in influencing the outcomes of planning decisions. Anecdotal evidence suggests that political power, relative affluence, and property-owner status all affect the amount of influence wielded by a particular community. There are few forums for proactive community planning, and there is nothing within the formal public participation process that requires the city to act on the community's advice. Thus, the status quo is generally maintained. And the status quo seems to be that M zones, which are typically neighborhoods that are poorer than average and with a higher percentage of minorities and renters than average, get "dumped on," with very little recourse in the formal structure of decision making.

The land use attorneys Kintish and Shapiro (1993) make some interesting observations about the relationship between the level of enforcement efforts and the level of affluence and influence of various communities in New York City, as well as the level of effectiveness of public participation. They mention the Bathgate industrial district in the Bronx as an example.

> Enforcement problems compound the issue: zoning regulations only work if there is an ability and will to enforce them. In neighborhoods where well-organized, well-informed, and well-connected community groups demand enforcement, zoning and other rules tend to be enforced. In more troubled neighborhoods, residents tend to be less influential, they are less likely to be familiar with city regulations, and they often view public officials with mistrust. Consequently, the city is less likely to express concern about violations to industrial performance standards in these areas. Similarly, in such neighborhoods, the city is more likely to ignore abandoned cars or sweatshops and is less likely to determine that an environmental impact statement is required for a proposal project. For example, no EIS [environmental impact statement] was prepared when the city established the Bathgate Industrial Park in what had been a residentially zoned portion of the South Bronx [p. 174].

It should also be noted that rezoning an area is costly in both time and money, thus making market forces an even more likely influence on rezoning efforts.

IS ZONING EQUITABLE?

After looking at the general issue of equity in zoning, researching the particular case of New York City, and analyzing the data, we are left trying to answer the question, Is zoning equitable? Zoning, as a body of law, is supposed to be applied and enforced so as to protect all portions of the population equally. Other studies have determined that many environmental laws are applied and enforced differentially depending on the characteristics of the affected populations, with facilities in poor and minority communities subject to less rigorous enforcement and less stringent penalties for noncompliance than facilities in predominantly White communities (Lavelle and Coyle, 1992; Bullard, 1994). Do New York City's zoning regulations succumb to this unfortunate predilection? Does zoning protect some areas, and therefore some people, better than it does others? Some quotes from the zoning experts interviewed for this study:[14]

> No question that zoning protects some people better than others. Zoning is responsive to wealth, property, political power, and those areas or communities that are more politically empowered or connected clearly will be able to get done the zoning changes that they desire and to prevent the zoning changes they don't desire. Less politically or economically empowered communities, even though you have a formal structure [for public participation], will be less able to impact on changes that are taking place to them or around them. (ZI 6)

> Of course zoning doesn't protect equally—but this is just part and parcel of our negative attitudes towards both industry and poor people. Zoning segregates not just land use, but also people. Zoning protects areas of home ownership. It protects areas of higher land values. These areas need to be protected because, reading between the lines, these are presumably the people who need and deserve to be most protected. (ZI 1)

> Zoning, which looks like a very egalitarian system, really isn't. The critical element being enforcement. In pre-1961 zoning, 60 to 70 percent of the city was unrestricted zones, they didn't impose rules on things. . . . [Today] there are no unrestricted zones—every zone is subject to enforcement under zoning laws, building laws, noise laws, environmental laws, etc. But in fact, these laws are only enforced in areas where people have the clout to make the complaints count. When you look at those areas and you overlay them against the rest of the city, you may come up with the same ratios as you had in 1930, when you had 60 to 70 percent of the city in unrestricted zones in terms of use. Areas of low enforcement today correspond to the old unrestricted areas. So maybe there was less hypocrisy in governing land use then. We have this fiction of zoning protecting everyone equally. (ZI 5)

It is often argued that these effects are unintentional and coincidental, but even if coincidence is assumed:

> [a] society that allows such a pattern of coincidence to persist has failed to equally protect its citizens. This failure, itself, constitutes an environmental injustice. . . . Whether the result of overt or covert racism, putting economic profits over the health of people, or benign neglect, this disproportionate risk can and does lead to disastrous results. An injustice exists even if it is merely a coincidence that
>
> - the food, air, and water that people of color and those who are poor consume are more contaminated;
> - nonwhite workers are 50 percent more likely to be exposed to hazards in the workplace; and
> - hazardous waste facilities are located disproportionately in communities where people of color and the poor live [White, 1998, p. 75].

THE IMPLICATIONS OF ZONING CHANGES

Understanding the zoning change process is important because zoning changes can have a significant effect on neighborhoods and neighborhood health. A land use planning tool that governs where things may go should come under more scrutiny than it has. Zoning is the gatekeeper in terms of noxious uses and therefore requires comprehensive, rather than piecemeal, planning. The zoning change process should take into account that a zoning change in one part of the city may have far-reaching consequences for other parts of the city. For instance, reducing industrial zones in the Lower West Side of Manhattan (SoHo, Tribeca, and the Far West Village neighborhoods) in the late 1960s and 1970s was not isolated from the need to increase industrial zones in the South Bronx in the late 1970s and early 1980s. Neither was the reduction of Manhattan's industrial zones isolated from the increasing intensification of industrial land use in other industrial parts of the city.

It is not possible to isolate the effects of the city's land use policies from the many other factors affecting the demographic makeup, economic status, and land use conditions of particular neighborhoods. However, although the results of rezoning may be unintentional, zoning changes and associated city policies are reducing some people's quality of life and improving that of others, while undermining the ideal of equal protection under the law of zoning.

Zoning is not a benign or neutral process. Decisions about the best locations for noxious uses have racial and classist implications, since industrial zones are the only places in New York City where noxious uses can be located and the people living in and near industrial zones have a much higher than average likelihood of being poor and minority. Zoning tends to concentrate noxious uses in poor and minority industrial neighborhoods as more affluent industrial neighborhoods with lower minority populations are rezoned to other uses.

As long as "market forces" govern zoning, and therefore planning, the concentration of noxious uses in poor neighborhoods is inevitable. When planning tries to address quality-of-life issues in low-income populations, this concentration is less inevitable.

NOT IN ANYBODY'S BACKYARD

The problem of the disproportionate distribution of noxious land uses is not just a siting issue: it is not just about distributing unwanted land uses more evenly or equitably, but about eliminating or reducing the need for these noxious uses. "Not in my backyard" must become "not in anybody's backyard": "the not-in-anybody's-backyard stand forces the debate away from the suitability [or fairness] of specific waste treatment facilities or locations, and toward a more fundamental reassessment of the propriety of a production system under private control where, in the quest for profit, the public is exposed to known risks" (Heiman, 1990, p. 351).

By taking a not-in-anybody's-backyard stand against locally unwanted land uses, we change the debate from an either-or debate—either a technical siting solution for a hazardous facility or a selfish, parochial, "not in my backyard" response—to one forcing the government and providers of private capital to deal with broader issues, "such as waste production, community control, and the process of policy making" (Lake, 1993, p. 90).

Much of noxious industry need not exist at all, and the rest could be made less injurious by means of altered consumption patterns, technological solutions, pollution prevention strategies, more robust enforcement, and more community involvement with industry (such as the use of good-neighbor agreements and community environmental audits). Many adverse impacts could be ameliorated or eliminated altogether by the use of industrial best-management practices, application of waste reduction measures at the source, more enlightened consumer choices, improved recycling initiatives and market development strategies for using recycled materials in consumer goods, updated environmental and land use regulations, and rigorous enforcement.

Balancing economic development, community sustainability, and environmental and health conditions in industrial areas is a tremendous undertaking that will require planners, public health professionals, and experts from many other disciplines to work together. The public health community has been largely absent from or made marginal in these discussions. Public health professionals could help immensely just by adding their thoughts and voices in addressing some of the structural changes that will be required to solve these problems.

Just as New York City took a bold lead in the then radical experiment called zoning, it is now beginning to grapple with some of these issues. However, effective and just solutions cannot be formulated on a city-by-city, or even a country-by-country, basis. As the world continues its rapid urbanization, the problems of waste production and waste disposal will continue to increase, both in extent and in the level of disparity among places. Noxious land uses have been expanded and concentrated in the poorer places on the earth, as well as in the poorer places within the relatively more affluent countries. The waste and pollution process has been globalized into one system.

These problems are exacerbated by widespread poverty, poor governments, and unwise development in many cities in the relatively less affluent countries, such as Mexico City, Mexico; Rio de Janeiro, Brazil; Calcutta, India; Manila, Philippines; Istanbul, Turkey; and Lagos, Nigeria. The burgeoning populations of these cities are among the world's most vulnerable in terms of health, so accepting additional waste and noxious land uses magnifies the existing health problems in many less affluent places. To avoid simply shifting the problem from one place to a poorer place, the connections between land use planning and public health must be forged on a worldwide basis.

Notes

1. Ninety-seven percent of all U.S. cities with populations over 5,000 had zoning laws by 1967.

2. The 1961–1998 time frame was selected for the study because December 1961 marks the date of the last major overhaul of the New York City Zoning Resolution. Data for actions prior to 1961 would not be directly comparable to data for later actions owing to significant changes in zoning categories, procedures, and record keeping. October 1998 marks the time the archival data were researched and compiled for this study and thus represents the end point of the time frame.

3. As defined by the New York City Department of City Planning in its *Citywide Industry Study: Geographical Atlas of Industrial Areas,* January 1993a. The determination of "major" industrial zones was based on the department's analysis of employment data, land use, and transportation access. The boundaries for these major industrial districts were based on neighborhood boundaries, major geographic or physical features, historic and present-day functions, and census tract boundaries (where feasible).

4. Based on comparison of archival zoning change maps, map sections 1–35, New York City Department of City Planning, 1961–1998.

5. Population characteristics (race, ethnicity, income, and homeownership status) were obtained from census data from 1960, 1970, 1980, and 1990. Digital data sources were used so that census data could be mapped and analyzed through a geographic information system (GIS) on the computer.

6. An extensive search of archival planning policy documents was conducted including those at the New York City Municipal Archives, Municipal Library, the New York Historical Society, the New York City Public Library's Map Room, and the Department of City Planning. Information from archival project files at the Department of City Planning was obtained through the Freedom of Information Law (FOIL)(Public Officers Law, art. 6, secs. 84–90).

7. Additionally, the city's Fair Share guidelines apply only to city-owned or -operated facilities, and many of the waste-related facilities are privately owned.

8. These cases have been documented predominantly outside the realm of traditional epidemiology.

9. New York City Planning Commission/Sanborn Company, *Land Use Maps of New York City,* 1956, 1980, and 1990. New York Public Library 42nd Street Map Archives. Five case-study industrial areas were selected for detailed land use analysis.

10. The term *minority people* refers to the population that is not non-Hispanic White. Many people consider the term *minority* to be a misnomer, because in many U.S. urban areas, as in New York City, people classified as minorities actually constitute the majority. For this study I used a derived variable of "minority" based on the census definitions and the guidelines established in Federal Statistical Directive No. 15, issued by the Office of Management and Budget in 1992, which provides standards on ethnic and racial categories for statistical reporting to be used by all federal agencies. This category is a summation of Hispanic; non-Hispanic Black; non-Hispanic American Indian; non-Hispanic Asian or Pacific Islander, Eskimo, or Aleut; and non-Hispanic other race. Other federal agencies, such as the U.S. Environmental Protection Agency, construct a similar "minority" category for their research on environmental justice issues.

    Because this study required a longitudinal analysis, census data from 1960 through 1990 were used. One of the problems with cross-census comparisons is the lack of consistency in many census attribute data categories over the years, especially with data on race and ethnicity. Variables, methods of data aggregation, types of information collected, and census policies on issues such as confidentiality differ from one census to the next, potentially affecting the validity of cross-census comparisons.

11. An inventory of industrial rezoning actions was compiled from the New York City Department of City Planning archival zoning maps from 1961 through 1998. A database of rezonings was created and then mapped with a GIS. The rezonings were classified by type and magnitude and were aggregated both by decade and by borough.

12. To examine the pattern of industrial zones and zoning changes, I used a GIS to map the major M zones and the rezoning actions. These locations were overlaid with a spatial database of census tracts linked to attribute data of population characteristics. New York City was divided into 2,218 census tracts for the 1990 census. Census attribute data from 1960, 1970, 1980, and 1990 were mapped and compared by a standard deviation classification method to allow longitudinal

comparison of deviation from the average, since absolute numbers for income and percentage minority changed drastically over the four-decade period. For each of the four census periods, population information was aggregated at the following geographic levels: citywide, boroughwide, census tracts within major M zones, census tracts within 0.5 mile of large and very large M zone increases, and census tracts within 0.5 mile of large and very large M zone decreases.

13. Analysis of policy trends is based on a review of archival documentation such as zoning amendment applications, city planning commission calendars, uniform land use review procedure applications, urban renewal plans, environmental impact assessments, planning studies, and letters and other documents obtained through New York State's Freedom of Information Law (Public Officers Law, art 6, §§ 84–90) for the years 1961 through 1999. Documents from 1916 through 1961 were also consulted, as available, for context and background on later policy developments. A complete list of archival sources appears in Maantay (2000, app. C), *Industrial Zoning Changes* (see note 3).

14. To gain a wider perspective on zoning policy and decision making, past and present, I interviewed a number of zoning experts for this study. This was not a representative sample of New York City's planners; the intention was to obtain as wide a range of opinions and experiences as possible. The interviewees included former city planning commissioners, land use attorneys, past and current staff at the Department of City Planning, academics, and planners for nonprofit, community, economic development, and good-government groups. Since most of those interviewed are still active in New York City planning and politics, they requested that they not be quoted by name. Therefore, quotations are attributed to "ZI 2," for example, meaning zoning interviewee 2. The complete list of names and professional affiliations of those interviewed appears in Maantay (2000, app. B), *Industrial Zoning Changes* (see note 3).

References

Adams, T. K. *Census of Population and Housing, 1960, 1970. and 1980 Extract Data.* Ann Arbor, Mich.: Inter-University Consortium for Political and Social Research, 1992.

Albion. R. G. *The Rise of New York Port, 1815–1860.* New York: Scribner, 1939.

Babcock, R. *The Zoning Game.* Madison: University of Wisconsin Press, 1966.

Bassett, E. M. *Zoning.* New York: Russell Sage Foundation, 1936.

Blackmar, E. *Manhattan for Rent, 1785–1850.* Ithaca, N.Y.: Cornell University Press, 1989.

Board of Estimate and Apportionment of the City of New York. *New York City Zoning Regulations.* New York: Board of Estimate and Apportionment of the City of New York, 1916.

Branfman, E., Cohen, B., and Trubek, D. "Measuring the Invisible Wall: Land Use Controls and Residential Patterns of the Poor." In D. Listokin (ed.), *Land Use Controls: Present Problems and Future Reform.* New Brunswick, N.J.: Center for Urban Policy Research, Rutgers University, 1974.

Bryant, R.W.G. *Land: Private Property, Public Control.* Montreal, Canada: Harvest House, 1968.

Bullard, R. "Overcoming Racism in Environmental Decision-Making." *Environment,* 1994, *36,* 11–40.

Buttenwieser, A. *Manhattan Waterbound: Planning and Developing Manhattan's Waterfront from the Seventeenth Century to the Present.* New York: New York University Press, 1987.

Caro, R. *The Power Broker: Robert Moses and the Fall of New York.* New York: Vintage, 1974.

Castells, M., and Hall, P. *Technopoles of the World: The Making of the Twenty-First-Century Industrial Complexes.* London: Routledge, 1994.

Citizens' Association of New York. *Report of the Council of Hygiene and Public Health upon the Sanitary Condition of the City.* New York: Arno Press, 1970. (Originally published 1866)

Committee on City Planning. *The Report of the Commission on the Height and Arrangement of Buildings.* New York: Board of Estimate and Apportionment of the City of New York, 1913.

Commoner, B. "The Hazards of Risk Assessment." *Columbia Journal of Environmental Law,* 1989, *14,* 365–378.

Costner, P., and Thornton, J. "We All Live Downstream: The Mississippi River and the Toxics Crisis." *Greenpeace,* Dec. 1989, pp. 11–13.

De Forest, R., and Veiller, L. *The Tenement House Problem.* 2 vols. New York: Macmillan, 1903.

Elias, E. "Significant Developments and Trends in Zoning Litigation: Exclusionary Zoning Perspective." In D. Listokin (ed.), *Land Use Controls: Present Problems and Future Reform.* New Brunswick, N.J.: Center for Urban Policy Research, Rutgers University, 1974.

Fitch, R. *The Assassination of New York.* New York: Verso, 1993.

Ford, J. *Slums and Housing.* 2 vols. Cambridge, Mass: Harvard University Press, 1936.

Freund, E. *The Police Power: Public Policy and Constitutional Law.* Chicago: Callaghan, 1904.

Haar, C., and Wolf, M. *Land Use Planning: The Use, Misuse, and Reuse of Urban Land.* New York: Little, Brown, 1989.

Haggerty, M. "Crisis at Indian Creek." In R. Bullard (ed.), *Unequal Protection: Environmental Justice and Communities of Color.* San Francisco: Sierra Club Books, 1996.

Head, R. A. "Health-Based Standards: What Role in Environmental Justice?" In B. Bryant (ed.), *Environmental Justice: Issues, Policies, and Solutions.* Washington, D.C.: Island Press, 1995.

Hearne, S. A. "Tracking Toxics: Chemical Use and the Public's 'Right to Know.'" *Environment,* 1996, *38,* 6–33.

Heiman, M. "From 'Not in My Backyard!' to 'Not in Anybody's Backyard!': Grassroots Challenge to Hazardous Waste Facility Siting." *Journal of the American Planning Association,* 1990, *56,* 359–362.

Hoover, E., and Vernon, R. *Anatomy of a Metropolis: The Changing Distribution of People and Jobs Within the New York Metropolitan Region.* Cambridge, Mass: Harvard University Press, 1959.

Kintish, B., and Shapiro, J. "The Zoning of Today in the City of Tomorrow." In T. Bressi (ed.), *Planning and Zoning in New York City.* New Brunswick, N.J.: Center for Urban Policy Research, Rutgers University, 1993.

Lake, R. "Rethinking NIMBY." *Journal of the American Planning Association,* 1993, *59,* 87–94.

Lauber, D. "Recent Cases in Exclusionary Zoning." In D. Listokin (ed.), *Land Use Controls: Present Problems and Future Reform.* New Brunswick, N.J.: Center for Urban Policy Research, Rutgers University, 1974.

Lavelle, M., and Coyle, M. "Unequal Protection: The Racial Divide in Environmental Law." *National Law Journal,* Sept. 21, 1992, pp. S1–S2.

Lubove, R. *The Progressive and the Slums: Tenement House Reform in New York City.* Pittsburgh: University of Pittsburgh Press, 1962.

Maantay, J. A. *Urban Air Pollution, Respiratory Disease, and Environmental Justice: Making the Links in the South Bronx.* Bronx, N.Y.: Center for a Sustainable Urban Environment, Hostos Community College, 1996.

Maantay, J. A. "Industrial Zoning Changes and Environmental Justice in New York City: A Historical, Geographical, and Cultural Analysis." Dissertation, Rutgers University, 2000.

Maantay, J. A., and others. *The Bronx Toxic Release Report.* New York: Center for a Sustainable Urban Environment/United States Environmental Protection Agency, 1997.

Makielski, S. J., Jr. *The Politics of Zoning: The New York Experience.* New York: Columbia University Press, 1966.

Mandelker, D. R. *The Zoning Dilemma: A Legal Strategy for Urban Change.* Indianapolis: Bobbs-Merrill, 1971.

Miller, D., and de Roo, G. "Integrated Zoning: An Innovative Dutch Approach to Measuring and Managing Environmental Spillovers in Urban Regions." *Journal of the American Planning Association,* 1996, *62,* 373–380.

National Committee Against Discrimination in Housing/Urban Land Institute. *Fair Housing and Exclusionary Land Use*. Urban Land Institute Research Report no. 23. Washington, D.C.: National Committee Against Discrimination in Housing/Urban Land Institute, 1974.

New York City Department of City Planning. *New York City Zoning Resolution*. New York: New York City Department of City Planning, 1961.

New York City Department of City Planning. *Master Plan for New York City*. Vol. 1. New York: New York City Department of City Planning, 1969.

New York City Department of City Planning. *Locating City Facilities: A Guide to the "Fair Share" Criteria*. New York: New York City Department of City Planning, 1991.

New York City Department of City Planning. *Citywide Industry Study: Geographical Atlas of Industrial Areas*. New York: New York City Department of City Planning, 1993a.

New York City Department of City Planning. *Citywide Industry Study: Zoning Technical Report*. New York: New York City Department of City Planning, 1993b.

New York City Department of Health. *Asthma Facts*. New York New York City Department of Health, 1999.

Nienaber-Clarke, J., and Gerlak, A. "Environmental Racism in Southern Arizona: The Reality Behind the Rhetoric." In D. E. Camacho (ed.), *Environmental Injustices, Political Struggles: Race, Class, and the Environment*. Durham, N.C.: Duke University Press, 1998.

Nossiter, A. "Asthma Common and on the Rise in Crowded South Bronx." *New York Times*, Mar. 5, 1995, p. A1.

Novotny, P. "Popular Epidemiology and the Struggle for Community Health in the Environmental Justice Movement." In D. Faber (ed.), *The Struggle for Ecological Democracy*. New York: Guilford Press, 1998.

O'Neill, H., and Moss, M. *Reinventing New York: Competing in the Next Century's Global Economy*. New York: Urban Research Center, New York University, 1991.

Office of the Bronx Borough President. *Solid Waste Management Plan*. Bronx, N.Y.: Office of the Bronx Borough President, 1997.

Oliver, P. R. "Living on a Superfund Site in Texarkana." In R. Bullard (ed.), *Unequal Protection: Environmental Justice and Communities of Color*. San Francisco: Sierra Club Books, 1996.

Perin, C. *Everything in Its Place: Social Order and Land Use in America*. Princeton, N.J.: Princeton University Press, 1977.

Perlin, S. A., and others. "Distribution of Industrial Air Emissions by Income and Race in the United States: An Approach Using the Toxic Release Inventory." *Environmental Science and Technology*, 1995, 29, 69–80.

Plan for Re-Zoning the City of New York. New York: Harrison, Ballard & Allen, 1950.

Platt, R. *Land Use Control: Geography, Law, and Public Policy.* Upper Saddle River, N.J.: Prentice Hall, 1991.

Plotkin, S. *Keep Out: The Struggle for Land Use Control.* Los Angeles: University of California Press, 1987.

Plunz, R. (ed.). *Housing Form and Public Policy in the United States.* New York: Praeger, 1983.

Regeski, D. "GIS and Risk: A Three-Culture Problem." In M. Goodchild, B. Parks, and L. Steyaert (eds.), *Environmental Modeling with GIS.* Oxford: Oxford University Press, 1993.

Robinson, R. "West Dallas Versus the Lead Smelter." In R. Bullard (ed.), *Unequal Protection: Environmental Justice and Communities of Color.* San Francisco: Sierra Club Books, 1996.

Shenkel, W. "The Economic Consequences of Industrial Zoning." In R. Andrews (ed.), *Urban Land Use Policy: The Central City.* New York: Free Press, 1972.

Siegan, B. H. *Land Use Without Zoning.* Lanham, Mass.: Lexington Books, 1972.

Toll, S. *Zoned American.* New York: Grossman, 1969.

U.S. Bureau of the Census. *1980 Summary Tape File 3a: Technical Documentation.* Washington, D.C.: U.S. Department of Commerce, 1980.

U.S. Bureau of the Census. *Census of Population and Housing, 1990 Summary Tape File on CD-ROM: Technical Documentation.* Washington, D.C.: U.S. Department of Commerce, 1990.

Weaver, C. L., and Babcock, R. F. *City Zoning. The Once and Future Frontier.* Washington, D.C.: Planners Press, American Planning Association, 1979.

White, H. L. "Race, Class, and Environmental Hazards." In D. E. Camacho (ed.), *Environmental Injustices, Political Struggles: Race, Class, and the Environment.* Durham, N.C.: Duke University Press, 1998.

Williams, N., Jr. and Norman, T. "Exclusionary Land Use Controls: The Case of Northeastern New Jersey." In D. Listokin (ed.), *Land Use Controls: Present Problems and Future Reform.* New Brunswick, N.J.: Center for Urban Policy Research, Rutgers University, 1974.

Willis, C. "How The 1916 Zoning Law Shaped Manhattan's Central Business Districts." In T. Bressi (ed.), *Planning and Zoning in New York City.* New Brunswick, N.J.: Center for Urban Policy Research, Rutgers University, 1993.

Wright, B., Bryant, P., and Bullard, R. "Coping with Poisons in Cancer Alley." In R. Bullard (ed.), *Unequal Protection: Environmental Justice and Communities of Color.* San Francisco: Sierra Club Books, 1996.

Zoning New York City: A Proposal for a Zoning Resolution for the City of New York. New York: Voorhees, Walker, Smith & Smith, 1958.

CHAPTER NINE

The Changing Structure of Work in the United States

Implications for Health and Welfare

Sarah Kuhn
John Wooding

In an earlier work (Kuhn and Wooding, 1997), we presented some of the significant features of the rapidly changing structure of work in the United States. We argued that these phenomena derive from the maturation of the American economy, the application of new technologies, intense foreign competition, the rapid expansion of global trade, and extensive international interdependence. These features and their impact are intensified by a new international division of labor and the extensive and rapid movement of capital.

Clearly, the changing character of the U.S. economy has altered the nature and experience of work for many Americans. It also has enormous axial and political implications. The decrease in heavy manufacturing, the expansion of the service sector, and the concomitant changes in benefits and unionization have all contributed to changes in the overall welfare of working people. But the structural changes we described have had a profound impact on the complexion of employer–employee relations that goes well beyond the restructuring of work and the availability and extent of benefits such as health coverage and vacation time.

What we will argue here is that these changes have resulted in some clearly identifiable problems that shape the overall welfare of Americans and have

The authors would like to thank the following for many helpful comments and suggestions in the writing of this chapter: Barbara Baran, Charles Levenstein, Charles Richardson, and three anonymous reviewers for *New Solutions*.

251

important health consequences in and outside of the workplace. In broad terms, we suggest that technological and economic changes place an increasing burden on workers, including but not limited to new chemical and ergonomic hazards. Further, working now takes up more and more time for those in full-time work, resulting in a significant reduction of leisure time and a negative impact on the quality of life for many working Americans.

We relate these problems not only to the issue of the restructuring of work as a response to global economic changes of the 1970s and 1980s but also to the decreasing ability of many workers to resist these changes. This results, in particular, from the decline in trade union power in the workplace and the dominance of an ideology that promotes the rights of corporations and limits the acceptability and legitimacy of state interventions to protect worker and environmental health. In the final part of this chapter, we propose a number of areas in which solutions to these problems might be pursued.

CHANGING WORK, CHANGING HAZARDS

The change in work and work organization, reflecting international economic changes, accompanies significant transformations of technology and production. While the impact of technology on work has been discussed extensively elsewhere (see Bright, 1958; Woodward, 1965; Bell, 1973; Braverman, 1974; Gable, 1978; and Hirschhorn, 1984), the overall effects may be briefly noted here.

The literature of the 1970s was divided between those who saw technology as upgrading jobs and skill requirements on the one hand, and those who believed that technology "deskilled" the majority of jobs. The literature of the 1980s and 1990s, however, delivers a consistent message: work organization, skill requirements, autonomy, and other features of the automated workplace are not predetermined. Instead, they are the outcome of a host of factors such as organization size and culture, the design of hardware and software, organization politics, industry, and so forth (Karasek and Theorell, 1990; Hartmann, Kraut, and Tilly, 1986; Office of Technology Assessment, 1985).

Effects on jobs include "job enrichment" (in which task variety, skill, and often autonomy are increased), "deskilling" (the removal of these features, creating narrower and more repetitive work), and "job enlargement" (an increased workload) (9to5, 1985). Furthermore, the effects on jobs are not static, since the organization and content of work may change significantly before, during, and after the implementation phase of a new technology. Early inefficiencies may give way to increased efficiency, varied and nonroutine work may become tedious as "bugs" are removed from the system, and so forth (Office of Technology Assessment, 1985; Greenbaum, Pullman, and Szymanski, 1985).

Even though the effect of technology is indeterminate, technology is not neutral. The impact technology and automation will have in the workplace will depend on the social organization of work, the amount of control workers have over their working conditions, the availability of alternative employment, and the extent of competitive economic pressures. Increasing use of technology in the rapidly expanding service sector—particularly in clerical and office work—raises a number of significant issues for the health and autonomy of workers.

We have tended to think of the office, for example, as a safe place, by contrast to the dirty, noisy, and physically hazardous industrial shop floor. This perception is generally accurate and is borne out by industrial statistics on the incidence of illness and accidents, which show that industries like finance, insurance, and real estate, as well as consumer services, have significantly below average incidence of illness and injuries. Service sector work is far from free of health hazards, however, although they tend to be less visible and dramatic than those in manufacturing settings. A number of problems, such as eye strain, musculo-skeletal problems, reproductive hazards, other exposures (including chemicals and other pollutants in the air), noise, poor light, overcrowding, and stress-related illness, have been associated with office work and many other service occupations (for example, janitors and garbage collectors).

Many jobs now generate a host of ergonomic problems as technology and automation force prolonged periods of sitting and standing in front of computers, check-out scanners, automated systems, and the like. The frequent and repetitive motions required by these jobs strain the musculo-skeletal system and have created a wide range of repetitive motion injuries.

STRESS

Perhaps the most significant human health consequence of many of the changes we have discussed is the increase in stress felt by most workers across a range of occupations. Stress-related illness is prevalent in the automated workplace, the offices of private and public corporations, small and large retail outlets, and a host of service industries. The state of chronic heightened arousal characteristic of those under stress can lead to lowered immune function, ulcers, cardiovascular problems, anxiety, and depression. Stress on the job is exacerbated as organizations frequently respond to increased competitive pressures by passing this pressure along to employees. The U.S. Office of Technology Assessment (1985) predicts that stress-related illness may be the greatest public health problem faced by office workers in the future.[1]

Autonomy on the job bears an important relationship to stress and health outcomes, since the ability of a worker to control her or his work environment can make the difference between experiencing added workload as a challenge or as a source of negative stress. Control over the pace and methods of work is repeatedly cited as key to worker health, satisfaction, and well-being (Karasek and Theorell, 1990; U.S. Office of Technology Assessment, 1985; 9to5, 1985). To offer just a single example: women who reported having a heavy workload and limited job control were at three times greater risk for coronary heart disease than women who had heavy workloads combined with control over their work (U.S. Office of Technology Assessment, 1985). Lack of work autonomy is particularly prevalent in lower-level service occupations and is characteristic of much part-time, temporary, and contingent work.

WORKPLACE MONITORING

In addition to the stress problems resulting from work speed-up, longer hours, and increased responsibility, technology used to monitor employee performance adds to the burdens placed on workers. Monitoring of employee performance acts as a constraint on worker autonomy. In the United States, the controversy over employer monitoring of workers is framed as a conflict between the right of employers to manage the enterprise, to act to reduce costs, and to avoid potential liability on the one hand, and employees' right to privacy and individual freedom on the other (U.S. Office of Technology Assessment, 1985). Computerized information technology has increased the speed and scope of potential employee monitoring, expanding the detail and comprehensiveness of information available to management about employee performance (Hartmann, Kraut, and Tilly, 1986), and created new tensions and conflicts between employer and employee.[2]

Some evidence exists to suggest that the use of electronic monitoring contributes to negative stress and deteriorating quality of work life. Nearly half of those monitored by computer report their work "very stressful," compared to less than one-third of those not so monitored, and excessive supervision or monitoring was found to be most highly correlated with stress-related medical problems (9to5, 1985). The U.S. Office of Technology Assessment (1987) asserts, however, that there is still very little research that allows us to differentiate the effects of electronic monitoring from those of job and equipment design, machine pacing, and so forth.

The impact of such monitoring, in combination with competitive pressures that force management to seek myriad methods to increase worker productivity, not only increases the stress felt by the individual worker but also exacerbates the tensions deriving from alienation at work and job insecurity (Attewell, 1987).

LESS TIME, MORE WORK

American workers are now working longer and harder than at any time in the postwar period. Juliet Schor (1991) calculates that the average employed person in the United States today works 163 hours more a year than she or he would have 20 years ago. These extra hours are worked in all industries and by many kinds of workers. This expansion of work not only adds to overall stress in the workplace but clearly reduces the amount of time available for relaxation, family, recreation, and leisure pursuits. Longer work hours for those Americans in full-time employment obviously reduce leisure time, as the demands of family life, work, and self-improvement have burgeoned with two-earner families and a decrease in real incomes since the 1970s. Automation and technological sophistication seem to have resulted not, as much of the sociological literature of the 1950s and 1960s predicted, in increased leisure time for workers, but rather quite the reverse.

WORK, POWER, AND TRADE UNIONS

The restructuring of work has also brought about a restructuring of power in the workplace. The increase in nonunion service-sector employment, heightened economic competition, and the changed demographic characteristics of the work force have significantly reduced the ability of workers to resist demands for speed-up, and monitoring, and to fight against the introduction of technologies that create new occupational hazards. In particular, the decline in union power limits the ability of workers to resist pressures for wage cutbacks and to gain long-term employment security.

Organized labor in the United States is now weaker numerically and politically than at any time in its postwar history. This decline began in the 1970s and increased precipitously by the late 1970s, and early 1980s. It is reflected across the whole range of union activity: loss of negotiating strength at the bargaining table, the decrease in union membership, the decline in strike activity, and the vast increase in the number of "concessionary" collective bargaining agreements between unions and industry.

A flavor for the magnitude of this change can be gained by just looking at a few figures. In 1982, 45 percent of all workers covered by collective bargaining agreements had their wages frozen or reduced. In 1983, 37 percent of workers suffered a similar fate, and 22 percent in 1984. These concessions dropped off as the economy moved out of recession, but they left workers in major industries (particularly textiles, rubber, lumber, metal fabrication, transportation, and mining—in other words, in most of the traditional manufacturing sector) with a significant decrease in standard of living. Industrial actions for better wages or conditions—strikes—have also declined: the number of work stoppages involving more than one thousand workers reached a peak in 1974 (424 stoppages) and dropped steadily until 1984 (Wren, 1985).

The decline in union membership is also significant. In 1969, unions represented about one quarter of the total labor force. By 1993, union membership was 16.6 million in both public and private sectors (reflecting an increase from 16.4 million in 1992—the first increase in fourteen years). In 1993, approximately 11.2 percent of workers (7 million workers) were organized in the private sector, a further 6.6 million were organized in the public sector, the only area experiencing an increase in union memberships (Bureau of Labor Statistics, 1993).

Absolute numbers are even more dramatic: in the ten years between 1979 and 1989, some unions lost enormously. For example, the United Steelworkers (USWA) lost 408,000 members; the Oil, Chemical and Atomic Workers (OCAW) 75,000; and the International Ladies Garment Workers (ILGWU) lost 161,000 members. While some unions (predominantly in the service and public sectors, notably Service Employees International [SEIU] and the American Federation of State, County and Municipal Employees [AFSCME]), made gains, the overall membership picture for American unions remains bleak.

Along with these problems, organized labor has suffered from the antilabor pronouncements of both the Reagan and Bush administrations that have built up a public antagonism to labor unions. Cuts in the "social wage" (unemployment insurance, welfare programs, food stamps, and so forth) have also hit workers in America (the social wage functions to reduce the impact of the reserve army of unemployed labor on employed workers). Without such programs, the competition for jobs becomes more fierce and the bargaining strength of employed workers is further reduced.

The decline of unionization has many causes and would require a long discussion, but one contributing factor has been the changing industrial mix in the U.S. economy. Industries with high levels of unionization are the infrastructural industries (transportation, communication, and public utilities), government, and the goods-producing sector. Service sector industries, the growth areas of the economy, have low rates of unionization. Furthermore, part-time workers in all industries are rarely organized (just over 7 percent in 1985), while temporary workers and independent contractors are also rarely represented by unions (Applebaum and Gregory, 1988). The opportunity for organizing exists, and some unions and locals are pursuing it actively. Because unions can make the adjustments necessary to appeal to service employees, as some have already done, there seems reason to believe that more workers can gain union protection:

40 percent of service workers told a Harris poll that they would welcome a union, as opposed to 25 percent in manufacturing (Green and Tilly, 1987).

Unions and other forms of protection for workers—such as protective labor legislation and a strong social welfare infrastructure—are important because much of the change in work, as well as in the nature of the employment contract in the last decade or so, seems to have taken place at the behest of management rather than as a result of worker preference (Applebaum and Gregory, 1998; Christopherson and Noyelle, 1988).

NEW PROBLEMS, NEW SOLUTIONS

In the changing American workplace, much is made of leaner, meaner production. In many workplaces, management has achieved remarkable productive gains and improved the bottom line. That this was possible in the 1980s had much to do with new technologies, increased automation, and capital flight to countries where labor is cheap and the government regulation weak. But it also reflects a changing set of beliefs about how management's (and the state's) responsibilities to workers are defined. Stressing the virtues of trickle-down economics and emphasizing the need of capital to be free from governmental, that is to say, social, constraints (environmental and health and safety regulation in particular, taxation in general) created a new ethic of personal responsibility and reaffirmed the seeming virtues of the market. What little sense of obligation there had been of employer to employee (to provide relatively secure employment over the long term, to provide steadily increasing income, to offer some rudimentary set of benefits) has broken down as the structural pressures for change are played out in the form of ideological assertions of the rights of capital over those of workers and citizens. Attacks on government regulation and organized labor, often spearheaded by business, have exacerbated job instability and insecurity. There is no longer a commitment by the government to full employment.

In spite of this, there have been some positive developments in the structure of work in the last several decades. Workers in the new, service-based jobs are at less risk from life-threatening industrial injuries, and are generally safer at work than those working in heavy industry. Although the glass ceiling and job segregation are still pervasive, there is more economic opportunity for women and some members of minority groups. There is some evidence that jobs are becoming more skilled, and perhaps, therefore, more interesting. To reinforce these positive changes and reduce the negative ones, what might be done to ameliorate the problems we have outlined above? Our review suggests that what is required is the development of a basic political program essential to public health.

Full Employment or a Superfund for Workers?

At one time, this country (like many in western Europe) made a commitment to maintaining a level of full employment for its citizens. That commitment was predicated on government's willingness to use public investment, monetary, and fiscal policies to ensure that most Americans had a job sufficient to provide a minimal standard of living. Since unemployment weakens workers' economic and political voice and, therefore, the ability to protect public health, the political demand for full employment remains a powerful and important strategy.

Since, however, a rapidly changing economy will necessitate redundancies and layoffs, and some types of work and production are dangerous to the health of workers and the environment, it may be preferable to provide programs for workers temporarily facing unemployment. The demand for a Superfund for workers has merit. It should provide income, training, and security for workers from a wide range of industries and professions.

A National Health Program

Some system of guaranteed publicly funded health care is not only necessary as a replacement for the employer-based, high-cost private system currently in crisis but is indispensable if workers are to regain any kind of security about the availability and quality of health care. Further, a system of guaranteed health care would prevent "job-lock," where workers remain tied to an employer because of health insurance. It also would provide coverage for the increasing number of Americans in part-time and contingent work who have no health benefits.

Labor Law Reform

Organized labor should seek to expand its efforts to build union membership in the new industries and among younger workers, minorities, and women. Unions also should seek support from members of communities affected by plant closings, environmental threats, and the consequences of investment decisions. But the development of traditional unions under the economic and political conditions we have described is and will be extremely difficult. The broader public must be convinced to strengthen labor laws, including OSHA. Effective public health efforts require a strong labor movement.

Reform of Corporate Governance

It is clear that public control over investment decisions must be broadened. The increasing mobility of all forms of capital and the enormous economic and social consequences of capital flight need to be addressed. Workers and communities should not be held hostage to investment decisions. Without some control over investment, security of employment, environmental health, and community identity are constantly threatened. Some form of return to the original meaning of a "corporate charter," reinforcing the idea that corporations are social creations and exist at the pleasure of the public, is necessary, and it must outline the obligations that companies have to workers and communities (see Grossman and Adams, 1996).

Community-Based Political Organizing

New groups of workers (immigrants and minorities, part-timers, temporary workers, and professionals working independently) are not linked by the commonalty of their work; rather they may be linked by the commonalty of their community. This suggests that organizing efforts for change and struggles to resist the impact on general health and welfare of the restructuring of the U.S. economy might more profitably be pursued in the context of community and neighborhood rather than within the confines of the rapidly eroding "traditional" workplace. Unions need to develop new community-based forms to be responsive to these changed circumstances. The enormously successful Right-to-Know coalitions of local labor organizations, environmental, and public interest groups suggest the shape of a new popular political form of organizing. The rise of the environmental justice movement further suggests that such new forms hold promise for meaningful change.

Reduce Income Inequality

The dramatic income inequality resulting from the changes we describe must be lessened. Many of the physical, mental, and emotional ills we discuss above can arguably be called "diseases of poverty" or "diseases of powerlessness" and can be attributed to increased income inequality.[3] While well-paid professionals are not immune to stress and ergonomic hazards, to name two examples, their ability to avoid these problems is far greater, both because of professionals' greater power in the workplace and because their high income and class status provide them with more options. Furthermore, many other social problems, such as the maldistribution of health care, can arguably be traced to income inequality.

A steeply progressive income tax is one possible measure to reduce income inequality while also helping to fund improved health care for all and other vital social services; this measure does not, however, address the underlying causes of increased inequality.

The American economic landscape has changed considerably. Some of these changes are beneficial. Many of the new industries and jobs are less dangerous than those in the heavy manufacturing sector. There are now more opportunities for women and some minorities to obtain decent work and occupational mobility. Yet accompanying these changes is a decline in security, living standards, and access to meaningful work for many. What we have described in this chapter reflects permanent and structural changes in the economic system. Protecting the health of Americans requires, therefore, a political response—that labor and the public health movement turn to political action.

Notes

1. A major survey on workplace stress, conducted by 9to5, National Association of Working Women (1984), found that two-thirds of respondents who worked with automated equipment reported that it made their job more interesting and enjoyable than before (while 9 percent said it made their jobs more boring and monotonous). A slight majority (54 percent) said that their work was easier and less stressful than before automation. The findings of the U.S. Office of Technology Assessment (1985), consistent with this, are that automation can either increase or decrease workload, depending on a host of factors.

2. The U.S. Office of Technology Assessment (1987) identifies three types of electronic monitoring of office activities: computer-based monitoring (the use of a computer to automatically record data about the work activity, such as number of keystrokes, time per transaction, and nature of transaction), service observation (supervisors listen electronically to employee interaction with customers; new technology allows this to be done completely silently, without the knowledge of the worker or customer), and telephone call accounting (records origin, destination, and length of telephone calls; this is generally used for reducing telephone costs, sometimes by limiting or prohibiting personal calls).

3. For a discussion of the ethical dimension of the health care system and the link between unfairness and income inequality, see Dworkin (1994).

References

Applebaum, E., and Gregory, J. "Union Responses to Contingent Work: Are Win-Win Outcomes Possible?" In Women's Bureau, *Flexible Workstyles: A Look at Contingent Labor.* Washington, D.C.: U.S. Department of Labor, 1988.

Attewell, P. "Big Brother and the Sweatshop: Computer Surveillance in the Automated Office." *Sociological Theory,* 1987, *5,* 87–99.

Bell, D. *The Coming of Postindustrial Society: A Venture in Social Forecasting.* New York: Basic Books, 1973.

Braverman, H. *Labor and Monopoly Capital.* New York: Monthly Review Press, 1974.

Bright, J. R. "Does Automation Raise Skill Requirements?" *Harvard Business Review,* 1958, *36,* 85–98.

Bureau of Labor Statistics. Washington, D.C.: U.S. Department of Labor, 1993.

Christopherson, S., and Noyelle, T. *The Contingent Worker: New Employment and Benefit Options for the Year 2000.* Quarterly Report, Conservation of Human Resources, Columbia University, Oct. 1988.

Dworkin, R. "Will Clinton's Plan Be Fair?" *New York Review of Books,* Jan. 13, 1994, p. 20.

Gable, D. *In Search of the New Working Class: Automation and Social Integration Within the Capitalist Enterprise.* Cambridge: Cambridge University Press, 1978.

Green, J., and Tilly, C. "Service Unionism: Directions for Organizing." *Labor Law Journal,* 1987, *38*(8), 486–495.

Greenbaum, J., Pullman, S., and Szymanski, S. "Effects of Office Automation on the Public Sector Workforce: Case Study." Report to the Office of Technology Assessment, Apr. 1985.

Grossman, R., and Adams, F. T. "Taking Care of Business: Citizenship and the Charter of Incorporation." *New Solutions,* 1996, *3*(3), 7–18.

Hartmann, H. I., Kraut, R. E., and Tilly, L. A. *Computer Chips and Paper Clips: Technology and Women's Employment.* Washington, D.C.: National Academy Press, 1986.

Hirschhorn, L. *Beyond Mechanization: Work and Technology in a Postindustrial Age.* Cambridge, Mass.: MIT Press, 1984.

Karasek, R., and Theorell, T. *Healthy Work.* New York: Basic Books, 1990.

Kuhn, S., and Wooding, K. "The Changing Structure of Work in the United States: Part 1. The Impact on Income and Benefits." In C. Levenstein and J. Wooding (eds.), *Work, Health, and Environment: Old Problems, New Solutions.* New York: Guilford Press, 1997.

9to5, National Association of Working Women. *The 9to5 National Survey on Women and Stress.* Cleveland, Ohio: 9to5, National Association of Working Women, 1984.

9to5, National Association of Working Women. *Hidden Victims: Clerical Workers, Automation, and the Changing Economy.* Cleveland, Ohio: 9to5, National Association of Working Women, 1985.

Office of Technology Assessment. *Automation of America's Offices.* Washington, D.C.: U.S. Government Printing Office, 1985.

Office of Technology Assessment. *The Electronic Supervisor: New Technology, New Tensions.* Washington, D.C.: U.S. Government Printing Office, 1987.

Schor, J. *The Overworked American: The Unexpected Decline of Leisure.* New York: Basic Books, 1991.

Woodward, J. *Industrial Organization: Theory and Practice.* Oxford: Oxford University Press, 1965.

Wren, R. "The Decline of American Labor." *Socialist Review,* 1985, *15*, 89–101.

PART TWO

THEORY, IDEOLOGY, AND POLITICS: CRITICAL PERSPECTIVES

The debate on health inequities in the United States has become domesticated, bogged down in the search for medical solutions, psychological analysis of social capital, programs to educate the poor, and avoiding long-term continuing injustices. The contributors to Part Two explore the theoretical and ideological conceptions that limit the ability to think critically about health inequities. They examine some of the basic concepts and ideas that dominate the way in which researchers and policymakers narrow the scope of the possible in how we think about or avoid the issue of health inequities. A lot is at stake in the perspectives adopted to explain inequality because they will determine the effectiveness of given strategies. A perspective that incorporates principles of social justice might draw attention to the connection between hierarchies of power, systems of production, and inequalities in health status, thereby suggesting much broader forms of social transformation.

In a classic article from the mid-1970s, Dan Beauchamp argues that our basic attention in public health policy should be directed toward ethical and political barriers associated with achieving justice, rather than technology in seeking to minimize death and disability. In particular, he considers how the most critical social ethic—"market justice"—unfairly protects the most powerful from the burdens of prevention.

With the recent interest in the construct of social capital, Carles Muntaner, John Lynch, and George Davey Smith review hypotheses on the link between social capital and health, the empirical evidence, and the implications for health policy. They argue that the construct, as it is applied, is an unfortunate use of an idealist social psychology, which represents a privatization of economics and politics.

Paula Braveman examines the meaning of equity as applied to health status and critiques the ideological elements of the *World Health Report 2000's* measure of health inequalities as a guide to national policy. Specifically, the author points out how the report removes equity and human rights considerations from the routine measurement and reporting of health disparities within nations.

Alexandra Bambas and Juan Antonio Casas note that although the relationship between health inequities and living conditions is receiving more consideration in public health thinking, insufficient attention continues to be given to why inequalities in health or health resources might be unfair and the implications of labeling them as unfair. Demonstrating the importance of language and categories of analysis, they argue for a more organic and systematic process for assessing fairness in the distribution of resources for health.

Analyzing the social context of income inequality, David Coburn argues for paying more attention to the causes of income inequality itself, beyond its consequences. He links neoliberal, market-oriented political doctrines with both income inequality and lowered social cohesion. Neoliberal theory has undermined the welfare state, in his view, and therefore produces negative effects on health. In addition, he further argues that recognizing the contextual causes of inequality may influence our understanding of the causal pathways associated with inequality in health status.

John Lynch picks up where David Coburn leaves off and further explains why income inequality cannot be the starting point for a theory of health inequalities. Lynch responds to Coburn's call to expand the terms of reference for the debate over interpreting the link between income inequality and health to include an analysis of neoliberalism and global capitalism in the discourse. He maintains that income inequality cannot be the starting "social fact" of a theory of health inequalities. Instead, building on the discussion of neomaterial conditions begun in Chapter Seven, he considers the concept of institutionalized social connectedness of marginalized groups and their control over health resources as a way to understand the context of health inequities.

Richard Levins asks why health professionals were caught off guard by the return of many infectious diseases they thought had been eliminated. He suggests that a misplaced belief in technology and economic development as a solution to poverty, along with assumptions made in Western science and epidemiology, provides part of the answer. In addition, he argues that attention to evolution, the changing ecosystem, social circumstances, and class differences results in a more powerful explanation of contemporary inequities in health. He presents an ecological proposal that considers how changes in the way of life of populations will cause changes in pathogens and the vectors of disease. He also argues for a movement that will incorporate the insights of the environmental justice movement, knowledge of ecosystem health, the social determinants of health, and alternative medicine.

Jennie Popay, Gareth Williams, Carol Thomas, and Anthony Gatrell offer a theoretical framework for researching social inequalities in health. They critique some recent research that emphasizes risk and risk behavior and argue for the integration of macrosocial analysis with microsocial decisions of individuals. They ask why individuals who receive information about health risks cannot easily change their lives and how social structures influence behavior. A greater reliance on lay knowledge and ways to express it, in their view, would offer a way to link personal experience with social structure and the organization of time and place.

Dennis Raphael and Toba Bryant examine the definition of population health as developed by the Canadian Institute for Advanced Research and express concern about the way it has influenced the shape and direction of Canadian public health policy and its potential to do the same in the United States and elsewhere. They argue that because population health is rooted in epidemiology, a militantly quantitative discipline, population health eschews analysis of societal structures as determinants of health and elevates scientific understanding over health promotion action. Its lack of an explicit values base is also problematic. Policymakers should recognize these and other limitations as they consider models for a new public health.

Nancy Krieger contends that we require innovative theory to explain the causal connections that link biology and the material world. She suggests that dealing with causation involves not only difficult philosophical issues but also questions of accountability and agency—the responsibility for populations' patterns of health, disease, and well-being. A major tension, Krieger argues, historically and today, is between theories that seek causes of social inequalities in health in innate versus imposed or as individual versus societal characteristics. She evaluates psychosocial theory, social production of disease, and political economy and ecosocial theory and their related frameworks in order to generate testable principles for guiding scientific theory and action.

CHAPTER TEN

Public Health as Social Justice

Dan E. Beauchamp

Anthony Downs (1970) has observed that our most intractable public problems have two significant characteristics. First, they occur to a relative minority of our population (even though that minority may number millions of people). Second, they result in significant part from arrangements that are providing substantial benefits or advantages to a majority or to a powerful minority of citizens. Thus solving or minimizing these problems requires painful losses, the restructuring of society and the acceptance of new burdens by the most powerful and the most numerous on behalf of the least powerful or the least numerous. As Downs notes, this bleak reality has resulted in recent years in cycles of public attention to such problems as poverty, racial discrimination, poor housing, unemployment or the abandonment of the aged; however, this attention and interest rapidly wane when it becomes clear that solving these problems requires painful costs that the dominant interests in society are unwilling to pay. Our public ethics do not seem to fit our public problems.

It is not sufficiently appreciated that these same bleak realities plague attempts to protect the public's health. Automobile-related injury and death;

This chapter is a slightly revised version of a paper presented at the annual meeting of the American Public Health Association in Chicago, November 18, 1975, entitled "Health Policy and the Politics of Prevention: Breaking the Ethical and Political Barriers to Public Health."

tobacco, alcohol and other drug damage; the perils of the workplace; environmental pollution; the inequitable and ineffective distribution of medical care services; the hazards of biomedicine—all of these threats inflict death and disability on a minority of our society at any given time. Further, minimizing or even significantly reducing the death and disability from these perils entails that the majority or powerful minorities accept new burdens or relinquish existing privileges that they presently enjoy. Typically, these new burdens or restrictions involve more stringent controls over these and other hazards of the world.

This somber reality suggests that our fundamental attention in public health policy and prevention should not be directed toward a search for new technology, but rather toward breaking existing ethical and political barriers to minimizing death and disability. This is not to say that technology will never again help avoid painful social and political adjustments (Etzioni and Remp, 1987). Nonetheless, only the technological Pollyannas will ignore the mounting evidence that the critical barriers to protecting the public against death and disability are not the barriers to technological progress—indeed the evidence is that it is often technology itself that is our own worst enemy. The critical barrier to dramatic reductions in death and disability is a social ethic that unfairly protects the most numerous or the most powerful from the burdens of prevention.

This is the issue of justice. In the broadest sense, justice means that each person in society ought to receive his due and that the burdens and benefits of society should be fairly and equitably distributed (Jonsen and Hellegers, 1974). But what criteria should be followed in allocating burdens and benefits: Merit, equality or need? (Outka, 1974). What end or goal in life should receive our highest priority: Life, liberty or the pursuit of happiness? The answers to these questions can be found in our prevailing theories or models of justice. These models of justice, roughly speaking, form the foundation of our politics and public policy in general, and our health policy (including our prevention policy) specifically. Here I am speaking of politics not as partisan politics but rather the more ancient and venerable meaning of the political as the search for the common good and the just society.

These models of justice furnish a symbolic framework or blueprint with which to think about and react to the problems of the public, providing the basic rules to classify and categorize problems of society as to whether they necessitate public and collective protection, or whether individual responsibility should prevail. These models function as a sort of map or guide to the common world of members of society, making visible some conditions in society as public issues and concerns, and hiding, obscuring or concealing other conditions that might otherwise emerge as public issues or problems were a different map or model of justice in hand.

In the case of health, these models of justice form the basis for thinking about and reacting to the problems of disability and premature death in society. Thus, if public health policy requires that the majority or a powerful minority accept their fair share of the burdens of protecting a relative minority threatened with death or disability, we need to ask if our prevailing model of justice contemplates and legitimates such sacrifices.

MARKET-JUSTICE

The dominant model of justice in the American experience has been market-justice.[1] Under the norms of market-justice people are entitled only to those valued ends such as status, income, happiness, etc., that they have acquired by fair rules of entitlement, e.g., by their own individual efforts, actions or abilities. Market-justice emphasizes individual responsibility, minimal collective action and freedom from collective obligations except to respect other persons' fundamental rights.

While we have as a society compromised pure market-justice in many ways to protect the public's health, we are far from recognizing the principle that death and disability are collective problems and that all persons are entitled to health protection. Society does not recognize a general obligation to protect the individual against disease and injury. While society does prohibit individuals from causing direct harm to others, and has in many instances regulated clear public health hazards, the norm of market-justice is still dominant and the primary duty to avert disease and injury still rests with the individual. The individual is ultimately alone in his or her struggle against death.

Barriers to Protection

This individual isolation creates a powerful barrier to the goal of protecting all human life by magnifying the power of death, granting to death an almost supernatural reality (Marcuse, 1959). Death has throughout history presented a basic problem to humankind (Illich, 1974), but even in an advanced society with enormous biomedical technology, the individualism of market-justice tends to retain and exaggerate pessimistic and fatalistic attitudes toward death and injury. This fatalism leads to a sense of powerlessness, to the acceptance of risk as an essential element of life, to resignation in the face of calamity, and to a weakening of collective impulses to confront the problems of premature death and disability.

Perhaps the most direct way in which market-justice undermines our resolve to preserve and protect human life lies in the primary freedom this ethic extends to all individuals and groups to act with minimal obligations to protect the common good. Despite the fact that this rule of self-interest predictably fails to protect adequately the safety of our workplaces, our modes of transportation, the physical environment, the commodities we consume, or the equitable and effective distribution of medical care, these failures have resulted so far in only half-hearted attempts at regulation and control. This response is explained in large part by the powerful sway market-justice holds over our imagination, granting fundamental freedom to all individuals to be left alone—even if the "individuals" in question are giant producer groups with enormous capacities to create great public harm through sheer inadvertence. Efforts for truly effective controls over these perils must constantly struggle against a prevailing ethical paradigm that defines as threats to fundamental freedoms attempts to assure that all groups—even powerful producer groups—accept their fair share of the burdens of prevention.

Market-justice is also the source of another major barrier to public health measures to minimize death and disability—the category of voluntary behavior. Market-justice forces a basic distinction between the harm caused by a factory polluting the atmosphere and the harm caused by the cigarette or alcohol industries, because in the latter case those that are harmed are perceived as engaged in "voluntary" behavior (Brotman and Suffet, 1975). It is the radical individualism inherent in the market model that encourages attention to the individual's behavior and inattention to the social preconditions of that behavior. In the case of smoking, these preconditions include a powerful cigarette industry and accompanying social and cultural forces encouraging the practice of smoking. These social forces include norms sanctioning smoking as well as all forms of media, advertising, literature, movies, folklore, etc. Since the smoker is free in some ultimate sense to not smoke, the norms of market-justice force the conclusion that the individual voluntarily "chooses" to smoke; and we are prevented from taking strong collective action against the powerful structures encouraging this so-called voluntary behavior.

Yet another way in which the market ethic obstructs the possibilities for minimizing death and disability, and alibis the need for structural change, is through explanations for death and disability that "blame the victim (Ryan, 1971)."[2] Victim-blaming misdefines structural and collective problems of the entire society as individual problems, seeing these problems as caused by the behavioral failures or deficiencies of the victims. These behavioral explanations for public problems tend to protect the larger society and powerful interests from the burdens of collective action, and instead encourage attempts to change the "faulty" behavior of victims.

Market-justice is perhaps the major cause for our over-investment and over-confidence in curative medical services. It is not obvious that the rise of medical science and the physician, taken alone, should become fundamental obstacles to collective action to prevent death and injury. But the prejudice found in market-justice against collective action perverts these scientific advances into an unrealistic hope for "technological shortcuts" (Etzioni and Remp, 1972) to painful social change. Moreover, the great emphasis placed on individual achievement in market-justice has further diverted attention and interest away from primary prevention and collective action by dramatizing the role of the solitary physician-scientist, picturing him as our primary weapon and first line of defense against the threat of death and injury.

The prestige of medical care encouraged by market-justice prevents large-scale research to determine whether, in fact, our medical care technology actually brings about the result desired—a significant reduction in the damage and losses suffered from disease and injury. The model conceals questions about our pervasive use of drugs, our intense specialization, and our seemingly boundless commitment to biomedical technology. Instead, the market model of justice encourages us to see problems as due primarily to the failure of individual doctors and the quality of their care, rather than to recognize the possibility of failure from the structure of medical care itself (Freidson, 1971). Consequently, we seek to remedy problems by trying to change individual doctors through appeals to their ethical sensibilities, or by reshaping their education, or by creating new financial incentives.

Government Health Policy

The vast expansion of government in health policy over the past decades might seem to signal the demise of the market ethic for health. But it is important to remember that the preponderance of our public policy for health continues to define health care as a consumption good to be allocated primarily by private decisions and markets, and only interferes with this market with public policy to subsidize, supplement or extend the market system when private decisions result in sufficient imperfections or inequities to be of public concern. Medicare and Medicaid are examples. Other examples include subsidizing or stimulating the private sector through public support for research, education of professionals, limited areawide planning, and the construction of facilities. Even national health insurance is largely a public financing mechanism to subsidize private markets in the hope that curative health services will be more equitably distributed. None of these policies is likely to bring dramatic reductions in rates of death and disability.

Our current efforts to reform the so-called health system are little more than the use of public authority to perpetuate essentially private mechanisms for allocating curative health services. These reforms are paraded as evidence that the system is capable of functioning equitably. But, as Barthes (1972) points out (in a different context), reform measures may merely serve to "inoculate" the larger society against the suspicion that it is the model itself (in our case, market-justice) that is at fault. In fact, the constant reform efforts designed to "save the system" may better be viewed as an attempt to expand the hegemony of the key actors in the present system—especially the medical care complex. As McKnight (1975) says, the medical care complex may need the hot air of reform if its ballooning empire is to continue to inflate.

Public Health Measures

I have saved for last an important class of health policies—public health measures to protect the environment, the workplace, or the commodities we purchase and consume. Are these not signs that American society is willing to accept collective action in the face of clear public health hazards?

I do not wish to minimize the importance of these advances to protect the public in many domains. But these separate reforms, taken alone, should be cautiously received. This is because each reform effort is perceived as an isolated exception to the norm of market-justice; the norm itself still stands. Consequently, the predictable career of such measures is to see enthusiasm for enforcement peak and wane. These public health measures are clear signs of hope. But as long as these actions are seen as merely minor exceptions to the rule of individual responsibility, the goals of public health will remain beyond our reach. What is required is for the public to see that protecting the public's health takes us beyond the norms of market-justice categorically and necessitates a completely new health ethic.

I return to my original point: Market-justice is the primary roadblock to dramatic reductions in preventable injury and death. More than this, market-justice is a pervasive ideology protecting the most powerful or the most numerous from the burdens of collective action. If this be true, the central goal of public health should be ethical in nature: The challenging of market-justice as fatally deficient in protecting the health of the public. Further, public health should advocate a "counter-ethic" for protecting the public's health, one articulated in a different tradition of justice and one designed to give the highest priority to minimizing death and disability and to the protection of all human life against the hazards of this world.

SOCIAL JUSTICE

The fundamental critique of market-justice found in the Western liberal tradition is social justice. Under social justice all persons are entitled equally to key ends such as health protection or minimum standards of income. Further, unless collective burdens are accepted, powerful forces of environment, heredity or social structure will preclude a fair distribution of these ends (Tawney, 1964; Hobhouse, 1964; Rawls, 1971). While many forces influenced the development of public health, the historic dream of public health that preventable death and disability ought to be minimized is a dream of social justice.[3] Yet these egalitarian and social justice implications of the public health vision are either still not widely recognized or are conveniently ignored.

Seeing the public health vision as ultimately rooted in an egalitarian tradition that conflicts directly with the norms of market-justice is often glossed over and obscured by referring to public health as a general strategy to control the "environment." For example, Canada's *New Perspectives on the Health of Canadians* (Government of Canada, 1974) correctly notes that major reductions in death and disability cannot be expected from curative health services. Future progress will have to result from alterations in the "environment" and "lifestyle." But if we substitute the words *market-justice* for *environment* or *lifestyle*, *New Perspectives* becomes a very radical document indeed. Ideally, then, the public health ethic[4] is not simply an alternative to the market ethic for health—it is a fundamental critique of that ethic as it unjustly protects powerful interests from the burdens of prevention and as that ethic serves to legitimate a mindless and extravagant faith in the efficacy of medical care. In other words, the public health ethic is a *counter-ethic* to market-justice and the ethics of individualism as these are applied to the health problems of the public.

This view of public health is admittedly not widely accepted. Indeed, in recent times the mission of public health has been viewed by many as limited to that minority of health problems that cannot be solved by the market provision of medical care services and that necessitate organized community action.[5] It is interesting to speculate why many in the public health profession have come to accept this narrow view of public health—a view that is obviously influenced and shaped by the market model as it attempts to limit the burdens placed on powerful groups (Beauchamp, 1975c).

Nonetheless, the broader view of public health set out here is logically and ethically justified if one accepts the vision of public health as being the protection of all human life. The central task of public health, then, is to complete its unfinished revolution: The elaboration of a health ethic adequate to protect and preserve all human life. This new ethic has several key implications which are referred to here as "principles":[6] (1) controlling the hazards of this world (2) to prevent death and disability (3) through organized collective action (4) shared equally by all except where unequal burdens result in increased protection of everyone's health and especially potential victims of death and disability.

These ethical principles are not new to public health. To the contrary, making the ethical foundations of public health visible only serves to highlight the social justice influences at work behind pre-existing principles.

Controlling the Hazards

A key principle of the public health ethic is the focus on the identification and control of the hazards of this world rather than a focus on the behavioral defects of those individuals damaged by these hazards. Against this principle it is often argued that today the causes of death and disability are multiple and frequently behavioral in origin (Brotman and Suffet, 1975). Further, since it is usually only a minority of the public that fails to protect itself against most known hazards, additional controls over these perilous sources would not seem to be effective or just. We should look instead for the behavioral origins of most public health problems (Sade, 1971), asking why some people expose themselves to known hazards or perils, or act in an unsafe or careless manner.

Public health should—at least ideally—be suspicious of behavioral paradigms for viewing public health problems since they tend to "blame the victim" and unfairly protect majorities and powerful interests from the burdens of prevention (Ryan, 1971; see also Terris, 1968). It is clear that behavioral models of public health problems are rooted in the tradition of market-justice, where the emphasis is upon individual ability and capacity, and individual success and failure.

Public health, ideally, should not be concerned with explaining the successes and failures of differing individuals (dispositional explanations)[7] in controlling the hazards of this world. Rather these failures should be seen as signs of still weak and ineffective controls or limits over those conditions, commodities, services, products or practices that are either hazardous for the health and safety of members of the public, or that are vital to protect the public's health.

Prevention

Like the other principles of public health, prevention is a logical consequence of the ethical goal of minimizing the numbers of persons suffering death and disability. The only known way to minimize these adverse events is to prevent the occurrence of damaging exchanges or exposures in the first place, or to seek to minimize damage when exposures cannot be controlled.

Prevention, then, is that set of priority rules for restructuring existing market rules in order to maximally protect the public. These rules seek to create policies and obligations to replace the norm of market-justice, where the latter permits specific conditions, commodities, services, products, activities or practices to pose a direct threat or hazard to the health and safety of members of the public, or where the market norm fails to allocate effectively and equitably those services (such as medical care) that are necessary to attend to disease at hand.

Thus, the familiar public health options:[8]

1. Creating rules to minimize exposure of the public to hazards (kinetic, chemical, ionizing, biological, etc.) so as to reduce the rates of hazardous exchanges

2. Creating rules to strengthen the public against damage in the event that damaging exchanges occur anyway, where such techniques (fluoridation, seat-belts, immunization) are feasible

3. Creating rules to organize treatment resources in the community so as to minimize damage that does occur since we can rarely prevent all damage

Collective Action

Another principle of the public health ethic is that the control of hazards cannot be achieved through voluntary mechanisms but must be undertaken by governmental or non-governmental agencies through planned, organized and collective action that is obligatory or non-voluntary in nature. This is for two reasons.

The first is because market or voluntary action is typically inadequate for providing what are called public goods (Olson, 1965). Public goods are those public policies (national defense, police and fire protection, or the protection of all persons against preventable death and disability) that are universal in their impacts and effects, affecting everyone equally. These kinds of goods cannot easily be withheld from those individuals in the community who choose not to support these services (this is typically called the "free rider" problem). Also, individual holdouts might plausibly reason that their small contribution might not prevent the public good from being offered.

The second reason why self-regarding individuals might refuse to voluntarily pay the costs of such public goods as public health policies is because these policies frequently require burdens that self-interest or self-protection might see as too stringent. For example, the minimization of rates of alcoholism in a community clearly seems to require norms or controls over the substance of alcohol that limit the use of this substance to levels that are far below what would be safe for individual drinkers (Beauchamp, 1975b).

With these temptations for individual noncompliance, justice demands assurance that all persons share equally the costs of collective action through obligatory and sanctioned social and public policy.

Fair Sharing of the Burdens

A final principle of the public health ethic is that all persons are equally responsible for sharing the burdens—as well as the benefits—of protection against death and disability, except where unequal burdens result in greater protection for every person and especially potential victims of death and disability.[9] In practice this means that policies to control the hazards of a given substance, service or commodity fall unequally (but still fairly) on those involved in the production, provision or consumption of the service, commodity or substance. The clear implication of this principle is that the automotive industry, the tobacco industry, the coal industry and the medical care industry—to mention only a few key groups—have an unequal responsibility to bear the costs of reducing death and disability since their actions have far greater impact than those of individual citizens.

DOING JUSTICE: BUILDING A NEW PUBLIC HEALTH

I have attempted to show the broad implications of a public health commitment to protect and preserve human life, setting out tentatively the logical consequences of that commitment in the form of some general principles. We need, however, to go beyond these broad principles and ask more specifically: What implications does this model have for doing public health and the public health profession?

The central implication of the view set out here is that doing public health should not be narrowly conceived as an instrumental or technical activity. Public health should be a way of doing justice, a way of asserting the value and priority of all human life. The primary aim of all public health activity should be the elaboration and adoption of a new ethical model or paradigm for protecting the public's health. This new ethical paradigm will necessitate a heightened consciousness of the manifold forces threatening human life, and will require thinking about and reacting to the problems of disability and premature death as primarily collective problems of the entire society.

The Right to Health

What concrete steps can public health take to accomplish this dramatic shift? Perhaps the most important step that public health might take to overturn the application of market-justice to the category of health protection would be to centrally challenge the absence of a right to health. Historically, the way in which inequality in American society has been confronted is by asserting the need for additional rights beyond basic political freedoms. (By a right to health, I do not mean anything so limited as the current assertion of a right to payment for medical care services.) Public health should immediately lay plans for a national campaign for a new public entitlement—the right to full and equal protection for all persons against preventable disease and disability.

This new public commitment needs more than merely organizational and symbolic expression; ultimately, it needs fundamental statutory and perhaps even constitutional protection. I can think of nothing more helpful to the goal of challenging the application of market-justice to the domain of health than to see public health enter into a protracted and lengthy struggle to secure a right-to-health amendment.[10] This campaign would in and of itself signal the failure of market-justice to protect the health of all the public. Once secured, this legislation could serve as the basic counterpoise to our numerous and countless policies sanctioning unreflecting growth, uncontrolled technology or unrelenting individualism. Such an amendment could enable public health in all of its activity to constantly, relentlessly, stubbornly, militantly confront and resist all efforts to dishonor the integrity of human life in the name of progress, convenience, security and prosperity, as well as assist public health in challenging the dubious stretching of the principle of personal freedom to protect every corner of social life.[11]

A second step on the path to a fundamental paradigm change is the work of constructing collective definitions of public health problems (Friedmann, 1973). Creating and disseminating collective definitions of the problems of death and disability would clearly communicate that the origins of these fates plainly lie beyond merely individual factors (but, as always, some individual factors cannot be totally ignored), and are to be found in structural features of the society such as the rules that govern exposure to the hazards of this world. These new collective descriptions, as they create more accurate explanations of public health problems, would in and of themselves expose the weakness of the norm of individual responsibility and point to, the need for collective solutions.

These new definitions of public health problems are especially needed to challenge the ultimately arbitrary distinction between voluntary and involuntary hazards, especially since the former category (recently termed "lifestyle") looms so large in terms of death and disease (see Government of Canada, 1974). Under the current definition of the situation, more stringent controls over involuntary risks are acceptable (if still strenuously resisted by producer groups), while controls over voluntary risks (smoking, alcohol, recreational risks) are viewed as infringements of basic personal rights and freedoms.

These new definitions would reveal the collective and structural aspects of what are termed voluntary risks, challenging attempts to narrowly and persuasively limit public attention to the behavior of the smoker or the drinker, and exposing pervasive myths that "blame the victim."[12] These collective definitions and descriptions would focus attention on the industry behind these activities, asking whether powerful producer groups and supporting cultural and social norms are not primary factors encouraging individuals to accept unreasonable risks to life and limb, and whether these groups or norms constitute aggressive collective structures threatening human life.

A case in point: Under the present definition of the situation, alcoholism is mostly defined in individual terms, mainly in terms of the attributes of those persons who are "unable" to control their drinking. But I have shown elsewhere (Beauchamp, 1975a) that this argument is both conceptually and empirically erroneous. Alcohol problems are collective problems that require more adequate controls over this important hazard.

This is not to say that there are no important issues of liberty and freedom in these areas. It is rather to say that viewing the use of, for example, alcohol or cigarettes by millions of American adults as "voluntary" behavior, and somehow fundamentally different from other public health hazards, impoverishes the public health approach, tending, as Terris (1968) has suggested, to divorce the behavior of the individual from its social base.

In building these collective redefinitions of health problems, however, public health must take care to do more than merely shed light on specific public health problems. The central problems remain the injustice of a market ethic that unfairly protects majorities and powerful interests from their fair share of the burdens of prevention, and of convincing the public that the task of protecting the public's health lies categorically beyond the norms of market-justice. This means that the function of each different redefinition of a specific problem must be to raise the common and recurrent issue of justice by exposing the aggressive and powerful structures implicated in all instances of preventable death and disability, and further to point to the necessity for collective measures to confront and resist these structures.

Political Struggle

Doing public health involves more than merely elaborating a new social ethic; doing public health involves the political process and the challenging of some very important and powerful interests in society. The public health model involves at its very center the commitment to a very controversial ethic—the radical commitment to protect and preserve human life. To realize and make visible this commitment means challenging the embedded arid structured values—as well as sheer political power—of dominant interests. These interests will not yield their influence without struggle.

This political struggle for a *truly* public health policy crucially involves bringing the medical care complex under the control of a new public health ethic. The medical care industry, like other powerful groups, must bear its fair share of the burdens of minimizing death and disability. Of all the perils presently confronting the public health community, there is none greater than that of gradually limiting and diminishing its mission to that of public medical care. I am deeply concerned that national health insurance will become a vehicle to be used by what Alford (1972) has labeled the "corporate rationalizers" to further finance, extend, solidify and entrench the power of the medical care complex. The nation's leading medical care issue is not to expand the medical care service market; the central issue is to control a powerful and expansionist medical care industry. Challenging medical dominance could go a long way toward reclaiming health as a public concern and an issue of social justice.

Challenging these centers of power in order to incarnate the priority of human life requires not only a new ethic but a supporting base of power. I believe that while professional prestige is an important attribute in the modern-day public policy process, public health is ultimately better understood as a broad social movement. There is simply no way that we can hope to capture public health under a defining set of competences, skills and professional backgrounds. The political potential of public health goes beyond professionalism; at its very heart is advocacy of an explosive and radical ethic. Doing public health should be a ubiquitous, pervasive, common and routine activity accomplished in every public and private agency, at every level of government, among all peoples, and at every moment of our common history. Health policy is most decidedly not the sole preserve of physicians, schools of public health, health educators, consumer groups or any other special interest group; rather it is a fundamental concern of all human activity and a distinguishing sign of a just community. By stressing the pervasive character of public health and the problems of death and disability, the foundation for a broad social movement can be established.

At the same time, public health should always hold in mind that this power struggle is meant to be not only instrumental but also dialectical, informative and symbolic. The point of the struggle is not merely to ensure that producer interests accept their fair share of the costs of minimizing death and disability, but also—and once again—to reveal through the process of confrontation and challenge the structured and collective nature of the problems of death and disability and the urgency for more adequate structures to protect all human life.

I also believe that the realism inherent in the public health ethic dictates that the foundation of all public health policy should be primarily (but not exclusively) national in locus. I simply disagree with the current tendency, rooted in misguided pluralism and market metaphors, to build from the bottom up. This current drift will, in my opinion, simply provide the medical care industry and its acolytes (to cite only one powerful group) with the tools necessary to further elaborate and extend its hegemony. Confronting organizations, interests, ideologies and alliances that are national and even international in scope with such limited resources seems hopelessly sentimental. We must always remember that the forces opposed to full protection of the public's health are fundamental and powerful, deeply rooted in our national character. We are unlikely to successfully oppose these forces with appeals or strategies more appropriate for an earlier and more provincial time.

Finally, the public health movement must cease being defensive about the wisdom or the necessity of collective action. One of the most interesting aspects of market-justice—and particularly its ideological thrusts—is that it makes collective or governmental activity seem unwise if not dangerous. Such rhetoric predictably ignores the influence of private power over the health and safety of every individual. Public health need not be oblivious to the very real concerns about a proliferating bureaucracy in the emergent welfare state. In point of fact, however, the preventive thrust of public health transcends the notion of the welfare or service state and its most recent variant, the human services society. Much as the ideals of service and welfare are improvements over the simple working of market-justice, the service society frequently functions to spread the costs of public problems among the entire public while permitting the interests, industries, or professions who might remedy or prevent many of these problems to operate with expanding power and autonomy.

CONCLUSION

The central thesis of this chapter is that public health is ultimately and essentially an ethical enterprise committed to the notion that all persons are entitled to protection against the hazards of this world and to the minimization of death and disability in society. I have tried to make the implications of this ethical vision manifest, especially as the public health ethic challenges and confronts the norms of market-justice.

I do not see these goals of public health as hopelessly unrealistic or destructive of fundamental liberties. Public health may be an "alien ethic in a strange land" (Beauchamp, 1975c). Yet if anything, the public health ethic is more faithful to the traditions of Judeo-Christian ethics than market-justice is.

The image of public health that I have drawn here does raise legitimate questions about what it is to be a professional, and legitimate questions about reasonable limits to restrictions on human liberty. These questions must be addressed more thoroughly than I have done here. Nonetheless, we must never pass over the chaos of preventable disease and disability in our society by simply celebrating the benefits of our prosperity and abundance, or our technological advances. What are these benefits worth if they have been purchased at the price of human lives?

Nothing written here should be construed as a per se attack on the market system. I have, rather, surfaced the moral and ethical norms of that system and argued that, whatever other benefits might accrue from those norms, they are woefully inadequate to ensure full and equal protection of all human life.

The adoption of a new public health ethic and a new public health policy must and should occur within the context of a democratic polity. I agree with Terris (1968) that the central task of the public health movement is to persuade society to accept these measures.

Finally, it is a peculiarity of the word *freedom* that its meaning has become so distorted and stretched as to lend itself as a defense against nearly every attempt to extend equal health protection to all persons. This is the ultimate irony. The idea of liberty should mean, above all else, the liberation of society from the injustice of preventable disability and early death. Instead, the concept of freedom has become a defense and protection of powerful vested interests, and the central issue is viewed as a choice between freedom on the one hand, and health and safety on the other. I am confident that ultimately the public will come to see that extending life and health to all persons will require some diminution of personal choices but that such restrictions are not only fair and do not constitute abridgment of fundamental liberties, they are a basic sign and imprint of a just society and a guarantee of that most basic of all freedoms—protection against humanity's most ancient foe.

Notes

1. Some readers might object to the marriage of the terms *market* and *justice*. One theory of the market holds that it is a blind hand that rewards without regard to merit or individual effort. For this point of view, see Friedman (1962) and Hayek (1960). But Kristol (1970) argues that this is a minority view; most accept the marriage of the market ideal and the merits of individual effort and performance. I agree with this point of view—which is to say I see the dominant model of justice in America as a merger of the notions of merit-based and market norms.

2. See Barry (1975) for an excellent discussion of "victim-blaming" in the field of injury-control. Also see Beauchamp(1975a, 1976) for discussion of the process of victim-blaming in the area of alcoholism policy.

3. I am aware that I am passing too quickly over a very complex subject: the formative influences for public health. I am simply asserting that the dream of eliminating or minimizing preventable death and disability involves a radical commitment to the protection and preservation of human life and that this vision ultimately belongs to the tradition of social justice. Further, one can clearly find social justice influences in the classics of the public health literature. For example, see Smith (1973) and Winslow (1929).

   There are several reasons why public health has seldom been treated as standing in the tradition of social justice. Public health usually entails public or collective goods (such as clean air and water supplies) where the question of distributive shares seems unimportant. However, for collective goods and in the case of death and disability, the key distributive questions are the *numbers* or *rates* of persons who suffer these fates, that no group or individual be unfairly or arbitrarily excluded from protection, and that the *burdens* of collective policies be fairly distributed. Writers in the tradition of social justice (such as Rawls) do not pay sufficient attention to the social justice implications of public or collective goods. This helps explain in part why many in the public health movement seldom saw themselves as involved in a drive for social justice—their work was defined as protection for the entire community (and often the entire community, rather than a minority, seem threatened in the age of acute infectious epidemics or in the drive for sanitary reform). Further, while there was opposition to even these reforms, the question of distributing the burdens of collective action did not arise so acutely as it does in the present period.

4. By "public health ethic" I mean several things: The assignment of the highest priority to the preservation of human life, the assurance that this protection is extended maximally (consistent with maintaining basic political liberties; see Rawls, 1971, and note 12), that no person or group should be arbitrarily excluded, and that all persons ought accept these burdens of preserving life as just.

5. Let me cite two examples of this point. First, a standard text in health administration, John Hanlon's *Public Health Administration and Practice* (1974), does reference very broad definitions of public health but quickly settles down to discussing public health in terms of the various programs designed to deal with market fail-

ures or inadequacies. Nowhere does Hanlon seem to view the concept of public health as an ethical concept standing as a fundamental critique of the existing measures to protect human life.

6. I hasten to add that I am not arguing that there are exactly four principles of the public health ethic. Actually, the four offered here can be easily collapsed to two: controls over the hazards of this world and the fair sharing of the burdens of these controls. However, the reason for expanding these two key principles is to draw out the character of the public health ethic as a counterethic or counterparadigm to the market model and to demonstrate that the public health ethic focuses on different aspects of the world, asserts different priorities, and imposes different obligations than the market ethic.

7. See Brown (1963) for an excellent discussion of the limitations of dispositional explanations in social science. Also see Beauchamp (1976) for further discussion of the pitfalls of dispositional explanations in the specific area of alcohol policy.

8. For excellent discussions of the strategies of public health, see Haddon (1968, 1973) and Terris (1974).

9. This principle is similar to Rawls's "difference principle"; see Rawls (1971).

10. I must confess a certain ambivalence about the expression "right to health." It is not only easily confused with a right to payment for medical care services, but it suffers the further limitation of not conveying the full intent of the public health ethic, which, at least as I see it, is to give the highest priority to life and to ensure collective rules and arrangements that embody and incarnate that priority. The expression "right to health" could easily be construed as something far less ambitious than these goals.

11. I realize that I have not begun to clarify the issue of just how far a society can go in protecting life and limb without jeopardizing political liberty. I agree with Rawls (1971) as to the priority of liberty. However, I tend to think of liberty in terms of specific constitutional guarantees (freedom of speech, religion, due process, and so on) rather than in the more extensive sense of a positive freedom to act as one chooses except where one's actions bring harm to others. Also, shedding light on this issue of the conflict between liberty and the protection of the public's health would help shed light on just what "minimizing" death and disability specifically entails. I am satisfied at this point, however, that the public health ethic would move us much further toward protecting all of the public's health without relinquishing the basic liberties and freedoms that are the attributes of a just political community and without which the very notion of social justice itself would be in jeopardy.

12. Destroying these "myths" could be a major task of public health activity. See Ryan (1971) for the best discussion of "victim-blaming" myths. See Beauchamp (1975a) for a foray against the "myth" of alcoholism. I am using the word *myth* here very specifically to mean the confusion and false definitions that arise when we discuss a *public* problem in an individual idiom. For a good discussion of the concept of myths in general, see Ryle (1949).

References

Alford, R. "The Political Economy of Health Care: Dynamics Without Change." *Politics and Society,* 1972, *2,* 127–164.

Barry, P. "Individual Versus Community Orientation in the Prevention of Injuries." *Preventive Medicine,* 1975, *4,* 45–56.

Barthes, R. *Mythologies.* New York: Hill & Wang, 1972.

Beauchamp, D. E. "The Alcohol Alibi: Blaming Alcoholics." *Society,* 1975a, *12,* 12–17.

Beauchamp, D. E. "Federal Alcohol Policy: Captive to an Industry and a Myth." *Christian Century,* 1975b, *92,* 788–791.

Beauchamp, D. E. "Public Health: Alien Ethic in a Strange Land?" *American Journal of Public Health,* 1975c, *65,* 1338–1339.

Beauchamp, D. E. "Alcoholism as Blaming the Alcoholic." *International Journal of Addictions,* 1976, *11,* 41–52.

Brotman, R., and Suffet, F. "The Concept of Prevention and Its Limitations." *Annals of the American Academy of Political and Social Science,* 1975, *417,* 53–65.

Brown, R. *Explanation in Social Science.* Hawthorne, N.Y.: Aldine de Gruyter, 1963.

Downs, A. "The Issue-Attention Cycle and the Political Economy of Improving Our Environment." Paper presented as part of the Royer Lectures at the University of California, Berkeley, Apr. 13–14, 1970.

Etzioni, A., and Remp, R. "Technological 'Shortcuts' to Social Change." *Science,* 1972, *175,* 31–38.

Freidson, E. *Professional Dominance.* Hawthorne, N.Y.: Aldine de Gruyter, 1971.

Friedman, M. *Capitalism and Freedom.* Chicago: University of Chicago Press, 1962.

Friedmann, J. *Retracking America: A Theory of Transactive Planning.* New York: Anchor/Doubleday, 1973.

Government of Canada. *A New Perspective on the Health of Canadians.* Ottawa, Canada: Ministry of National Health and Welfare, 1974.

Haddon, W., Jr. "The Changing Approach to the Epidemiology, Prevention, and Amelioration of Trauma." *American Journal of Public Health,* 1968, *58,* 1431–1438.

Haddon, W., Jr. "Energy Damage and the Ten Countermeasure Strategies." *Journal of Trauma,* 1973, *13,* 321–331.

Hanlon, J. *Public Health Administration and Practice.* St. Louis, Mo.: Mosby, 1974.

Hardin, G. *Exploring New Ethics for Survival.* New York: Penguin Books, 1972.

Hayek, F. *The Constitution of Liberty.* Chicago: University of Chicago Press, 1960.

Hobhouse, L. T. *Liberalism.* New York: Oxford University Press, 1964.

Illich, I. "The Political Uses of Natural Death." *Hastings Center Studies,* 1974, *2,* 3–20.

Jonsen, A. R., and Hellegers, A. E. "Conceptual Foundations for an Ethics of Medical Care." In L. R. Tancredi (ed.), *Ethics of Health Care.* Washington, D.C.: National Academy of Sciences, 1974.

Kapp, W. *Social Costs of Business Enterprise.* (2nd ed.) New York: Asia Publishing House, 1964.

Kristol, I. "When Virtue Loses All Her Loveliness." *Public Interest,* 1970, *21,* 3–15.

Marcuse, H. "The Ideology of Death." In H. Feifel (ed.), *The Meaning of Death.* New York: McGraw-Hill, 1959.

McKnight, J. "The Medicalization of Politics." *Christian Century,* 1975, *92,* 785–787.

Mishan, E. *The Costs of Economic Growth.* New York: Praeger, 1967.

Olson, M. *The Logic of Collective Action.* Cambridge, Mass.: Harvard University Press, 1965.

Outka, E. "Social Justice and Equal Access to Health Care." *Journal of Religious Ethics,* 1974, *2,* 11–32.

Rawls, J. *A Theory of Justice.* Cambridge, Mass.: Harvard University Press, 1971.

Ryan, W. *Blaming the Victim.* New York: Vintage Books, 1971.

Ryle, G. *The Concept of Mind.* New York: Barnes & Noble Books, 1949.

Sade, R. "Medical Care as a Right: A Refutation." *New England Journal of Medicine,* 1971, *285,* 1288–1292.

Tawney, R. *Equality.* London: Allen & Unwin, 1964.

Terris, M. "A Social Policy for Health." *American Journal of Public Health,* 1968, *58,* 5–12.

Terris, M. "Breaking the Barriers to Prevention." Paper presented at the annual health conference, New York Academy of Medicine, Apr. 26, 1974.

CHAPTER ELEVEN

Social Capital and the Third Way in Public Health

Carles Muntaner
John W. Lynch
George Davey Smith

Within the last few years, we have witnessed the rapid appearance of the concept of social capital in public health discourse. Before 1995, there was only one reference to the term *social capital* in the Medline database, and that was in regard to so-called "family social capital" and its effect on educational and occupational aspirations (Marjoribanks, 1991). Though the basic ideas encapsulated in the current use of *social capital* can be traced to the origins of classical sociology and political science, the appearance of the term itself in the mid-1990s was largely stimulated by Robert Putnam's work on civic participation and its effect on local governance (Putnam, Leonardi, and Nanetti et al., 1993). He popularized this thesis by discussing the decline of social capital using the metaphor that America was "bowling alone" (Putnam, 1995a)—a powerful image that propelled Putnam to an audience with President Clinton to discuss the fraying of the social fabric in America. Since then, the concept of social capital has also appeared in other fields such as sociology (Portes, 1998) and development economics (Grootaert, 1997; Ostrom, 1999). In these fields, there has been a good deal of debate about the definition, operationalization, and the theoretical and practical utility of the concept for improving human welfare, especially in regard to alleviating poverty and stimulating economic growth in less industrialized countries (Collier, 1998; Knack and Keefer, 1997). In fact, the World Bank sponsors a Web site devoted exclusively to the topic of social capital, where information is exchanged and issues actively debated. Despite all this activity, one of the leading scholars in this field, Michael Woolcock, has argued that the concept of social capital "risks trying to explain too much with too little" (1998, p. 155). He says that the term *social capital* is being "adopted indiscriminately, adapted uncritically, and applied imprecisely" (p. 196).

SOCIAL CAPITAL AND ITS USE IN PUBLIC HEALTH

We believe Woolcock's critique is especially true for many of the ways that the term *social capital* has been used in relation to health. To date there has been very little systematic theoretical, empirical, or practical appraisal of the concept in the public health literature, although more critical accounts are beginning to appear. (Muntaner and Lynch, 1999a; Muntaner, Nieto, and O'Campo, 1997; Lynch and others, 2000; Hawe and Shiell, 2000). Nevertheless, the term has slipped effortlessly into the public health lexicon as if there were a clear, shared understanding of its meaning and its relevance for improving public health. The term *social capital* and its close cousin, *social cohesion,* have been used as multipurpose descriptors for all types and levels of connections among individuals, within families, friendship networks, businesses and communities (Wilkinson, 1996; Aneshensel and Sucoff, 1996; Kawachi and Kennedy, 1997; Kawachi, Kennedy, and Lochner, 1997; Kawachi, Kennedy, and Prothrow-Stith, 1997; Fullilove, 1998; Baum, 1997, 1999; Kennedy, Kawachi, and Brainerd, 1999). In addition, it has been the subject of theme conferences (Eleventh National Health Promotion Conference, Perth, Australia) and government-sponsored discussion papers (Jenson, 1998; Lavis and Stoddart, 1999); it has been the topic of million-dollar calls for research proposals funded by the Centers for Disease Control in the United States, and on the basis of highly dubious comparisons between observational studies and clinical trials of such things as anti-thrombolytic therapy, it has even been proposed as an important avenue of public health intervention. Lomas (1998) has argued that "interventions to increase social support and/or social cohesion in a community are at least as worthy of exploration as improved access or routine medical care. Certainly they are more worthwhile than public health's traditional risk factor modification approach to cardiovascular disease" (p. 1184). These are impressive, yet completely untested, claims.

Similarly, in a recent book published by the Health Education Authority in Britain, the authors state that "there is a consensus in recent literature that the construct of 'social capital' may be usefully applied to the study of health and health-related behavior" (Cooper, Arber, and Ginn, 1999, p. 4). They leave the impression that we know much more about the theoretical and practical value of social capital than an examination of the actual evidence would suggest. Furthermore, they go on to say that "researchers have measured social capital in terms of the social, collective, economic and cultural resources available to a family, neighbourhood or community" (p. 4). There are a myriad of indicators of social, collective, economic and cultural resources across the levels of families, neighbourhoods and communities—are they all markers of levels of social capital? We are not concerned about the multi-dimensionality of the concept, but we are concerned that this multi-dimensionality has received so little theoretical exploration in regard to public health. Consequently it provides little guidance about the importance of the particular mechanisms that might link these different dimensions to health. Stated in this undifferentiated way, the laundry list of measurement strategies outlined above merely suggests that there may be a little something for everyone in social capital. Hawe and Shiell (2000) have commented that the health-related applications of social capital have often involved measuring "all that is good in a community." Conflating the political, cultural and economic aspects of a community under the one umbrella of social capital, may mask important conceptual distinctions as to the origins of those group resources and may obscure the fact that these dimensions are not necessarily equally important as determinants of health. It would seem that under this kind of undifferentiated approach to social capital, establishing an arts festival (the cultural dimension) and a job creation program (the economic dimension) are both interventions to improve social capital—but are they likely to have an equal impact on public health? This in no way denies the importance of improving the cultural life of a community through programmes of arts and music. The question is whether tossing all these dimensions into the grab bag of social capital can inform strategies to improve public health.

The reasons for the easy and almost completely uncritical acceptance of social capital into public health discourse is of interest in itself. Discussion of the concept would appear to come from at least three main sources within the public health community—from those concerned with community-based health promotion (Baum, 1999; Cooper, Arber, and Ginn, 1999), from those in the social support field (Cooper, Arber, and Ginn, 1999; Tijhuis and others, 1995), and from those who have claimed that social capital and social cohesion are the main mediators of the link between income inequality and population health (Wilkinson, 1996; Kawachi, Kennedy, and Lochner, 1997; Kawachi, Kennedy, and Prothrow-Stith, 1997). One factor that perhaps links these diverse areas of public health research and practice is that they are all motivated to some extent, by the underlying idea that there is something about the connections among individuals that is important for public health. Levels of population health may be more than the arithmetic sum of the health of the individuals in those populations, and the determinants of population health are both individual and contextual. In this view there is something inherently "social" about improving public health that cannot be reduced to studying and changing discrete individuals. This idea is not new (Rose, 1985) and there have been many critiques of an overly individualistic approach to public health research and intervention (Krieger, 1994; Lynch, Kaplan, and Salonen, 1997; Muntaner and O'Campo, 1993). The concept and language of social capital have perhaps been seen as offering a new and exciting way to invigorate supra-individual public health research and to provide support for a non-individualized, social science approach to improving public health (Baum, 1999).

PUBLIC HEALTH AND THE CONNECTIONS AMONG INDIVIDUALS

The goal of moving beyond individualistic theory and practice in public health is laudable and as one of us has recently argued, the connections among individuals are an important and neglected research area in epidemiology and public health. In that paper, Koopman and Lynch (1999) showed how the different arrangement of connections among individuals can produce very different patterns of infectious disease transmission in a population. Infectious disease transmission depends on who is connected to whom, and it is possible that other disease processes are also influenced by the pattern of connections within a population. This disease transmission perspective perhaps provides another language for understanding how social support has sometimes been found to protect against certain poor health outcomes. High levels of social support block the transmission of the pathogenic agent, in this case, usually hypothesized as stress.

Populations are not just unrelated heaps of individuals, whose patterns of connections can be ignored. However, overly simplistic interpretations of the patterns of connections among people may mask, not reveal determinants of population health. For example, strong links among individuals can both increase and decrease the risk of certain health outcomes. Tight connections among infants in a day-care centre may increase their risk of otitis-media. In one context, strong friendship networks of peers can increase the risk of smoking, drinking or use of illicit drugs, while in a different situation these same sorts of links may decrease the risk of suicide. Tight networks among the Mafia, neo-Nazi parties, or semi-clandestine business organizations such as the Trilateral Commission, the World Trade Organization, or GATT increase health risks for other members of the population. Scratch beyond a superficial level and the public health consequences of how individuals and groups are connected rapidly becomes very complicated.

As we have stated above, we are advocates of the idea that the way individuals and groups get connected to form friendship networks, neighbourhoods, communities and populations can be important for public health. However, we are less convinced that the concept of social capital, in its present form, can provide an adequate basis to understand how these connections may be linked to population health. We believe that social capital has been under-theorized in its public health usage, and that it is time to engage in serious debate about its definition, measurement, and application in public health research and practice. It is within this broader framework of appreciating how both the formal and informal connections among individuals, and the connections among population sub-groups are linked to population health, that we must critically evaluate the concept of social capital. We think that some of the issues for public health research and practice are (1) to explore the sources of the connections among different individuals and groups—i.e., what determines who gets connected to whom; (2) to understand what is transmitted over those networks that might be plausibly linked to health outcomes; and (3) to understand how the health-relevant aspects of the connections among individuals and groups can be changed to improve public health.

THEORETICAL DIFFERENCES WITH SOCIAL SCIENCE

"When I use a word," Humpty Dumpty said, in a rather scornful tone, "it means just what I choose it to mean—neither more nor less." "The question is," said Alice, "whether you can make words mean so many different things." "The question is," said Humpty Dumpty, "which is to be the master, that's all."
(Lewis Carroll's *Alice Through the Looking Glass*)

Because the scant empirical literature on social capital and health has been accompanied by enthusiastic expectations about social capital's future relevance to public health (Kawachi, Kennedy, and Lochner, 1997; Kawachi, Kennedy, and Prothrow-Stith, 1997; Marmot, 1998; Mustard, 1996), social capital often conveys the authoritarian arbitrariness of Alice's famous exchange with Humpty Dumpty. Powerful institutions, actors and funding agencies have a lot to say about what a concept means and what concepts are considered legitimate for empirical research (Muntaner, Nieto, and O' Campo, 1997; Muntaner, 1999a, 1999b; Wing, 1998). Nevertheless, because public health is a science, and thus has adjacent disciplines, we can examine the compatibility of its social capital construct with regard to the social capital theories that have been developed in contiguous disciplines (e.g., sociology, demography, and international development). Almost exclusively, the construct of social capital adopted by public health researchers has been the most psychological, the communitarian view (Putnam, Leonardi, and Nanetti, 1993). This conception emphasizes civic engagement, as in membership in local non-governmental organizations, or norms of reciprocity and trust among community members. Communitarians, who often favour minimal government and self-reliance (Etzioni and George, 1999), present their position as a "third way" between laissez-faire neoliberalism and social democracy (Etzioni and George, 1999), and have been supported by the New Labour and New Democrat administrations in the United Kingdom and the United States (Muntaner and Lynch, 1999a). The "small government" communitarian view, with its emphasis on civic organizations (third sector, not-for-profit institutions, and non-governmental organizations), not only undermines government intervention in the social democratic European welfare state but also undermines political representation, since national class-based parties that strive for state control are substituted with idealized notions of small-scale political organizing at the community level (Muntaner and Lynch, 1999a). Thus it is possible that in public health, social capital may function as a health policy alternative to large-scale government redistribution (dismantling or reducing the post–World War II welfare state) (Wainwright, 1996; Muntaner and Lynch, 1999a). In social epidemiology more specifically, social capital presents a model of the social determinants of health that does not include any analysis of structural inequalities (e.g., class, gender or racial relations) in favour of a horizontal view of social relations based on distributive inequalities in income (Muntaner and Lynch, 1999b). As a consequence, class, race or gender-based political movements are also ignored as explanations for reducing social inequalities in health (Muntaner and Lynch, 1999a).

In spite of the confusion regarding the referents of social capital (Coleman, 1990; Woolcock, 1998), there is no justification as to why public health scholars should restrict their conception of social capital to the communitarian notion of civic participation and its indicators (e.g., organization membership, newspaper readership). In social science—in particular, in sociology, demography, and developmental economics—social capital has at least two other conceptualizations that have a larger sociological content: one is that of network analysis (Granovetter, 1973; Portes, 1998; Woolcock, 1998). This view of social capital derives from the Weberian tradition in sociology and acknowledges the existence of stratification as well as the negative effects of strong networks for communities (e.g., in Mafia "families"). For example, Granovetter (1973) showed the differences in the networks of professionals and non-professionals—weak ties among professionals facilitate access to information about job opportunities. Portes (1998) showed the conditions under which strong networks among immigrants have facilitated the enrichment of ethnic businessmen in the United States. Another sociological approach to social capital emphasizes the role of institutions, including the state. Following the seminal work of Evans (1995) on economic development, this institutional approach considers both a community's social capital—its internal cohesion, ties and networks—and the type of relation that the state has with communities (Szreter, 1999). This "embeddedness" or institutional support dictates how the state co-operates with civil society to foster economic development via interaction between private and public institutions, legal and democratic systems, and citizen rights (Woolcock, 1998). As we will show below, and have argued earlier (Lynch and others, 2000), this notion of social capital is more encompassing and allows greater explanatory potential and integration with other sociological traditions in social epidemiology and public health (e.g., the study of the health effects of class, gender and race relations).

IDEALIST SOCIAL PSYCHOLOGY: "BOWLING WITH DE TOCQUEVILLE" AND OTHER EXAGGERATIONS

Social capital in public health is coined in terms of a lay or commonsense social psychology that has great appeal in the United States and elsewhere (Cooper, Arber, and Ginn, 1999; Baum, 1999; Kawachi, Kennedy, and Lochner, 1997). Who would oppose the notion that civic participation, trust in communities, and good neighbourly relations are good for health? In the United States, the "mom and apple pie" idea that good community relations are desirable is part of the collective wisdom among communitarians, liberals and social conservatives alike (Putnam, 1995a, 1995b; Etzioni and George, 1999).

Behind this conventional aspiration for achieving "healthy communities" also lies an idealized view of past community life that is seldom warranted (Lynch and Kaplan, 1997). A particular form of historical imprecision is the selective reading of Alexis de Tocqueville, a French aristocrat known for his observations on the high degree of civic participation in American communities during his nineteenth-century journey in the United States (e.g., Kawachi, Kennedy, and Lochner, 1997; Kawachi, Kennedy, and Prothrow-Stith, 1997; Kawachi and Berkman, 2000). Leaving aside the contradictions in *Democracy in America* (Elster, 1993), Tocqueville displayed a sharp critical view, for example, when reflecting on the individualism and self-sufficiency that is so dear to communitarians: "Individualism is a calm and considered feeling which disposes each citizen to isolate himself from the mass of his fellows and withdraw into the circle of family and friends; with this little society formed to his taste he gladly leaves the greater society to look after itself" (Tocqueville, [1835] 1969, p. 506). This sentence highlights the perils of narrow associationism, or a negative effect of social capital which is largely absent from current public health and social policy writings on the subject (Muntaner and Lynch, 1999a). A negative appraisal of vibrant, local associationism in the United States is not new, however. Multiple local interest group associations are part of "American exceptionalism" (Muntaner, 1999b) and these strongly localized associations may be seen as both potential barriers and supports to creating public policies aimed to improve population health. For example, the failure of creating a broad working class political party capable of establishing a strong welfare state, including the lack of universal access to health care (Navarro, 1994), has been a barrier to improvements in public health in the United States. Furthermore, a recent analysis of voter participation data in American cities circa 1880 lends no support to the social capital perspective whereby civic associations would have a beneficial impact on broad-based political participation (Kaufman, 1999). Rather, these analyses reveal that civic associations functioned as powerful interest groups that lobbied for specific party platforms that were not necessarily in the broader public interest (Kaufman, 1999).

Another inaccuracy of the received wisdom in current public health accounts of social capital is the uncritical acceptance of Putnam's "bowling alone" thesis on the decline of social capital in the United States (Kawachi and Kennedy, 1997; Kawachi, Kennedy, and Prothrow-Stith, 1997; Kawachi, Kennedy, and Wilkinson, 1999; Wilkinson, Kawachi, and Kennedy, 1998). The available evidence in the United States suggests that there has not been a decline in associations over the last two decades (Smith, 1997; Paxton, 1999). Furthermore, older forms of civic participation that have perhaps declined have been transformed over time (Skocpol, 1999). In addition, Putnam's analysis of social capital as the key factor underlying economic development in several Italian regions (e.g., Emilia-Romagna) has also been challenged (e.g., the neglect of class relations or 19th century socialist and Catholic political traditions in the creation of contemporary social capital; Warren, 1994). The notion that social capital drives political and economic performance has been refuted with new analyses of data from Italian regions and other industrial democracies (Jackman et al., 1996). Our overall point here is that the discourse around social capital in public health has tended to focus on its upside. We believe a more complete reading of the literature relevant to understanding the likely health effects of social capital reveals that the concept has been portrayed narrowly and has focused on more optimistic appraisals of its relevance to population health.

COMMUNITARIANS OF THE WORLD UNITE! IGNORING THE CLASS, GENDER AND RACE STRUCTURE

Given the scant support for the social capital hypotheses reviewed above, one would expect that policy makers and researchers alike would be more sanguine in their approach to the subject. At least, some acknowledgement of alternative mechanisms driving the political, economic and health performance of nations (e.g., political movements, and class relations) might be expected from objective scholars. Unfortunately, in the enthusiastic entourage of social capital, this is not the case (e.g., Kawachi, Kennedy, and Prothrow-Stith, 1997). The field is indeed inundated with paradoxes and omissions. For example, although communitarians such as Vaclav Havel (1999) accept the "end of the nation-state"—that is, of its welfare policies (universal health care, public education, subsidized housing, poverty relief, unemployment compensation, etc.), they are often accepting of international military interventions under the umbrella of powerful nation-states (e.g., NATO's war in the former Yugoslavia; Chomsky, 1999a).

Even the most erudite scholars seem to dismiss competing alternatives to social capital. For example, in the fields of comparative political sociology and economic development, dependency and world-system theories are far from exhausted, contrary to what Woolcock (1998) claims in his exhaustive review and integration of social capital studies (Woolcock, 1998). The early dependency (e.g., Andre Gunder-Frank, Fernando-Henrique Cardoso) and world-system theories (e.g., Immanuel Wallerstein, Christopher Chase-Dunn), which were a spinoff of the Marxian tradition in sociology, have de facto evolved into stronger research programs that retain some of their ideas. This has happened for several reasons, including, (1) in recent years there has been a number of empirical articles on these theories in the leading sociological journals (*American Journal of Sociology, American Sociological Review*); (2) hypotheses arising from these theories of development (e.g., that receiving aid from the International Monetary Fund and the World Bank is associated with increased income inequality) have been confirmed by researchers coming from different perspectives (e.g., Boswell, who comes from the Marxian tradition, and Nielsen, who does not; see Muntaner and Lynch, 1999a); and (3) controversies in this field have reached such a degree of sophistication that the issue is less whether IMF or WB aid is associated with increases in a nation's income inequality (it is), but rather the timing of these income inequalities (Dixon and Boswell, 1996; Kentor, 1998; Alderson and Nielsen, 1999). In other areas of social science, social capital has been integrated with research on social inequalities (e.g., class, gender and race). For example, in historical sociology, Gould (1991, 1993) explains social class mobilization in the Paris Commune with network analysis and pre-existing levels of social cohesion. Another area of integration between stratification and social capital is the sociology of gender. Brines (1999), for example, has shown how earnings equality among cohabiting couples reinforces cohesion and stability, making couples more likely to remain together than in conditions where one of the members of the couple (most notably the woman in heterosexual couples) earns more than her male partner. In addition to class and gender (Erikson, 1996; Muntaner, Oates, and Lynch, 1999; Persell, Catsambis, and Cookson, 1992; Zweigenhaft, 1993), racial and ethnic segregation has also been linked to social capital (Borjas, 1992). Contrary to the "law and order" view of social capital often portrayed in public health, Pattillo (1998) has shown the difficulty of separating networks of "law-abiding" and "criminal" residents in cohesive African American neighbourhoods characterized by dense networks. Recently, researchers have also found that educational networks (Coleman's original notion of social capital) are class and racially segregated (Schneider et al., 1997).

Thus, in social science the fields of class, gender and race/ethnic inequalities are often integrated with social capital (mostly its network and institutional versions). However, with few exceptions (Matthews, Stansfeld, and Power, 1999) the mostly communitarian approach to social capital in public health shies away from these mechanisms (Muntaner and Lynch, 1999a, 1999b).

FAMILIAR HEALTH POLICY IMPLICATIONS:
"THE IMPORTANCE OF SUBJECTIVITY"

One implication of social capital in public health is the role of individual subjectivity in mediating the relation between inequality and health (Wilkinson, 1996, 1999). The breakdown in social cohesion occurs because individuals perceive their relative position in the social distribution of income, which creates anxiety and other psychosocial injuries which, in turn, affect health (Wilkinson, 1999). As no explanations for the causes of income inequalities are provided, this psychosocial mechanism becomes the central explanation of social cohesion models in public health (Muntaner and Lynch, 1999b; Lynch et al., 2000). This is not surprising as individuals look for explanations and they hold to those that are offered (Muntaner and Lynch, 1999b). The move towards psychosocial explanations on the effects of social cohesion (e.g., the culture of inequality; Wilkinson, 1996, 1999) is rather surprising, as just a few years ago the field of social inequalities in health was still materialist (Kaplan, 1995). Even researchers that had been relatively sympathetic to materialist explanations such as social class and working conditions (Marmot and Theorell, 1988), seem suddenly convinced by social capital/psychosocial environment explanations for health inequalities (Marmot, 1998).

The "culture of inequality" mechanism underlying the social capital-health association is not, however, all that innovative. For example, the "culture of poverty" hypothesis popularized by Oscar Lewis ([1963] 1998) is strikingly similar to the social capital/social cohesion formulations by Wilkinson and colleagues, albeit more psychologically reductionist and "victim-blaming" than the latter (Muntaner and Lynch, 1999a). The culture of poverty states that some poor communities bring poverty onto themselves because of few community ties and little community heritage (i.e., social capital). Perceptions and subjectivity are all-important, as it is not objective inequalities that ultimately determine the well-being of populations but the subjective response to those inequalities.

One of the implications of the social capital/social cohesion hypothesis for public health is that communities may be seen as responsible for their crime rates (Sampson, Raudenbush, and Earls, 1997) or aggregated health rates, an idea that nicely justifies the privatization of health services, such as managed care (Stoto, 1999). Another possible direction for public health may be that we take a step back from the structural sources of health inequalities ("the impor-tance of subjectivity," Wilkinson, 1999, p. 540)—after all, if they are not an inte-gral part of our theories of health inequalities and are so difficult to change, then perhaps an achievable alternative is to retreat to mass psychotherapy for the poor to change their perceptions of place in the social hierarchy (e.g., Proud-foot and Guest, 1997). Again, this idea is not new. In the 1960s the functional-ist sociologist W. Lloyd Warner revealed his hopes for his book called *Social Class in America* (1960): "The lives of many are destroyed because they do not understand the workings of social class. It is the hope . . . that this book will provide a corrective instrument which will permit men and women better to evaluate their social situations and thereby better adapt themselves to social reality and fit their dreams and aspirations to what is possible" (Warner, 1960, p. 5). Elsewhere, we have labelled this new set of public health implications associated with the idea of a loss of social capital "blaming the community" (Muntaner and Lynch, 1999a). The problem with subjectivity as an explanation for health inequalities is not only that it has little empirical support but also that it may yield anti-egalitarian public health policies (Muntaner and Lynch, 1999a, 1999b). Such anti-egalitarian public policy outcomes are not desired by any of the proponents of the social capital/psychosocial environment approach to health inequalities, or for that matter, anyone in the broader public health com-munity. This is because social egalitarianism constitutes one of public health's core values (Muntaner, 2000).

The "perceptions of relative inequality" approach implies a psychophysical dualism that is at odds with scientific psychology since Sechenov and Pavlov (Muntaner and Lynch, 1999a). The "culture of inequality" view implies that cul-ture is non-material (a subjective invention of people's minds that is not tied to the material world), while economics is material (Wilkinson, 1999). There is no basis for this assumption in modern science: ideology, technology, and art are as material as political representation or production of goods and services. The process of writing an article on anarchism is a cultural activity, selling it is an economic activity and censoring it because of its content is a political activ-ity—all of them material processes, as they take part in a social system, which is a material, albeit not physical, system (Muntaner and Lynch, 1999a).

EXPLAINING THE GROWING INTEREST IN SOCIAL CAPITAL

The literature on different approaches to social capital (e.g., communitarian, network, institutional) has been growing for the last three decades, from Loury, Bourdieu and Coleman, to Portes, Evans and Putnam (Coleman, 1990; Putnam, 1995b). However, not until the 1990s has the concept of social capital/social cohesion gained popularity in public health (e.g., Wilkinson, 1996) and devel-opment studies (Woolcock, 1998).

To understand the timely emergence of social capital from a psychosocial construct in the sociology of education (Coleman, 1990) to the next research "paradigm" in developmental economics at the World Bank (Stiglitz, 1996, 1997), we need to understand the difficult position of international lending institutions in the current decade. After the demise of the Soviet Union, the so-called Washington Consensus rhetoric of minimal governments, austerity measures, debt repayment, and neo-classical (e.g., rational choice) economics pervaded unchallenged (Chomsky, 1999b). Maybe the clearest example of this attitude is the now famous 1991 memorandum attributed to Lant Pritchett and to Larry Summers, formerly U.S. secretary of the treasury and then chief economist at the World Bank. This unique historical document provides a testimony of the policies of the Bank's ideology that has been replaced by the language of social capital at the end of the decade (e.g, Stiglitz, 1996, 1997; Woolcock, 1998):

"Dirty" Industries: Just between you and me, shouldn't the World Bank be encouraging MORE migration of the dirty industries to the LDCs [less developed countries]? I can think of three reasons:

1) The measurements of the costs of health impairing pollution depends on the foregone earnings from increased morbidity and mortality. From this point of view a given amount of health impairing pollution should be done in the country with the lowest cost, which will be the country with the lowest wages. I think the economic logic behind dumping a load of toxic waste in the lowest wage country is impeccable and we should face up to that.

2) The costs of pollution are likely to be non-linear as the initial increments of pollution probably have very low cost. I've always thought that under-populated countries in Africa are vastly UNDER-polluted, their air quality is probably vastly inefficiently low compared to Los Angeles or Mexico City. Only the lamentable facts that so much pollution is generated by non-tradable industries (transport, electrical generation) and that the unit transport costs of solid waste are so high prevent world welfare enhancing trade in air pollution and waste.

3) The demand for a clean environment for aesthetic and health reasons is likely to have very high income elasticity. The concern over an agent that causes a one in a million change in the odds of prostate cancer is obviously going to be much higher in a country where people survive to get prostate cancer than in a country where under 5 mortality is 200 per thousand. Also, much of the concern over industrial atmosphere discharge is about visibility impairing particulates. These discharges may have very little direct health impact. Clearly trade in goods that embody aesthetic pollution concerns could be welfare enhancing. While production is mobile the consumption of pretty air is a non-tradable.

The problem with the arguments against all of these proposals for more pollution in LDCs (intrinsic rights to certain goods, moral reasons, social concerns, lack of adequate markets, etc.) could be turned around and used more or less effectively against every Bank proposal for liberalization [Valette, 1999].

This economic "logic," that if applied to interpersonal, rather than international relations, would be considered psychopathic, had to change once a series of economic crises in part fuelled by IMF and WB policies started to creep up around the globe (e.g., Mexico, Russia, Brazil, and East Asia; Galbraith, 1999). Criticism of IMF austerity policies escalated (Kolko, 1999) even at WB headquarters where the Bank's new chief economist began using more social democratic language where a positive role for governments was acknowledged, including references to social capital as a key factor in economic development (Stiglitz, 1996, 1997). The Bank's interest in social capital thus marked a departure from economic imperialism, rational choice and public choice models, and a growing attention to integrating economics with sociology (Woolcock, 1998; World Bank, 1999a). Recent annual reports from the Bank also include the social dimension of economic development, including the need for government intervention in reducing international inequalities in science and technology (Stiglitz, 1997; World Bank, 1999b).

Sceptical observers argue that economic development happens precisely when countries do not follow IMF policies (Chomsky, 1999b); that countries that receive IMF and WB payments suffer increases in social inequalities (Kentor, 1998); and that social democracy has already been successfully tested in some European countries during part of the World War II period, without the need for social capital explanations. On close scrutiny, now that communism and big bureaucratic states cannot be blamed, social capital allows for a different kind of criticism of debtor countries (e.g., Woolcock, 1998). Social capital allows for the characterization of countries as "corrupt" or "developmental," according to the character of the ties between state, private sector, and civil society (Evans, 1995). For example, after the crisis of 1997, South Korea, a country formerly praised for its Asian values and Confucian capitalism, became an example of "crony capitalism," while the role of the deregulation of Korean financial markets in the crisis was ignored (Galbraith, 1999).

In the case of Russia, the economic policy dictated by Harvard and the IMF (Wedel, 1998) is not to blame for its failure to develop, it is Russian corruption ("Fuelling Russia's Economy," 1999). Thus, in the WB's post–Washington Consensus documents, the interpretation of what happened to Russia in the 1990s is thought of as capitalism without proper social capital (i.e., deficient governmental regulation), rather than communism's inevitable heritage (World Bank, 1999a, 1999b). Russian events such as the 30% GDP decline and unregulated monopolies are explained as the outcome of a deliberate hurry to privatize before any institutional capability to regulate could be put in place. Russian events are used as an example of social capital failure that provides a rationale for the Bank's retreat from neo-liberalism and its attempt to build a new development theory. Social capital is used to inform a supposedly new comprehensive and participatory approach to development, which avoids small government and authoritarian top-down neo-liberalism (Stiglitz, 1997; Woolcock, 1998). The underlying notion is that with adequate levels of social capital (proper civil and state guidance and regulation), the internationalization of markets and private property are optimal policies for the welfare of nations (World Bank, 1999a, 1999b). Social capital thus represents a leaner version of previous proposals on various degrees of state intervention in capitalist economies. There is thus a correspondence between the World Bank's approach to social capital and its public health applications (less state interventions, emphasis on civic life, "blaming the community," sharing responsibility with the community). This should not be surprising as there is a strong interdependence between the World Bank and the U.S. government ("The Holy Trinity," 1999).

WHAT IS NOT TO BE DONE: A "THIRD WAY" FOR COMPARATIVE HEALTH RESEARCH

Social capital has been explicitly associated with Third Way social policies in the United States and in the European Union as well (Szreter, 1999). The Third Way, as in the New Labour or New Democrat governments and their intellectuals (Robert Reich, Anthony Giddens) has been associated with the reduced role of the state, privatization of social services, labour market flexibility, nongovernmental organizations, modern philanthropy and the demise of the welfare state (Muntaner and Lynch, 1999a). Critics of the Third Way have argued that instead of representing a new set of policies by social-democratic parties, it represents a capitulation to the political right that leads to greater social inequalities (Albo and Zuege, 1999; Muntaner and Lynch, 1999a, 1999b). Albo and Zuege (1999) have argued that the failures of European social democracy in the seventies (e.g., Sweden's Meidner plan) and early eighties (e.g., Mitterrand's "U turn") sent them into a path of retreat, accommodation and confusion from which they still have to recover. The Third Way rhetoric, more often defined by what it is not than by what it is (Giddens, 1994), would be part of a search for a "big idea" that would ensure a durable political base for social-democratic parties in the new European capitalism. It is this potential role for social capital in public health that we think should be avoided (Muntaner and Lynch, 1999b).

In the wake of recent elections in Europe, some analysts are arguing that support for Third Way policies is fading, most notably in Germany (Singer, 1999). If that were to be the case, the fortunes of social capital in public health could follow, at least in the European Union, where governments have been more responsible to egalitarian pressures from working class parties (Navarro, 1999). This is less likely to occur in the United States, where government is more insulated from egalitarian working class politics (Navarro, 1994). Within public health, rather than discarding structural inequalities such as gender, race and class as outmoded materialism, in favour of psychosocial constructs such as social cohesion (Wilkinson, 1999), a much more fruitful strategy would be to seize the opportunity that social capital brings to integrate sociology and economics into the field of social inequalities in health. For example, the Marxian tradition of class inequality (Wright, 1997) could be integrated with the Weberian tradition of institutional social capital (Evans, 1995). The institutional view of social capital stresses how states operate: some states are efficient or inefficient, others are strong or weak. The role of political institutions such as parties, the judicial system, how the executive and legislative branches of governments operate (e.g., the rationalization of state bureaucracies) become central to understanding how states are formed (Evans, 1995). From a Marxian perspective on the other hand, class inequality guides the analysis of the state. How does the capitalist class influence the legislative, administrative and executive branches of government? What are the class alliances (capitalist vs. working class) and splits among different segments of the capitalist class (financial vs. industrial) that affect government function or the relationship between the capitalist class and state elites? (Kadushin, 1995). At least the institutional approach to social capital favoured by Woolcock (1998) seems to be open to this kind of integration (e.g., Evans, 1995). But then, as public health scholars and activists, should we place false hopes on initiatives heralded by institutions (Amin, 1997) that have helped generate the health inequalities that we want to eliminate?

References

Albo, G., and Zuege, A. "European Capitalism Today: Between the Euro and the Third Way." *Monthly Review,* 1999, *51*(3), 100–119.

Alderson, A. S., and Nielsen, F. "Income Inequality, Development, and Dependence: A Reconsideration." *American Sociological Review,* 1999, *64,* 606–631.

Amin, S. *Capitalism in the Age of Globalization: The Management of Contemporary Society.* Atlantic Highlands, N.J.: Zed Books, 1997.

Aneshensel, C. S., and Sucoff, C. A. "The Neighborhood Context of Adolescent Mental Health." *Journal of Health and Social Behavior,* 1996, *37,* 293–310.

Baum, F. "Public Health and Civil Society: Understanding and Valuing the Connection." *Australian Journal of Public Health,* 1997, *21,* 673–675.

Baum, F. "Social Capital: Is It Good for Your Health? Issues for a Public Health Agenda." *Journal of Epidemiology and Community Health,* 1999, *53,* 195–196.

Borjas, G. J. "Ethnic Capital and Intergenerational Mobility." *Quarterly Journal of Economics,* 1992, *107,* 123–150.

Brines, J. "The Ties That Bind: Principles of Cohesion in Cohabitation and Marriage." *American Sociological Review,* 1999, *64,* 333–355.

Carroll, L. *Alice Through the Looking-Glass.* 1872.

Chomsky, N. "The New Military Humanism: Lessons from Kosovo." *In These Times,* September 1999a, pp. 7–11.

Chomsky, N. *Profit over People: Neoliberalism and Global Order.* New York: Seven Stories Press, 1999b.

Coleman, J. *Foundations of Social Theory.* Cambridge, Mass.: Harvard University Press, 1990.

Collier, P. *Social Capital and Poverty.* Washington, D.C.: World Bank, 1998.

Cooper, H., Arber, S., and Ginn, J. *The Influence of Social Support and Social Capital on Health.* London: Health Education Authority, 1999.

Dixon, W. J., and Boswell, T. "Dependency, Disarticulation, and Denominator Effects: Another Look at Foreign Capital Penetration." *American Journal of Sociology,* 1996, *102,* 543–562.

Elster, J. *Political Psychology.* New York: Cambridge University Press, 1993.

Erikson, B. H. "Culture, Class, and Connections." *American Journal of Sociology,* 1996, *102,* 217–251.

Etzioni, A., and George, R. P. "Virtue and the State: A Dialogue Between a Commmunitarian and a Social Conservative." *Responsive Community,* 1999, *9*(2), 54–56.

Evans, P. *Embedded Autonomy.* Princeton, N.J.: Princeton University Press, 1995.

"Fuelling Russia's Economy." [Editorial.] *Economist,* Aug. 28, 1999.

Fullilove, M. T. "Promoting Social Cohesion to Improve Health." *Journal of the American Medical Women's Association,* 1998, *53*(2), 72–76.

Galbraith, J. K. "The Crisis of Globalization." *Dissent,* Spring 1999, pp. 13–19.

Giddens, A. *Beyond Left and Right.* Stanford, Calif.: Stanford University Press, 1994.

Gould, R. V. "Multiple Networks and Mobilization in the Paris Commune, 1871." *American Sociological Review,* 1991, *56,* 716–729.

Gould, R. V. "Trade Cohesion, Class Unity, and Urban Insurrection." *American Journal of Sociology,* 1993, *98,* 721–754.

Granovetter, M. "The Strength of Weak Ties." *American Journal of Sociology,* 1973, *78,* 1360–1380.

Grootaert, C. "Social Capital: The Missing Link?" In World Bank, *Expanding the Measure of Wealth: Indicators of Environmentally Sustainable Development.* Washington, D.C.: World Bank, 1997.

Havel, V. "Beyond the Nation-State." *Responsive Community,* 1999, *9*(3), 26–33.

Hawe, P., and Shiell, A. "Social Capital and Health Promotion: A Review." *Social Science and Medicine,* 2000, *51,* 871–885.

"The Holy Trinity: Rubin, Greenspan, Summers." *Left Business Observer,* 1999, *90,* 6–7.

Jackman, R. W., and others. "A Renaissance of Political Culture." *American Journal of Political Science,* 1996, *40,* 632–659.

Jenson, J. *Mapping Social Cohesion: The State of Canadian Research.* Ottawa: Canadian Policy Research Networks, 1998.

Kadushin, C. "Friendship Among the French Financial Elite." *American Sociological Review*, 1995, *60*, 202–221.

Kaplan, G. A. "Where Do Shared Pathways Lead? Some Reflections on a Research Agenda." *Psychosomatic Medicine*, 1995, *57*, 208–212.

Kaufman, J. "Three Views of Associationalism in 19th-Century America: An Empirical Examination." *American Journal of Sociology*, 1999, *104*, 1296–1345.

Kawachi, I., and Berkman, L. F. "Social Cohesion, Social Capital, and Health." In L. F. Berkman and I. Kawachi (eds.), *Social Epidemiology*. New York: Oxford University Press, 2000.

Kawachi, I., and Kennedy, B. P. "Health and Social Cohesion: Why Care About Income Inequality?" *British Medical Journal*, 1997, *314*, 1037–1039.

Kawachi, I., Kennedy, B. P., and Lochner, K. "Long Live Community. Social Capital as Public Health." *American Prospect*, Nov.-Dec. 1997, pp. 56–59.

Kawachi, I., Kennedy, B. P., and Prothrow-Stith, D. "Social Capital, Income Inequality, and Mortality." *American Journal of Public Health*, 1997, *87*, 1491–1498.

Kawachi, I., Kennedy, B. P., and Wilkinson, R. G. "Crime: Social Disorganization and Relative Deprivation." *Social Science and Medicine*, 1999, *48*, 719–731.

Kennedy, B. P., Kawachi, I, and Brainerd, E. "The Role of Social Capital in the Russian Mortality Crisis." *World Development*, 1999, *26*, 2029–2043.

Kentor, J. "The Long-Term Effects of Foreign Investment Dependence on Economic Growth, 1940–1990." *American Journal of Sociology*, 1998, *103*, 1024–1046.

Knack, S., and Keefer, P. "Does Social Capital Have an Economic Pay Off? A Cross-Country Investigation." *Quarterly Journal of Economics*, 1997, *112*, 1251–1288.

Kolko, G. "Ravaging the Poor: The International Monetary Fund Indicted by Its Own Data." *International Journal of Health Services*, 1999, *29*, 51–57.

Koopman, J. S. and Lynch, J. W. "Individual Causal Models and Population Systems Models in Epidemiology." *American Journal of Public Health*, 1999, *89*, 1170–1175.

Krieger, N. "Epidemiology and the Web of Causation: Has Anyone Seen the Spider?" *Social Science and Medicine*, 1994, *39*, 887–903.

Lavis, J. N., and Stoddart, G. L. *Social Cohesion and Health*. Toronto: Canadian Institute for Advanced Research, 1999.

Lewis, O. "The Culture of Poverty." *Society*, 1998, *35*, 7–9. (Originally published 1963)

Lomas, J. "Social Capital and Health: Implications for Public Health and Epidemiology." *Social Science and Medicine*, 1998, *47*, 1181–1188.

Lynch, J. W., and Kaplan, G. A. "Wither Studies on the Socioeconomic Foundations of Population Health?" *American Journal of Public Health*, 1997, *87*, 1409–1411.

Lynch, J. W., Kaplan, G. A., and Salonen, J. T. "Why Do Poor People Behave Poorly? Variations in Adult Health Behaviour and Psychosocial Characteristics, by Stage of the Socioeconomic Lifecourse." *Social Science and Medicine*, 1997, *44*, 809–820.

Lynch, J. W., and others. "Social Capital: Is It a Good Investment Strategy for Public Health?" *Journal of Epidemiology and Community Health*, 2000, *54*, 404–408.

Marjoribanks, K. "Family Human and Social Capital and Young Adults' Educational Attainment and Occupational Aspirations." *Psychological Reports,* 1991, *69,* 237–238.

Marmot, M. G. "Improvement of the Social Environment to Improve Health." *Lancet,* 1998, *351,* 57–60.

Marmot, M. G., and Theorell, T. "Social Class and Cardiovascular Disease: The Contribution of Work." *International Journal of Health Services,* 1988, *18,* 659–674.

Matthews, S., Stansfeld, S., and Power, C. "Social Support at Age 33: The Influence of Gender, Employment Status and Social Class." *Social Science and Medicine,* 1999, *49,* 133–142.

Muntaner, C. "Social Mechanisms, Race, and Social Epidemiology." *American Journal of Epidemiology,* 1999a, *150,* 121–126.

Muntaner, C. "Teaching Social Inequalities in Health: Barriers and Opportunities." *Scandinavian Journal of Public Health,* 1999b, *27,* 161–165.

Muntaner, C. "Applied Epidemiology." *Journal of Public Health Policy,* 2000, *21,* 99–102.

Muntaner, C., and Lynch, J. "Income Inequality and Social Cohesion Versus Class Relations: A Critique of Wilkinson's Neo-Durkheimian Research Program." *International Journal of Health Services,* 1999a, *29,* 59–82.

Muntaner, C., and Lynch, J. "The Social Class Determinants of Income Inequality and Social Cohesion: Part 1. Further Comments on Wilkinson's Reply." *International Journal of Health Services,* 1999b, *29,* 699–715.

Muntaner, C., and O'Campo, P. "A Critical Appraisal of the Demand/Control Model of the Psychosocial Work Environment: Epistemological, Social, Behavioral and Class Considerations." *Social Science and Medicine,* 1993, *36,* 1509–1517.

Muntaner, C., Nieto, J., and O' Campo, P. "Additional Clarification re 'On Race, Social Class, and Epidemiologic Research.'" *American Journal of Epidemiology,* 1997, *146,* 607–608.

Muntaner, C., Oates, G., and Lynch, J. "The Social Class Determinants of Income Inequality and Social Cohesion: Part 2. Presentation of an Alternative Model." *International Journal of Health Services,* 1999, *29,* 715–732.

Mustard, J. F. *Health and Social Capital in Health and Social Organization: Toward a Health Policy for the 21st Century.* New York: Routledge, 1996.

Navarro, V. *The Politics of Health Policy.* Amityville, N.Y.: Baywood, 1994.

Navarro, V. "The Political Economy of the Welfare State in Developed Capitalist Countries." *International Journal of Health Services,* 1999, *29,* 1–50.

Ostrom, E. "Revisiting the Commons: Local Lessons, Global Challenges." *Science,* 1999, *284,* 278–282.

Pattillo, M. E. "Sweet Mothers and Gangbangers: Managing Crime in a Black Middle-Class Neighborhood." *Social Forces,* 1998, *76,* 747–774.

Paxton, P. "Is Social Capital Declining in the United States? A Multiple Indicator Assessment." *American Journal of Sociology,* 1999, *105,* 88–127.

Persell, C. H., Catsambis, S., and Cookson, P. W. "Differential Asset Conversion: Class and Gendered Pathways to Selective Colleges." *Sociology of Education,* 1992, *65,* 208–225.

Portes, A. "Social Capital: Its Origins and Applications in Contemporary Sociology." *Annual Review of Sociology,* 1998, *24,* 1–24.

Proudfoot, J., and Guest, D. "Effect of Cognitive-Behavioural Training on Job-Finding Among Long-Term Unemployed People." *Lancet,* 1997, *350,* 96–100.

Putnam, R. "Bowling Alone: America's Declining Social Capital." *Journal of Democracy,* 1995a, *6,* 65–78.

Putnam, R. "The Prosperous Community: Social Capital and Public Life." *American Prospect,* Spring 1995b, pp. 27–40.

Putnam, R., Leonardi, R., and Nanetti, R. *Making Democracy Work: Civic Traditions in Modern Italy.* Princeton, N.J.: Princeton University Press, 1993.

Rose, G. "Sick Individuals and Sick Populations." *International Journal of Epidemiology,* 1985, *14,* 32–38.

Sampson, R. J., Raudenbush, S. W., and Earls, F. "Neighborhoods and Violent Crime: A Multilevel Study of Collective Efficacy." *Science,* 1997, *277,* 918–924.

Schneider, M., and others. "Networks to Nowhere: Segregation and Stratification in Networks of Information About Schools." *American Journal of Political Science,* 1997, *41,* 1201–1223.

Singer, D. "Third Way—Dead End?" [Editorial.] *Nation,* July 5, 1999.

Skocpol, T. "Associations Without Members." *American Prospect,* August 1999, pp. 66–73.

Smith, T. "Factors Relating to Misanthropy in Contemporary American Society." *Social Science Research,* 1997, *26,* 170–196.

Stiglitz, J. "Some Lessons from the East Asian Miracle." *World Bank Research Observer,* 1996, *11,* 151–178.

Stiglitz, J. "An Agenda for Development for the Twenty-First Century." In B. Pleskovic and J. Stiglitz (eds.), *Annual Bank Conference on Development Economics, 1997.* Washington, D.C.: World Bank, 1997.

Stoto, M. A. "Sharing Responsibility for the Public's Health." *Public Health Reports,* 1999, *114,* 231–235.

Szreter, S. "A New Political Economy for New Labour: The Importance of Social Capital." *Renewal,* 1999, *7,* 30–44.

Tijhuis, M. A., and others. "Social Support and Stressful Events in Two Dimensions: Life Events and Illness as an Event." *Social Science and Medicine,* 1995, *40,* 1513–1526.

Tocqueville, A. de. *Democracy in America.* New York: Anchor/Doubleday, 1969. (Originally published 1835)

Valette, J. "Larry Summer's War Against the Earth." *Counterpunch.* 1999. [http//:www.counterpunch.org/summers.html].

Wainwright, D. "The Political Transformation of the Health Inequalities Debate." *Critical Social Policy,* 1996, *16,* 67–82.

Warner, W. L. *Social Class in America.* New York: HarperCollins, 1960.

Warren, M. R. "Exploitation or Cooperation? The Political Basis of Regional Variation in the Italian Informal Economy." *Politics and Society,* 1994, *22,* 89–115.

Wedel, J. R. *Collision and Collusion: The Strange Case of Western Aid to Eastern Europe 1989–1998.* New York: St. Martin's Press, 1998.

Wilkinson, R. G. *Unhealthy Societies: The Afflictions of Inequality.* New York: Routledge, 1996.

Wilkinson, R. G. "Income Inequality, Social Cohesion, and Health: Clarifying the Theory—A Reply to Muntaner and Lynch." *International Journal of Health Services,* 1999, *29,* 525–543.

Wilkinson, R. G, Kawachi, I., and Kennedy, B. P. "Mortality, the Social Environment, Crime, and Violence." *Sociology of Health and Illness,* 1998, *20,* 578–597.

Wing, S. "Whose Epidemiology, Whose Health?" *International Journal of Health Services,* 1998, *28,* 241–252.

Woolcock, M. "Social Capital and Economic Development: A Critical Review." *Theory and Society,* 1998, *27,* 151–208.

World Bank. *Social Capital for Development.* Washington, D.C.: World Bank, 1999a.

World Bank. "World Bank Calls for a Narrowing of the Knowledge Gap Between Rich and Poor." [Press release.] Washington, D.C.: World Bank, 1999b.

Wright, E. O. *Class Counts. Comparative Studies in Class Analysis.* New York: Cambridge University Press, 1997.

Zweigenhaft, R. L. "Accumulation of Cultural and Social Capital." *Social Spectrum,* 1993, *13,* 365–376.

CHAPTER TWELVE

Measuring Health Inequalities

The Politics of the World Health Report 2000

Paula A. Braveman

The World Health Organization's *World Health Report* for the year 2000 ranked countries on several indicators intended to reflect the performance of their health systems; the WHO defined health systems as all actions whose primary purpose is to improve health. Welcome elements in the report were the principle that the distribution of health within a population, and not just a population's average levels of health, is an important criterion for judging health policies and also the notion that the distribution of health within countries, and not just between countries, is of major significance. Much as the Gini coefficient reflects variation in income, the *World Health Report 2000* (*WHR 2000*) inequality measure reflects variation in health, without taking into consideration how health is distributed according to other population characteristics (such as occupation, race or ethnic group, urban or rural residence, age, or sex). Thus the *WHR 2000* health inequality measure can tell you how much total variation there is in child mortality within a country but not whether child mortality varies between the rich and poor, between residents of slums, shantytowns, or rural areas compared with residents of relatively affluent areas, or between dominant and nondominant racial or ethnic groups in a country.

Portions of this chapter are based on Braveman, Krieger, and Lynch (2000). The author thanks Susan Egerter and Catherine Cubbin for their suggestions and Jennie Kamen for assistance with research and preparing the chapter.

In the first journal article presenting this approach to measuring health inequalities (Murray, Gakidou, and Frenk, 1999), the report's authors explained the need to replace standard approaches to measuring health inequalities, which compare different social groups (for example, socioeconomic or racial or ethnic groups) who are specified a priori. Their argument was based both on social values and on technical grounds. Regarding values, they questioned whether more importance should be given to addressing ill health among socially disadvantaged than among more advantaged people. On technical grounds, they contended that measuring health inequalities in the "traditional" manner—by comparing social groups—is inherently flawed. Debates ensued in scientific forums on the ethical and technical issues (Braveman, Krieger, and Lynch, 2000; Braveman, Starfield, and Geiger, 2001; Murray, 2001; Almeida and others, 2001; Landmann Szwarcwald, 2002; Gakidou and King, 2002). This chapter reviews the debates, discussing how the positions taken by the *World Health Report 2000* authors reflect strong contemporary ideological currents that, despite good intentions on the part of the *Report*'s authors, generally tend to oppose efforts to achieve greater equity in health and its key determinants.

A CONCEPTUAL AND ETHICAL FRAME OF REFERENCE

This discussion can only be understood in light of an explicit conceptual framework for considering health inequalities and why one would want to measure them. The expressions "health inequalities" and "health disparities" have become widely used as a concise substitute for more precise terminology, such as "social inequalities in health," which is somewhat more cumbersome, or "health inequities," which tends to sound judgmental and emotionally charged. The literal meaning of health inequalities or disparities is any difference in health, without specifying the kinds of differences that might be of interest. However, in common public health and medical parlance over the past two decades in Europe and the past several years in the United States, "health disparities or inequalities" has been used to refer to social inequalities in health— differences in health between different social groups. The implicit understanding in using "health inequalities" to reflect social inequalities in health has been that the social inequalities of interest were disparities between social groups that differ with respect to their relative positions in a social hierarchy, that is, their levels of underlying social advantage or privilege, reflecting differences in wealth, power, or prestige. In Europe, the main interest has been in socioeconomic differences in health. In the United States, although there is a growing literature on socioeconomic inequalities in health, the main focus of federal agencies, private foundations, and professional organizations has been on health and health care differences between persons of European ancestry and light-colored skin ("Whites") and other racial and ethnic groups; in fact, unless otherwise specified, the term "health disparities" in the United States is generally assumed to mean racial/ethnic disparities.

Why would one want to compare the health of more and less socially privileged groups of people? In Europe (but not in the United States), there has been considerable public discussion of the social values underlying a commitment to reduce social inequalities in health (Dahlgren and Whitehead, 1992; Whitehead, 1990; World Health Organization, 1994; Mackenbach and Bakker, 2002). Whitehead's *Concepts and Principles of Equity in Health* (1990) articulated the notion that health inequities were differences in health that were "unavoidable, unjust, and unfair." That definition has been extremely useful in public debates about equity in many different countries. I have argued that being unjust or unfair implies avoidability and that avoidability should not be used as a separate criterion for judging whether a given health difference is inequitable (Braveman and Gruskin, 2003). Significantly reducing some of the greatest inequities in health will probably require fundamental changes in underlying social structures, the feasibility of which many people would question; one would not want to make the extent of avoidability a criterion for judging how inequitable a situation is. I have offered a definition that is less useful than Whitehead's for communicating with nontechnical audiences but may more easily lend itself to measurement: pursuing equity in health means striving to eliminate systematic (Starfield, 2001) disparities in health between more and less advantaged social groups; health inequities put already disadvantaged groups at further disadvantage with respect to their health (Braveman and Gruskin, 2003).

A commitment to health equity, that is, to reduce social inequalities in health, rests on ethical values, specifically the principle of distributive justice; it also is consonant and closely related with human rights principles (Braveman and Gruskin, 2003). As noted, the authors of the *WHR 2000* explicitly questioned whether ill health in a socially disadvantaged (say, uneducated) person should be of more concern than ill health in a socially advantaged (say, highly educated) person. Of course, on an individual basis, in a given clinical setting, faced with two individuals seeking medical care, one a highly educated person who has an acute, life-threatening emergency and the other a poorly educated person with a minor, nonurgent problem, a health caregiver should not adversely discriminate against the more socially advantaged individual. But individual behavior is not the relevant concern when defining equity in health and how it should be measured; the concern is public policies and how those policies allocate resources, which cannot be on an individual basis but must be according to systematic criteria. Criteria define social groups. While individual caregivers should not discriminate based on underlying social advantage, public policy should actively seek to remove obstacles to achieving optimal health, giving highest priority and devoting additional resources to removing obstacles for those with more barriers to health to begin with because of underlying social disadvantage.

Based on ethical principles and consistent with human rights concepts, public policy should actively seek to equalize opportunities to be healthy. Determining whether progress is being made toward greater health equity requires ongoing monitoring of social inequalities in health. The *World Health Report 2000* authors' implicit ethical rationale for abandoning the measurement of social inequalities in health appears to be an anti–affirmative action position, contending that selectively allocating resources in ways that will reduce social inequalities in health discriminates against socially advantaged individuals; this position is profoundly ideological and not defensible on ethical grounds.

ADDRESSING THE TECHNICAL CRITICISMS MADE BY THE *WHR 2000* AUTHORS

The ethical justification provided by the *World Health Report 2000* authors was that the traditional approach is unfair because it presumes a commitment to affirmative action for historically disadvantaged groups. They also presented a number of technical arguments with the goal of establishing that "traditional" approaches (methodologies in line with those taken by recognized experts in the field) to examining health inequalities were scientifically inferior to and should be replaced by the new and improved method they were propounding. The report authors contended that the "social group" approach to the measurement of health inequalities—that is, the measurement of social inequalities in health—is fundamentally flawed. This is so, they claimed, because by categorizing the population into groups that are specified a priori—such as different socioeconomic groups—one is prejudging the causation of the inequalities. This, they argued, inevitably leads to masking intragroup variation and blinds the investigator to other possible causal agents that might be important, perhaps even more important than the factors that were selected a priori to define the social groups (Murray, Gakidou, and Frenk, 1999).

It is ironic to label the approaches taken in the past to study social inequalities in health as "traditional," given that this work has received relatively little attention from the research community until very recently and is so new that it hardly has deeply entrenched "traditions." Indeed, until recently, and particularly in the United States, research on social inequalities in health was marginalized; individuals who did it were few in number and had great difficulty obtaining funding and finding journals that would publish their work. Implying that rigid traditions in health inequalities research exist and are resistant to change is misleading.

The standard approach that has been taken to measuring social inequalities in health involves systematically disaggregating health data according to markers of social factors with demonstrated relevance to health. Relevant social factors include differences in income, accumulated economic assets (for example, ownership of a house, automobile or other vehicle, or household amenities), education, occupation, geographical residence, and being a member of a socially or politically dominant or marginalized ethnic or religious group. The choice of such social variables is not arbitrary. It derives from an understanding that these factors reflect differences in underlying social position—wealth, power, or prestige—and on a concern based on ethical values about how social groups with different levels of wealth, power, or prestige may be at an underlying disadvantage with respect to health. It is not based on assuming that every health outcome in every population and setting will always be differentially distributed across social groups categorized by all a priori social variables. Choosing social variables depends on a massive body of evidence showing strong associations between social position and health for many outcomes and many settings.

And most centrally, the choice of social variables to serve as the basis for comparisons among social groups is based on a commitment to distributive justice; that commitment requires answering this question: How is the health of disadvantaged social groups faring with respect to their more advantaged counterparts? The health of the most advantaged social group in a society indicates what should be possible for everyone. The concept in the World Health Organization constitution (1946), also appearing in various human rights instruments, of the right to health defines it as the right to the highest attainable standard of health. This notion has been widely criticized for the difficulty of operationalizing it. I believe that the notion of the highest attainable standard of health can be operationalized insofar as it is reflected by the health status achieved by the most socially advantaged groups in a society. The health of the most socially advantaged group indicates what is biologically possible. It probably underestimates what is possible because scientific advances may lead to further improvements in health not yet reflected in the health of the most privileged members of a society.

Furthermore, the "social group approach" is useful because it provides practical information for designing policies and programs. For example, the reason for choosing given social variables as the basis for stratifying by socioeconomic position typically concerns, in part, their utility for targeting interventions. They indicate identifiable population groups that require particular attention because their social and economic characteristics, such as poverty, hinder their ability to reduce their health risks without help.

Studying and monitoring social inequalities in health does not mean prejudging the causation of observed inequalities, any more than comparing health statistics for different geographical areas prejudges the causes of disparities by spatial location. Nor does it mean obscuring intragroup variation, any more than comparing health between different geographical areas prevents one's studying variations within the areas. The *WHR 2000* authors deliberately chose examples involving spatial location here because at the same time that they were attempting to discredit the scientific basis for examining social inequalities in health, they also suggested the value of comparing aggregate levels of health in different geographical areas.

Observing gaps in life expectancy according to education, for example, cannot be interpreted to mean that education per se is the cause of the observed disparities in survival. But it points in a promising direction by prompting the following questions: Why is educational level persistently associated with diverse health status measures, over time and across diverse settings? And how are people with different levels of educational attainment different from each other in ways that could potentially explain the observed disparities in mortality? Moving from bivariate description toward explanation requires in-depth inferential analyses that seek to understand differential risks of poor health outcomes not only between but also *within* specified social groups. Contrary to the *World Health Report 2000* authors, comparing groups in no way imposes any conceptual or methodological limitation on examining variation *within* those groups; indeed, it can only be understood as a first step, identifying promising issues to focus on in searching for explanatory factors by conducting within-group analyses. Learning about likely causal factors in studying social inequalities in health requires proceeding from comparisons identifying "at-risk" groups to in-depth within-group analyses of the likely causal or contributory factors among those groups.

Proponents of the *World Health Report 2000* approach also have argued on technical grounds, as justification for discontinuing prior WHO work on social inequalities in health, that cross-national comparisons cannot be made using social inequalities in health. My colleagues and I disagree (Braveman, Krieger, and Lynch, 2000; Kunst and Mackenbach, 1994a, 1994b; Kunst and others, 1998a, 1998b, 1999; Mackenbach and others, 1997, 1999). The *World Health Report* for 1999 (World Health Organization, 1999), reflecting WHO work and leadership before the *WHR 2000* authors assumed their posts, included comparisons among forty-nine countries of the ratio of several health indicators among the poor versus the nonpoor populations of those countries, labeled "Country performance on equity." The World Bank has issued a series of reports examining similar cross-national comparisons on a wide array of maternal and child health indicators, using the ratio of each indicator among the poorest and wealthiest population quintiles, as well as a more complex measure of inequality, the concentration index, which takes into account more information than a poor-to-nonpoor ratio or a ratio of the extremes (Gwatkin and others, 2000). The comparisons in the World Bank reports are intended to provide guidance for developing strategies for and monitoring the success of Bank-supported poverty reduction initiatives in many of the poorest countries. The health inequality measures used in the 1999 WHO report and in the World Bank reports contain limitations for making cross-national comparisons over time. This is not an insoluble problem in measuring social inequalities in health, however. The additional methodological work needed to permit broader, cross-national comparisons over time using social inequalities in health would require relatively modest support that could and should be provided by the WHO.

DOES IT REALLY MATTER WHICH MEASURE IS USED?

One might ask, however, whether this dispute is primarily academic hair-splitting. Does it matter in practical terms whether one uses the "social group" approach or the *World Health Report 2000* approach to defining and measuring health inequalities? The answer is unequivocal: it matters greatly, for empirical, practical, and political reasons.

Empirically, my colleagues and I have demonstrated, using data on countries analyzed by the World Bank, that one would come to very different conclusions about the extent of socioeconomic inequality in child mortality in a country using the *WHR 2000* approach than if one used accepted measures of social inequalities in health (Braveman, Starfield, and Geiger, 2001; Wagstaff, Paci, and van Doorslaer, 1991; Mackenbach and Kunst, 1997). We examined, for countries with data available from the World Bank (Gwatkin and others, 2000) on socioeconomic inequalities in child survival, rankings for each country first based on the *WHR 2000* measure of inequalities in child survival and then based on three different indices extensively examined and used in the measurement of social inequalities in health (Wagstaff, Paci, and van Doorslaer, 1991; Mackenbach and Kunst, 1997). These indices are the *poor/rich ratio,* comparing child mortality rates for the poorest 20 percent versus the wealthiest 20 percent of a country's population; the *poor/rich rate difference,* the absolute difference between child mortality rates in the poorest and the richest groups; and the *concentration index,* an inequality measure that reflects the extent of inequalities across the entire population, including the groups between the extremes as well as the contrast between the two groups at the extremes. We first examined the ranking of each country among all one hundred ninety-one countries examined in the *WHR 2000* and its relative ranking within the forty-four-country subset, in both cases using the *WHR 2000* inequalities measure. Next we examined the relative rankings for each of the countries using the poor/rich ratio, the poor/rich rate difference, the concentration index, and for additional comparison, the average child mortality rate, which of course does not reflect disparities or distribution but does give the mean level for an entire population.

We consistently found poor correspondence between relative rankings based on the *WHR 2000* measure and the poor/rich ratio, poor/rich rate difference, and the concentration index. Additional analyses actually revealed modest *negative* correlations between the *WHR 2000* child morality inequalities measure and the accepted measures of socioeconomic inequalities in child mortality. Rankings based on the *WHR 2000* inequalities measure corresponded moderately well to rankings based on average rates of child mortality in the countries examined, raising questions about the former measure's additional contribution to knowledge of the distribution of child health. One would come to very different conclusions about the extent of health inequalities in a country, based on whether one used the *WHR 2000* inequalities measure or measures considered more appropriate by scholars in the field of health inequalities.

In addition to the empiric concerns, this debate matters because the *WHR 2000* measure of health inequality lacks practical meaning for guiding policy. Because it gives no information about the social distribution of ill health—for example, whether ill health is more likely to be experienced by the poor or the rich, rural or urban dwellers, or disadvantaged racial or ethnic groups versus others—the *WHR 2000* measure provides no information to guide resource allocation or target policies. A minister of health whose country ranked poorly on the *WHR 2000* inequalities measure might well attribute this difference to factors beyond the reach of policies, such as more diverse terrain, climate, or natural resources.

Because there is no identification of who needs additional attention when using the *World Health Report 2000* inequalities measure, there is no guidance for determining where and how to direct policies and programs. Furthermore, the *World Health Report 2000* approach would circumvent advocacy efforts; because there is no identification of who benefits adequately from policies and programs, there is no way to mobilize sympathetic constituencies who might advocate on behalf of disadvantaged groups.

In other words, reliance on the *WHR 2000* measure of health inequality removes consideration of ethics and human rights from the measurement of health disparities. Because it does not measure differences in health between different social groups, reliance on the *WHR 2000* measure rather than measures of social inequalities in health to assess inequality in health within a country would remove from the public health monitoring agenda questions such as these: Is progress being made over time in closing gaps in nutritional status between children in poor and nonpoor families? Are racial/ethnic disparities in infant mortality being reduced? Are the large gender gaps in child mortality and immunization rates in many countries being reduced? In a world with wide and widening disparities in wealth (United Nations Development Programme 1996; World Bank 2001) and strong evidence linking disparities in wealth to disparities in health (Feinstein, 1993; Townsend, 1990; Egbuono and Starfield, 1982;

Evans, Barer, and Marmor, 1994; Evans and others, 2001; Kaplan and Keil, 1993; Kaplan and others, 1996; Marmot and others, 1991; Hahn and others, 1996), as well as widespread ethnic conflicts and gender discrimination, these questions should remain on the public policy agenda—and hence the routine monitoring agenda.

WHY DID A NEW "HEALTH INEQUALITIES" APPROACH EMERGE AT THIS TIME?

Is it an accident that the *World Health Report 2000* approach to health inequalities emerged at this particular time in history? It may seem surprising to connect an analytical approach taken by researchers at an international agency with ideological currents, but in this case, striking links emerge on reflection.

The *World Health Report 2000* health inequalities approach fits well with dominant political and economic trends generally opposing redistribution of resources in favor of disadvantaged groups. A dramatic redistribution of wealth in favor of the already advantaged occurred globally over recent decades. According to the World Bank's *World Development Report* for 2000–2001 (2001), the average income in the richest twenty countries is thirty-seven times the average in the poorest twenty—a gap that doubled over the preceding four decades. In seventy countries, average incomes in the mid-1990s were less than they were in 1980; in forty-three countries, they were less than in 1970 (United Nations Development Programme, 1996). Per capita water supply in lower-income countries dropped by two-thirds between 1970 and the mid-1990s (United Nations Development Programme, 1996). While poverty has decreased in East Asia, the numbers of poor people (defined conservatively as those living on less than U.S.$1 a day) has increased in Latin America, South Asia, and sub-Saharan Africa. In the former Soviet countries and Central Asia, there has been a twentyfold rise in the numbers of people living on less than $1 a day (World Bank, 2001). The world's richest 1 percent of people now have as much income as the poorest 57 percent (United Nations Development Programme, 2002).

At the same time, when one might expect the need for public services to increase because of increasing numbers of poor people, there has been a strong movement toward government "downsizing," dismantling public services and infrastructure and privatizing a range of formerly public functions, including provision of water. In the wake of the demise of centrally planned economies in the former Soviet Union, a market-driven model has been widely touted as the only sensible alternative and the previously extensive network of social protections has been abruptly withdrawn, in most cases without substituting any alternative (World Health Organization and Braveman, 1996).

The justification given for these trends is that only through achievement of a certain level of overall wealth can a society provide for all of its citizens, that the amassing of private wealth, regardless of its distribution, advances everyone because its benefits will inevitably reach everyone. However, this "trickle-down" theory has been widely discredited (United Nations Development Programme, 1996), as the UNDP and World Bank statistics demonstrate. For example, examining associations between child survival and per capita GDP reveals that while overall strong relationships exist between these two factors, numerous examples do not follow the general trend. Countries such as Costa Rica, Cuba, Singapore, and Sri Lanka, with relatively high child survival rates for their levels of GDP per capita, have made major investments in public services, redistributing national wealth to provide high levels of education, health care, and other social services on a populationwide basis (United Nations Development Programme, 1996; World Health Organization and Braveman, 1996; World Health Organization, 2001). Even the World Bank (2001) is now calling for the need for pro-growth policies that are systematically "pro-poor."

Against the current background of the dismantling of government infrastructure and services, privatization, and the deregulation accompanying globalization of trade and services, it is particularly important to monitor the health of social groups likely to experience different results. Only the interests of the wealthiest and most powerful benefit from the absence of documentation regarding trends in the health of those likely not to fare so well, in comparison with those likely to benefit most from the status quo. And regardless of the *World Health Report 2000* authors' good intentions or elaborate justifications, the WHO's approach to public health monitoring ensures that information required to compare the health of vulnerable societal groups to that of the more privileged is unavailable. Merely comparing the health and health care of different social groups cannot definitely reveal the role played by any particular policy or how it was implemented. However, health comparisons between more and less privileged social groups can indicate whether overall policies and programs appear on or off target in moving toward more equitable distribution of health and suggest the need for more intensive research on particular issues.

The *World Health Report 2000* approach to defining and measuring health inequalities both reflects the underlying assumptions of neoliberalism and reinforces its hegemony (see Chapter Fourteen). *Neoliberalism* is a term sometimes used to refer to the now globally dominant economic and political order, in which the "free" market is sovereign within the context of a Western-style political democracy. The assumptions on which it rests are that aggregate economic growth is the ultimate measure of societal development and that optimal growth can be attained only when market forces are unimpeded by policies designed to redistribute wealth and protect the disadvantaged (see Chapter Five). According to this perspective, efforts at progressive taxation to support social programs and regulatory initiatives to protect workers from hazardous working conditions or to protect the environment from contamination serve only to hurt everyone, including the disadvantaged, because they provoke job flight, with the inevitable accompanying domino effects on the economy as a whole. A neoliberal approach generally favors privatization of services traditionally provided by governments, under the notion that the private sector can always perform better than the public sector. The private sector is seen as having inherent incentives for productivity and innovation lacked by the public sector, and the latter is seen as hampered by inherent rigidity, due in part to protections and benefits for government workers. This view argues that lack of incentives for investment and productivity—rather than historically unfair relationships between the rich and the poor—are the main obstacles to economic growth, which will automatically improve living standards for everyone. The neoliberal view either assumes fair opportunity for everyone to compete in the marketplace or does not perceive such fairness as a priority.

What is the relevance of these political and economic issues to a controversy over research methods? For centuries, strong links between health and socioeconomic status or position have been demonstrated across diverse settings and health measures. Although the precise mechanisms are not well understood in many cases, few analysts question the strong associations. Given the compelling evidence of links between health and wealth, and given the wide and in some cases widening disparities in wealth occurring in countries of all income levels, many have argued for routine reporting and analysis of health information disaggregated (broken down) into socioeconomic subgroups, in contrast with standard public health data reporting, which is in the form of population averages for a specified territory (Krieger, Williams, Moss, 1997; Whitehead, 1990; Culyer, 1991; Culyer and Wagstaff, 1993; Daniels, 1985; Anand, 2002; World Health Organization and Braveman, 1996; Braveman, 1998). Many recognize that social advantage and disadvantage are distributed along other dimensions in addition to wealth—by gender, by race or ethnic group, by religion, or by other characteristics; these other characteristics often interact with socioeconomic characteristics to greatly increase overall social disadvantage. Without making specific assumptions about causal mechanisms, recognition of the strong associations between social position and health supports the need for ongoing monitoring of social inequalities in health within countries, that is, health disparities between subnational population groups defined by social factors such as poverty or wealth or other markers of social advantage.

With the goal of ensuring the ongoing availability of data needed to guide policies to reduce such disparities, a 1995–1998 World Health Organization initiative with support from the Swedish government (Swedish International Development and Cooperation Agency, the Swedish equivalent of the Agency for International Development in the United States) focused in part on developing capacity within lower-income nations for assessing social inequalities in health. The WHO viewed the data not as an end in themselves but as a crucial tool to guide policy and stimulate public debate (Evans and others, 2001; Anand, 2002). However, as noted, in contrast to the "social group" approach to monitoring, the *World Health Report 2000* measures the magnitude of inequalities between all (ungrouped) individuals in a population and does not compare the magnitude of health inequalities between the rich and the poor or between other social groups.

The *World Health Report 2000* choice to measure ungrouped health inequalities and to abandon previous work on the measurement of health inequalities is linked with the prevailing neoliberal economic order in that (1) using the *World Health Report 2000* approach is inherently more compatible conceptually with the basic assumptions underlying neoliberalism and (2) in practical terms, information based on the *World Health Report 2000* measure is far less likely to challenge the prevailing conditions of neoliberalism. Indeed, substitution of the *World Health Report 2000* measure of "health inequalities" for measuring social inequalities in health removes the capability to produce crucial evidence indicating deleterious health effects on disadvantaged population groups from discussion of the impact of neoliberal policies. This lack of specificity is not a problem in the eyes of the proponents of the ungrouped approach; rather, they view it as an advantage, because, as noted, they have argued that policymakers should not necessarily be more concerned about ill health in socially disadvantaged persons than in their more advantaged counterparts (Murray, Gakidou, and Frenk, 1999).

Choosing to monitor social inequalities in health implicitly acknowledges that some population groups are at an underlying disadvantage and assumes that policies should place a high priority on reducing health disparities between more and less advantaged social groups. Indeed, the express intent of monitoring social inequalities in health is to guide policies designed to reduce differences in social advantage or its health effects (or both). Proponents of the use of social inequalities in health for monitoring health inequalities have argued that while on a personal and clinical level one should be equally concerned about everyone who suffers, public policies must preferentially protect those whose circumstances put them at an inherent disadvantage for attaining good health on their own (Braveman, Krieger, and Lynch, 2000).

Because the use of the *World Health Report 2000* measure in place of monitoring social inequalities in health limits the extent to which countries can document widening disparities in health between different social groups within their national populations, it leaves policymakers and advocates without evidence that could suggest detrimental impacts of national and international policies on the health of socially disadvantaged groups. One might surmise that the *World Health Report 2000* measure could perhaps be used as a proxy for social inequalities health, but this clearly was not its proponents' intention (Murray, Gakidou, and Frenk, 1999), and my colleagues and I have demonstrated, as described, that results of applying the different approaches do not correspond (Braveman, Starfield, and Geiger, 2001).

CONCLUSION

The *WHR 2000* approach to measuring health inequalities removes the consideration of social justice from the measurement of health disparities, reducing it to an exercise devoid of practical meaning. A high level of "health inequalities" between ungrouped individuals in a society could suggest an array of possible ways to distribute those inequalities, including patterns that would not necessarily be inequitable. Investment in the *WHR 2000* health inequalities approach is a diversion of resources needed to build capacity to measure, monitor, and understand social inequalities in health in order to guide policies to reduce the gaps.

In their most recent publication on this topic, some *World Health Report 2000* authors (Gakidou and King, 2002) have for the first time presented their approach as an adjunct to measuring social inequalities in health, not a substitute. This is welcome. However, in practical terms, they continue to devote the resources of the World Health Organization to work on their approach and do not appear to believe in strengthening global and national capacity to monitor social inequalities in health. Efforts toward those ends were under way at the WHO in the late 1990s but were discontinued by the *World Health Report 2000* authors when they assumed their posts (World Health Organization, 1999; World Health Organization and Braveman, 1996; Braveman, 1998). Furthermore, replacing the earlier WHO efforts to build lower-income countries' capacity to monitor social inequalities in health with the more recent work focused on cross-national comparisons using the *World Health Report 2000* measure has the additional serious practical consequence of reinforcing control of expertise and information in international organizations rather than developing monitoring capacity within countries themselves.

In the example discussed here, proponents of measuring "health inequalities" between ungrouped individuals have called into question both the scientific basis and the importance of studying *social inequalities in health,* and resources formerly devoted to studying social inequalities have been reallocated to their very divergent agenda. This unfortunate circumstance should not detract from credit due to the *World Health Report 2000* authors for important contributions to work on social inequalities in health that they have made in the past (Murray and others, 1998), and recently by calling for distribution of health within and not just between countries, to be a major criterion for judging health policies (World Health Organization, 2000). It should not be surprising that scientific methods would tend to mirror (in more or less subtle ways) the prevailing ideological perspectives of the society in which the scientists live and work. We cannot escape this tendency entirely, but we can strive to be more aware of the assumptions that underlie our analytical methods and to expose those assumptions to more rigorous scrutiny and open debate.

References

Almeida, C, and others. "*World Health Report 2000:* Methodologic Concerns and Recommendations Considering Policy Consequences." *Lancet,* 2001, *357,* 1692–1697.

Anand, S. "The Concern for Equity in Health." *Journal of Epidemiology and Community Health,* 2002, *56,* 485–487.

Braveman, P. A. *Monitoring Equity in Health: A Policy-Oriented Approach in Low- and Middle-Income Countries.* Geneva: World Health Organization, 1998.

Braveman, P. A., and Gruskin, S. "Defining Equity in Health." *Journal of Epidemiology and Community Health,* 2003, *57,* 254–258.

Braveman, P. A., Krieger, N., and Lynch, J. W. "Health Inequalities and Social Inequalities in Health." *Bulletin of the World Health Organization,* 2000, *78,* 232–234.

Braveman, P. A., Starfield, B., and Geiger, H. J. "The *World Health Report 2000's* 'Health Inequalities' Approach Removes Equity from the Agenda for Public Health Monitoring and Policy." *British Medical Journal,* 2001, *323,* 678–680.

Braveman, P.A., and Tarimo, E. "Avoidable Social Inequalities in Health Within Countries: Not Only an Issue for Affluent Nations." *Social Science and Medicine,* 2001, *54,* 1621–1635.

Culyer, A. J. "The Promise of a Reformed NHS: An Economist's Angle." *British Medical Journal,* 1991, *302,* 1253–1256.

Culyer, A. J., and Wagstaff, A. "Equity and Equality in Health and Health Care." *Journal of Health Economics,* 1993, *12,* 431–457.

Dahlgren, G., and Whitehead, M. *Policies and Strategies to Promote Equity in Health.* Copenhagen: World Health Organization Regional Office for Europe, 1992.

Daniels, N. *Just Health Care.* New York: Cambridge University Press, 1985.

Egbuono, L., and Starfield, B. "Child Health and Social Status." *Pediatrics,* 1982, *69,* 550–557.

Evans, R. G., Barer, M. L., and Marmor, T. R. *Why Are Some People Healthy and Others Not? The Determinants of Health of Populations.* Hawthorne, N.Y.: Aldine de Gruyter, 1994.

Evans, T., and others (eds.). *Challenging Inequities in Health: From Ethics to Action.* New York: Oxford University Press, 2001.

Feinstein, J. S. "The Relationship Between Socioeconomic Status and Health: A Review of the Literature." *Milbank Quarterly,* 1993, *71,* 279–322.

Gakidou, E. E., and King, G. "Measuring Total Health Inequality: Adding Individual Variation to Group-Level Differences." *International Journal of Equity in Health,* 2002, *1*(1), 3.

Gwatkin, D. R., and others. *Socioeconomic Differences in Health, Nutrition, and Population.* Washington, D.C.: World Bank, 2000.

Hahn, R. A., and others. "Poverty and Death in the United States." *International Journal of Health Services,* 1996, *26,* 673–690.

Kaplan, G. A., and Keil, J. E. "Socioeconomic Factors and Cardiovascular Disease: A Review of the Literature." *Circulation,* 1993, *88,* 1973–1998.

Kaplan, G. A., and others. "Inequality in Income and Mortality in the United States: Analysis of Mortality and Potential Pathways." *British Medical Journal,* 1996, *312,* 999–1003.

Krieger, N., Williams, D. R., Moss, N. E. "Measuring Social Class in U.S. Public Health Research: Concepts, Methodologies, and Guidelines." *Annual Review of Public Health,* 1997, 18, 341-378.

Kunst, A. E., and Mackenbach, J. P. "International Variation in the Size of Mortality Differences Associated with Occupational Status." *International Journal of Epidemiology,* 1994a, *23,* 742–750.

Kunst, A. E., and Mackenbach, J. P. "The Size of Mortality Differences Associated with Educational Level in Nine Industrialized Countries." *American Journal of Public Health,* 1994b, *84,* 932–937.

Kunst, A. E., and others. "Mortality by Occupational Class Among Men 30–64 Years in Eleven European Countries." *Social Science and Medicine,* 1998a, *46,* 1459–1476.

Kunst, A. E., and others. "Occupational Class and Cause-Specific Mortality in Middle-Aged Men in Eleven European Countries: Comparison of Population-Based Studies." *British Medical Journal,* 1998b, *316,* 1636–1642.

Kunst, A. E., and others. "Occupational Class and Ischemic Health Disease Mortality in the United States and Eleven European Countries." *American Journal of Public Health,* 1999, *89,* 47–53.

Landmann Szwarcwald, C. "On the World Health Organization's Measurement of Health Inequalities." *Journal of Epidemiology and Community Health,* 2002, *56,* 177–182.

Mackenbach, J. P., and Bakker, M. (eds.). *Reducing Inequalities in Health: A European Perspective.* London: Routledge, 2002.

Mackenbach, J. P., and Kunst, A. E. "Measuring the Magnitude of Socio-Economic Inequalities in Health: An Overview of Available Measures Illustrated with Two Examples from Europe." *Social Science and Medicine,* 1997, *44,* 757–771.

Mackenbach, J. P., and others. "Socioeconomic Inequalities in Morbidity and Mortality in Western Europe." *Lancet,* 1997, *349,* 1655–1659.

Mackenbach, J. P., and others. "Socioeconomic Inequalities Among Women and Among Men: An International Study." *American Journal of Public Health,* 1999, *89,* 1800–1806.

Marmot, M. G., and others. "Health Inequalities Among British Civil Servants: The Whitehall II Study." *Lancet,* 1991, *337,* 1387–1393.

Murray, C. "Commentary: Comprehensive Approaches Are Needed for Full Understanding." *British Medical Journal,* 2001, *323,* 680–681.

Murray, C., Gakidou, E. E., and Frenk, J. "Health Inequalities and Social Group Differences: What Should We Measure?" *Bulletin of the World Health Organization,* 1999, *77,* 537–543.

Murray, C., and others. *U.S. County Patterns of Mortality by Race, 1965–1994.* Cambridge, Mass.: Harvard Center for Population and Development Studies, 1998.

Starfield, B. "Improving Equity in Health: A Research Agenda." *International Journal of Health Services,* 2001, *31,* 545–566.

Townsend, P. "Widening Inequalities of Health in Britain: A Rejoinder to Rudolph Klein." *International Journal of Health Services,* 1990, *20,* 363–372.

United Nations Development Programme. *Human Development Report, 1996.* New York: Oxford University Press, 1996.

United Nations Development Programme. *Human Development Report, 2002.* New York: Oxford University Press, 2002.

Wagstaff, A., Paci, P., and van Doorslaer, E. "On the Measurement of Inequalities in Health." *Social Science and Medicine,* 1991, *33,* 545–557.

Wagstaff, A., and van Doorslaer, E. "Equity in the Finance of Health Care: Some International Comparisons." *Journal of Health Economics,* 1992, *11,* 361–387.

Wagstaff, A., van Doorslaer, E., and Paci, P. "Horizontal Equity in the Delivery of Health Care." *Journal of Health Economics,* 1991, *10,* 251–256.

Whitehead, M. *The Concepts and Principles of Equity in Health.* Copenhagen: World Health Organization Regional Office for Europe, 1990.

World Bank. *World Development Report 2000/2001: Attacking Poverty.* New York: Oxford University Press, 2001.

World Health Organization. *Constitution of the World Health Organization.* Official Records of the World Health Organization, no. 2. Geneva: World Health Organization, 1946.

World Health Organization Regional Committee for Europe. *Technical Discussions.* Copenhagen: World Health Organization Regional Office for Europe, 1994.

World Health Organization. *World Health Report 1999: Making a Difference.* Geneva: World Health Organization, 1999.

World Health Organization. *World Health Report 2000.* Geneva: World Health Organization, 2000.

World Health Organization. "World Health Chart, 2001." 2001. [http://www.whc.ki.se/files/basicinfo.php].

World Health Organization and Braveman, P. A. *Equity in Health and Health Care: A World Health Organization Initiative.* Geneva: World Health Organization, 1996.

CHAPTER THIRTEEN

Assessing Equity in Health

Conceptual Criteria

Alexandra Bambas
Juan Antonio Casas

Fifty years ago, the framers of the Universal Declaration of Human Rights (UDHR) established a benchmark of standards against which to assess equity in health, both in terms of equity in health and well-being and in access to medical care.[1] They wrote:

> Article 25. Everyone has the right to a standard of living adequate for the health and well-being of himself and of his family, including food, clothing, housing and medical care and necessary social services, and the right to security in the event of unemployment, sickness, disability, widowhood, old age or other lack of livelihood in circumstances beyond his control.

The UDHR also states:

> Article 2. Everyone is entitled to all the rights and freedoms set forth in this Declaration, without distinction of any kind, such as race, colour, sex, language, religion, political or other opinion, national or social origin, property, birth or other status.

This chapter is based on a larger work by Alexandra Bambas, entitled "An Interpretation of Equity in Health for Latin America and the Caribbean" (working title), which examines conceptual and programming issues for equity in health in the context of the region. The chapter was also supported by the Division of Health and Human Development's Health Equity Interprogrammatic Group, with inputs from various other Pan American Health Organization technical units.

Unfortunately, those ideals for human health and well-being set forth in that document have not become a reality for every citizen in the world. In fact, given the competition for resources among different aspects of human well-being, attaining these standards is unfeasible for the present. Consequently, we must now attempt to develop a more organic process for assessing fairness in the distribution of resources for health that takes into consideration our organizational and technical abilities, personal autonomy, and reasonable expectations for action.

In recent decades, important authors have devoted themselves to study, define, and interpret the concepts of equity and social justice, as well as that of health equity. The works of John Rawls (1971), Amartya Sen (1992), and Margaret Whitehead (1991) stand out. In the region of the Americas, several authors and public health leaders have contributed to the understanding of health equity as a public health issue,[2] and since 1995, under the leadership of its director, Sir George Alleyne, the Pan American Health Organization has identified the reduction of health inequities as the main goal of its technical cooperation (see for example, Pan American Health Organization, 1996; Alleyne, 1999). Other leading development institutions, such as the Rockefeller Foundation and the World Bank, also have launched important initiatives that consider health equity as a priority issue for human development.

The persistence of infectious diseases among the poor; the growing proportion of the burden of disease that is due to non-infectious, behavior-related causes; and the growing inequalities within and between countries that have accompanied the globalization process and its worldwide expansion of free trade, market economies and liberal democracy, have added urgency to the need to address the growing health inequities. As a result, national and international health authorities have increasingly addressed the macrodeterminants of health inequities. The issue of health inequities and their relation to living conditions is now in the mainstream of public health thinking. And yet, although the technical aspects of measuring inequalities in health have evolved, insufficient attention is given to the explanation of why inequalities in health or health resources might be unfair or what the larger implications of labeling them as unfair might be. Moreover, the term *equity* often is used loosely, making it unclear how the term should be interpreted in a given context.

Many of the discussions about health equity make reasonable claims that there are inequalities in health status and access to care for different categories of people, whether identified by social class (as measured by income, wealth, and/or formal education), spatial distribution, gender, or ethnicity. Those who work in the public policy sector take this a step further, often referring to these inequalities in health as "inequities," casually using the term as shorthand for describing differences between better- and worse-off groups. Implicit to these discussions is an assumption that any difference is unacceptable and requires attention and intervention, but such discussions rarely provide an explanation for that value judgment or make distinctions between different kinds and levels of inequalities.

Asserting that these inequalities are inequities makes a forceful claim about justice—the normative implication of the word is useful. Confusing *equity* with *equality,* a common implication of comparisons between the best-off and worst-off, can result in a much higher standard than we might agree to under a more careful examination, however. The failure to distinguish between philosophical and pragmatic decisions regarding equity concerns in health could confuse the assessment of resource allocation or other policy decisions. This, in turn, would undermine the transparency of the process, making it difficult to generate public support.

At least three emerging empirical findings commonly drive the claim that inequalities in health between socioeconomic groups should be a development issue, and specifically a public health concern, particularly in Latin America and the Caribbean:

1. The poor use fewer public resources than middle and upper income groups.

2. There are vast and patterned health inequalities between socioeconomic groups, as well as between gender and ethnic origin categories, suggesting links between health outcomes and a variety of material and social living conditions.

3. Inequalities in the impact of these macro-determinants on health and overall well-being are growing.

These observations are often associated with the effects of globalization, and imply that intervention is required to prevent market distributions of resources from creating large discrepancies in health. These concerns also suggest that past interventions have not sufficiently compensated for these market effects.

DEFINITIONS OF EQUITY

Dictionary definitions of *equity* are fairly consistent. The term is defined as "justice according to natural law or right; specifically, freedom from bias or favoritism," or "the state, ideal, or quality of being just, impartial, and fair."

Inequity, then, is the linguistic opposite: the state, ideal, or quality of being unjust, partial, or unfair. Most importantly, notice that not *equality of distributions* but rather *fairness of distributions* is central to the definition. Although *equality* and *equity* are often conflated, the words have two distinct meanings and are conceptually very different. *Equality* is sameness, and *equity* is fairness. In any particular situation, *equal* may not be *equitable,* or *equal* may be precisely *equitable,* but we must present an ethical justification for why a certain distribution constitutes an *inequity.*

Vertical and Horizontal Equity

In describing an equitable situation, distinctions must be made between the appropriateness of equal and unequal distributions—or horizontal and vertical equity—either of which may constitute "even-handed treatment," depending on the situation. Equity simultaneously requires that relevantly similar cases be treated in similar ways, and relevantly different cases be treated in different ways. As noted in the *Oxford Dictionary of Philosophy* (Blackburn, 1994), controversy arises from the delineation of relevant similarity—*horizontal equity* is the allocation of equal or equivalent resources for *equal need; vertical equity* is the allocation of different resources for *different levels of need.*

These two conceptions of equity have dramatically different policy implications and cannot be applied randomly to problems. Rather, their application must appeal to some principle or special feature of the problem that justifies the choice of one over the other. For example, a universal health care plan might appeal to horizontal equity on the basis that *everyone* needs health care at some point. On the other hand, targeted programs for the poor would appeal to vertical equity. The distinction between these situations turns on the interpretation of *need:* in the first case, the justification is that everyone needs health care in the biological sense, while the second case appeals to a sense of financial need of the poor which doesn't apply to the non-poor.

Vertical equity has a higher potential for redistributing resources, and therefore often faces more political obstacles. However, in the current political climate, which challenges the legitimacy of public provision of services in areas thought to have market potential, vertical equity has gained momentum as a mechanism for constraining claims of need to those based on severe financial deprivation. For instance, where market mechanisms have been introduced into national health systems in the process of health sector reform, publicly funded basic packages or focalization strategies were instituted to provide for the needs of the worst-off. This approach has been criticized as having an overly narrow interpretation of need, which left large segments of the population vulnerable once again. On the other hand, some focalized strategies based on vertical equity are seen as quite reasonable and successful, such as in immunization programs.

Equity in Access to Health Care Services

An operational definition of health equity that focuses on need as the appropriate distribution mechanism specifically addresses equity in access to health care services. Aday and Andersen's definition, which has pervaded thinking in the health field, often is taken for granted and seldom questioned. They define an equitable distribution of health care services as "one in which illness (as defined by the patient and his family or by health-care professionals) is the major determinant of the allocation of resources" (Aday and Andersen, 1981).

The crux of the argument is that health resources are special goods that should not be distributed strictly as normal market commodities according to economic resources, because their social worth is significant. But this service-oriented approach has been found to be insufficient in reducing inequalities in health status and access to health between socioeconomic groups. For instance, the Black and Acheson reports examined the British National Health System, a prime example of universal coverage in health, and concluded that the effect of approaching health using a medical services strategy did not address concerns of reducing health inequalities and achieving fairness.

"Access to medical services" historically has been used as a measure of a fair distribution, partly because it is easier to measure and to improve access to services than to achieve more ambitious goals—say, securing a certain level of well-being in a population—and because of the historical compartmentalization of the social sectors within government, which provided focal advantages, but may at times limit the activities seen as appropriate for any one sector.

Additionally, there is an implicit assumption that services are a means to improve the population health, an assumption that has not been sufficiently confirmed (McKeon, 1976). Recent attention to inequalities in health status, especially with regard to socioeconomic categories, underlies a certain dissatisfaction with approaches strictly focused on access to services. This is due in part to the recognition that medical services may not be the most important determinant of health status and certainly are not the only means to improving health status. Insofar as access to services is supposed to be a means to higher level goals, such as better health, or even more opportunities in life, it is a limited measure of health equity. Various other sectors and aspects of life affect one's health status, including living conditions, working conditions, environmental issues such as air quality, education level, and access to cultural, social, and political participation.

By limiting our evaluation of health equity to "access to medical services," we ignore the importance of other sectors in determining health and effectively exclude their incorporation into an equity strategy. Such an approach tends to value these services for their own sake rather than emphasizing the role of medical services as *one of many means* to health.

If our consideration of health equity is widened to include inequalities in health outcomes, it becomes necessary to measure health status directly (rather than using only access to services) and to incorporate the analysis of access to other basic services, and the level of satisfaction of other basic needs, into the assessment of equity in health. The expansion from a medical services approach to a health outcomes approach involves the recognition that people do not get sick randomly, but in relation to their living, working, environmental, social, and political contexts, as well as with regard to biological and environmental factors that are unevenly distributed in the population. This broader concept is also much more conducive to considering the improvement of health status as part of the larger work of human development.

EQUITY IN HEALTH OUTCOMES

Based on the broad concept of health equity, as developed by Margaret White-head and adopted by the World Health Organization Regional Office for Europe, the government of the United Kingdom has taken the policy position that all health differences between the best-off and worst-off in different socioeconomic groups constitute inequities in health. Whitehead (1991) defines health inequities as "differences in health which are not only unnecessary and avoid-able but, in addition, are considered unfair and unjust"(p. 5).

If this were the complete definition, people with different life perspectives and even different political ideologies might be able to agree to it in principle, which would make it useful in the larger political forum to generate a working consensus on the matter. However, it entails reaching agreement on two poten-tially controversial parameters, i.e., determining what is unnecessary and unfair vis-à-vis what is inevitable and unavoidable.

Whitehead (1991) does go on to specify that there are seven determinants of health inequalities that can be identified:

1. Natural, biological variation
2. Health-damaging behavior that is freely chosen, such as participation in certain sports and pastimes
3. The transient health advantage of one group over another when that group is first to adopt a health-promoting behavior (as long as other groups have the means to catch up fairly soon)
4. Health-damaging behavior in which the degree of choice of lifestyles is severely restricted
5. Exposure to unhealthy, stressful living and working conditions
6. Inadequate access to essential health and other basic services
7. Natural selection or health-related social mobility involving the ten-dency for sick people to move down the social scale

Health inequalities determined by the first three categories would not be con-sidered unfair nor unjust, while the last four would be "considered by many to be avoidable and the resultant health differences to be unjust" (p. 6).

Although Whitehead's definition includes adequate access to health services as a condition of justice, it extends far beyond that—and beyond the more procedural standard related to access to services—to a much broader set of conditions that can affect health and establish a health advantage of one group over another. It's a robust concept of equity, encompassing a range of situations including outcomes, exposures, risks, living conditions, and social mobility.

CRITERIA FOR ASSESSING HEALTH EQUITY

The burden of proof lies in demonstrating that a situation is inequitable (rather than equitable), because making a social argument to change the present order requires justifying the allocation of public resources for interventions to redress the inequality. But to make this claim, we must give contextual and concrete meaning to the operational definitions of equity to determine when the judgment would apply. These meanings are reflected in the criteria that are repeatedly referred to in discussions regarding fair distributions of goods.

To establish a situation as inequitable, differences in distributions of a good, such as health resources or even the larger determinants of health status, must satisfy each of the following criteria:

- The differences in distribution must *be avoidable.*
- The difference must *not reflect free choice.*
- The claim must *link the distribution to a responsible agent.*

As the claimants, we must be able to argue how these criteria relate to particular claims of inequity.

Although these criteria might be applied to either individual distributions or to social distributions, their implications will take on somewhat different tones with each. For the purposes of policy development, we are concerned with social distributions, and therefore the interpretation of each of these criteria will relate not to equity judgments of any particular person's situation, but to trends in the health of the population and its subgroups. Some might argue that distributions are *politically necessary*—that sufficient support cannot be generated to support redistribution. But political will should be driven by justice; it should not constrain justice. If political will is lacking but equity criteria are present, mobilizing civil society to create political pressure becomes a technical issue.

Avoidability

"Avoidability" is a key criterion for equity, because if a distribution is not avoidable, it cannot be interpreted to be unfair in a social sense. While we emotionally respond by feeling that the universe or life is not just—and we may even have a will to intervene to change such distributions—to make a social claim based on equity is quite a different matter in that it *requires* action.

A proposal for redistribution, whether it be of health services or of macro-determinants of health, must show the current distribution to be avoidable in several senses.

- It must be *technically avoidable* because current scientific and organizational knowledge provides a solution for successful intervention.

- It must be *financially avoidable* because sufficient resources do exist either within the public sector or more generally to satisfy fair conditions.

- And it must be *morally avoidable* because the proposed redistribution would not violate some other, greater, sense of justice.

The subcategories of avoidability are highly relevant to claims of socioeconomic health inequities. Certainly there are individual cases of "technically unavoidable" health differences, such as in the case of health harms linked to naturally occurring genetic variations. But unless given reason to believe the contrary, we would not expect such occurrences to be patterned according to socioeconomic groups, thereby eliminating one source of "technically unavoidable" health inequalities and strengthening claims that patterned distributions of health may constitute inequities. Assuming that genetically related differences in health are not used to define our groups, the health standard of best-off groups demonstrates that those health indicators are indeed technically feasible. That is, in *technical terms,* there is no reason why all groups could not achieve health levels similar to those of best-off groups.

However, the setting of standards according to best-off groups may be prohibitively expensive, at least above a certain level of health. Diminishing margins of utility certainly do not argue against *any* redistribution or investment, but may place a limit on what might be financially possible in reducing health inequalities given resource constraints. Therefore, such studies contribute significantly to our understanding of financial avoidability, and therefore to reasonable and fair differences, even if absolute equality proves unfeasible. Finally, the evaluation of financial feasibility and the effect of re-distributions cannot be restricted to current public spending levels, but must necessarily include an economic evaluation of the availability of external resources based on the potential to increase fiscal base, since the question at issue is whether the financial resources exist at a macroeconomic level, not only within the institutional confines of the health sector.

At some point, we may determine that a certain redistribution level is technically and financially feasible, but impinges on other social values to the extent that the redistribution itself becomes unjust, either by severely restricting civil liberties or by prioritizing health to the unjustifiable detriment of other social goods. Analyses must therefore include not only studies of diminishing margins of utility, but also the larger social effect of such redistributions. Hypothetically, if, for a particular country, we found that we could bring inequalities of infant mortality rates, maternal mortality rates, and communicable diseases within "an acceptable range" only by instituting tax rates of 90 percent of income, we may decide that personal freedoms would be compromised to an extent that the social injustices created are more important than those that existed under conditions of larger health inequalities. If we accomplished the task by directing public spending for health activities by virtually eliminating other important national programs, not only might we find greater injustices than health inequalities, but also the actions might prove counter-productive if certain other programs (such as education or environmental protection) were to be affected.

If an argument that inequities exist is able to respond to each of these issues, it has succeeded in establishing that such inequalities are in fact avoidable, perhaps the most difficult of the criteria to secure.

Choice

Choice is particularly relevant to interpreting justice in health in terms of the protection of individual autonomy. Therefore *health behaviors* are better at indicating possible choice issues than health outcomes. The application of choice as a criterion might range from an individual electing to (1) engage in an activity, to (2) buy a product, to (3) prioritize needs. We hope that given sufficient information and opportunity, people will opt for activities and behaviors that enhance their health. Even when such activities and behaviors may not always be chosen, justifications for health-enhancing interventions may be limited by concerns for autonomy and preservation of civil liberties.

Free choices may, in fact, create acceptable differences between *individuals'* health, as some persons may choose behaviors that lead to worse health outcomes. But if the choice was in fact made under perfect, or even reasonably high conditions of choice, including adequate information and free will, claims of an injustice would be more difficult to sustain.

Particularly in the context of population-based analyses, protecting autonomy and promoting health often are more complimentary goals rather than competing interests. While individuals might make free choices based on their own particular wants or needs, we would not expect to see strong patterns of such behavior stratified in socioeconomic groups, unless an additional correlation that explains the concentration of risky behavior were presented.

A case for socioeconomic inequities in health must be built on the presumption that population *groups* would not freely choose lesser levels of health. In fact, some studies have shown that health behaviors do not differ significantly between population groups, and when they do, such as in the case of high fat diets among some minority groups in the United States or the urban poor in Latin America and the Caribbean, culture and lack of health information can be seen to clearly diminish the role of free choice. Further, when health behaviors are controlled for income, differences between groups dissolve, and income is not usually considered a "chosen" socioeconomic category. Consequently, choice as a justification for health differences tends to fall away in population studies. Therefore, when we do see such patterns, there is reason to believe that low levels of choice, or a thin sense of choice, might better describe those behaviors or decisions. Investigation into causality, whether through physical or social science, can bolster the argument that choice is limited.

Opponents of redistribution sometimes try to limit the scope of challenges to choice by depending on claims of economic choices in prioritizing goods or procedural interpretations of legal entitlement (in the case of public programs), as sufficient conditions for establishing free choice. Such conclusions generally rely on assumptions of equal opportunity for individuals within a society, at least at some level, although little attention is given to elaborating on the conditions of equal opportunity or a practical demonstration that such opportunity exists. Failure of the poor to "protect their health," for instance, is seen as due to their own negligence, or to the life situation that they have put themselves in (e.g., "choosing" to work in a dangerous factory), rather than any larger social, economic, or political disadvantages over which they had little control.

Some might argue that the poor or other vulnerable groups "choose" poor health, when they fail to seek care when they are ill. However, the priorities that intervene to prevent such utilization of care are often not only equally basic and necessary for survival, but also often contribute to the family's health in some other way, as when financial resources are used to purchase food or support the survival of the family business. Such arguments gain by conflating "decision making," which can include prioritizing certain needs over other needs, with a richer meaning of "free choice." Further, if we can demonstrate that health is strongly linked to other social sectors, the argument that the poor can "choose" to invest in health by financially prioritizing health care services over, say, housing or nutrition, loses its weight, since the areas are interrelated, and that "choice" simply becomes a decision, with little real meaning in terms of improving one's well-being.

Insofar as access to health services is concerned, proponents of resource redistributing have succeeded in expanding the narrow, but commonly used interpretation of "choice"—the *legal right to utilize resources*. They include more socially embedded issues that are needed to access health resources, such as support services, including transportation. Recognizing the social context of a situation demonstrates how real "choices" can be thwarted by the reality of people's daily lives. Removal of those barriers, then, actually enhances individual autonomy in a meaningful sense, rather than detracting from it.

Transportation is only one of many barriers to free choice. While individuals often do make choices about their own health, decisions are also made by groups at the national, community, and family levels. Such situations can be used against the politically disenfranchised in a democracy, if the assertion is made that all citizens have agreed to certain conditions, and therefore have "chosen" those conditions. The recognition of macrodeterminants of health, including social and economic factors that influence health status, has greatly broadened the social meaning of health resources, and consequently has expanded the list of relevant resources involved in the choice claim. Lack of access to education and access to information, for instance, can ground a health inequity claim related to choice. Though more difficult to empirically demonstrate, psychological issues are also basic to a conception of choice. Elements of social control and influence, actual and perceived locus of control, and the larger implications of certain health-related choices on one's life become very important to identify in order to establish that choice is more limited than it might appear.

Agency

The third criterion for establishing that an inequity exists is that the claim be linked to a responsible agent. To make this determination, either of two meanings of *responsible* may be used. We may establish that there is a *culpable* entity who caused direct or indirect harm, as we might apply in cases of damage to health due to environmental degradation or occupational hazards. One of the difficulties in identifying and establishing the culpable agent is that culpability can be masked. The externalization of health harms in industry or manufacturing, for instance, would first have to be recognized, then traced. In the absence of empirical studies linking problems to their sources, our ability to perceive the culpability of a particular agent will be impaired, even if there is a very direct cause-and-effect relationship. Further, for the purposes of socioeconomic differences in health, discrete instances of culpability are less relevant than larger systematic patterns of harms that would be generated through responses to policy, or its absence.

Alternatively, we might make a claim that there is an *accountable* entity, one who is responsible for rectifying the unfair distribution. In the case of health equity, claims often center on the responsibility of the government to ensure certain rights or provide a certain amount of protection to all citizens, which justifies state intervention. A claim of lax or unenforced government regulations, or governmental assistance in externalizing health harms, makes a particularly strong claim. Although a government might not be responsible for creating a health-harming situation, once an issue has been publicly discussed, lack of response by government must be interpreted as a decision affecting the public to which it, as a presumably just institution, must be held accountable. The level of governance then, will also affect perceptions of the responsibility (and the ability to respond) of the government.

The Spectrum of Inequalities

If any one of these criteria is absent, or is present only weakly, the argument that a difference is an inequity begins to lose power. In addition to the empirical verification that inequalities in health status or access to resources exist, scientific research can assist in demonstrating that these criteria apply, thereby greatly strengthening the political claim that inequities also exist. Because scientific knowledge is constantly growing, our interpretation of whether criteria apply to specific issues also changes over time. For instance, in relation to "free choice," alcoholism and smoking are not seen as much as lifestyle *choices* as they once were because of increasing evidence on the biological basis of addiction. Social science research also contributes to our interpretations, as when we attend to the effect of targeted advertising on alcohol consumption and smoking rates.

When we make the claim that differences in health are inequitable, the strength of the evidence or the argument, according to the above criteria, will determine the level of inequity. We might think of this as a spectrum, with each of the criteria moving our assessment of the situation either closer to "misfortune" or to "inequity" (see Figure 13.1).

To be sure, we must be willing to recognize some differences as "fair" differences; otherwise, the criteria would not be meaningful. Genetic birth defects and deaths due to "old age" may be very unfortunate but not necessarily unfair if little could have been done to prevent them; that is, they were not avoidable. Therefore, it will also be important for a clear analysis to identify those differences that do not fit into the criteria.

CONCLUSION

The framework presented here must now be supplemented with quantitative and qualitative information that applies each of these criteria to the health conditions and broader societal abilities and resources in order to set priorities and targets for equity in health. Research should be supported not only by traditional epidemiological studies but also by social science research, including methodologies that are continuing to be developed. The particular resources

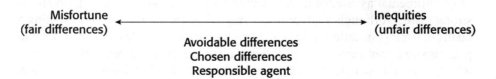

Figure 13.1. The Spectrum of Inequalities.

and challenges will differ among countries, and the quest for health equity should be recognized as a development process, and one that must alter its goals on occasion to adjust to the changing environment.

An equity-driven approach in health policy requires a broad vision of the determinants of population health and an understanding of how both health policy and wider social policy will affect those determinants. To the extent that health and other socioeconomic factors are interdependent, health policy must consider how other sectoral policies and actions as well as societal trends, can be directed to promote health equity. Similarly, health policy must take into consideration how health policy can contribute to broader equity goals in health development.

Finally, the pursuit of equity is necessarily linked to issues of governance, which includes accountability, transparency, decision-making procedures, and the ability of the political sphere to allow for broad representation and the effective exercise of choice by all social groups and members of society (Gilson, 1998). Leadership in health equity requires both a high level of capacity for managing resources and developing policy and a strong political society. Once a society embraces a political foundation of egalitarianism, whereby all citizens of a country are due equal regard under the law and have equal political voices, societies themselves become the ultimate arbitrators of equity, in health or any other sphere.

Notes

1. The complete text of the Universal Declaration of Human Rights (1948) is available at http://www.un.org/Overview/rights.html.

2. These Latin American public health figures include Jaime Breilh, Juan Cesar Garcia, Asa Cristina Laurell, Cristina Possas, Mario Testa, Naomar de Almeida Filho, Pedro Luis Castellanos, Juan Samaja, Carlos Montoya, Jeanette Vega, among others.

References

Aday, L. A., and Andersen, R. M. "Equity of Access to Medical Care: A Conceptual and Empirical Review." *Medical Care*, 1981, *19*(12 Suppl.), 4–27.

Alleyne, G.A.O. "Equity and Health." Speech presented at the Eleventh World Congress of Psychiatry, Hamburg, Germany, Aug. 1999.

Blackburn, S. *Oxford Dictionary of Philosophy.* Oxford: Oxford University Press, 1994.

Gilson, L. "In Defense and Pursuit of Equity." *Social Science and Medicine*, 1998, *47*, 1891–1896.

McKeon, T. *The Role of Medicine: Dream, Miracle or Nemesis?* Oxford: Oxford University Press/Nuffield Provincial Trust. 1976.

Pan American Health Organization. *Annual Report of the Director, 1995: In Search of Equity.* Washington, D.C.: Pan American Health Organization, 1996.

Rawls, J. *A Theory of Justice.* Cambridge, Mass.: Harvard University Press; 1971.

Sen, A. K. *Inequality Reexamined.* Cambridge, Mass.: Harvard University Press; 1992.

Whitehead, M. *The Concepts and Principles of Equity and Health.* Copenhagen: World Health Organization Regional Office for Europe, 1991.

CHAPTER FOURTEEN

Income Inequality, Social Cohesion, and the Health Status of Populations

The Role of Neo-Liberalism

David Coburn

There has been a recent upsurge of interest in the relationships between socio-economic status (SES) and health. Numerous papers in *Social Science and Medicine,* the *International Journal of Health Services,* recent special editions of such journals as the *Sociology of Health and Illness* and the *Milbank Quarterly* and a variety of books (Evans, Barer, and Marmor, 1994; Amick et al., 1995; Blane, Brunner, and Wilkinson, 1996) have focused directly or indirectly on the social determinants of health generally and on the SES and health status relationship specifically.

It has long been known that there are historically persistent inverse relationships between SES and health status within nations. In most developed countries health inequalities have not decreased despite rising national wealth (as measured by increasing GNP per capita) and improvements in longevity. Recently attention has turned to analysis of the relationships between levels of inequality and longevity amongst the economically advanced nations rather than only within them. In his interesting and provocative book *Unhealthy Societies: The Afflictions of Inequality* (1996), a central writer in the area, Richard

This chapter arose from ideas stimulated by discussion in the Critical Social Science and Health Group at the University of Toronto (Joan Eakin, Richard Edwards, Rhonda Love, Blake Poland, Ann Robertson and others). I owe much to discussions in that group and with participants in a reading course on social cohesion and health (Blake Poland, Rhonda Love, Ann Robertson, Sylvia-Ann Brooker, Robert Rose, Lyn Talbot). The reviewers' comments were helpful.

Wilkinson, proposes that after certain absolute levels of GNP per capita are attained (about U.S.$5,000), the major determinant of differing levels of health status amongst nations lies in their degree of income inequality. In the developed nations, controlling for such factors as GNP per capita, the greater a nation's income inequality, the poorer the average national health status. That is, it is inequality rather than wealth that is important for health.

Wilkinson also cites support for his findings about international differences in research on differences in health status between states in the United States (Kaplan et al., 1996; Kennedy, Kawachi, and Prothrow-Stith, 1996; Daly et al., 1998; Lynch et al., 1998). The U.S. analyses support the Wilkinson hypothesis in indicating that inter-state and inter-city differences in health status are more closely related to the income inequality of these areas than to their average level of income.

A focus on absolute levels of income as determinants of health does not explain why some rich countries show lower levels of health than do some poorer, but more egalitarian countries. It has also been frequently pointed out that within countries, there are differences in health status across the SES gradient. That is, it is not simply those at the low end of the SES continuum that are the issue. Even SES groups quite high in income and SES show poorer health than those immediately above them. Attention has thus turned to the more indirect influence of psycho-social factors on health status rather than simply the direct and immediate effects of material life circumstances. If indeed relative status is related to health up and down the SES hierarchy, then it is likely that psycho-social factors, and not only absolute material conditions, are a major influence on health (Wilkinson, 1997b—but see Coburn, 2003).

Though the psycho-social channels relating inequality to health status within countries are numerous and rather general, many observers argue that those lower in SES show lowered self-esteem, lack of control, more harmful emotional reactions to life events, higher stress or the like. Attempting to explain between-country differences, Wilkinson, Kawachi and others (Kawachi and Kennedy, 1997; Kawachi et al., 1997; Wilkinson, 1996) have drawn on the work of Putnam (1993) to argue that social cohesion/trust is one of the main mechanisms linking the national degree of income inequality with health. Putnam had contended that northern Italy was more socially and economically successful than southern Italy because the north had developed greater "social capital," that is, more extensive social networks and greater social "trust," than had the south. Drawing on these findings, the "inequality" theorists argue, with some supporting evidence, that higher income inequality produces lowered social cohesion/lower trust, which in turn produces lowered health status. It is also implied that between-country differences are explained by the fact that elongated status hierarchies exacerbate the status effects noted within countries. Thus there is a more or less linear income inequality–social cohesion/trust/esteem, etc., health status linkage.

Wilkinson's contention that the health differences amongst countries are explained by their differing degrees of income inequality has been critiqued on methodological grounds by Judge (1995; and Judge, 1996) and by Gravelle (1998). In this chapter, I do not question the income inequality–health status relationship, nor will I analyze in any depth the rather vague use of the concept of social cohesion, which requires separate analysis. Rather, I initially assume that income inequalities amongst nations are related to national levels of health status partly through the vehicle of social cohesion/social disorganization. I discuss the Wilkinson hypothesis on between-country differences to provide a focus for discussion; the analysis that follows has obvious relevance also for within-country SES–health status relationship.

BACKGROUND

As a number of analysts note, almost all the attention within the SES–health status tradition has been devoted to attempts to explain why and how SES is related to health (Bartley, Blane, and Davey Smith, 1998; Daly et al., 1998; Popay et al., 1999). There has been an overwhelming tendency to focus on the possible social/psycho-biological mechanisms through which social factors might be tied to health rather than on examination of the basic social causes of inequality and health. With only a few exceptions (Muntaner and Lynch, 1999; Navarro, 1999a, 1999b; Scambler and Higgs, 1999), there has been a startling lack of attention to the social/political/economic context of SES or income inequality–health status relationships. It is striking that in various summaries of the literature relating SES to various negative outcomes, and in those proposing or studying various measures to "prevent" these negative outcomes, the possible causes of inequalities are seldom, if ever, mentioned. For example, a good deal of attention is now centered on low-income children in the belief that enriching their environments will help prevent health or other difficulties later in life. Seldom, however, is there any discussion of the causes of SES differences themselves.

The neglect of putative causes is justified on the basis that we should focus our research attention on something we can actually do something about (Syme, 1998). SES or income inequalities are apparently viewed as beyond the reach of reform activities. A focus on "meso" or "micro" levels of amelioration of health inequalities is valuable. It might also be argued that bringing about relatively small changes in the consequences of inequality might lead, in time through feedback mechanisms, to changes in inequality itself, as Syme implies (Syme, 1998). Nevertheless, it is troublesome that assumptions of what is feasible or unfeasible are used as a justification for the failure to contextualize the income inequality–health status relationship. Such assessments may not, in fact, be correct. If the "contextualizing causes" of income inequality and social disorganization are not even examined, the notion of the feasibility of reform is premature. Moreover, if we assume, with Bhaskar and the "realists" (Bhaskar, 1975, 1989; Sayer, 1992), that social systems are "open" systems, then contextual factors may modify our notions of the causal model involved in the SES-health linkage itself. That is, it is misleading to simply draw out the relationships amongst particular social "variables" without consideration of the context within which such relationships exist (see Robertson, 1998). Finally, analysis of the income inequality–health relationship might be as useful for what it tells us about social structures as it is for the immediate concerns of public health. Health matters have for too long been viewed as somehow separate from the societies in which they are in fact embedded.

The general lack of attention to the possible determinants of SES and to income inequalities is doubly interesting given obvious international and national political and economic trends which one would assume have implications for our understanding of income inequality and, presumably, the health of populations. These trends include the "globalization" of the world economy as well as the rise of New Right political regimes and the concomitant "decline of the welfare state" (Stubbs and Underhill, 1994).

In this chapter, I use the income inequality (II)–lowered social cohesion (SC)–lowered health status (HS) sequence put forward by Wilkinson and others as a starting point for broadening discussion of the topic. In doing so, I hope only to make more explicit potential causal pathways and models which are implicit in Wilkinson's writings on the topic and to build on Wilkinson's work and explicit proposals which have appeared in recent studies in the area (Lynch et al., 1998; Muntaner and Lynch, 1999; Scambler and Higgs, 1999).

In analyzing the issues raised by the II-SC-HS relationships, I relate inequalities to their broader context, including their relationship to the welfare state and the class bases of different types of welfare state regime. The result of such a consideration does bring in processes involved in the relationships amongst markets, states and civil society and leads to a somewhat different causal picture about national and international differences in income inequality and in longevity than that usually implied by Wilkinson and others.

In broadening the discussion about the determinants of health, Wilkinson contends that income inequality produces social disorganization (or lowered social cohesion), which leads to lower average national health status. He is, however, somewhat equivocal about the nature of the causal pathways involving income inequality and social cohesion. In places, he suggests that it is possible that social cohesion produces lowered income inequality or that there is some form of reciprocal relationship between the two. That is, a highly cohesive community might "not permit" high levels of income inequality. Wilkinson also suggests that income inequality may directly produce both lowered social cohesion and lowered longevity; that is, social cohesion might not be the mediator between income inequality and health status. In a number of places, Wilkinson and particularly Kawachi and colleagues also imply that markets are at the source of the income inequality problem even though there are obviously differences amongst "market societies." Other writers point to the importance of welfare state measures or a version of social capital (referring to the social infrastructure) as possibly underlying social cohesion or as a major link between income inequality and longevity (Daly et al., 1998; Davey Smith, 1996; Kawachi and Kennedy, 1997; Kawachi et al., 1997).

Here, I extend the discussions linking income inequality and health by arguing that, rather than income inequality producing lowered social cohesion/trust leading to lowered health status, neo-liberalism (market dominance) produces *both* higher income inequality and lower social cohesion (a proposition suggested by Muntaner and Lynch, 1999) and, presumably, either lowered health status or a health status which is not as high as it might otherwise have been. Neo-liberalism has this effect partly through its undermining of (particular types of) welfare state. Discussion of this thesis, while focused on the income inequality–health status international literature, also has implications for the more widespread and substantial evidence of within country SES–health status relationships. It also draws in analyses of the "rise and fall" of the welfare state, as well as the presumed class causes and consequences of such a sequence, and thus broadens and contextualizes the topic.

I cannot here examine the history and consequences for health of the revival of neo-liberalism. Simply as a first step, I show that the fundamental postulates or assumptions of neo-liberalism are congruent with a "neo-liberalism produces both inequality and lowered social cohesion" conclusion. That is, there is an affinity between neo-liberal doctrines, inequality, and social fragmentation. While I cite evidence supporting this proposition, this chapter does not constitute a test of the neo-liberalism–inequality/lower social cohesion–health status linkages, but is simply a first step in opening up neglected areas for exploration. (For a second step, see Coburn, 2003). I hope to help "bring the social back in" by pointing to possible linkages between national and international studies of SES-HS differences and broader social processes. Such a consideration involves a theoretical and empirical literature often viewed as at some distance from the health field, such as the literature on welfare state theory, globalization and class dynamics.

In asserting a particular affinity between neo-liberalism, inequality and low-ered social cohesiveness, I point out:

1. "Ideal-type" neo-liberal tenets are congruent with the production of, or at least acceptance of, greater socio-economic inequalities (and selective examples support that contention).

2. There are striking parallels between "ideal" or pure neo-liberal ideology or tenets and factors related to, or constituent of, social disorganization/lowered trust.

3. Neo-liberalism and economic globalization are associated with the decline of the welfare state. This decline is one of the causes both of increased inequality and lowered social cohesion.

In making these arguments, for the sake of clarity and simplicity I omit the numerous caveats that might modify or make more complex the linkages I suggest. Obviously, societal inequalities and changes in health status have complex, multifaceted causes. I am not trying to posit a single-cause explanation. Rather, I point to neo-liberalism as a major, if complex, set of causes amongst others. Although I equate neo-liberalism with the dominance of markets, the comparisons made are not between market versus nonmarket societies but amongst capitalist societies with varying degrees of market domination.

At the end of the chapter, I note and briefly respond to some of the more obvious objections to the thesis proposed and outline a possible causal pathway between such macro forces as globalization, changes in the balance of class forces, neo-liberalism and health status.

GENERAL TENETS OF NEO-LIBERALISM

I assume that neo-liberalism refers to the dominance of markets and the market model. Though composed of a complex combination of characteristics, the basic assumptions of neo-liberalism, the "philosophy" of the New Right, are:

1. That markets are the best and most efficient allocators of resources in production and distribution

2. That societies are composed of autonomous individuals (producers and consumers) motivated chiefly or entirely by material or economic considerations

3. That competition is the major market vehicle for innovation

Neo-liberalism is distinguished from neo-conservatism by the fact that the latter contains a particular social component supportive of traditional family values, particular religious traditions, and not only a free-enterprise economic doctrine.

The essence of neo-liberalism, its pure form, is a more or less thoroughgoing adherence, in rhetoric if not in practice, to the virtues of a market economy, and, by extension, a market-oriented society. While some neo-liberals appear to assume that one can construct any kind of society on any kind of economy, the position taken here is that the economy, the state and civil society are in fact inextricably interrelated.

THE RELATIONSHIP BETWEEN NEO-LIBERAL DOCTRINES AND INEQUALITY

Neo-liberals, I contend, are not particularly concerned about inequality or regard it either as a positive virtue or as inevitable or necessary. That is, if the market is the best or most efficient allocator of goods and resources, neo-liberals are inclined to accept whatever markets bring. Certainly, political parties which espouse neo-liberal principles have been the mainspring behind attacks on the Keynesian welfare state (KWS), whose functions included not only the correction of market fluctuations but also the amelioration of market-produced inequalities. The welfare state, in the neo-liberal view, interferes with the "normal" functioning of the market. Neo-liberals oppose any form of "intervention" in markets because they feel that such intervention damages the operation of the "invisible hand," which most efficiently aligns production, consumption and distribution (while they at the same time deny that markets themselves are "structured" by state action).

reinforces the idea of deserving and undeserving

Neo-liberals contend not only that market inequalities are the necessary by-product of a well-functioning economy but that these inequalities are just, because what one puts into the market one gets out. That is, the invisible hand doctrine implies some reasonable relationship between one's activities and subsequent rewards. Moreover, as noted, there is a resistance to "correcting" market-produced inequalities through various welfare state measures, since these are assumed to lead to "market distortions." State actions, then, are not only inefficient but may also be unethical (while some feel markets are ethical, e.g., Hendrickson, 1996, others radically disagree; see McMurtry, 1998).

The whole ideological and political spectrum is now so skewed towards market solutions that even previously social democratic governments have moved towards market-oriented policies of varying degrees. Neo-liberalism is not confined to political jurisdictions in which the New Right actually forms the government. Some might assert that this is so because there are no alternatives to increasing neo-liberal policies because of the internationalization of markets or "globalization." We return to this argument later.

Given the focus on markets and inequality any discussion of neo-liberalism, inequalities and health in the contemporary era has to be tied to discussion of the welfare state. After all, the rise of the welfare state was viewed as either preventing or ameliorating the unwanted excesses or problems produced by the market system.

NEO-LIBERALISM, THE WELFARE STATE AND INEQUALITY

The contemporary rise of neo-liberalism and of inequality following the 1970s is historically tied to the decline of the welfare state. While markets produce inequalities, these may be prevented (through labor market policies) or ameliorated (through social welfare measures or the decommodification of education, health and welfare). Decommodification meant that access to social resources was not completely determined by market criteria (i.e., income or wealth) or by power in the market (the ability of some groups to bargain for private welfare benefits; see Esping-Andersen, 1999). Both health, through the effects of the welfare state on the social determinants of health, and health care, through various forms of national health care systems, are tied to the fate of the welfare state. Any consideration of the social determinants of health would have to take account of welfare state dynamics. Whether or not the effects of welfare state measures are direct and material or indirect and psycho-social is a matter of dispute. Nevertheless, as Popay et al. (1999), Bartley, Blane, and Davey Smith (1998) and Daly et al. (1998) and others note there may be critical periods of the life cycle in which the buffering effects of the "social wage" or of social policies generally are crucially important. Daly et al. even contend that "political units that tolerate a high degree of income inequality are less likely to support the human, physical, cultural, civic, and health resources needed to maximize the health of their populations" (p. 319). Bartley, Blane and Montgomery (1997) feel that the welfare state has both material and psychosocial effects "by preventing dramatic falls in living standards and by a wider effect on the degree to which citizens experience a sense of control of their lives" (p. 1195). Redistributive policies are important materially and psycho-socially. Davey Smith (1996, p. 988) contends that "cross nationally, higher levels of both social expenditure and taxation as a proportion of gross domestic product are associated with longer life expectancy, lower maternal mortality, and a smaller proportion of low-birthweight deliveries" (see also Kaplan et al., 1996; Kennedy, Kawachi, and Prothrow-Stith, 1996). There are thus many suggestions that the welfare state provided the material base for a more cohesive society and/or more or less directly influences health status.

Neo-liberals opposed or only reluctantly accepted the post–World War II establishment of the major attributes of the KWS as expressed in various pension, social insurance, health care, labor market or welfare measures involving government actions. Nevertheless, the example of the KWS was used to argue that capitalism had "solved" one of its major problems through ameliorating the inequalities produced by market mechanisms. Whereas in the 19th century, inequality had been viewed as legitimate or perhaps inevitable, within the KWS, issues of inequality seemed no longer a major concern—first, because through the notion of "social citizenship," inequalities in the market were ameliorated and second, because fluctuations of boom and bust were reduced by Keynesian counter-cyclical economic policies (demand stimulation in times of downturn, restriction of demand in times of boom).

Most welfare state analysts attribute the formation of welfare state measures directly or indirectly to some form of working class pressure or, in more complex formulations, to various class coalitions and class strength (Esping-Andersen, 1990; O'Connor and Olsen, 1998; Korpi, 1989; Quandango, 1987). Ross and Trachte (1990) and others have implied a lessened resistance to working class pressures for welfare state measures from dominant classes in an era of monopoly capital because of divisions between the competitive and monopoly sectors of capital. The KWS, however, is not a unitary phenomenon. As Esping-Andersen (1990, 1999) has indicated, there are various types of welfare state of which the ones involving the least state action, and the greatest dominance of market-related solutions were the liberal welfare states of the Anglo-American nations (as opposed to social democratic or corporate welfare states developed elsewhere). In fact, it can be argued that the liberal welfare states did the least to either prevent (particularly because of the absence of labor-market policies) or to rectify (through social welfare and health care) the depredations of the capitalist marketplace and the inequalities it tended to produce. Within liberal welfare states, social policies were most generally designed to supplement market provision, to reflect participation in the market, or generally, to be targeted or "means-tested" rather than universal in application. That is, these measures are less decommodifying (Korpi and Palme, 1998).

Most recently, given globalization, in which finance and, to a lesser extent, industrial capital has escaped from national controls while labor has not, has come a return to neo-liberal doctrines (Ross and Trachte, 1990; Stubbs and Underhill, 1994; Teeple, 1995). Economic globalization was aided by neo-liberals, and neo-liberalism benefited from economic globalization. Hence a "restructuring" of society, including markets and the welfare state. In a global era it is claimed that higher degrees of inequality are inevitable or that inequalities are an inescapable adjunct to economic growth or to the realities of international competition. Inequality is also viewed as a key motivational factor aiding a productive economy i.e., through lowering the costs of labor. Any measures to alter market-produced motivations simply deform the operation of markets and, furthermore, are unjust or at least inefficient. Inequality, then, is more to be welcomed or at least accepted than it is to be prevented or ameliorated by state or other forms of welfare. (See Kenworthy, 1998, for a summary and rebuttal of many of these arguments.)

Much contemporary neo-liberal policy, in fact, involves "recommodifying" aspects of society that were decommodified or taken out of the market during the rise of the KWS. The rise of neo-liberal political regimes has meant an increased focus on means testing regarding various income support measures, on reducing entitlements, or on undermining the power of labor unions or other organizations opposing the strict application of market mechanisms.

The data produced by Wilkinson, but also more general analyses of international differences in income inequality, do suggest that most social democratic or even corporate welfare state regimes, such as the Scandinavian countries, have been much less unequal than more neo-liberal regimes such as the United States, Britain, and the former British colonies (Atkinson, 1995; Gottschalk and Smeeding, 1997, 2000; Korpi and Palme, 1998; Smeeding, 1997). Some analysts have also argued that the more social democratic or corporate welfare state regime types have also been more successful in resisting the trend towards a dismantling or restructuring of the welfare state than have the market-oriented Anglo-democracies (Mishra, 1990). Certainly, welfare states have both causes and consequences. Evidence indicates, for example, that less market-based social welfare measures in fact reinforce support for the welfare state. Universal plus earnings-related welfare measures have the effect of reinforcing working and middle class coalitions in support of the welfare state (Korpi and Palme, 1998).

Redistributive policies in the less neo-liberal states have been important in reducing inequalities (see Bartley, Blane and Montgomery, 1997; Kenworthy, 1998). Welfare states did tend to do what they were supposed to do. Inequalities are thus more or less directly related to the class structure because class pressure tends to reduce the degree to which markets predominate.

The most recent evidence from the United States, Britain, Australia, Canada, New Zealand and the Organization for Economic Cooperation and Development countries generally, indicates that neo-liberalism in action, while obviously a far from perfect neo-liberalism, is associated with more or less rapidly increasing inequality. The United States and the United Kingdom, but also Canada and Australia, show much higher inequality than do such countries as Switzerland, Germany or the Netherlands, which in turn show higher inequality than do the Scandinavian countries (Atkinson, 1995; Smeeding, 1997; Korpi and Palme, 1998; Kenworthy, 1998; Gottschalk and Smeeding, 2000). It is not that inequalities did not exist before recent neo-liberal regimes or doctrines, simply that inequality was and is exacerbated under neo-liberalism. As many of the working papers emanating from the Luxembourg Income Study (2003) indicate, the welfare state did ameliorate market inequalities and inequalities were higher in countries with less decommodifying welfare state systems. With the rise of neo-liberal policies and the decline of the welfare state, inequality is rising in most countries; however, inequality is much more noticeable in countries characterized by neo-liberal political and welfare regimes than in less market-oriented systems (Smeeding, 1997; Korpi and Palme, 1998; Kenworthy, 1998; Gottschalk and Smeeding, 2000).

Arguably then markets produce income inequalities, and neo-liberalism opposes measures to redistribute income resources—therefore the proposition that *the more market-oriented or neo-liberal the regime, the greater the income inequality.*

A major possible empirical exception to the higher neo-liberalism–higher inequality scenario amongst the developed nations appears to be Japan. That country seems, on the face of it, to show relative income equality (and very high population longevity) yet to be highly market-oriented.

It might, however, be argued that Japan was, and is, less market-oriented than previously thought. Although at the time when Japan was rapidly growing economically in the 1960s to 1980s, most observers viewed Japan as more "capitalist" or market-oriented than other developed countries, many now have begun to retract that earlier judgment. Economic observers of a Japan in the late 1980s and 1990s, which shows signs of prolonged economic turbulence, now contend that that country, and other Asian Tigers, is characterized not by the dominance of markets but by close (nonmarket) ties between business and the state and/or by various forms of capitalist cronyism. Furthermore, Japan, with its earlier emphasis on lifetime employment (for employees of large corporations at least) and by a subordinate and service role for women, was far from being a thoroughgoing market-oriented economy. Rather, markets in Japan were considerably modified, constrained or shaped by business-state elite ties and by various cultural or normative practices. In sum, Japan might not be as much of a counter-example as is first assumed, although it is obviously worthy of further study.

Finally, the Japanese example raises the more general issue of the nature of the relationship between economies and national jurisdictions and boundaries (Poland et al., 1998). In an era of global trade, metropolitan or core nations like Japan have economic footprints which extend far beyond their national boundaries. Perhaps a core economy can preserve particular levels of equality at the expense of its periphery. What are the units of analysis where economies and inequality are concerned?

THE RELATIONSHIP BETWEEN NEO-LIBERALISM AND SOCIAL COHESION/TRUST

A strong argument can be made that neo-liberal doctrines are antithetical to social cohesion or to social trust. The image of society which neo-liberalism carries with it is that of voluntaristic "possessive individualism" (Macpherson, 1964). The most appropriate relationship is that embodied in contracts reflecting varied material self-interests. In the neo-liberal view, societies are not more than the sum of their parts. As former British Prime Minister Margaret Thatcher asserted, there is no such thing as "society," only individuals or families. Whereas in previous liberal theory the state is viewed as at least partially representative of the general interests of society, in the neo-liberal perspective the state should have as small a role as possible. Not much is said by many neo-liberals, however, about how markets themselves are constructed or about corporate monopolies or oligopolies, although thoroughgoing neo-liberals i.e., libertarians (utopian capitalists) claim to want to break up such market hindrances.

As noted, the neo-liberal vision is individualistic rather than collectivist or communitarian. There is a stark divide between collectivist views of society, including the notion that goods can be held in common, and market ideology. Thus the first act of many contemporary neo-liberal regimes has been to "privatize" state organizations or functions and those which might be said to have been included in the commons. Privatization in fact means the individual ownership of what were once possessions or functions of the state as representative of society, or of those things which were previously viewed as the possession of everyone (including natural products, land, fish, etc.). As noted earlier, even in the era of the welfare state, the "liberal" versions of the KWS were characterized by "insurance" or targeted versus universal or citizenship-oriented social or other programs. In that sense, then, they bracketed or excluded low-income groups from the rest of society.

The very notion of citizenship as carrying with it particular rights, social as well as political, is an inclusionary concept. The implication of universal citizenship measures is that we are all members of the same society and we should all benefit. The more neo-liberal targeted programs are exclusionary· in "privatizing" the negative effects of market mechanisms. The implication of targeted programs is that it is individuals and families which are the problem, not the structure of opportunities within that society. Yet as noted earlier, during the life-course, decommodification makes critical periods less likely to have negative consequences. These crises include periods of inability to earn an income. Wilkinson himself remarks that "indeed, integration in the economic life of society, reduced unemployment, material security, and narrower income differences provide the material base for a more cohesive society" (Wilkinson, 1997b, p. 319).

Neo-liberals generally view anything in the "public" sphere as something which would benefit from privatization. Some of the results of these individualist notions may be reflected in attitudes towards private versus public property or goods. That is, what is private is valued and what is public is denigrated. What is mine is valuable; the rest is not mine and not "ours" either and hence is of little concern.

Given the absence of a broader sense of community, neo-liberals advocate individualistic market-based solutions to problems. Thus gated communities and private security guards are a response to crime, and private health insurance is a response to the increased health needs of an aging population. There is an emphasis on private versus public transportation, private versus public schooling, private versus public health care. Reducing the size of government means reducing government expenditures. Neo-liberals strongly favor lower taxes (see Raphael, 1999). Given the use of government revenues to redistribute income, lower taxes imply increased inequality but also connote a privatizing or individualizing of societal risks and opportunities. Even given obvious societal inefficiencies. as, for example, in the U.S. health care system, neo-liberals prefer private to public expenditures (Drache and Sullivan, 1999). Wilkinson neatly captures the essence of neo-liberalism in the notion of a "cash and keys" economy (Wilkinson, 1996, p. 266):

> Increasingly we live in what might be called a "cash and keys" society. Whenever we leave the confines of our own homes we face the world with the two perfect symbols of the nature of social relations on the street. Cash equips us to take part in transactions mediated by the market, while keys protect our private gains from each other's envy and greed. Although we are wholly dependent on one another for our livelihoods, this interdependence is turned from being a social process into a process by which we fend for ourselves in an attempt to wrest a living from an asocial environment. Instead of being people with whom we have bonds and share common interests, others become rivals, competitors for jobs, for houses, for space, seats on the bus, parking places.

In light of this quote, it is interesting that income inequality and social trust have been found to be highly related to homicide and violent crimes (Wilkinson, Kawachi, and Kennedy, 1998), as well as to a whole range of other social indicators ranging from library books per capita to high school graduation rates (Lynch et al., 1998).

The absence of any concept of the social in neo-liberalism is related to neo-liberal views which imply the universalizing of market characteristics to all areas of human existence. Even the self comes to be viewed in terms of its market use. In an enterprise culture, the self is seen in terms of its usefulness on the market as an instrument for economic advancement. Social development or even social capital becomes individual human capital. The importance of those aspects of social capital, aspects of the social environment which benefit everyone, are downplayed or ignored (Coleman, 1988; Evans, 1996; Heller, 1996). Society is thus reduced to a collection of individuals in which the whole is viewed simply as the sum of the individual voluntary actions—social structure disappears.

Privatization and the lack of (noncontractual) connections amongst citizens implies a generalized increase in skepticism or distrust towards one's fellows. If everyone is legitimately seeking their own economic self-interest, as neo-liberalism implies, then there is reason for widespread suspicion of the motives and intentions of others rather than trust. There might be an increasing emphasis on self-aggrandizement at the expense of collective goals, an increasing contempt for public institutions and a lack of support for those organizations through which collective notions are expressed, maintained or reproduced.

Furthermore, since markets are efficient (and just) allocators of rewards, economic or "social" problems are attributed to individual failings. If markets give people what they deserve, there is likely to be an increase in individual blame and an inclination to punish rather than help others. Thus recipients of social welfare measures are "welfare bums." As Sennett and Cobb indicate, there are many relatively invisible "injuries of class" (Sennet and Cobb, 1973).

While it has been asserted that neo-liberalism produces a lowered sense of community, it might also be argued that the rise of neo-liberalism is itself a signifier of the decline of more widespread feelings of social solidarity. The political rise of neo-liberalism is freighted with a more individualistic view of society and perhaps itself reflects a decline in the notion that we are all in the same boat. Not only do neo-liberal policies undermine the social infrastructure underlying social cohesion, but neo-liberal movements themselves are partial causes of the decline of a sense of social cohesion.

Thus the proposition that *the more market-oriented the society, the higher the social fragmentation and the lower the social cohesion and trust.*

NEO-LIBERALISM, INCOME INEQUALITY AND SOCIAL COHESION/TRUST

Bringing the two major areas together leads to our general hypothesis that neo-liberalism produces *both* higher levels of inequality *and* lower levels of social cohesion (see Muntaner and Lynch, 1999). Rather than an inequality–social cohesion–health status sequence, neo-liberalism produces both inequality and social fragmentation, which may, if Wilkinson and others are right, have negative consequences in lowered health status.

I have argued that a focus on the relationship between neo-liberalism, income inequality, and health leads to a somewhat different understanding of income inequality and health relationships than previously discussed. The emphasis on neo-liberalism as a political movement and as a signal of attacks on the power of the working class to negotiate within the market or on the welfare state generally is supported by recent examinations of globalization, neo-liberalism, inequality and the welfare state by Navarro (1998, 1999a, 1999b) and by analyses of trends in income inequality and the redistributive effects of the welfare state (Kenworthy, 1998). Moreover, it might be argued that social cohesion and the related concept of social capital themselves have dual meanings. On the one hand, some view social capital as "social infrastructure," and others see it more in terms of social networks or trust, its area of greatest overlap with the concept of social cohesion. Even so, much of the discussion about social cohesion seems to measure its effects rather than the actual existence of social networks. That is, "trust" is an assumed consequence of social networks rather than a measure of the extensiveness of social networks. The question arises whether at least some attention should be paid to the social infrastructural arrangements as embedded in the welfare state, which might underlie income inequality–life expectancy relationships. In this light, the explosion of interest in social cohesion seems to again signal attention to the mechanisms of income inequality rather than to its causes. There does seem a contradiction between an increasing emphasis on social capital and social cohesion under regimes which are actually undermining these processes.

DISCUSSION

After putting forward the proposition that neo-liberalism is a major contextual factor regarding II-SES-HS relationships, I briefly noted some objections to, or modifications of, these arguments before discussing possible underlying causal mechanisms.

First, there might be an efficiency-equity trade-off—that in fact it is prosperity rather than lowered inequality that is the most highly related to improved health status and that market societies are associated with higher levels of wealth production than others. Prosperity trumps equality. Certainly, there is evidence that increased wealth production is associated with improved health (see Wilkinson, 1996, 1997a, 1997b). That is, as noted by Wilkinson and others, below a particular level of GNP per capita (around U.S.$5,000), GNP rather than income inequalities seems to be the major determinant of health status amongst nations. However, contra the prosperity argument, over this level there is little or no relationship between per capita GNP and health status amongst nations. Again, as noted, some less developed countries have much better health statistics than others—many of these seem to have a more equal social infrastructure than the others. Moreover, there are as many suggestions that income equality facilitates economic growth as there are that it harms economic growth.

In the popular literature generally, there has been an unwarranted tendency to equate economic development with human well-being. In fact, in the advanced capitalist countries, national wealth seems to have relatively little to do with national well-being. Broad indicators of social well-being show considerable divergence from purely economic indicators. Interestingly, there are some data that indicate that during the welfare state era, indices of well-being more or less tracked indices of per capita GNP. With the decline of the welfare state, these indices of social well-being began to markedly decline as compared to purely economic indices (Brink and Zeesman, 1997). The economy, after all, is presumably only the means to an end and not an end in itself.

There is, however, still some debate about the relationship between wealth, inequality, and health, even in Wilkinson's account. That is, Wilkinson notes (1996) that there has been a general increase in levels of health status over the past decades in the developed countries despite variations in the degree of inequality over that time. Wilkinson thus is describing fluctuations about a baseline rather than the baseline increases themselves. Higher inequality is thus associated with relative decreases in the trend towards greater longevity. Wilkinson attributes the secular increase itself to improvements in the quality of life which are somehow related to higher income levels. The secular rise of e.g., longevity, in Wilkinson's account, however, does deserve further consideration even though it might be argued that long-term inequality might eventually produce decreases in health status.

A second objection to the neo-liberalism–health status/social cohesion proposition might be that there is no alternative to neo-liberal policies. That in fact these are simply outcomes of increased global competition over which no single nation or political regime has much control. The change from nationally based monopoly to global capitalism ensures that whether we like it or not, neo-liberal policies are our only choice. That this is not the case, however, is indicated by the differences in economic policy and in income inequality and health that exist amongst the developed nations and even amongst particular areas within nations. There are local, national and international examples of more or less successful resistance to neo-liberal policies, one of the most recent and most prominent being opposition to the Multilateral Agreement on Investment. There are in fact choices to be made. Even so, one might agree that the spread of neo-liberalism on a world-wide basis has somewhat constrained national differences and that alternatives to neo-liberal perspectives other than simply a defense of the remnants of the KWS are not widely debated.

The issue of the inevitability of market-oriented policies does bring up the distinction between neo-liberal tenets, political rhetoric and reality. The principles or general philosophy of neo-liberalism are not always, or perhaps never, actually put into practice. We still have, some might claim, insufficient markets rather than an excess of these. Furthermore, some would contend that neo-liberal political regimes have not, for example, actually reduced the power of the state. The state may have retained a role, as exemplified by increased general state expenditures within countries having neo-liberal governments. Certainly, a number of neo-liberal regimes have, despite their emphasis on individual "liberty," shown a good deal of evidence of centralizing or authoritarian tendencies. Strong (authoritarian) state policies are viewed as necessary to "break" opposition to the restructuring of society, but as noted, these are not state collective policies but policies, often punitive, which are aimed at supporting or enforcing markets.

It might be argued that under neo-liberalism, the welfare state has not disappeared but has simply changed its form. Some authors contend that we now have not a directly involved state but the "regulative state" (Ruggie, 1996). In the new globalizing era, states do not carry out actions themselves but simply regulate private agencies in civil society to do so. Whatever the ultimate merits of such an argument, it is clear that under neo-liberal regimes, entitlements have been reduced or undermined, not simply structured in a different way.

An important question is how to begin to understand the mechanisms underlying the rise of neo-liberalism and how this might influence our understanding of rising SES inequalities. While there is not the space here to fully describe a possible sequence, Ross and Trachte (1990) have pointed to one explanatory pathway through their analysis of the change from monopoly to global capitalism. Extending their argument to the welfare state and to neo-liberalism permits a provisional explanation of increasing SES inequalities in class terms (for a more extended discussion, see Coburn, 1999, 2003, and compare Muntaner and Lynch, 1999).

Ross and Trachte (1990) claim that the globalization of capital has created a new balance of power in which the "relative autonomy of the state" prevalent under nationally based monopoly capitalism has declined. Under monopoly capital, the working class had gained in power in confrontation with a business class divided between its monopoly and competitive fractions. The increasing globalization of financial and industrial capital gave business great political power in its interactions with national, regional and local authorities. The state, which monopoly capitalism had attained a relative autonomy because of the more equal balance of class power between capital and labor and because of the divisions within capital, in the new global phase is more directly shaped and constrained by business interests (see Navarro, 1998, 1999a, 1999b).

Global competition and the mobility of capital are real forces but are also employed rhetorically by the New Right to capture the ideological and political agenda (Navarro, 1999a, 1999b). Ross and Trachte's argument (1990) is that economic globalization brings a new phase of capitalism which produced dramatic changes in the "balance of class power." The "legitimation" as opposed to the "accumulation" functions of the state became largely irrelevant in the face of the escape of corporations from national control. Business power increased, and state autonomy decreased. The consequence is the overpowering dominance of market doctrines and policies and, as I assert, increased inequality.

The model which emerges based on this argument is thus that economic globalization is accompanied by and produces changes in the balance of class power. The decline of working class power in the face of a resurgent business class is marked by the domination of neo-liberal ideology and policies, by attacks on the welfare state, and by a dominance of employer interests in the market. The decline of the power of workers to bargain for benefits within markets (Esping-Andersen, 1999) or to politically force decommodification through state welfare measures produces higher income inequality and lowered social cohesion and, directly and indirectly, lowered health status. International differences in health status can thus be traced to different national class structures, national institutions and different national degrees of "marketization" within common international pressures (Esping-Andersen, 1999; Gough, 1978, 1979).

The argument presented here emphasizes a unique relationship amongst neoliberalism, income inequality, social fragmentation, and lower health status. It also raises issues about the generally unanalyzed contextual conditions of various hypotheses relating income inequality to health status between and within countries. Hopefully, it will help to draw back into discussion broader social, political and economic factors which to date have been largely ignored in the II-SES-HS literature. Inequality is not a necessary condition produced by extrahuman forces. Degrees of inequality are clearly influenced by international, national and local political policies, which are amenable to change. We can either ignore these processes or seek to understand and begin to change them.

References

Amick, B. C., III, and others (eds.). *Society and Health.* New York: Oxford University Press, 1995.

Atkinson, A. B. *Incomes and the Welfare State: Essays on Britain and Europe.* Cambridge: Cambridge University Press, 1995.

Bartley, M., Blane, D., and Davey Smith, G. "Introduction: Beyond the Black Report." *Sociology of Health and Illness,* 1998, *20,* 563–577.

Bartley, M., Blane, D., and Montgomery, S. "Socioeconomic Determinants of Health: Health and the Life Course: Why Safety Nets Matter." *British Medical Journal,* 1997, *314,* 1194–1196.

Bhaskar, R. *A Realist Theory of Science.* Leeds, England: Leeds Books, 1975.

Bhaskar, R. *Reclaiming Reality.* London: Verso, 1989.

Blane, D., Brunner, E., and Wilkinson, R. G. (eds.). *Health and Social Organization: Toward a Health Policy for the 21st Century.* London: Routledge, 1996.

Brink, S., and Zeesman. A. *Measuring Social Well-Being: An Index of Social Health for Canada.* Research Paper Series, no. R-97-9E. Hull: Applied Research Branch, Strategic Policy, Human Resources Development Canada, 1997.

Coburn, D. "Phases of Capitalism, Welfare States, Medical Dominance and Health Care in Ontario." *International Journal of Health Services,* 1999, *29,* 833–851.

Coburn, D. "Beyond the Income Inequality Hypothesis: Neo-Liberalism, the Welfare State and Health." *Social Science and Medicine,* 2003 (forthcoming).

Coleman, J. S. "Social Capital in the Creation of Human Capital." *American Journal of Sociology,* 1988, *94*(suppl.), S95–S120.

Daly, M., and others. "Macro-to-Micro Links in the Relation Between Income Inequality and Mortality." *Milbank Quarterly,* 1998, *76,* 315–402.

Davey Smith, G. "Income Inequality and Mortality—Why Are They Related? Income Inequality Goes Hand in Hand with Underinvestment in Human-Resources." *British Medical Journal,* 1996, *312,* 987–989.

Drache, D., and Sullivan, T. (eds.). *Health Reform: Public Success, Private Failure.* London: Routledge, 1999.

Esping-Andersen, G. *The Three Worlds of Welfare Capitalism.* Princeton, N.J.: Princeton University Press, 1990.

Esping-Andersen, G. *Social Foundations of Postindustrial Economies.* Oxford: Oxford University Press, 1999.

Evans, P. "Government Action, Social Capital, and Development: Reviewing the Evidence on Synergy." *World Development,* 1996, *24,* 1119–1132.

Evans, R. G., Barer, M. L., and Marmor, T. R. (eds.). *Why Are Some People Healthy and Others Not? The Determinants of Health of Populations.* Hawthorne, N.Y.: Aldine de Gruyter, 1994.

Gottschalk, P., and Smeeding, T. M. "Cross-National Comparisons of Earnings and Income Inequality." *Journal of Economic Literature,* 1997, *35,* 633–687.

Gottschalk, P., and Smeeding. T. M. "Empirical Evidence on Income Inequality in Industrialized Countries." In A. B. Atkinson and F. Bourgignon (eds.), *The Handbook of Income Distribution.* New York: North-Holland, 2000.

Gough, I. "Theories of the Welfare State: A Critique." *International Journal of Health Services,* 1978, *8,* 27–40.

Gough, L. *The Political Economy of the Welfare State.* London: Macmillan, 1979.

Gravelle, H. "How Much of the Relation Between Population Mortality and Unequal Distribution of Income Is a Statistical Artifact?" *British Medical Journal,* 1998, *316,* 382–385.

Heller, P. "Social Capital as a Product of Class Mobilization and State Intervention: Industrial Workers in Kerala, India." *World Development,* 1996, *24,* 1055–1071.

Hendrickson, M. W. (ed.). *The Morality of Capitalism.* (2nd ed.) New York: Foundation for Economic Education, 1996.

Judge, K. "Income Distribution and Life Expectancy: A Critical Appraisal." *British Medical Journal,* 1995, *311,* 1282–1285.

Judge, K. "Income and Mortality in the United States. Letter in Response to Kaplan et al." *British Medical Journal* 1996, *313,* 1206.

Kaplan, G. A., and others. "Inequality in Income and Mortality in the United States: Analysis of Mortality and Potential Pathways." *British Medical Journal,* 1996, *312,* 999–1003.

Kawachi, I., and Kennedy, B. P. "Socioeconomic Determinants of Health: Health and Social Cohesion: Why Care About Income Inequality?" *British Medical Journal,* 1997, *314,* 1037.

Kawachi, I., and others. "Social Capital, Income Inequality, and Mortality." *American Journal of Public Health,* 1997, *87,* 1491–1499.

Kennedy, B. P., Kawachi, I., and Prothrow-Stith, D. "Income Distribution and Mortality: Cross Sectional Ecological Study of the Robin Hood Index in the United States." *British Medical Journal,* 1996, *312,* 1004–1007.

Kenworthy, L. "Do Social-Welfare Policies Reduce Poverty? A Cross-National Assessment." *Social Forces,* 1998, *77,* 1119–1139.

Korpi, W. "Power Politics and State Autonomy in the Development of Social Citizenship: Social Rights During Sickness in Eighteen OECD Countries Since 1930." *American Sociological Review,* 1989, *54,* 309–328.

Korpi, W., and Palme, J. "The Paradox of Redistribution and Strategies of Equality: Welfare State Institutions, Inequality and Poverty in the Western Countries." Luxembourg Income Study, Working Paper no. 174. 1998. [http://www.lisproject.org/publications/liswps/174.pdf].

Luxembourg Income Study. 2003. [http://www.lisproject.org].

Lynch, J. W., and others. "Income Inequality and Mortality in Metropolitan Areas of the United States." *American Journal of Public Health,* 1998, *88,* 1074–1080.

Macpherson, C. B. *The Political Theory of Possessive Individualism.* Oxford: Oxford University Press, 1964.

McMurtry, J. *Unequal Freedoms: The Global Market as an Ethical System.* Toronto: Garamond Press, 1998.

Mishra, R. *The Welfare State in Capitalist Society.* Toronto: University of Toronto Press, 1990.

Muntaner, C., and Lynch, J. W. "Income Inequality, Social Cohesion, and Class Relations: A Critique of Wilkinson's Neo-Durkheimian Research Program." *International Journal of Health Services,* 1999, *29,* 59–81.

Navarro, V. "Neoliberalism, 'Globalization,' Unemployment Inequalities and the Welfare State." *International Journal of Health Services,* 1998, *28,* 607–682.

Navarro, V. "Health and Equity in the World in the Era of 'Globalization.'" *International Journal of Health Services,* 1999a, *29,* 215–226.

Navarro, V. "The Political Economy of the Welfare State in Developed Capitalist Countries." *International Journal of Health Services,* 1999b, *29,* 1–50.

O'Connor, J., and Olsen, G. M. (eds.). *Power Resources Theory and the Welfare State: A Critical Approach.* Toronto: University of Toronto Press, 1998.

Poland, B., and others. "Wealth, Equity and Health Care: A Critique of a 'Population Health' Perspective on the Determinants of Health." *Social Science and Medicine,* 1998, *46,* 785–798.

Popay, J., and others. "Theorizing Inequalities in Health: The Place of Lay Knowledge." *Sociology of Health and Illness*, 1999, *20*, 619–644.

Putnam, R. *Making Democracy Work: Civic Traditions in Modern Italy.* Princeton, N.J.: Princeton University Press, 1993

Quandango, J. "Theories of the Welfare State." *Annual Review of Sociology*, 1987, *13*, 109–128.

Raphael, D. "Health Effects of Economic Inequality." In Armstrong, P., Armstrong, H., and Coburn, D. (eds.) *Unhealthy Societies: The Political Economy of Health and Health Care in Canada.* Toronto: Oxford University Press, 1999.

Robertson, A. "Shifting Discourses in Health in Canada: From Health Promotion to Population Health." *Health Promotion International*, 1998, *13*, 155–166.

Ross, R.J.S., and Trachte, K. C. *Global Capitalism: The New Leviathan.* Albany: State University of New York Press, 1990.

Ruggie, M. *Realignments in the Welfare State: Health Policy in the United States, Britain, and Canada.* New York: Columbia University Press, 1996.

Sayer, A. *Method in Social Science: A Realist Approach.* (2nd ed.) London: Routledge, 1992.

Scambler, G., and Higgs, P. "Stratification, Class, and Health: Class Relations and Health Inequalities in High Modernity." *Sociology*, 1999, *33*, 275–296.

Sennett, R., and Cobb, J., 1973. *The Hidden Injuries of Class.* Knopf, New York.

Smeeding, T. M. "American Income Inequality in a Cross-National Perspective: Why Are We So Different?" Luxembourg Income Study, Working Paper no. 157. 1997. [http://www.lisproject.org/publications/liswps/157.pdf].

Stubbs, R., and Underhill, G.R.D. (eds.). *Political Economy and the Changing Global Order.* Toronto: McClelland & Stewart, 1994.

Syme, S. L. "Social and Economic Disparities in Health: Thoughts About Intervention." *Milbank Quarterly*, 1998, *76*, 492–505.

Teeple, G. *Globalization and the Decline of Social Reform.* Toronto: Garamond Press, 1995.

Wilkinson, R. G. *Unhealthy Societies: The Afflictions of Inequality.* New York: Routledge, 1996.

Wilkinson, R. G. "Comment: Income Inequality and Social Cohesion." *American Journal of Public Health*, 1997a, *89*, 1504–1506.

Wilkinson, R. G. "Socio-Economic Determinants of Health: Health Inequalities—Relative or Absolute Material Standards?" *British Medical Journal*, 1997b, *314*, 591–595.

Wilkinson, R. G., Kawachi, I., and Kennedy, B. P. "Mortality, the Social Environment, Crime and Violence." *Sociology of Health and Illness*, 1998, *20*, 578–597.

CHAPTER FIFTEEN

Income Inequality and Health

Expanding the Debate

John W. Lynch

David Coburn's paper on the role of neo-liberalism in influencing both income inequality and social cohesion, reprinted in this volume as Chapter Fourteen, is a welcome addition to the debate over interpretations of the link between income inequality and health. Coburn asked us to expand the terms of reference for this debate. He argued that a more complete understanding of the income inequality–health link would evolve by including neo-liberalism, global capitalism, market domination, class structure and welfare-state policies as central elements of the health inequalities discourse. Income inequality cannot be the starting "social fact" of a theory of health inequalities—a central point that Carles Muntaner and I made in our first critique of Wilkinson's "social cohesion" model of inequalities in health (Muntaner and Lynch, 1999). The extent of unequal income distribution comes from somewhere—it is the product of a complex mix of country and region-specific background and historical factors. Coburn's lesson in political-economic science has served to highlight some of the concepts with which to discuss this important background to income inequality, and helps to explain the unprecedented increases in inequality witnessed over the last 20 years, in political-economic terms. It is no accident that the Nordic countries have lower income inequality than Britain, Australia or the United States (Gottschalk and Smeeding, 1997), and the role that welfare-state policies have played in blunting market-driven income inequality is central to any interpretation of the link between income inequality and health.

THREE INTERPRETATIONS OF ASSOCIATIONS BETWEEN INCOME INEQUALITY AND HEALTH

In Chapter Seven we discussed three interpretations of the association between income inequality and health—the individual income, the psychosocial environment, and the neo-material. Under a neo-material interpretation, the effect of income inequality on health reflects both lack of resources held by individuals, and systematic under-investments across a wide range of community infrastructure (Kaplan, Pamuk, Lynch, Cohen and Balfour, 1996; Davey Smith, 1996; Davey Smith and Egger, 1996; Lynch and Kaplan, 1997; Lynch et al., 1998) These aspects of living conditions function to reduce health-damaging exposures and increase health-protective resources at the individual and community level. From this perspective, we argued that income inequality is but one, albeit important, manifestation of a set of background historical, political, cultural and economic factors. These background factors not only produce a particular pattern of income distribution, but also create a context of community infrastructure through policies that affect education, public health services, transportation, occupational health regulations, availability of healthy food, zoning laws, pollution, housing, etc. It is understanding patterns of strategic public and private investments in this matrix of what we called "neo-material living conditions" that is likely to provide the most complete interpretation of links between income inequality and health. While we focussed on interpretations of the mechanisms that may link income inequality to health, this neo-material approach is entirely consistent with, and extends Coburn's analysis of what he calls the "affinity between neo-liberal doctrines, inequality, and social fragmentation" (Chapter Fourteen).

Figure 15.1 attempts to show relationships between the basic elements of the neo-material approach to understanding health inequalities at the individual and population levels. In this case, I have included Coburn's contribution of neo-liberalism as an important specific element of the background factors that increase income inequality and decrease social cohesion. Coburn cogently argued that neo-liberalism increases income inequality through its reliance on less regulated labour and capital markets, and through reductions and privatization of welfare-state infrastructure (Muntaner and Lynch, 1999; Muntaner, Lynch and Oates, 1999). Simultaneously, the social and philosophical tenets of neo-liberalism reflect individualist rather than collectivist sentiments, and so foster a climate of economic self-interest by encouraging the view that those outside immediate family and friends should perhaps be viewed with some skepticism and distrust, as competitors for scarce resources. Thus, neo-liberalism influences income inequality, trust, reciprocity and social cohesion.

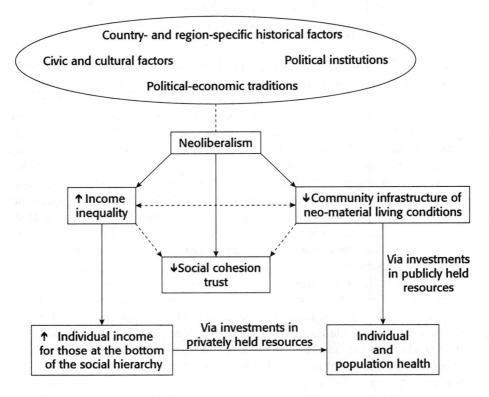

Figure 15.1. A Neo-material Interpretation of Income Inequality and Health.

Figure 15.1 also suggests that there is no necessary observable association between income inequality and health at the aggregate level. Associations between geographic variations in health and income inequality may depend upon the nature and distribution of community infrastructure, characterized by neo-material living conditions. However, the extent of income inequality will always be indirectly associated with variations in health at the individual level through its role in determining individual income and the health-related resources that income can buy. This idea is consistent with the large number of studies in different countries and time periods that have shown an association between low income and poor health at the individual level (Backlund, Sorlie and Johnson, 1996; Davey Smith, Neaton, Wentworth, Stamler and Stamler, 1996; Lynch, Kaplan, Cohen, Tuomilehto and Salonen, 1996; Ecob and Davey Smith, 1999).

The neo-material interpretation of the income inequality–health link can be contrasted with the psychosocial environment approach that has focussed on the role of shame, trust, social cohesion, and more recently social capital, as key determinants of health inequalities (Wilkinson, 1996, 1997, 1999; Kawachi, Kennedy, Lochner and Prothrow-Stith, 1997). The psychosocial environment interpretation views health inequalities as the result of perceptions of relative income. These perceptions produce negative emotions like shame and distrust that are translated into poorer health at the individual level through psycho-neuro-endocrine mechanisms, and health-damaging behaviours. Simultaneously, perceptions of relative social position and the negative emotions they foster are translated into anti-social behavior, reduced civic participation, and less social cohesion within the community. Thus, perceptions of social status have both negative biological consequences for individuals, and negative social consequences for how individuals interact, and serve as the conceptual link between individual and social pathology. Under this view, it is social rank per se that produces poorer individual and population health.

Results of social hierarchy experiments in monkeys and baboons have been used as evidence for the importance of social rank in generating health inequalities (Wilkinson, 1996). However, recent evidence on the potentially negative health consequences of rank is presenting a more complicated picture, in which the health effects of low social rank are contingent upon the availability of material resources that structure living conditions in those animal communities (Kaplan and Manuck, 1999). In fact, Sapolsky has proclaimed that "a prime revisionist emphasis of this chapter has been how *little,* in fact, rank *per se* predicts any of those (health-related) endpoints. Instead, it seems virtually meaningless to think about the physiological correlates of rank outside the context of a number of other modifiers—the sort of society in which the rank occurs" (emphasis in the original) (Sapolsky, 1999, p. 39). Moreover, there is some evidence that perceptions of relative disadvantage may not always have negative effects on psychological functioning (Diener, Sandvik, Seidlitz and Diener, 1993).

I am not arguing that greater income inequality has no detrimental psychosocial consequences or that these consequences are not important issues for public health in their own right (Muntaner, Eaton and Diala, 1999). But as Amartya Sen pointed out in his award speech for the 1998 Nobel Prize in economics, "Mental reactions, the mainstay of classical utility, can be a very defective basis for the analysis of deprivation. Thus, in understanding poverty and inequality, there is a strong case for looking at real deprivation and not merely at mental reactions to that deprivation" (Sen, 1999, p. 363). Although his comments were related to situations of gender inequality where some women reported less deprivation and discrimination than was obviously present, the fundamental point holds—that there are real-world living conditions that should be the basis for understanding and analyzing inequality. At one level, the psychosocial and neo-material interpretations of health inequalities are not necessarily in conflict if the psychosocial consequences of differences in neo-material living conditions are understood as precisely that—consequences of contextualized real-world living conditions. The idea that individuals and groups "embody" their social class position is an important lens through which to understand health inequalities (Bourdieu, 1984; Krieger, 1999; Lynch and others, 2000). It follows from this idea, that there are measurable individual-level psychological and biological responses to neo-material living conditions, expressed in such things as hostility, depression, sense of control, immune function, haemostatic factors or stress hormones—all of which have been shown to be patterned by socioeconomic position (Brunner, 1997; Lynch, Kaplan and Salonen, 1997). However, the bottom-line for public health is that it seems hard to understand how a theory of health inequalities built on a foundation of perceptions of social rank, shame, distrust, hostility and informal social support can form the basis for an effective policy agenda to improve overall levels of population health and to reduce health inequalities.

SOCIAL CONNECTEDNESS

In the same way that it is important to recognize the potentially negative psychosocial and biological consequences of social inequality in individuals, it is also important to recognize that there are aspects of the "social connectedness" of groups that may be important for population health and health inequalities. My use of the term "social connectedness" is deliberately broad and can be understood both as interpersonal, informal-horizontal links, and as formal-vertical links that characterize how individuals and groups are "connected" to institutional, legal, political and economic structures. In the context of debates about social capital, authors like Woolcock (1998) and Szreter (1999) have argued for the importance of these institutional links in terms of sustainable economic development and of considering both horizontal "bonding" and vertical "bridging" social connections (Granovetter, 1973). Indeed, a recognition of the public health importance of connections among individuals is also an emerging principle in epidemiologic science, especially in regard to infectious disease transmission (Koopman and Lynch, 1999), although the salience of these different sorts of social connections may vary according to the specific pathobiological processes involved.

The issue for public health is to understand what sorts of connections across individuals and groups are likely to have the most impact on levels of population health and health inequalities. Some of the most profound and deplorable inequalities in health in the United States exist between the African-American and white communities (National Center for Health Statistics, 1998). The same is true in countries like Australia where life expectancy for the indigenous Koori population is 13 years less for women and 14 years lower for men in the state of Victoria (Voss, 1999). Are the poorer health profiles of these disadvantaged communities better understood in terms of their levels of trust, reciprocity, hostility and quality of informal social relations, or through understanding the institutional "social connectedness" of these disadvantaged groups in terms of their political, economic, legal and other formal-vertical connections? Is the public health question better framed in terms of bonding or bridging social ties? The role of informal social networks should not be discounted, but their importance for public health and health inequalities needs to be placed in the broader context of institutional structures that place limits on the deployment of health-enhancing resources, knowledge and power across those informal networks.

CONCLUSION

Any theory of population health and health inequalities has to deal with the fact that the greatest absolute burden of poor health is borne at the bottom of the social hierarchy (see Figure 15.2). The fact that health differences can be observed between the top of the social hierarchy and the next level down, is surely important, but may be an incomplete basis for understanding why the largest burden of excess deaths occurs at the bottom of the social hierarchy.

In this light, it may be useful for health inequalities researchers to explore the institutional "social connectedness" of socially marginalized groups. It is likely that overall levels of population health and the extent of health inequalities may be driven by how these groups, marginalized by their educational, economic, racial/ethnic or gender status, have access to and control over the society's health-related resources, and how this access and control have been developed and sustained over successive generations. In the United States, the most marginalized social groups have no health care, a pitifully low minimum wage, underfunded schools, poor transportation links between where they live and where they work, low levels of neighborhood resources and poor housing. The most marginalized groups in countries like Sweden or Norway experience a different set of neo-material living conditions. It is also true that absolute health inequalities in these countries are smaller and average levels of population health higher than in the United States (Kunst, Groenhof and Mackenbach, 1998).

Perhaps the most useful approaches to understanding health inequalities will be built around a combination of understanding the influence of private and community neo-material living conditions, the accumulation of these socially patterned conditions over the lifecourse, and the effects of public policies that influence the degree of "social connectedness" of marginalized groups. The neo-material interpretation of health inequalities is an explicit recognition that political–economic processes, discussed by Coburn in terms of neo-liberalism,

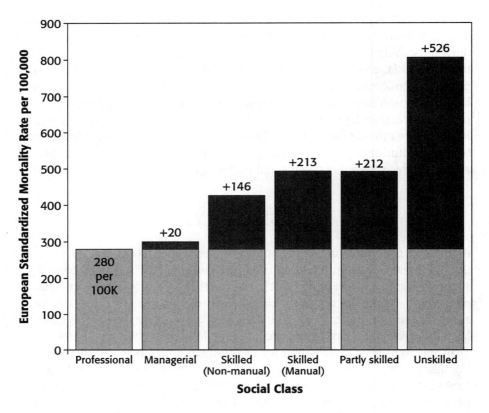

Figure 15.2 Excess Mortality per 100,000 by Social Class Among Men Aged 20–64 Years, England and Wales, 1991–1993.

Source: Adapted from Acheson and others, 1998.

generate income inequality, influence individual economic resources, and also impact community resources such as schooling, health care, social welfare, and working conditions. It is strategic investments in aspects of these neo-material living conditions via more equitable distribution of publicly and privately held health-related resources that are likely to have the most impact on improving overall population health and reducing health inequalities in the 21st century.

References

Acheson, D., and others. *Independent Inquiry into Inequalities in Health.* London: Stationery Office, 1998.

Backlund, E., Sorlie, P. D., and Johnson, N. J. "The Shape of the Relationship Between Income and Mortality in the United States: Evidence from the National Longitudinal Mortality Study." *Annals of Epidemiology,* 1996, *6,* 1–9.

Bourdieu, P. *Distinction: A Social Critique of the Judgment of Taste.* Cambridge, Mass.: Harvard University Press, 1984.

Brunner, E. "Stress and the Biology of Inequality." *British Medical Journal,* 1997, *314,* 1472–1476.

Coburn, D. "Income Inequality, Social Cohesion and the Health Status of Populations: The Role of Neo-Liberalism." *Social Science and Medicine,* 2000, *51,* 139–150.

Davey Smith, G. "Income Inequality and Mortality: Why Are They Related? Income Inequality Goes Hand in Hand with Underinvestment in Human Resources." *British Medical Journal,* 1996, *312,* 987–988.

Davey Smith, G., and Egger, M. "Commentary: Understanding It All—Health, Meta-Theories and Mortality Trends." *British Medical Journal,* 1996, *313,* 1584–1585.

Davey, Smith G., and others. "Socioeconomic Differentials in Mortality Risk Among Men Screened for the Multiple Risk Factor Intervention Trial: 1. White Men." *American Journal of Public Health,* 1996, *86,* 486–496.

Diener, E., and others. "The Relationship Between Income and Subjective Well-Being: Relative or Absolute?" *Social Indicators Research,* 1993, *28,* 195–223.

Ecob, R., and Davey Smith, G. "Income and Health: What Is the Nature of the Relationship?" *Social Science and Medicine,* 1999, *48,* 693–705.

Gottschalk, P., and Smeeding, T. M. "Cross-National Comparisons of Earnings and Income Inequality." *Journal of Economic Literature,* 1997, *35,* 633–686.

Granovetter, M. "The Strength of Weak Ties." *American Journal of Sociology,* 1973, *78,* 1360–1380.

Kaplan, G. A., and others. "Inequality in Income and Mortality in the United States: Analysis of Mortality and Potential Pathways." *British Medical Journal,* 1996, *312,* 999–1003.

Kaplan, J. R., and Manuck, S. B. "Status, Stress, and Atherosclerosis: The Role of Environment and Individual Behavior." *Annals of the New York Academy of Sciences,* 1999, *896,* 145–161.

Kawachi, I., and others. "Social Capital, Income Inequality, and Mortality." *American Journal of Public Health,* 1997, *87,* 1491–1499.

Koopman, J. S., and Lynch, J. W. "Individual Causal Models and Population Systems Models in Epidemiology." *American Journal of Public Health,* 1999, *89,* 1170–1175.

Krieger, N. "Embodying Inequality: A Review of Concepts, Measures, and Methods for Studying Health Consequences of Discrimination." *International Journal of Health Services,* 1999, *29,* 295–352.

Kunst, A. E., Groenhof, F., and Mackenbach, J. P. "Mortality by Occupational Class Among Men 30–64 Years in 11 European Countries. EU Working Group on Socio-Economic Inequalities in Health." *Social Science and Medicine,* 1998, *46,* 1459–1476.

Lynch, J. W., and Kaplan, G. A. "Understanding How Inequality in the Distribution of Income Affects Health." *Journal of Health Psychology,* 1997, *2,* 297–314.

Lynch, J. W., Kaplan, G. A., and Salonen, J. T. "Why Do Poor People Behave Poorly? Variations in Adult Health Behaviour and Psychosocial Characteristics, by Stage of the Socio-Economic Lifecourse." *Social Science and Medicine,* 1997, *44,* 809–820.

Lynch, J. W., and others. "Do Cardiovascular Risk Factors Explain the Relation Between Socioeconomic Status, Risk of All-Cause Mortality, Cardiovascular Mortality, and Acute Myocardial Infarction?" *American Journal of Epidemiology,* 1996, *144,* 934–942.

Lynch, J. W., and others. "Income Inequality and Mortality in Metropolitan Areas of the United States." *American Journal of Public Health,* 1998, *88,* 1074–1080.

Lynch, J. W., and others. "Social Capital—Is It a Good Investment Strategy for Public Health?" *Journal of Epidemiology and Community Health,* 2000, *54,* 404–408.

Muntaner, C., Eaton, W. W., and Diala, C. C. "Social Inequalities in Mental Health: A Review of Underlying Assumptions." *Health,* 1999, *4,* 82–106.

Muntaner, C., and Lynch, J. W. "Income Inequality and Social Cohesion Versus Class Relations: A Critique of Wilkinson's Neo-Durkheimian Research Program." *International Journal of Health Services,* 1999, *29,* 59–81.

Muntaner, C., Lynch, J. W., and Oates, G. "The Social Class Determinants of Income Inequality and Social Cohesion." *International Journal of Health Services,* 1999, *29,* 699–732.

National Center for Health Statistics. *Health, United States, 1998, with Socioeconomic Status and Health Chartbook.* Hyattsville, Md.: National Center for Health Statistics, 1998.

Sapolsky, R. M. "Hormonal Correlates of Personality and Social Contexts: From Non-Human to Human Primates." In C. Panter-Brick and C. M. Worthman, *Hormones, Health and Behaviour: A Socio-Ecological and Lifespan Perspective.* Cambridge: Cambridge University Press, 1999.

Sen, A. K. "The Possibility of Social Choice." *American Economic Review,* 1999, *89,* 349–378.

Szreter, S. "A New Political Economy for New Labour: The Importance of Social Capital." *Renewal,* 1999, *7,* 30–44.

Voss, T. *The Victoria Burden of Disease Study: Mortality.* Melbourne, Australia: Public Health and Development Division, Department of Human Services, 1999.

Wilkinson, R. G. *Unhealthy Societies: The Afflictions of Inequality.* New York: Routledge, 1996.

Wilkinson, R. G. "Socio-Economic Determinants of Health: Health Inequalities—Relative or Absolute Material Standards?" *British Medical Journal,* 1997, *314,* 591–595.

Wilkinson, R. G. "The Culture of Inequality." In I. Kawachi, B. P. Kennedy, and R. G. Wilkinson (eds.), *The Society and Population Health Reader: Income Inequality and Health.* New York: New Press, 1999.

Woolcock, M. "Social Capital and Economic Development: Toward a Theoretical Synthesis and Policy Framework." *Theory and Society,* 1998, *27,* 151–208.

CHAPTER SIXTEEN

Is Capitalism a Disease?

The Crisis in U.S. Public Health

Richard Levins

The scientific tradition of the West, of Europe and North America, has had its greatest success when it has dealt with what we have come to think of as the central questions of scientific inquiry: "What is this made of?" and "How does this work?" Over the centuries, we have developed more and more sophisticated ways of answering these questions. We can cut things open, slice them thin, stain them, and answer what they are made of. We have made great achievements in these relatively simple areas, but have had dramatic failures in attempts to deal with more complex systems. We see this especially when we ask questions about health. When we look at the changing patterns of health over the last century or so, we have both cause for celebration and for dismay. Human life expectancy has increased by perhaps thirty years since the beginning of the twentieth century, and the incidence of some of the classical deadly diseases has declined and almost disappeared. Smallpox presumably has been eradicated, leprosy is very rare, and polio has nearly vanished from most regions of the world. Scientific technologies have advanced to the point where we can give very sophisticated diagnoses, distinguishing between kinds of germs that are very similar to each other.

But the growing gap between rich and poor makes many technical advances irrelevant to most of the world's people. Public health authorities were caught by surprise by the emergence of new diseases and the reappearance of diseases believed to be eradicated. In the 1970s, it was common to hear that infectious disease as an area of research was dying. In principle, infection had been licked; the health problems of the future would be degenerative diseases, problems of aging and chronic diseases. We now know this was a monumental error. The public health establishment was caught short by the return of malaria, cholera, tuberculosis, dengue, and other classical diseases. But it was also surprised by the appearance of apparently new infectious diseases, the most threatening of which is AIDS, but also Legionnaire's disease, Ebola virus, toxic shock syndrome, multiple-drug-resistant tuberculosis, and many others. Not only was infectious disease not on the way out, but old diseases have come back with increased virulence and totally new ones have emerged.

How did this happen; why was public health caught by surprise? Why did the health professions assume that infectious disease would disappear, and why were they so wrong? In fact, infectious disease had been declining dramatically in Europe and North America for the last 150 years. One of the simplest kinds of predictions is that things will continue the way they have been going. Health professionals argued that infectious disease would disappear because we were inventing all kinds of new technologies for coping with them. We now can carry out diagnoses so rapidly that some diseases that might kill a person in two days can be identified in the laboratory soon enough to permit treatment. Instead of spending weeks culturing bacteria, we can use DNA to distinguish between pathogens that may have very similar symptoms. More important, we had developed a new arsenal of antimicrobial weapons, drugs, and vaccines, as well as pesticides to get rid of mosquitoes and ticks that are disease carriers. We came to understand that through mutation and natural selection, micro-organisms can present a recurring threat.

We assumed that whatever the microbial changes, the disease-causing mechanism would remain the same while we developed ever-newer weapons against it. It was, we believed, a war between us and the microbes in which we would have the upper hand because our weapons were growing stronger and ever more effective. Another cause for optimism—at least this was the argument put forth by the World Bank and the International Monetary Fund—was that economic development would eliminate poverty and produce affluence, making all the new technologies universally available. Finally, the demographers noted that while most infectious diseases are most deadly to children, we have an aging population, so the proportion of people likely to catch such illnesses will be smaller. One thing missing from this hypothesis was that one reason children are so vulnerable is that they have not developed the immunities that go along with exposure; older people have reduced susceptibility precisely because they have been exposed. But if there are fewer children, older people will have a lower level of immunity and will contract diseases at an older age. Indeed, some diseases, like mumps, are more serious in adults than they are in children.

So what was wrong with our epidemiological assumptions? We need to recognize that the historical mindset in medicine and related sciences was dangerously—and ideologically—limited. Nearly all who engaged in public health prediction took too narrow a view, both geographically and temporally. Typically, they looked only at a century or two instead of the whole sweep of human history. Had they looked at a wider time-frame, they would have recognized that diseases come and go when there are major changes in social relations, population, the kinds of food we eat, and land use. When we change our relations with nature, we also change epidemiology and the opportunities for infection.

THE PLAGUE IN EUROPE

Plague erupted in Europe for the first time in the sixth century during the decline of the Roman Empire under Justinian. Europe suffered from social disruption and declining production. The sanitary facilities of the great ancient cities were crumbling; under those circumstances, when plague was introduced it swept through the population with devastating effects. Plague reappeared in the fourteenth century during a developing crisis of feudalism, causing a population decline even before plague became widespread. The standard history of this plague occurrence is that sailors landing in ports along the Black Sea brought plague with them from Asia in 1338; it then spread westward and in a short time reached Rome, Paris, and London. In other words, plague spread because it had been introduced from elsewhere. But it seems more likely that plague had entered Europe many times before but really didn't take off. It only became successful when the population became more vulnerable, when the human ecosystem could not confront a disease spread by rats at a time when the social infrastructure that would have controlled rats had crumbled.

AN ECOLOGICAL PROPOSAL

When we at look at other diseases, we see that they rose and fell with historical change and circumstance. So instead of a doctrine of the epidemiological transition, which held that infectious disease would simply disappear as countries developed, we need to substitute an ecological proposal: that with any major change in the way of life of a population (such as population density, patterns of residence, or means of production), there will also be a change in our relations with pathogens, their reservoirs, and with the vectors of diseases. The new hemorrhagic fevers appearing in South America, Africa, and elsewhere almost all seem to be related to increased contact with rodents that humans don't normally meet, caused by the clearing of land for the production of grain in particular. Grain is also rodent food; rodents survive by eating seeds and grasses. When a forest is cleared and grain is planted, we also eliminate the coyotes, jaguars, snakes, and owls that eat rodents. The net result is an increase in rodent food and a reduction in rodent mortality. The rodent population grows. Now these disease-deliverers are social animals. They nest and build communities; when a new generation emerges, the young adults go out looking for homes elsewhere—often wandering into warehouses and people's homes, facilitating the transmission of diseases.

Another human activity, irrigation, is especially related to the breeding of snails, who transmit liver fluke disease, and mosquitoes, who spread malaria, dengue, and yellow fever. When irrigation proliferates, as it did, for example, after the construction of Egypt's Aswan Dam, habitats for mosquitoes were created. Rift Valley fever, which had occasionally erupted in Egypt, can now be found fulltime. The development of giant cities in the Third World has created new environments for the spread of dengue, transmitted by the same mosquito that transmits yellow fever (*Aedes aegypti*). It has adapted to life around the edges of cities. A poor competitor against other varieties of mosquito in the forest, these mosquitoes are able to breed in abandoned lots, puddles, water barrels, and old tires—in the special environment that we create in the giant cities in the tropics. Dengue and yellow fever are particularly threatening because of the growth of urbanization in the tropics with megacities like Bangkok, Rio de Janeiro, Mexico City, and others with populations of ten to twenty million. As human population grows, there are new opportunities for diseases. For instance, you need a few hundred thousand in a population before it can sustain measles. If there are fewer, measles can infect the entire population; those who survive will be resistant. But if there aren't enough new babies to maintain the disease, it will disappear and have to be reintroduced. But in a population of a quarter million people, there will be enough new babies who are not resistant that the disease can sustain itself in the population. Consider this: if we know there are diseases that require a quarter million people to be self-sustaining, what diseases will emerge in crowded populations of ten or twenty million? Clearly, as life conditions change, so do opportunities for disease.

Yet another kind of myopic thinking in the public health community arose from the fact that doctors are concerned with human diseases but have not paid much attention to diseases of wildlife or of domestic animals or plants. Had they done this, they would have had to confront the reality that all organisms carry diseases. Diseases come from the invasion of an organism by a parasite. When an infection takes place, it may or may not produce symptoms. But all organisms deal with parasites and, from the point of view of the parasite, invading an organism is a way of escaping from competition in the water or in the soil. For instance, the bacteria that causes Legionnaire's disease lives in water. It is found all over the world but is never very common because it is a poor competitor. It has very finicky dietary requirements, so normally humans don't encounter it. However, it has two things going for it. It can tolerate high temperatures and is resistant to chlorine. It withstands chlorine by hiding out inside an amoeba. In a convention center, hotel, or truck stop, water is both heated and chlorinated. And if it's a good hotel, we may find a showerhead that gives a fine spray of tiny droplets, perfect for carrying the bacteria into the furthest corners of your lungs. What we've done is create the ideal environment for Legionnaire's disease. The chlorine and the high temperature kill their competitors, the remains of which form a coating on the inside of the pipes that is marvelously rich in the food that the Legionnaire's bacterium loves.

If we look at other organisms, we see a constant jockeying for position between parasites and hosts. The more common a species is, the more attractive it is to new invasions by parasites. Humans are very common and thus offer wonderful opportunities for invasion. When we observe disease patterns, we see that cholera, for example, spread from the Eastern Hemisphere into the Americas, entering Peru and then traveling up to Central America. But a similar route was followed by a disease of orange trees, by viruses of beans and tomatoes, as well as by wildlife diseases. What we see, then, is a constant coevolution between pathogens and hosts across all animal and plant life rather than a situation unique to humans. Surely, we would have a much better understanding of potential dangers if we understood human illness from this perspective.

TRANSMISSION OF DISEASES

What kinds of insects spread viruses to people? Nearly all of them are mosquitoes or flies or belong to a second group, which includes ticks, fleas, and lice. These are the two main groups that overwhelmingly spread human virus diseases, even though there are hundreds of thousands of other kinds of insects. There are very few diseases spread by beetles, none that I know of by butterflies or dragonflies. Why? Are there circumstances under which they might become transmitters of diseases? Among plants, the major distributors of plant viruses belong to a totally different group of insects—aphids. However, both groups have similar mouths and subsist by sucking liquid from their hosts: the mosquito sucking blood, the aphid sucking sap. If you have ever sucked something through a straw, you know that after a while, a vacuum builds up and in order to be able to continue slurping the liquid, you have to be able to return liquid. Similarly, the salivary glands of mosquitoes and of aphids return liquid to their hosts when they take up the blood or the sap, and in that liquid you find the viruses. That's why when we study viruses, we look at the salivary glands of mosquitoes or of ticks or anything else. We can begin to encounter these generalizations when we step back from looking at the particular details of a given disease and try to get a broad picture. But this wasn't done.

THE FAILURE TO STUDY EVOLUTION AND SOCIETY

Another kind of scientific narrowness—really a self-imposed intellectual constriction—is the failure to study evolution. Evolution tells us immediately that organisms respond to the challenges of their environment. If the challenge is, for example, an antibiotic, organisms will respond by adapting to those antibiotics. In agriculture, we know of hundreds of cases of insects that have become pesticide-resistant; in medicine, increasing numbers of micro-organisms have become resistant to antibiotics meant to fight them. Some microbes have become resistant to antibiotics even before they are used! This happens when an antibiotic is released on the market with a new trade name, but in fact is hardly different from its predecessor. It may look different, but if it acts on the bacteria in the same way, it will be met by the same defenses. It is not enough to look at the agent of disease; we have to look at what makes populations vulnerable. Conventional public health failed to look at world history, to look at other species, to look at evolution and ecology, and finally, to look at social science. There is a growing body of literature that says that the poor and oppressed are more vulnerable to nearly all health hazards. But we still don't recognize class differences in the United States. Researchers discuss differences in income or a mother's education level or even socioeconomic status. But U.S. epidemiology does not deal with class, even when class is the best predictor of life expectancy, of old-age disability, or the frequency of heart attacks. As a predictor of coronary disease, it is better to measure class position than to measure cholesterol.

OTHER EXPLANATIONS

Why do we wear these intellectual blinders that have so hobbled the study and practice of public health in this country? First, there are a multiplicity of long-term intellectual biases. Take, for example, American pragmatism. Americans pride themselves on their practicality. *Theory* is almost a dirty word. When we are overwhelmed with the urgency of a population that is sick, of kids that are dying, it becomes a luxury to ask about evolution. This overwhelming sense of urgency is one of the reasons why doctors don't look at diseases of tomatoes, don't ask about competition between different kinds of mosquitoes, and certainly don't look at historical factors. There is an inevitable tunnel vision built into the urgency of carrying out applied clinical or epidemiological work.

A second reason is the Western scientific tradition of reductionism, which says that the way to understand a problem is to reduce it to its smallest elements and change things one at a time. This is very successful when the question is "What is this made of?" Then we can isolate it, cut it out of an organism, put it in the blender or under the microscope. In fact, we have been marvelously successful at identifying what things are made of. That is why we have had a growing, if irrational, sophistication about small phenomena and events throughout the whole of scientific enterprise. Why is it we are so successful at giving individual emergency treatment and so ineffectual in stopping or preventing malaria, in anticipating its return, or dealing broadly with the health of whole populations? We are marvelously successful at breeding a wheat plant that can better use nitrogen to produce more grain but much less successful at alleviating hunger in the countryside.

FOUR HYPOTHESES

So the typical failure has been a refusal to look at complexity. The successes have been successes of the small, where we could focus on isolated elements. In the United States, even though we spend more than any other country on health care, we have among the worst results among the industrial countries; certainly we are behind the Europeans and in many ways also behind the Japanese when the usual indicators of health are considered. This is something that worries public health people; why, they ask, do we spend so much and have so little to show for it compared to other countries?

Here are four hypotheses:

One, we don't actually get more health care; we just spend more for it. We know that something like 20 percent of our health care bill is in administration, that is, the cost of billing and the like. The rate of profit of the pharmaceutical industry is greater than that of capitalism as a whole, and much of that is in the United States. Doctors' salaries are huge, as are charges for hospital rooms. The consequence is that "investment" per patient is enormous.

Two, even when we do get more health care, it is not always good health care. Now, this seems paradoxical because we have more MRIs and more CT scanners and more dialysis machines than most other countries. So why is our health not better? Medical decisions are not always made for medical reasons. There are a lot of incentives for making decisions as to which kinds of techniques to use, what kinds of interventions—when to carry out heart surgery, for example—which give rise to differences in medical procedure among countries. We do a lot more implanting of pacemakers than Europe and perform more cesarean sections and hysterectomies. A hospital buys an expensive machine to attract both doctors and patients. But once on hand, it has to be used. You can't allow an MRI machine to sit idle in the hospital, so doctors are encouraged to use it if only to amortize the institution's investment. Another is that in order to keep the "batting average" of a surgeon high, the surgeon has to perform enough operations (several hundred a year) to keep skill levels up. An isolated hospital with only one heart transplant every three or four months is not a safe place to go. The wise patient will seek out a hospital with a highly regarded cardiac service equipped with the latest technology. But to win that prestige, skills must be maintained, so there's an incentive to keep both surgeons and machines working. Since the service is also an expensive thing to have, it needs to be kept busy if only to bring in surgical fees. But does it make sense to have all that expensive equipment? Hospital administrators will tell you it does because the hospital down the road has it. If Mass General is in competition with Beth Israel and both compete with Mount Sinai, all of them need the most advanced machines. Then there are the HMOs, which have their accountants making medical decisions, effectively rationing health care. Both approaches are meant to maximize profit. What happens is that sometimes people get too much care, sometimes too little. But in both cases, our health is a side effect of the obsession with making money. The irrationality of the system extends even to the rich, who are overtreated. We kill nearly two hundred thousand people a year through improper medical interventions. Many more die due to misuse of heavily advertised prescription medications, over-the-counter remedies, and other preparations.

The third hypothesis is that the healthcare system is built on a foundation of inequality. Only some of us actually receive or have access to the health care we need, while most don't.

Finally, the fourth hypothesis: we have created a sick society, even as we invest more and more to repair the damage. We are exposed to more pollution and increasing levels of stress and are therefore exposed, ironically, to more opportunities to display our cardiac surgery skills. We make more people miserable, so we spend more on psychiatry and on psychotropic drugs. This is clearly evident in the public health situation in contemporary Russia, where the collapse of universal health coverage exposed the population to all the ills of incipient capitalism. They have had waves of epidemics, diphtheria, whooping cough, and the completely novel situation in modern times of declining life expectancy—from about sixty-four years to about fifty-nine years. Ours is a sick society that demands ever-greater expenditure to repair the damage to public health that it has itself inflicted.

RESPONSES TO THE CRISIS

The condition of health care has not gone unnoticed; in fact, there is widespread and growing dissatisfaction. And there have been a number of responses to address the situation.

Ecosystem Health

Ecologists looking at the problem have derived an approach they call ecosystem health. They posit that there are ecosystems under stress for multiple causes: from pollutants, contaminated food and water, high stress, and changes in the daily rhythm of life. For example, with nearly universal electrical light, people sleep less, and our physiology changes. If we examine human biology as a socialized biology, we notice that there are things that appear as constants of human biology that really are not. For instance, it has long been conventional wisdom that as a natural part of the aging process, blood pressure increases with age. But it turns out that among the !Kung Bushmen of the Kalahari, blood pressure increases with age only up through puberty and then levels off. Our blood pressure pattern is a function of the kind of society in which we live. We can see this in the pattern of stress reaction hormones, which vary with one's social location. Recent studies have shown that among groups of teenagers from high school, all of whom are doing equally well academically, working-class kids showed prolonged rises in cortisol under any kind of stress while upper-class kids showed a quick spike and then a decline. The physiology of working-class youngsters was altered by their social location, whether or not they acknowledged their working status. Evidently one's body knows one's class position no matter how well one has been taught to deny it. Human physiology, then, is a socialized physiology, and differing social locations create different relationships with the environment. This knowledge has led to the ecosystem health concept, bringing together environmentalists and public health people to examine questions about how we rate the health of the whole ecosystem.

The Environmental Justice Movement

This movement arose from the observation—by others—that the best way to find an incinerator or a toxic waste dump is to look for an African-American neighborhood. With lower real-estate values in minority neighborhoods, it is cheaper to put the incinerator there. Zoning rules, made by the powerful, are more lax there. So the health risks from pollution and industrial waste become yet another facet of oppression. Exposure to pollutants doesn't affect everybody equally. Exposure to occupational health hazards—the exposure of somebody who makes a living sandblasting buildings, for example—is very different from someone who works at a desk totaling up actuarial tables. Exposure to environmental insult also varies with class and the condition of oppression. The environmental justice movement has been a response to this, fighting the dumping of pollutants and attempting to equalize the risks of an industrial society.

Social Determination of Health

This approach has been growing among epidemiologists, partly due to the rediscovery of what Rudolph Wirchow and Frederick Engels pointed out in the nineteenth century: that capitalism itself can undermine health. This is important to keep in mind when conservative and reactionary commentators assert that there isn't any real poverty anymore. They argue that while some people make more money than others and can afford a bigger color television, the poor are not without their TVs. The car of a poor family is a little bit older or perhaps they do not eat in restaurants as often, but this inequality does not negate the real truth as the right-wing pundits see it: basically, there is no longer any poverty. Of course, an answer is easily found in the numerous studies that show that in fact black people pay for racist oppression with life spans ten years shorter than that of whites. Poor and oppressed minorities have 25 percent fewer successful encounters with the health care system than more privileged groups. Meanwhile, the rate of death or other harmful outcomes increases with the level of poverty in illnesses like coronary heart disease, cancer of all forms, obesity, growth retardation in children, unplanned pregnancies, and maternal mortality.

Those interested in the social determination of health include some English scholars, such as Richard Wilkinson, who has looked at the life expectancies of different ranks in the English civil service. He found there was a difference even among those groups that are better off than those exposed to obvious dire need. He noticed that mere social hierarchy, social differentiation, makes your health worse everywhere, not only among those in extreme poverty. Now this can be interpreted in two opposing ways, but both of them are operative. One is to say that inequality per se, rather than the level of poverty, can make a person sick. Another is to say, quite literally, that it is all in your head. In support of the latter, baboon studies are cited that seem to indicate that those with higher rank in their troupe have better health. Their arteries are cleaner, they respond to stress like upper-class people; their cortisol level shoots up under stress and then comes right down again. Lower-ranking baboons tend to have the effects of stress lasting longer; their life expectancies are lower. But if you intervene in animal communities and alter their social hierarchy, within a few months the baboon's physiology will take on the characteristics of its new social location. This leads some people to say that it is how people perceive their situation in society—and therefore that people must be taught to cope with where they are, that after all we create our own realities. That's a common phrase in some of the growth and therapy movements: we create our own realities. It's not so much that you're underpaid and poor, but that you feel lousy about it. And so we have devised cheer-up pills: the cure for depression is not to get rid of the depressing situation, but to help people feel better about it. Another way to look at this so-called social determination of health is to see it not as a simple result of inadequate incomes that need to be raised, but as a consequence of a profoundly stratified, class-based society. Those who emphasize the latter feel that it is a more radical position than simply talking about how absolute deprivation is bad for your health, because the remedy for that would seem to be to increase income. Instead, they say, you have to eliminate the inequalities of class. Since the same studies can give rise to opposite conclusions, we need to emphasize that inequality affects your health in many different ways. When rich people think about poverty, they think about it only in the sense of having a little bit less, without examining the underlying structure of impoverishment. Poverty affects people, first of all, as chronic deprivation, actually having less food or worse food. Kids who live in damp, moldy apartments have worse health than kids who live in dry apartments. There are many other ways in which chronic deprivation itself is a menace to health.

There are what we call low-frequency, high-intensity threats, meaning those experiences that do not happen to everybody, but that could and therefore are a constant threat to a sense of well being. Robert Fogel, a right-wing, Chicago-school economist, pointed out in his book *Time on the Cross: The Economics of American Negro Slavery* (1974) that most slaves were not whipped. He went on to say that slavery was not what we would imagine from reading *Uncle Tom's Cabin*, that it had a certain economic rationality. What he neglects to say is that physical abuse of slaves, even when not employed, was a constant threat. Most slaves, perhaps, weren't whipped but all of them witnessed or knew about beatings. Similarly, most kids in impoverished neighborhoods are not shot, but getting shot is a constant menace every time you go to the store or go outside. These are examples of medium- and low-frequency but very high-intensity threats.

There also are high-frequency, low-intensity insults, the daily harassment one can see, for instance, in African-American communities. There, one is constantly forced to make strategic decisions. Am I walking so slowly that the cop is going to think I'm loitering? Or am I walking so fast that he or she will think that I'm running away from the scene of a crime? If I come onto campus at night to work in my laboratory, will I first be stopped by the police who think that I'm a thief? I remember once when Ramos Antonini, the resident commissioner of Puerto Rico, was stopped by police on the way to his office in Washington. They laughed when he said he was a member of Congress and the resident commissioner. Antonini was black.

We are learning now from the study of neurotransmitters that our brain is not the only locus of social experience. The cerebrum gathers social experience and transmits it through many branches of the nervous system into the neurotransmitters. The neurotransmitters are chemically similar to substances in our immune system, in the white blood cells. In a certain sense, we think with our whole bodies, we feel with our whole bodies, and so the whole body is the locus of social experience that comes with these patterns of chronic conditions, of low-frequency threats or high-frequency insult. There are many dimensions to the experience of deprivation, but they are often lost in the hands of the statisticians, who simply see poverty as a quantitative difference in income.

The "Health Care for All" Movement

This group champions a national health insurance system and has done much work comparing the American system to the Canadian system; many progressive physicians are active in this movement.

Alternative Medicine

The alternative health movement deals mostly with individual health. It stresses diet, exercise, homeopathy, chiropractic, and naturopathic remedies—areas where people feel that they have not been treated adequately by the established medical system. They draw on a holistic approach to health rather than the targeted, magic-bullet approach of traditional allopathic medicine. They seem to be particularly effective in dealing with long-term chronic conditions rather than acute emergencies. For instance, for those who need radiation and chemotherapy for cancer, alternative practices are helpful in modulating the negative side-effects. The strategy of modern medicine is that cancerous tissue is sufficiently fragile and can in effect be poisoned in the hope that the radiation or chemotherapy will kill the cancer more than it kills you. The approach employed by alternative therapies is not to attack the cancer directly, but to try to build up the body's defenses. So the two approaches complement each other. Alternative medicine is very attractive and very powerful, but its primary appeal is to people who have control over their lives and access to the resources and techniques of alternative health care. It is not a mass movement; the holism it advocates stops at the edge of your skin. It is not a societal holism. Nonetheless, it is a powerful antidote to those movements that simply demand health care for all, without asking what kind of health care.

A RADICAL CRITIQUE

A radical critique of medicine has to deal with the things that make people sick and the kind and quality of health care people get. A Marxist approach to health would attempt to integrate the insights of ecosystem health, environmental justice, the social determination of health, "health care for all," and alternative medicine. One aspect of my approach to the issues of health care comes from my background as an ecologist. I looked at variability in health across geographic locations, occupational groups, age groups, or other socially defined categories. Just how variable, I asked, is the outcome in health care in different states in the United States, different counties in Kansas, different provinces in Cuba, different health districts in a Brazilian state or in a Canadian province? Very interesting patterns emerged from that work. My colleagues and I examined the rate of infant mortality in each of these regions, both as an average and how, in each place, the rates varied, reflecting the quality of health care, among other factors, from the best to the worst. What we saw was that infant mortality rates in the

United States were more or less comparable to Cuba, that Kansas had a rate a little higher than the U.S. average while Rio Grande do Sur in Brazil had a more typical, and much higher, Third World infant mortality rate. That Cuba scored so high was not very surprising.

However, when we viewed the same data from the perspective of the range from the best to the worst rates of infant mortality, that is, the variability within given populations, an effective measure of fairness, much more was revealed. The numbers for counties in Kansas showed the greatest variation, while the numbers that compared U.S. states showed somewhat less difference. The difference across health districts of Rio Grande was even less, and the least variation was in Cuba. Similar things happen when we look at all causes of death. Once again, we observed average rates as well as the disparity; we divided the variation, the difference between best and worst, by the average. For Kansas, the range divided by the average is .85, but in Cuba it was .34. We saw that the cancer rates in Kansas and in Cuba are comparable, but the variability is higher in Kansas than in Cuba. When we examined Canadian data, we found that Saskatchewan was somewhere between Kansas and Cuba.

The reason we chose these places is that on the one hand Brazil, Canada, and Kansas all have capitalist economies in which investment decisions are based on maximizing profit rather than any social imperative meant to equalize economic circumstance. Saskatchewan and Rio Grande do Sur along with Cuba have national health systems that provide fairly uniform coverage over a given geographic area. The Canadian and Brazilian regions have the advantage of a better and more just health care system, but unlike Cuba, they have the disadvantages of capitalism, giving them an intermediate location in the variability of health outcomes.

This method can also be applied when comparing different diseases. One question we want to answer is whether variability will be greater across states and other large geographic regions or across small areas like counties. There are good reasons why it might go either way. For example, weather could impact the data in large areas like states. But weather is not the only variable; others may vary greatly over smaller geographic units, only to be lost in the averages we develop for large areas. When we are able to look at smaller areas, for example, like different neighborhoods within the city of Wichita, Kansas, we find a threefold variation in infant mortality. We also notice that unemployment in Kansas averages 9 or 10 percent in most Kansas counties but is 30 percent in northeast Wichita. Why? Because neighborhoods are not simply random pieces of environment. They're structured. Wherever there is a rich neighborhood, you need a poor neighborhood, like northeast Wichita, to serve it. And so whenever we can get data across neighborhoods, we see very large variations in social conditions and, as a consequence, in the quality and quantity of health care— clearly unnecessary from the point of view of any limitation in our medical knowledge or resources.

Another interesting case can be found in Mexico, where a study was conducted of several villages, ranking them according to how marginalized they were from Mexican life. Examined were such variables as whether there was running water or what proportion of the people spoke Spanish. The research showed that the more marginal communities had worse health outcomes. But unexpectedly, the data also showed that there was tremendous difference among the outcomes in poor villages that you didn't get among the villages that were integrated into the Mexican economy.

It is an as yet unrecognized ecological principle in public health that when a community or an individual organism is stressed for any reason (low income, a very severe climate, for example), it will be extremely sensitive to other disparities. So if people have very low income, changing seasonal temperatures become very important. For example, in late autumn and early winter, emergency rooms have a lot of people coming in with burns from kerosene stoves, ovens, and other dangerous means used to compensate for inadequate heat in their houses. For such people, a small difference in temperature can have a big effect on their health—one that doesn't affect the more affluent. The same is true in relation to food. When people are unemployed or if the prices go up, they cut back on food and other kinds of expenditures with an immediate impact on nutrition. If you are a superb shopper, and if you clip all the coupons and scrutinize the supermarket ads, you might just get by on the Department of Agriculture poverty-level basket; the people who dream up these baskets assume you are a whiz at finding bargains. But suppose you are not so good or that you read the ads but cannot get away for two hours for comparison shopping. Or that you live in a neighborhood where the local supermarket was not as profitable as the national chain that owned it thought it should be and is gone, and with it your opportunity to get quality food. Or suppose that you would love to eat organic food for lunch but what you have is a half-hour break to go down to the vending machines. Under those circumstances, individual differences in where you work, how much energy you have, whether you can have a babysitter available or not can have a big impact on your health.

THE ILLUSION OF CHOICE

Poor health tends to cluster in poor communities. Conservatives will say, "Well, obviously, poverty is not good for you, but after all, not all kids turn out badly. I made it, so why can't you? Some people have become CEOs of corporations who came out of that neighborhood." What they miss is the notion of increased vulnerability. The apparently trivial difference in experience can have a vast effect on the health of someone who is marginal. Suppose a pupil is a bit nearsighted but, because she is tall, is seated at the back of the classroom. The teacher is overworked and does not notice that the student cannot see the black-board. She fidgets; she gets into a fight with the kid at the next desk. Suddenly she has become someone with a "learning problem" and is transferred to a vocational course even though she might have been a great poet. In a more affluent community, where the classes are smaller and teachers pay attention, this kid would simply end up with glasses. Individual differences can come from anything, from personal experiences growing up, even from genetics. But even when genetics is responsible for a given human characteristic, it is only respon-sible within a particular context. For instance, in a factory emitting toxic fumes, people will develop cancer at a higher rate; those most likely to develop the can-cer have livers that are not able to effectively process a particular chemical as well. This is a genetic variable and thus a genetic disease, but it occurs only with exposure to those fumes. The cancer is not a result of genetics alone; it is also caused by the environment.

Trivial biological differences can become the focus around which important life outcomes are located; the most obvious is pigmentation. The difference in melanin between Americans of African and European origin is, from the point of view of genetics and physiology, trivial. It is simply the way in which a pigment is deposited in the skin. Yet this difference can cost you ten years of life. So is this a lethal gene? Is this a gene for a higher spread of pigmentation—one that also makes you more vulnerable to arrest? A standard geneticist would look at family histories and determine that if your uncle was arrested, there would be a higher probability of your being arrested as well. Conclusion: the cause of crim-inality is genetic. Following the rules of genetics in this mechanistic way, he or she will have "proved" that crime is hereditary. This makes as much sense as the notion that black people get more tuberculosis because they have bad genes. Genetics is not an alternative explanation of social conditions; it a component of an investigation of causal factors. There is an intimate interdependence among biological, genetic, environmental, and social factors.

Behavior is one of the areas where public health workers want to intervene, arguing that much that differentiates health outcomes in poor neighborhoods from rich ones can be associated with behavior, such as smoking, exercise, and diet. Conservatives, finally forced to concede that there are big differences in health outcomes between rich and poor, now say, "Ah, yes, this is because the poor make unwise decisions. The appropriate remedy is education. We know that kids do better if their mothers have had more schooling, so what we need are education programs to teach people to make the best of their situation." In fact, some health education programs are valuable. Safety orientation within factories does help people cope with unsafe conditions. But let us take a closer look at this question of choice. The Centers for Disease Control and Prevention, and others that deal with these issues, say only some things can be chosen, while others are imposed by the environment. They would have us distinguish between disadvantages imposed on us, that may be unfair and/or can be eliminated, from those that were freely chosen and for which we can only blame ourselves. A Marxist confronted with choices among mutually exclusive categories like choice versus environment, heredity versus experience, or biological versus social knows that the categories themselves must be challenged. Choice also implies the lack of choice. Choices are always made from a set of alternatives that are presented to you by somebody else. We know this from elections and from shopping. We choose food, but only from the products a company has chosen to make available to us. The choice is distinguished by the lack of choice, that is, unchoice. The same is true with respect to the opportunity to exercise choice. There are always preconditions to the exercise of choice. If the conditions of life are very poor or oppressive, some of the things that are unwise choices under other circumstances become the lesser evil.

Public health people, like nearly everyone else, worry a great deal about teen pregnancies, which generally are not a good idea. Teen mothers are not experienced; they may have difficulty taking care of their babies; and the babies are more likely to be underweight. Nevertheless, it turns out that the health of a baby born to an African-American teenager is on the average better than the health of a baby born to an African-American woman in her twenties. Why? The environment of racism erodes health to such an extent that it makes a certain amount of sense to have your babies early if you're going to have them. This is something that is not obvious when you simply say, "Teen pregnancy is a danger to people." We need to look at teen pregnancy in a much broader social context before we can think about making it simply a public health issue.

Smoking is another example. Smoking increases inversely with the degree of freedom one has at work. People who have few choices in life at least can make the choice to smoke. It is one of the few legitimate ways in some jobs to take a break and step outside. So there are people who choose: "Yes," they say, "it might give me cancer in twenty years, but it sure keeps me alive today." The unhealthy choices people make are not irrational choices. We have to see them as constrained rationality, making the best of a bad situation. Most of the apparently unwise decisions people make have a relative rationality to them when their circumstance is taken into account, so it is unlikely their behavior will change simply by lecturing to them. You have to change the context within which choice is made.

Yet another dimension of choice is found in the way we perceive time. When making a choice about health, we assume that something we do now will have an impact later on. That may seem obvious, but it is not the experience of everyone. Most people, in fact, do not experience the kind or quality of freedom that gives them control over their own lives that would allow them to say, "I will quit smoking now so that I won't get cancer in twenty years." Not everyone can organize their lives along an orderly annual time scale. In the inner city of San Juan, in Puerto Rico, the life pattern is such that one can work unloading a ship for twenty-three hours a day for two days, then sleep for three days, then unexpectedly work in a restaurant for another two days because his or her cousin has to go to a funeral in the mountains. Time does not have the same structure when you can't make solid plans now for what is going to happen to you later.

On the other hand, the lives of, say, academics are notable for the way time is organized. Students can and do choose courses of study that in two or three years will prepare them for a career. On a shorter time scale, a professor may conveniently order his or her teaching schedule around patterns of Monday, Wednesday, and Friday or Tuesday and Thursday. Physicians decide when to see patients, when to be in the library, when to go to seminars. So some people can actually structure their lives in such a way that we can make predictions. Not absolute predictions, obviously. Things can come up; we can be hit by a car. But basically, the more control you have over your life and your experience of life, the more it makes sense to make the kind of decisions that public health experts recommend, the more the possibility, then, of exercising choice. So the answer to those who talk about decision-making and choice is to tell them, first of all, to expand the range of choices. Secondly, they need to provide the tools for making those choices. Third, of course, people need to control their own lives so that they can exercise all their faculties to make meaningful choices. In taking each of these steps, we directly challenge the false dichotomies that rule thinking about public health and constrain it within predetermined societal boundaries.

WHAT CAN BE DONE?

At a recent meeting I attended, a paper was distributed that posed the following dilemma: Why, living in a democracy, where all citizens have the vote, do we permit policies that create inequalities that have such a negative impact on our health? How do we explain this? We have schemes to improve agriculture, but they increase hunger. We create hospitals, and they become the centers for the propagation of new diseases. We invest in engineering projects to control floods, and they increase flood damage. What has gone wrong? One answer might be that we are just not smart enough. Or the problems are just too complicated, or we are selfish, or we have some defect. Or after having failed to eliminate hunger, improve people's health, and do away with inequalities, and failed, perhaps we need to face facts and conclude that it just cannot be done. Or perhaps we're just the kind of species that is incapable of living a cooperative life in a sensible relation to nature.

We should reject any of these unduly pessimistic conclusions. The history of struggle is long and not without achievements. But struggle is also difficult. For example, it is easy to depend on the illusion of democracy and a beneficent government to solve our problems. But when we look at the policies that emerge from those institutions of democracy, we see that those ostensibly aimed at improving the people's lives are nearly always hobbled by some hidden side condition. For instance, I am sure that on the whole, President Clinton would rather have people covered by health insurance than not. But that is subject to the side condition that insurance industry profitability must be protected. He probably would like medicines to be cheaper, but only if the pharmaceutical industry continues to make high profits. Abroad, the United States would like peasants to have land, but only if not expropriated from plantation owners. The basic reason that programs fail is not incompetence, ignorance, or stupidity, but because they are constrained by the interests of the powerful. Sometimes we discover that part of a program is carried out successfully and part not. An enterprise zone might be established in an inner city that actually brings in investment, but there is no impact on poverty because the assumption that benefits would trickle down was an illusion. A reasonable return on investment was the goal of the developers. When that was achieved, nothing else mattered.

A good way to see how these hidden constraints, these systemic barriers, operate is in the delivery of health services elsewhere. Health care in the United States exists against the background of this country's unrestrained capitalism. We have described at length both the prospects and problems of that system. But in Europe, social democrats historically have taken a different approach—one that acknowledges inequality as an obstacle. They have treated unemployment, for example, as a social problem rather than an inevitable by-product of a vigorous market. A town council will address it by financing a center for the unemployed, with counselors to advise them of their right to unemployment insurance and other benefit programs. The center may even organize a support group where people can deal with their feelings about not being able to bring home an income to the family. Local governments can address other social concerns. In London, there is a program to break down the isolation of young mothers, where they can meet one another, share experiences, and provide support. Of course, none of these measures affects profitability or challenges the market. So the council cannot create employment. Even the most farsighted programs initiated by European social democratic governments do not challenge the capitalist order in any way. What they do is to try to make things more equitable—for instance, through progressive income taxes or generous unemployment insurance. In Sweden, transport workers demanded improved food to reduce heart disease among truck drivers. They organized to improve the quality of food in the roadside canteens and collaborated with restaurant owners and canteen owners and food was improved. In other places, unions have negotiated collective agreements to change shift work, hours of work, and working conditions. The unions recognized that health concerns were but another aspect of class relations.

In some cases, improving on-the-job health is relatively cost-free. No employer will object to putting up a sign reminding workers to wear their hard hats on the construction site. But it begins to get a little tricky when you talk about the reorganization of work or the expenditure of money. If the expenditure of money comes from taxes, through government programs to improve health, we can expect the business class to object. And if after each new expenditure, they perceive some interference with their competitive position, their opposition may take some political form, for example, the repeal of some aspect of health and safety regulation. When an expenditure has to come from the individual employer, perhaps by way of a union demand, they will be even more resistant. They will say that it is bad for competition and threaten to close down and move somewhere else. If the union's demands deal with the organization of work itself, management will see workers impinging on the very core of class prerogative. In that situation, only a powerful and well-organized labor movement will be able to impose changes.

When health policy is looked at from the point of view of which issues involve a direct confrontation of fundamental, ruling-class interest, which ones involve simply relative benefits to a class, and which are relatively neutral, we can predict which kinds of measures are possible. This highlights the lie in the notion that society is trying to improve health for everybody. We need to see health care in a more complex way. Health is part of the wage goods of a society, part of the value of labor power, and therefore a regular object of contention in class struggle. But health is also a consumer good, particularly for the affluent, who can buy improvements in health for themselves. Rather than improve water quality, they buy bottled water; rather than improve air quality, they employ oxygen tanks in their living rooms. Health is also a commodity invested in by the health industries, including hospitals, HMOs, and pharmaceutical companies. They sell health care to as large a market as can afford to pay for it; they even push it on people who do not need it. Like any aggressive business, the health industries engage in public relations—the winning of hearts and minds. Some of the clinics that were established in Southeast Asia during the Vietnam War and earlier, during the Malayan insurrection, were for this purpose. Doctors, at great sacrifice, would go into the jungle and set up clinics and work very hard under very difficult conditions for low pay, seeing themselves either as bringing benefits to people who needed it or, more consciously, as trying to prevent communism. It was yet another reincarnation of the "white man's burden" that justified nineteenth-century imperialism.

If good health depends on one's capacity to carry out those activities that are necessary and appropriate according to one's station in life, it matters how that station is determined. Those who can determine for themselves what constitutes necessary and desirable activities are clearly different from the people who have that determination made for them. This distinction is clear when an employer negotiates health insurance for his or her employees; for the employer, the cost of the benefits package will always come before what employees may think they need. So health is always a point of contention in class struggle. So is medical and scientific research; knowledge and ignorance are determined, as in all scientific research, by who owns the research industry, who commands the production of knowledge. There is class struggle in the debates around what kind of research ought to be done. Increasingly, research in the health field is dominated by the pharmaceutical and electronic industries.

There are intellectual concerns about how to analyze data, about how to think about disease, about how widely we need to look at the epidemiological, historical, and social questions they raise; there are also issues of health service and health policy. But they are all part of one integral system that has to be our battleground in the future. We have to take up health as a pervasive issue as we do with problems of the environment; they are aspects of class struggle, not an alternative to it.

Reference

Fogel, R. W. *Time on the Cross: The Economics of American Negro Slavery.* New York: Little, Brown, 1974.

CHAPTER SEVENTEEN

Theorizing Inequalities in Health

The Place of Lay Knowledge

Jennie Popay
Gareth Williams
Carol Thomas
Anthony Gatrell

This chapter seeks to contribute to the development of a more adequate theoretical framework for future research on social inequalities in health. It begins by exploring some of the imitations in the existing largely quantitative research in this field, pointing in particular to the failure of this work adequately to address the relationship between human agency and social structure. We then explore at a conceptual level the contribution which lay knowledge—in its narrative form—may make to understanding this relationship.

We are not the first to have begun a discussion of research on health inequalities by highlighting the limits of existing research. However, our position is somewhat different from that of other critics. First, the ideas we describe below form the theoretical basis of a piece of empirical research. This chapter is unashamedly critical and conceptual in content, but empirical exploration and testing of the ideas we develop is under way and will form the basis for further papers. Second, our focus on the centrality of lay knowledge in the search for a better understanding of inequalities in health is unusual. Third, our critique of current research into inequalities in health is linked to the changing context in which theory, research and policy are being developed. At the level of social theory, the process of reflexive modernisation is creating growing pressure for

This study was part of the Economic and Social Research Council's program on social inequalities in health, contract number L 128 25 1020.

greater dialogue between "experts"—be they scientists, civil servants or social theorists—and lay publics—be they patients, members of self-help groups or community and neighbourhood pressure groups (Giddens, 1991). At the level of research, it is increasingly apparent that many stakeholders need to be brought into the processes whereby findings about public health are generated and then fed through into policy and practice in health and welfare. At the level of national policy there is a renewed interest, across Western Europe at least, in the development of interventions which might reduce, if not remove, inequalities in health—though there are those who remain understandably sceptical of the motives underlying recent "political transformations" of the inequalities debate (Wainwright, 1996).

It can be argued, therefore, that this is a particularly significant time for the development of theory and research on inequalities in health. We would also argue that this fertile ground will only yield new fruits if researchers are prepared to embrace the need for different frameworks of understanding as well as different research methods and are willing to use these frameworks in the context of a genuine dialogue across disciplines. It is an unfortunate outcome of the tendency to work within narrow disciplinary or subdisciplinary boundaries, and the limited view of "science" that often accompanies this, that historical, anthropological and philosophical literature on the nature of class, identity, social action, and well-being have rarely informed epidemiological or empirical social research on inequalities in health. Much of this latter work has focused on the categories of social class (occupation) and health (mortality and morbidity), but has tended to regard health, implicitly if not explicitly, as a category of the phenomenal world that is ontologically detachable from both power and experience. In contrast, we suggest there is much to be gained from adopting an historico-sociological perspective which defines inequalities in health neither as a category nor a structure but as an "historical phenomenon," something which in fact "happens (and can be shown to have happened) in human relationships" (Thompson, 1993, p. 9). On this basis, occupational social class is not necessarily the determining factor in the picture of inequalities in health.

We begin with a brief overview of conventional approaches to describing and explaining inequalities in health. We then consider some of the main criticisms of these approaches. Finally, building on recent studies which focus on place as a way of better understanding how structural inequalities work their way out in people's everyday lives and drawing on recent developments in social theory, we explore—at a conceptual level—the role lay knowledge may play in mediating the relationship between structural inequalities, individual or group action and health status. In so doing, we develop two linked but separate arguments. The first and main point is that lay knowledge, rooted in the places that people spend their lives, has theoretical significance for our understanding of the causes of health inequalities. The second, essentially political argument is that lay knowledge represents a privileged form of expertise about inequalities in health which may pose a challenge to those who claim the status of either research or policy expert in this field.

EXISTING APPROACHES TO STUDYING HEALTH INEQUALITIES

Whitehead (1995; see also Dahlgren and Whitehead, 1991) has constructed a graphical model attempting to capture the relationship between different modes of explanation in the inequalities field (Figure 17.1). Notwithstanding the criticisms of this model as a basis for action (Wainwright, 1996), it provides a convenient framework within which to discuss existing approaches to the study of these inequalities.

At the heart of the Whitehead/Dahlgren model are the "biological givens": not only our sex and age but also what is given to us by our biological parents. These are factors over which the individual has no control and include the environmental influences that shaped our parents' health when they were conceiving us or, indeed, when they themselves were conceived. These factors have been the focus of considerable research effort, and there is now a substantial body of evidence, much of which derives from the work of David Barker and

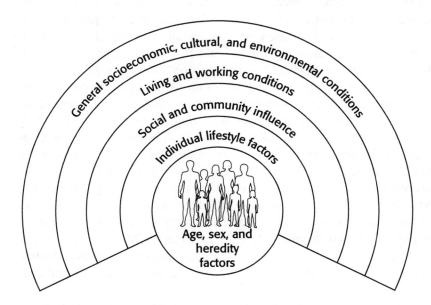

Figure 17.1. The Whitehead/Dahlgren Model.
Source: Dahlgren and Whitehead, 1991.

colleagues at Southampton University (see, for example, Barker, 1990, 1991, 1994). This suggests that experiences (such as nutrition) in utero determine or "programme" our risk of developing diseases later in life. Barker has, for example, demonstrated that mortality from cardiovascular disease is elevated among men whose birthweight was low or who were particularly thin.

Surrounding these biological determinants in the Whitehead/Dahlgren model are a set of factors that are theorised to impact upon our likelihood of developing disease or dying prematurely. These factors, that may be labelled lifestyle, embrace behaviours over which we may be said—though not without considerable argument—to have some degree of control. They include smoking, alcohol consumption, eating patterns, and propensity to exercise. Some of these are theorised to have direct effects on health outcome, while others are seen to operate indirectly. By far the most numerous of the studies directed at understanding inequalities in health have been focused on exploring the role of risk factors such as these. This body of work is widely referred to as *risk factor epidemiology.*

Much current epidemiological research has come in for criticism from those who see the outer layers of the Whitehead/Dahlgren model—the population level and the wider social context of individuals—as having more explanatory power than this body of research appears to allow. Such criticism includes that from social epidemiologists themselves (Syme, 1996; Shy, 1997). For example, Syme has noted that "epidemiologists tend to study individuals in order to find causes of disease even though it is clear that this will not be helpful in understanding the distribution of disease in the population. . . . Almost all epidemiologists study large numbers of individuals in communities. This is not epidemiology. It is clinical medicine in large groups" (1996, pp. 22, 23).

Syme's own solution to this problem is to address the social context of individuals through the set of factors identified in the second and third layer of the model—social and community influences and living and working conditions.(It is important to note that whilst these factors can be conceptualised as enveloping the lifestyle factors, they too operate at the individual level.) Syme gives prominence to the health implications of "control over one's destiny." This has been explored in considerable detail in relation to the workplace by Karasek and others who have developed and operationalised the notion of "job decision latitude" (Karasek and Theorell, 1990). Those working in occupations where there is the flexibility to structure one's own working day have been shown to suffer fewer health problems than those whose working practices are tightly defined and who have little or no discretion to influence the shape, schedule and content of their work.

A particularly important body of epidemiological work, which seeks to incorporate the social context of individual risks as well as aspects of individual lifestyle, has emanated from the Whitehall I and II studies (Marmot et al., 1978).

These studies have demonstrated clear gradients in mortality across the fine and distinct grades of employment amongst English civil servants. The differences in mortality identified between the various grades mirror national differences between social classes except that they are even more marked, with a greater than threefold difference in mortality being reported between the lowest and highest grades in the civil service.

The Whitehall studies have been important in drawing attention to the possibility that excess mortality is not just a matter of the cumulative effect of conventional risk factors. For example, they have shown that variations in risk factors (exercise, obesity, smoking and blood pressure) can explain only about a third of the variation among employment grades—although this approach to interpreting statistical findings has recently been criticized as misrepresenting the cumulative impact of risk factors. The Whitehall studies have also sought to incorporate psychosocial factors within and outside the world of work into the analysis (Marmot et al., 1991). Additionally, they have enabled Marmot and his colleagues to go beyond the presentation of aggregate, cross-sectional data and explore, in a "captive population," changes in mortality over time.

A considerable body of research, beside the Whitehall studies, supports the view that the structure and especially quality of social relations (layer two in the model) impacts on health and health inequalities. For example, a wide-ranging review of work on social ties and health (Seeman, 1996) suggests that social integration reduces the risk of mortality and leads to better mental health. Similarly, Oakley's (1992) review of research on the links between social support and motherhood points to many positive health outcomes related to social relationships. However, these reviews, and other work (Williams, Popay, and Oakley, 1998; Hall and Wellman, 1985) also point to negative health outcomes associated with social relationships.

The outermost level of the Whitehead/Dahlgren model represent the material aspects of the context within which individual and population health is located—aspects which are largely determined by national and international forces. Low income, poor housing and unemployment, for example, have been shown to be determinants of health inequalities. Research has demonstrated this relationship at an aggregate level, for example, by taking small-area data on ill health and attempting to account for variations using measures of material deprivation (Townsend, Phillimore, and Beattie, 1988). Townsend's composite index, described in Townsend et al. (1988), including census-based measures of car ownership, overcrowding, household tenure, and unemployment, has been used on numerous occasions as a predictor of mortality and limiting long-term illness.

More recently, researchers have begun to explore the relationship between patterns of mortality and morbidity and the macro socio-economic environment focusing in particular on the role of relative deprivation. This work has also begun to link different parts of the Whitehead/Dahlgren model—macro socio-economic circumstances and the nature and quality of social relationships, for example. Wilkinson (1996) has assembled a body of evidence, involving international comparisons, to demonstrate correlations between income inequality (as measured, for example, by the percentage of household income received by the least well-off households) and mortality and life expectancy. Others have pursued these associations at a national and small-area level (Kaplan et al., 1996; Kennedy, Kawachi, and Prothrow-Stith, 1996; Ben-Shlomo, White, and Marmot, 1996; Boyle, Gatrell, and Duke-Williams, 1999.

Wilkinson's explanation (1996) for this link between ill-health and relative deprivation extends the interest in the role of social relationships, drawing on work on the structure of civic society in Italy. He argues that involvement in community life (as measured, for example, by voting turnout and membership of local clubs and organisations) generates "social capital" that is conducive to good health. In effect, Wilkinson is suggesting an interaction between income inequalities, manifested in the outermost layer of the Whitehead/Dahlgren model and psychosocial factors operating within the second ring.

The potential theoretical leverage of the notion of social capital is generating growing research interest. It is, for example, prominent in the recently published research strategy for the English Health Education Authority (1996). A related but now neglected concept is that of the "social wage," prominent in social welfare research in the 1960s. This was developed in an attempt to capture the improved quality of life (in material and social terms) accruing to individuals and households as a result of public spending on common services such as education, health, housing and transport. Research has demonstrated that at some points during the postwar period the social wage was redistributive downwards to those living in poorer material circumstances, and over these periods there were major improvements in life expectancy (Charlton and Murphy, 1997). Ultimately, however, the main beneficiaries of welfare spending were the middle classes (Titmuss, 1958; Glennester, 1983).

The concept of a social wage is more materialist in its formulation and less psychological and relational than social capital. Although it may sound rather unfashionable in the wake of the 1980s and 90s critique of public welfare spending, it has not lost its salience for those concerned with understanding inequalities in health and the policies which might reduce these. Concepts such as "social capital" and the "social wage" may together have an important contribution to make to research in the health inequalities field. However, despite some empirical work seeking to operationalise them, these concepts remain somewhat ill-defined, and further work is required in order to demonstrate how these phenomena may impact upon health.

The final research tradition within the inequalities in health field we wish to highlight is that concerned with lifecourse or life-histories. There has been increasing academic interest in this approach in recent years, partly in response to the dominance of risk-factor epidemiology. For example, Power and colleagues (1996) have criticised Barker's work as being a narrow, biologically deterministic explanation of potential health inequalities. They argue instead for an approach that recognises that birthweight is itself influenced by socioeconomic circumstances (of the parents), and that socioeconomic experiences of individuals as they mature into and continue through adulthood are also crucial in drawing the contours of the relative risk of disease in later life. For instance, work using longitudinal data (Bartley et al., 1994) has shown that males of low birthweight are more likely to live as children and adolescents in poorer quality housing.

Although a lifecourse approach to inequalities research is sometimes presented as a recent methodological innovation, it actually has a long and honourable history. As reviews of this field have documented (Wadsworth, 1991, 1997), early and pathbreaking lifecourse work was begun in the 1940s in the field of social medicine and sociology at the MRC Sociology Unit in Aberdeen, Scotland (Illsley, 1955). This has been followed up in the decades since, as in the programme of work begun in the early 1980s at the MRC Medical Sociology Unit in Glasgow, Scotland.

The recent burgeoning of work using a lifecourse approach has been fuelled by the availability of new longitudinal datasets, such as the OPCS/ONS Longitudinal Study linking census data with mortality information over time for a 1% sample of the population of England and Wales, and the maturing of the samples involved in the British cohort studies begun in the 1940s, 50s and 70s. This type of research has also been stimulated by developments in computer hardware and statistical techniques, which have allowed for the easier handling of these complex longitudinal datasets. Wadsworth (1997) summarises the value of this type of research thus: "The overwhelming strengths of prospective studies are their information on the sequence and timing of events, and the opportunities they offer to study not only, in the conventional way, the relative predictive strengths of precursors of an outcome, but also the range of outcomes associated with a presumed risk factor or combination of risk factors which may either co-occur or be related sequentially or synergistically" (Wadsworth, 1997, p. 860).

Recognising these strengths of the lifecourse approach, Bartley and her colleagues have pointed to its significance for better targeting of policies to reduce inequalities: "a life course approach . . . is needed in order to take into account the complex ways in which biological risk interacts with economic, social and psychological factors in the development of chronic disease. Such an approach reveals biological and social 'critical periods' during which social policies that will defend individuals against an accumulation of risk are particularly important" (Bartley, Blane, and Montgomery, 1997, p. 1194). However, whilst lifecourse approaches to understanding inequalities in health have undoubted advantages, they are also characterised by many of the limitations of much other research in the inequalities field.

CRITIQUES OF CONVENTIONAL INEQUALITIES IN HEALTH RESEARCH

Having reviewed the dominant research approaches within the health inequalities field, we want now to examine some of the existing critiques of this work. We draw particularly, but not exclusively, on Kathryn Dean's critique of population health research in general (1993), Keith Paterson's critique of epidemiology (1981), Mike Kelly and Bruce Charlton's (1995) critique of the knowledge base of health promotion and Sally Macintyre's (1997) recent discussion of polarisation in explanatory modes in health inequalities research.

Three main linked points emerge from these and other critiques. First, existing theoretical frameworks (and by implication much empirical research) fail to capture the complexity of causal explanation in the health inequalities field. In particular, these writers point to the inadequate attention paid to the role of social organisations, processes and relationships at a macro level in the generation of inequalities. Second, and linked to the first point, there has been a lack of attention to the development of concepts which will help explain why individuals and groups behave in the way they do in the context of wider social structures—to link agency and structure, to use the sociological language. Third, the importance of developing work on the re-conceptualisation of the notion of place within explanatory models of inequalities in health is highlighted alongside the neglect of a robust historical perspective. We discuss these points in more detail below.

Missing Complexity

Dean (1993), Paterson (1981) and Macintyre (1997), in different ways, criticise much existing research on inequalities in health for failing to allow for the likely complexity of explanations. In her review of quantitative population health research, Kathryn Dean (1993) locates the difficulties in understanding the causal processes shaping health and illness in the failure of both epidemiology and social survey research to break free from positivistic philosophical foundations and empiricist methods. The problem, as Dean sees it, is that existing methods are simply not up to grasping the complexity inherent in the processes which shape health and illness: as she argues, health is "among the most complex of all dynamic systems" (1993, p. 26).

Dean traces the roots of this inadequacy back to the attempts made in both disciplines in the 1960s to overcome the acknowledged limitations of logical positivism. In resolving some of the methodological problems, she argues that these disciplines nevertheless remained wedded to positivism's empiricist tenets through the refinement of "single factor" studies and experimental design: "In spite of debates about empiricism and the limits of positivism, pressure grew in both fields for research approaches and methods which seek to predict the impact of specific factors on specific outcomes—factors separated from confounding influences by experimental design or its approximations" (1993, p. 21).

As we indicated in the last section, in epidemiology and social survey health research, the "risk factor" approach became, and remains, supreme and to a large extent continues its quest to isolate risk factors—carefully considering each in turn. Whilst there has been a clear move to incorporate aspects of social relationships in this type of work, the danger is that it simply adds another possible risk factor to the existing set, ignoring the complexity involved. Put crudely, social support, for example, becomes another covariate to enter into a regression model after adjustment for other risk factors. This atomistic approach disconnects individuals from their social context and destroys the structure of the social network within which they are embedded (Hall and Wellman, 1985). As Dean argues, "Risk factor methods have severe limitations for uncovering multicausal mechanisms. . . . This is because health and the influences that lead to its deterioration are multifaceted . . . and accumulate over the life course" (1993, p. 17). Dean goes on to argue that whilst social survey researchers have gone some way to overcoming the "factors" approach by developing techniques in causal modelling, they too exhibit a strong tendency to fall back into the search for single causes. One recent summary of the state of the epidemiological art illustrates the continuing dominance of positivist thinking in this field: "The aim of epidemiology is to decipher nature with respect to human health and disease" (Trichopoulos, 1996, p. 436).

For many of those working within conventional positivist epidemiology, the idea developed within modern philosophy that knowledge cannot simply be a "mirror of nature" (Rorty, 1980)—that there is no easy correspondence between what we know and what exists—is a challenge that has yet to be faced.

Dean suggests that the solution for quantitative population health researchers lies in the transfer to health research of some of the breakthroughs in knowledge in other scientific fields. In particular, she believes that theoretical developments in the study of dynamic systems, involving chaos and complexity theory, offer hope of new ways of thinking which could facilitate an understanding of the interplay of influences and processes shaping health and illness. Of key significance for Dean is the requirement for theory and empirical work to become more intimately related.

In his earlier critique, Keith Paterson (1981) also highlighted the lack of sophistication in epidemiological research in particular. However, unlike Dean, he was explicitly concerned with the neglect of structural issues, and his work is a critique of what might be called the political ontology of epidemiology. In his writing, he attempts to counterpoise a "materialist epidemiology" to the dominant positivistic one. Because they are embedded in a biological conception of disease, he argues, epidemiologists' empirical investigations of aetiological factors have left them dealing with surface appearances only—the result of an ideological stance which leaves the aetiological role of the social structure unquestioned. By giving primacy to the observable, privileging orthodox statistical techniques, and limiting its gaze to the "host," the "agent," and a limited number of environmental factors, he suggests, epidemiology fails to see the social relationships within which these factors are embedded: "By its focus on disease as a problem of incidence, conceived of as a product of a number of mechanically related risk factors, epidemiology denies that the structure of social relationships in society also has a primary determining role" (1981, p. 26). In contrast, for Paterson, a materialist epidemiology would "focus on these underlying structures and relationships and consider that the purpose of theory is to describe the fundamental processes that actually explain the observable regularities. Thus the aim of a materialist epidemiology would not be to deny the observed relationships between various diseases and different facets of the 'host,' 'agent,' and environment but rather to penetrate beneath the surface appearances described in statistical associations to the underlying socio-economic and historical context in which these associations are located" (1981, p. 27).

However, whilst a strong materialist/structural research tradition did develop in the health inequalities field through the 1980s and into the 1990s, in the wake of the Black Report (Department of Health and Social Security, 1980), this tended to be empiricist in nature, simply adding more social variables to an increasingly long list of risk factors. The more wide-ranging critique of positivism was largely lost until writers like Dean (1993) returned to theoretical matters. Today, a great deal of epidemiology and social survey work in the inequalities in the health field remains profoundly non-social in the sense that it does not explore the complex interactive relationship between individual experience, social action and the way in which societies are organised at a macro level.

Macintyre's critique of current research on inequalities in health provides a different but related perspective on the neglect of complexity, one focusing on the extent and nature of dualism in explanatory models in this field. In a recent research review (1997) she traces the continuities in modes of explanation of health determination and class differences in the patterning of death over the last 140 years in Britain. However, rather than focusing on positivism or the neglect of individual experience as key elements of these continuities, Macintyre explores explanatory discourses in their historical and political context and argues that for largely political and rhetorical reasons, explanations for inequalities in health have become unhelpfully polarised.

Of most significance for our purposes is the polarisation in explanatory approaches over the last 17 years along the lines of what Macintyre calls the "hard" versions of the four main categories of explanation for socioeconomic mortality differentials considered in the Black Report (DHSS, 1980): artifact explanations, theories of natural and social selection, materialist/structural explanations, and cultural/behavioural explanations. She argues that in research following the Black Report, there was "the sense that there were two or more opposing or polarised views, with proponents of each trying to convince the others, and an audience, of the correctness of their views" (Macintyre, 1997, p. 731). According to Macintyre, the proponents tended to adopt the position that explanatory approaches were mutually exclusive, setting up false antitheses: "selection versus causation," "artifact versus real differences," and "behaviour versus material circumstances" (1997, p. 740). She suggests that in more recent research the tendency to polarise positions has continued, noting, for example that "in the reaction to Barker's work (1991, 1994) on 'early life programming' the 'continued social disadvantage' theorists have rejected the former approach in its entirety; within the materialist/structural explanatory approach there has been a dichotomising into 'material' and 'psychosocial' factors such that these two components are seen to constitute competing and mutually exclusive explanations" (p. 737). Macintyre argues that health inequalities research now requires a move beyond this binary opposition so that a "more micro-level examination of the pathways by which social structure actually influences mental and physical health and functioning and life expectancy" (pp. 736–737) becomes possible. This, she suggests, would mean adopting a "more fine-grained" approach which explores not only the relative importance of categories of factors "but also their possible interactions or additive effects" (p. 740). Importantly, she notes that "the social context needs continually to be taken into account and is likely to result in more differentiated models (there is no a priori reason to suppose that the processes generating inequalities are the same at the top as at the bottom of the social scale, among men as compared with women, or in Northern Europe as compared with Mediterranean countries, the USA, or the Far East)" (p. 740).

Individuals and Social Structure

Neither Dean nor Macintyre explicitly addresses the neglect of individual agency within health inequalities research. It certainly does not figure in Macintyre's list of future research priorities. Paterson (1981) somewhat unusually does point to the potential theoretical significance of subjectivity, suggesting that by restricting science only to observables, positivism "specifically excludes any account of the experiences, perceptions, feelings and other subjective states of individuals," whereas a materialist epidemiology would "give consideration to subjective states and meanings" (pp. 26, 28). However, this is not a central issue in Paterson's work, nor does he explore the epistemological and methodological implications of this comment in detail. In contrast, recent sociological critiques of the conceptual foundations of health promotion (see, for example, Bunton, Nettleton, and Burrows, 1995) are centrally concerned with the neglect of the subjective—of individual lived experience—in much recent research and practice. Alongside Foucauldian analyses of epidemiology (Armstrong, 1983, 1993), these critiques suggest that the conceptualisation of the determinants of health found in health promotion, as in conventional epidemiology, are fundamentally modernist. Kelly and Charlton (1995) have argued, for instance, that despite being a product of postmodernism, health promotion's attachment to a social model of health does not signify a break with the tenets of "normal science." Rather, "the social model of health is, in this regard, no different to the medical model. In the medical model the pathogens are microbes, viruses or malfunctioning cellular reproduction. In the social model they are poor housing, poverty, unemployment and powerlessness. The discourse may be different but the epistemology is the same" (p. 82). This argument echoes that of Dean and Paterson. From a sociological perspective, however, Kelly and Charlton are concerned to point to a different set of problems which flow from a deterministic and dualistic stance: "Unemployment causes ill health. Deprivation causes disease. Society (the biggest system of all) is held to be at fault. . . . The individual is relegated to being nothing more than a system outcome, not a thinking and acting human being" (p. 83). Pointing to Giddens's structuration theory, they argue that developments in modern social theory may assist in resolving some of the difficulties in reconciling free will and determinism. In this body of work, they suggest, there may be concepts, or ways of thinking, which can help to enhance understanding of the interaction between the experience and action of individual human beings—seen potentially at least as creative agents acting on and shaping the world around them—and the structures of power and control within which they are embedded. As Kelly and Charlton note, "Such dynamic and reciprocal analysis of the individual set into context ought to be at the heart of health promotion. . . . Developing this, and making it work, is the task ahead" (p. 90). This task, daunting as it may be, is equally salient to health inequalities research in general.

Place and Time in Current Inequalities Research

Our earlier description of research within the inequalities field included a brief reference to studies which looked at the association between geographical area and patterns of mortality and morbidity. Much of this research has reproduced the same epistemological assumptions and methodological strategies evident in population health research. There has, for example, been relatively little work investigating the relationship between mortality and morbidity and the socioeconomic or cultural features of areas (Macintyre, MacIver, and Sooman, 1993). Nor is there much research which conceptualises "place" as the primary site for the impact of macro social structures to be played out in the daily lives of individuals.

In a recent review, Macintyre, MacIver, and Sooman (1993) divide existing research on place and health into two types: studies which focus on specific aspects of the physical environment and are concerned to provide information about the genesis of specific diseases and those which use area-level aggregate data to study the relationship between deprivation and mortality and/or morbidity. Focusing on these latter studies, Macintyre has further argued that whilst asset-based measures based on individuals, such as the car and home ownership variables used by Townsend and others in Britain, may do a good job of describing the social composition of an area, they do not describe other features of the area that may be health-promoting or health-damaging (1997, p. 173).

Phillimore (1993) similarly stresses the important conceptual and analytical distinction between characteristics of people and places, noting that "the characteristics of places may be as important as the characteristics of people for an understanding of particular patterns of health" (p. 176). As Jones and Moon (1993) argue in relation to research in the field of medical geography, "Seldom . . . does location itself play a real part in the analysis; it is the canvas on which events happen, but the nature of the locality and its role in structuring health status and health related behaviour is neglected" (p. 515).

The need for a re-conceptualisation of the notion of place is re-inforced by recent work demonstrating that places with similar socio-economic profiles can have very different population health profiles (Phillimore and Morris, 1991; Phillimore, 1993; Barker and Osmond, 1987). Similarly, Blaxter (1990) has noted that while men and women in manual occupations have worse health than those in non-manual occupations, the differences between them seem to be greater in "good" residential areas and industrial areas than in rural or resort areas. To understand these variations, we need a richer description of access to opportunity structures (good recreational and transport facilities, for example, as well as data on levels of crime and vandalism) that more adequately reflect an impoverished social topography (Macintyre, MacIver, and Sooman, 1993).

More profoundly, however, in re-conceptualising place it will be important to bring individuals into the analysis. What, for example, are the health consequences of being a materially deprived individual in a relatively prosperous place? How do individuals living in the most materially disadvantaged areas of societies make sense of and act upon their environments, with what consequences for their health and those they care for? What is the relationship between material risk, individual experience and action at the individual or group level? Much of this remains contested ground (see, for example, Sloggett and Joshi, 1994). Additionally, while new statistical techniques, such as multi-level modelling, may be brought to bear on such questions, the extent to which they offer good explanations, as opposed to good statistical descriptions, is a matter for theoretical debate.

There is some indication that research into health and place is beginning to include a focus on the experience and perspective of the people who live in the places being studied. In their recent research, for example, Macintyre and colleagues have given prominence to the importance of people's experience (Macintyre, MacIver, and Sooman, 1993). Sooman and Macintyre (1995) studied residents' perceptions of their local environment in four socially contrasting neighbourhoods in Glasgow. Six aspects of the areas—local amenities, local problems, area reputation, neighbourliness, fear of crime and general satisfaction—differed significantly between the neighbourhoods. They also found significant difference in levels of anxiety, depression and self-assessed health. The multivariate analysis they performed suggested that perceptions of the area acted independently of social class in influencing health differences between neighbourhoods. However, the quantitative, structured nature of this type of work means that it cannot explore the subjective—in the sense of capturing the meanings people themselves attach to experiences. In the words of Phillimore and Moffatt, "Whatever the methodological challenges involved, the voices of those living in local communities most at risk from possible environmental hazards must be heard" (1994, p. 150).

Any re-conceptualisation of place in health research must also pay more attention to the significance of time—both historical and biographical. The historical dimensions of place have been shown to be important in the work of Barker and Osmond (1987) exploring health variation in three Lancashire towns. This work highlights the significance of the socioeconomic history of places, pointing, in particular, to the contemporary health legacy of public housing initiatives begun at the end of the last century. Similarly, in his comparative work in Middlesborough and Sunderland, England, Phillimore (1993) has considered the role of a range of area characteristics, including economic/industrial history, pollution and cultural factors, in explaining area differences in patterns of mortality and morbidity. In the main, however, the historical dimension of places has been largely neglected in health inequalities research to date. As Mills (1959) argued, "Every social science—or better, every well considered social study—requires an historical scope of conception and a full use of historical material" (p. 145).

THE THEORETICAL SIGNIFICANCE OF PLACE AND LAY KNOWLEDGE IN INEQUALITIES RESEARCH

It is clear from the literature discussed so far that there is an urgent need for future research on inequalities in health to be more strongly informed by theory. We have also argued that the theoretical framework shaping future research in this field should give greater prominence than has hitherto been the case to the relationship between individual human agency and wider social structures. While the distinction between the layers of the Whitehead/Dahlgren model is a convenient one, these layers have thin membranes and interact in complex ways. As Tarlov has it, "the rings are porous. . . . [the model] is not like a game of pool wherein a ball in the outer ring strikes a stationary ball in the intermediate ring which in turn collides with a resting ball in the inner ring. . . . All of the balls are in motion most of the time" (1996, p. 83). This interaction or "porosity" between different layers of explanation is central to the work of social theorists such as Giddens (1984, 1991) and Bourdieu (1977, 1990). Both argue in effect for approaches to explanation in the social sphere that give due consideration to the combined effect of social structures and individual human agency. This argument is particularly relevant to future research on inequalities in health.

In this final section we suggest that two key developments are necessary to produce a richer and more dynamic framework for understanding the relationship between individual human agency, social structures and health inequalities. The first is to explore the conceptualisation and measurement of place within a historical context as the location in which macro social structures impact on individual lives. The second is to consider how places, conceptualised in this way, are understood within lay experience of the everyday life-world. In doing this we would be consciously exploring the connections between the sub-universes which people directly experience and the wider world which shapes those sub-universes (Schutz, 1962).

Reconceptualizing Place

The writings of social reformers in the last century provide fine detailed analyses of the relationship between health, wellbeing and place (broadly defined). The work of people like Engels, exploring the "ruinous and filthy districts" of Salford and Manchester, England, in 1842 (1969, p. 94), and of Mayhew (quoted in Hardy, 1993), revealing the places of work of the nineteenth century London labour force, is alluring because it focuses on particular features of the places in which people lived and worked: the effects of working in this occupation rather than that, or of living in this group of streets as compared with those half a mile away. In the absence of any theoretically sophisticated analysis of class and health, neighbourhoods and places were the natural focus for early public health analysis and in any event, epidemic infectious diseases did seem to strike particular localities, streets, and even households (Hardy, 1993; Chadwick, 1842).

Recent developments in research looking at place and health, briefly discussed above, suggest that a reconceptualisation of place is possible, recapturing and moving beyond the richness of this earlier work. There are, however, dangers in the seemingly innocent anthropological fascination with the particularities of places. It can, for instance, too readily lead to the stigmatising of neighbourhoods. Work on the "fear of crime," for example, shows that people's perceptions of personal safety in different neighbourhoods vary dramatically regardless of the actual differences in the likelihood of being mugged or burgled (Taylor, Evans, and Fraser, 1996). Particular areas of large cities, such as Moss Side in Manchester (Fraser, 1989), seem to retain a "reputation" long after the circumstances which gave rise to that reputation have changed. Research needs to be sensitive to these labelling processes.

These caveats notwithstanding, a refocusing on place in inequalities research may allow us to understand the dynamics of social class during a period when traditional class categorisations based on men's positions in the labour market are arguably less relevant than they have ever been. By looking at places with different social geographies and histories, we may be able to understand the "hidden injuries of class" (Sennett and Cobb, 1977), as well as their hidden sources of benefit, in a more sophisticated way than occupational classifications have allowed. The study of the places people inhabit may still allow us to explore the way in which structures work themselves through into the dynamics of everyday life. Places can be conceptualised as the locations for "structuration"—the interrelationship of the conscious intentions and actions of individuals and groups and the "environment" of cultural, social and economic forces in which people exist. Indeed, although the new interest in place can deflect attention from the continuing impact of the major social divisions of gender, class and ethnicity—encouraging the victim-blaming of particular working class households in places with "bad reputations"—it could equally provide a better context for exploring the dynamics of class in the context of the history and urban or rural geography of particular places.

In conventional studies of class and health, class is something that has become taken for granted both theoretically and in the methods that are used to measure it. As Macintyre, MacIver, and Sooman (1993) indicate, one of the implications of comparing places is that it allows for a much broader area-based definition of class. In addition to looking at the personal characteristics of individuals in households—income, occupation, and housing tenure—it is possible also to explore availability and price of good foods, recreational and sporting facilities, public transport, local health services and the safety and security of the local environment. In theorising place, we can gain much from looking at the writings of contemporary geographers and planners as they grapple with alternative notions of space and how we might collect information about place conceptualised in Aristotelian rather than Newtonian or Leibnizian terms (Curry, 1996). These approaches might allow for a theoretically and empirically more sophisticated approach to the operationalisation of concepts such as social capital and the social wage.

It is also necessary to develop a conception of both places and individuals in places that takes history and biography into account. Places have different histories, and the history and the present of a neighbourhood or locality will mean different things to individual people, who have their own temporal and historical associations with the area. People's relationships to places will be variable and diverse. For some people there will be one dominant place in which they spend much of their time. For others paid employment or education might involve extensive travel—and their relationship with the different places they inhabit might be more or less intense. The individual experience of place can be expected to be structured by gender, age, ethnicity, and other social factors—but individuals will be differentially and multiply positioned in relation to these aspects of social structures. Whilst some research has considered these issues in a spatial and quantitative way—mapping people's movement across physical space, time and social networks, for example—there is little, if any, work exploring the meanings people attach to their travels or how these meanings change over time.

Lay Knowledge, Narratives and Social Action

Places have histories, and people have biographies, which they articulate through stories or narratives. The history of sociology is replete with attempts to theorise this macro-micro link, to look at the intersection of history and biography, but the theoretical directions suggested by this work have rarely been taken up in empirical research on inequalities in health. Attention to the meanings people attach to their experience of places and how this shapes social action could provide a missing link in our understanding of the causes of inequalities in health. In particular, the articulation of these meanings—which we refer to as lay knowledge—in narrative form could provide invaluable insights into the dynamic relationships between human agency and wider social structures that underpin inequalities in health. As with the notion of place, however, the notion of lay knowledge requires re-conceptualisation if it is to fulfil this potential. Recent developments in social theory and research, in fields of study beyond those concerned with inequalities in health, point to possible directions for this reconceptualisation.

Williams and Popay (1998) have recently drawn a useful distinction between concepts which may help to link agency and structure and those which may link individuals to their capacity to act. In their discussion of a number of "mediating concepts," they also point to the substantive and methodological importance of narrative accounts of experience. In relation to the connection between structure and agency, for instance, Williams and Popay highlight the work of Janet Finch (1989). They discuss, in particular, the concepts of normative guidelines and time scales, which Finch develops out of people's narrative accounts of caregiving within families to help explain the non-material factors that shape people's action and how these change over time. Finch argues that these guidelines represent the "proper thing to do," but not in any simple way. Social norms and obligations shape individual behaviour, but in acting to "mobilize obligations," for example, people reproduce and mould these same norms and obligations in specific ways. In discussing the notion of "purposeful action," Finch points to the formative role of people's explanations for action: "People need to, and are able to, explain what they have done and why they have done it, and this in itself forms part of the action" (p. 88). In a similar way, developing the concept of "narrative reconstruction" as a means of understanding lay experiences of chronic illness, Williams (1984) has explored the way in which people living with chronic illness use this narrative knowledge, actively interpreting existing social norms and cultural values in order to pursue a virtuous course of action in response to the consequences of the illness (see also Williams, 1993).

In exploring ways in which individuals may be linked to their capacity for purposeful action, Williams and Popay (1998) point to the mediating potential of concepts such as autonomy, control and identity and to the central role of narratives in the construction of self-identity "An engagement with the understanding and structuring of self-identity is, according to Giddens, a characteristic of contemporary social life, not as a given but as something which individuals create and sustain through their own accounts (or narratives) of their life experience. . . . New circumstances, new risks, new identities (for example, created through divorce . . .) mean that people need to reassess the 'proper thing to do,' and one way they may do this is by recalling their experience and reconstructing their identities" (p. 15).

Williams and Popay (1998) further suggest that the concept of discourse, alongside that of identity, may also perform a bridging function because "it enables us to consider the structural and ideological influences upon people's lives in one frame" (p. 16). To illustrate this, they refer to research by Duncan and Edwards (1996), which explores the respective influence of discourses around motherhood and work on lone mothers' decisions about employment, compared to neo-liberal discourses around costs and benefits. In this work, too, the link between lone mothers' decision-making and discursive practices was drawn out from women's narrative accounts of their experiences.

Linking Narratives and Place

Until recently much of the work on people's narratives and stories has been empirical, but there has been a growing body of work at a theoretical level (see, for example, Hatch and Wisniewski, 1995; Hinchman and Hinchman, 1997; Somers, 1994). Somers's work is particularly interesting from the perspective of this chapter as it serves to link at a conceptual level lay knowledge in the form of narratives with our discussion above of place as the location for structuration.

Somers argues that recent research is revealing the substance of narratives as central to our understanding of social action, that social life is storied and that narrative is an ontological condition of social life . . . showing us that stories guide action; that people construct identities (however multiple and changing) by locating themselves or being located within a repertoire of emplotted stories; that 'experience' is constituted through narratives; that people make sense of what has happened and is happening to them by attempting to assemble or in some way to integrate these happenings within one or more narratives; and that people are guided to act in certain ways and not others on the basis of the projections, expectations and memories derived from a multiplicity but ultimately limited repertoire of available social, public and cultural narratives. [Somers, 1994, p. 614]

Narrative understanding, Somers argues, develops by connecting experience to structure in terms of a personal understanding of episodes rather than an abstract conceptualisation of events. Somers identifies four dimensions of narrative: ontological, public, conceptual, and "meta." Ontological narratives, she argues, are used to define who we are and are the basis for knowing what to do—akin to Finch's normative guidelines. It is through these that apparently disconnected sets of events are turned into meaningful episodes. Public narratives are those attached to cultural or institutional formations, such as families or workplaces, often by the mass media that transcend the individual. They often provide the legitimating context for ontological narratives. Metanarratives are "master" narratives of progress, decline and crisis which transcend the immediate context and are often used politically to construct a particular ideological position. Conceptual narratives are those which researchers construct using concepts that lie outside both ontological and public narratives, drawing on them both but introducing concepts, such as social class, behaviour change, mortality rate and so on which might not be found in either ontological or public narratives.

For Somers, the analytical challenge is "to develop concepts which will allow us to capture the narrativity through which agency is negotiated, identities are constructed and social action mediated" (1994, p. 620). She suggests that two central components here are narrative identity and relational settings, the latter being relations between people, narratives and institutions. These notions, she suggests, provide a conceptual bridge to (re)-introduce time, space, relationships and cultural practices into the process whereby people are categorised in research. In applying her arguments to an analysis of the relationship between social class and political action in the turbulent 18th century, Somers concludes that "from the narrative identity perspective, these same working classes would be seen as *members* of political cultures whose symbolic and relational *places* in a matrix of narratives and relationships are better indicators of action than their categorical classifications" (p. 625). This approach holds out the possibility of a deeper understanding of why different groups within the same class or social position can and do respond differently across the social and geographical landscape. Somers concludes her paper by arguing that as social scientists, "we need concepts that will enable us to plot over time and space the ontological narratives of historical actors, the public and cultural narratives that inform their lives, as well as the relevant range of other social forces—from politics to demographics—that configure together to shape history and social action" (p. 625).

The importance of seeing lay knowledge in its narrative form in this way is that it provides a different perspective on the relationship between individuals and the places, or "relational settings." in which they live. This perspective makes place more than a set of static environmental deficits or provisions, no matter how imaginatively these are operationalised, and it makes the life course more than a biological trajectory during which the individual is inertly exposed to various accumulating risks or benefits. It highlights the need to look not just at the statistical associations between significant events in people's lives as defined by researchers but at the meanings people give to the relationship between these events—how they translate events into meaningful episodes. In the context of inequalities in health it provides a strong case for looking at people's perceptions of episodes in their lives and the ways in which these may orient or fail to orient action at the individual or collective level. While narratives express a knowledge of the relationship between episodes over time, the relational settings which shape these narratives (and are shaped by them) also have a history and need to be explored in place and time.

CONCLUSION

Within the health inequalities field there is a widespread acceptance of the need for a deeper understanding of the relationship between individuals and their social context. What we are proposing here is a way in which the theoretical framework underpinning much of this work could be developed to provide this understanding. We have argued that the study of lay knowledge in the context of place and time should be central to this framework. It is the medium through which our understanding of the relationship between health and the places we inhabit is expressed. It is the means by which we locate ourselves within these places and determine how to act within and upon them. These places, in turn, are the site in which macro social structures impact upon individual lives. However, there are major barriers to the developments in inequalities research which would flow from this analysis.

First, major barriers flow from the way in which lay knowledge finds expression. Lay knowledge differs from expert knowledge in the sense that it has an ontological purpose, orienting behaviour in terms of an understanding to the individual's place in their life-world. It is, as we have argued, expressed in narrative form. This form is antithetical to traditional models of cause and effect, such as those given prominence within the inequalities research literature. Second, insofar as such narratives draw on or relate to wider public narratives (or discourses), they may also constitute a form of knowledge that challenges that of experts. Lay knowledge may stand not just as a different kind of knowledge but as knowledge which takes issue with the way in which media or experts characterise the relationships between events or the nature or needs and/or identity—on occasions forming what Nancy Fraser (1989) has described as "oppositional discourses." This challenge may hinder the developments in inequalities research we have argued for.

There is an on-going and welcome debate about the need for different and better research methods and techniques in the inequalities field and for greater collaboration between disciplines. However, to date this has largely failed to address the implications for future research which arise from the very different frameworks of understanding we have been discussing here.

What we are suggesting—to coin an old-fashioned phrase–is that people make their own history (and future)—but not always in conditions that they have themselves chosen. In order to further our understanding of the causes of health variations, we need to study directly the experiences of individuals and their biographies and link these to the social organisation of places and their histories. This analysis requires in turn an awareness of the influence of national and global socio-economic change. We would argue that this cannot be done without profound reconsideration of the scope and conception of social scientific investigations in the field of inequalities in health and its relationship to the work of other disciplines. What it means in practice is that the kind of social science we do should have four characteristics: it should ask questions about social structures and processes situated concretely in time and space, it should address processes over time and examine temporal sequences, it should look at the interplay of meaningful actions and social contexts and it should highlight the particular and varying features of specific structures and patterns (Skocpol, 1984).

References

Armstrong, D. *Political Anatomy of the Body: Medical Knowledge in Britain in the Twentieth Century.* Cambridge: Cambridge University Press, 1983.

Armstrong, D. "Public Health Spaces and the Fabrication of Identity." *Sociology,* 1993, *27,* 393–410.

Barker, D.J.P. "Fetal and Infant Origins of Adult Disease." *British Medical Journal,* 1990, *301,* 1111.

Barker, D.J.P. "The Foetal and Infant Origins of Inequalities in Health in Britain." *Journal of Public Health Medicine,* 1991, *13,* 64–68.

Barker, D.J.P. *Mothers, Babies and Disease in Later Life.* London: British Medical Journal Publications, 1994.

Barker, D.J.P., and Osmond, C. "Inequalities in Health in Britain: Specific Explanations in Three Lancashire Towns." *British Medical Journal,* 1987, *294,* 749–752.

Bartley, M., Blane, S. and Montgomery, S. "Health and the Life Course: Why Safety Nets Matter." *British Medical Journal,* 1997, *314,* 1194–1196.

Bartley, M., and others. "Birthweight and Later Socio-Economic Disadvantage: Evidence from the 1958 British Cohort Study." *British Medical Journal,* 1994, *309,* 1475–1478.

Ben-Shlomo, Y., White, I. R., and Marmot, M. G. "Does the Variation in the Socio-Economic Characteristics of an Area Affect Mortality?" *British Medical Journal,* 1996, *312,*1013–1014.

Blaxter, M. *Health and Lifestyles.* London: Routledge, 1990.

Bourdieu, P. *Outline of a Theory of Practice.* Cambridge: Cambridge University Press, 1977.

Bourdieu, P. *The Logic of Practice.* Cambridge: Polity Press, 1990.

Boyle, P. J., Gatrell, A. C., and Duke-Williams, O. "The Effect on Morbidity of Variability in Deprivation and Population Stability in England and Wales: An Investigation at Small-Area Level." *Social Science and Medicine,* 1999, *49,* 791–799.

Bunton, R., Nettleton, S., and Burrows, R. *The Sociology of Health Promotion: Critical Analyses of Consumption, Lifestyle and Risk.* London: Routledge, 1995.

Chadwick, E. *Report of an Enquiry into the Sanitary Conditions of the Labouring Population of Great Britain.* London: Poor Law Commission, 1842.

Charlton, D., and Murphy, M. (eds.). *Adult Health: Historical Aspects, 1850–1980.* London: Stationery Office, 1997.

Curry, M. "Space and Place in Geographic Decision-Making." In *Technical Expertise and Public Decisions,* Conference Proceedings, Princeton University, 1996, pp. 311–318.

Dahlgren, G., and Whitehead, M. *Policies and Strategies to Promote Social Equity in Health.* Stockholm: Institute for Futures Studies, 1991.

Dean, K. "Integrating Theory and Methods in Population Health Research." In K. Dean (ed.), *Population Health Research: Linking Theory and Methods.* Thousand Oaks, Calif.: Sage, 1993.

Department of Health and Social Security. *Inequalities in Health: Report of a Working Group Chaired by Sir Douglas Black.* London: Department of Health and Social Security, 1980.

Duncan, S., and Edwards, R. "Lone Mothers and Paid Work." *Social Politics,* 1996, *13,* 195–222.

Engels, F. *The Condition of the Working Class in England: From Personal Observation and Authentic Sources.* London: Panther, 1969. (Originally published 1842)

Fraser, N. *Unruly Practices: Power, Discourse, and Gender in Contemporary Social Theory.* Minneapolis: University of Minnesota Press, 1989.

Finch, J. *Family Obligation and Social Change.* Cambridge: Polity Press, 1989.

Giddens, A. *The Constitution of Society.* Cambridge: Polity Press, 1984.

Giddens, A. *Modernity and Self-Identity.* Cambridge: Polity Press, 1991.

Glennester, H. *The Future of the Welfare State: Remaking Social Policy.* London: Fabian Society, 1983.

Hall, A., and Wellman, B. "Social Networks and Social Support." In S. Cohen and S. L. Syme (eds.), *Social Support and Health.* London: Academic Press, 1985.

Hardy, A. *The Epidemic Streets: Infectious Disease and the Rise of Preventive Medicine, 1856–1900.* Oxford: Clarendon Press, 1993.

Hatch, J. A., and Wisniewski, R. *Life History and Narrative.* London: Falmer Press, 1995.

Health Education Authority. *Annual Report.* London: Health Education Authority, 1996.

Hinchman, L. P., and Hinchman, S. K. *Memory, Identity, Community: The Idea of Narrative in the Human Sciences.* Albany: State University of New York Press, 1997.

Illsley, R. "Social Class Selection and Class Differences in Relation to Stillbirth and Infant Deaths." *British Medical Journal,* 1955, *2,* 1520–1524.

Jones, K., and Moon, G. "Medical Geography: Taking Space Seriously." *Progress in Human Geography,* 1993, *17,* 515–524.

Kaplan, G. A., and others. "Inequality in Income and Mortality in the United States: Analysis of Mortality and Potential Pathways." *British Medical Journal,* 1996, *312,* 999–1003.

Karasek, R., and Theorell, T. *Healthy Work: Stress, Productivity, and the Reconstruction of Working Life.* New York: Basic Books, 1990.

Kelly, M., and Charlton, B. "The Modern and the Postmodern in Health Promotion." In R. Bunton, S. Nettleton, and R. Burrows (eds.), *The Sociology of Health Promotion: Critical Analyses of Consumption, Lifestyle and Risk.* London: Routledge, 1995.

Kennedy, B. P., Kawachi, I., and Prothrow-Stith, D. "Income Distribution and Mortality: Cross-Sectional Ecological Study of the Robin Hood Index in the United States." *British Medical Journal,* 1996, *312,* 1003–1007.

Macintyre, S. "The Black Report and Beyond: What Are the Issues?" *Social Science and Medicine,* 1997, *44,* 723–745.

Macintyre, S., MacIver, S., and Sooman, A. "Area, Class, and Health: Should We Be Focusing on Places or People?" *Journal of Social Policy,* 1993, *22,* 213–234.

Marmot, M. G., and others. "Employment Grade and Coronary Heart Disease in British Civil Servants." *Journal of Epidemiology and Community Health,* 1978, *3,* 244–249.

Marmot, M. G., and others. "Health Inequalities Among British Civil Servants: The Whitehall II Study." *Lancet,* 1991, *337,* 1387–1393.

Mills, C. W. *The Sociological Imagination.* New York: Oxford University Press, 1959.

Oakley, A. *Social Support and Motherhood: The Natural History of a Research Project.* Oxford: Blackwell, 1992.

Paterson, K. "Theoretical Perspectives in Epidemiology: A Critical Appraisal." *Radical Community Medicine,* Autumn 1981, pp. 23–34.

Phillimore, P. "How Do Places Shape Health? Rethinking Locality and Lifestyle in North East England." In S. Platt and others (eds.), *Locating Health: Sociological and Historical Explorations*. Aldershot, England: Avebury, 1993.

Phillimore, P., and Moffatt, S. "Discounted Knowledge: Local Experience, Environmental Pollution, and Health." In J. Popay and G. Williams (eds.), *Researching the People's Health*. New York: Routledge, 1994.

Phillimore, P., and Morris, D. "Discrepant Legacies: Premature Mortality in Two Industrial Towns." *Social Science and Medicine*, 1991, *33*, 139–152.

Power, C., and others. "Transmission of Social and Biological Risk Across the Life Course." In D. Blane, E. Brunner, and R. G. Wilkinson (eds.), *Health and Social Organization*. New York: Routledge, 1996.

Rorty, R. *Philosophy and the Mirror of Nature*. Oxford: Blackwell, 1980.

Schutz, A. *Collected Papers*. The Hague: Nijhoff, 1962.

Seeman, T. E. "Social Ties and Health: The Benefits of Social Integration." *Annals of Epidemiology*, 1996, *6*, 442–451.

Sennett, R., and Cobb, J. *The Hidden Injuries of Class*. Cambridge: Cambridge University Press, 1977.

Shy, C. M. "The Failure of Academic Epidemiology: Witness for the Prosecution." *American Journal of Epidemiology*, 1997, *145*, 479–487.

Skocpol, T. (ed.). *Vision and Method in Historical Sociology*. Cambridge: Cambridge University Press, 1984.

Sloggett, A., and Joshi, H. "Higher Mortality in Deprived Areas: Community or Personal Disadvantage?" *British Medical Journal*, 1994, *309*, 1470–1474.

Somers, M. R. "The Narrative Constitution of Identity: A Relational and Network Approach." *Theory and Society*, 1994, *23*, 605–649.

Sooman, A., and Macintyre, S. "Health and Perceptions of the Local Environment in Socially Contrasting Neighbourhoods in Glasgow." *Health and Place*, 1995, *1*, 15–26.

Syme, S. L. "To Prevent Disease: The Need for a New Approach." In D. Blane, E. Brunner, and R. G. Wilkinson (eds.), *Health and Social Organization*. New York: Routledge, 1996.

Tarlov, A. "Social Determinants of Health: The Sociobiological Translation." In D. Blane, E. Brunner, and R. G. Wilkinson (eds.), *Health and Social Organization*. New York: Routledge, 1996.

Taylor, L., Evans, K., and Fraser, P. *A Tale of Two Cities: Global Change, Local Feeling and Everyday Life in the North of England*. London: Routledge, 1996.

Thompson, E. P. *The Making of the English Working Class*. Harmondsworth, England: Penguin, 1993.

Titmuss, R. M. *Essays on the Welfare State*. London: Unwin, 1958.

Townsend, P., Phillimore, P., and Beattie, A. *Health and Deprivation: Inequality and the North*. London: Croom Helm, 1988.

Trichopoulos, D. "The Future of Epidemiology." *British Medical Journal,* 1996, *313,* 436–437.

Wadsworth, M. E. *The Imprint of Time: Childhood, History and Adult Life.* Oxford: Oxford University Press, 1991.

Wadsworth, M. E. "Health Inequalities in the Life Course Perspective." *Social Science and Medicine,* 1997, *44,* 859–869.

Wainwright, D. "The Political Transformation of the Health Inequalities Debate." *Critical Social Policy,* 1996, *49*(16), 67–82.

Whitehead, M. "Tackling Inequalities: A Review of Policy Initiatives." In M. Benzeval, K. Judge, and M. Whitehead (eds.), *Tackling Inequalities in Health.* London: King's Fund, 1995.

Whitehead, M., and Dahlgren, G. "What Can Be Done About Inequalities in Health?" *Lancet,* 1991, *338,* 1059–1063.

Wilkinson, R. G. *Unhealthy Societies: The Afflictions of Inequality.* New York: Routledge, 1996.

Williams, F., and Popay, J. "Developing a New Framework for Welfare Research." In F. Williams, J. Popay, and A. Oakley (eds.), *Welfare Research: A Critical Review.* London: University College Press, 1998.

Williams, F., Popay, J., and Oakley, A. (eds.). *Welfare Research: A Critical Review.* London: University College Press, 1998.

Williams, G. H. "The Genesis of Chronic Illness: Narrative Reconstruction." *Sociology of Health and Illness,* 1984, *6,* 175–200.

Williams, G. H. "Chronic Illness and the Pursuit of Virtue in Everyday Life." In A. Radley (ed.), *Worlds of Illness: Cultural and Biographical Perspectives on Health and Disease.* London: Routledge, 1993.

CHAPTER EIGHTEEN

The Limitations of Population Health as a Model for a New Public Health

Dennis Raphael
Toba Bryant

Population health has a variety of meanings, but in Canada it has come to signify the Canadian Institute for Advanced Research's (CIAR) analysis of how system-level variables influence the health of populations. The CIAR approach has influenced the direction of health policy in Canada, and there is evidence that it is poised to influence health policy in the United States. In this chapter, we argue that while CIAR concepts add to the debate concerning the determinants of health, its ascendence as a model for a new public health in Canada and elsewhere threatens progress in improving the health of populations.

Three propositions inform this analysis. The first is that while there are differing concepts of what constitutes population health—including differences in emphasis among CIAR adherents—an orthodoxy is arising of what constitutes the determinants of health and the means of examining their effects. The second proposition is that the CIAR version of population health limits consideration of various forms of evidence and means of improving health. The third proposition is that CIAR's lack of concern with social theory and values serves to conceal the potent social forces that influence the health of populations.

THE CIAR VERSION OF POPULATION HEALTH

The debate in Canada between health promoters and population health advocates is difficult for health workers to understand (Labonte, 1995, 1997; Coburn and Poland, 1996; Wong, 1997; Poland et al., 1998; Robertson, 1998). One barrier to understanding is that there has been little penetration of World Health Organization (WHO) concepts of health promotion into daily public health discourse, such that the term is limited to an emphasis on behavioural or lifestyle change. This has been less so in Canada, though a lifestyle emphasis continues to be the main focus of public health efforts (Raphael, 2000b). Another barrier to understanding is the complete paradigmatic dominance of epidemiology in public health research and planning in many nations. This epidemiological lens is the subject of much of this critique.

The CIAR population health approach was first described in the *Social Science and Medicine* paper "Producing Health, Consuming Health Care" (Evans and Stoddart, 1990) and further elaborated in the volume *Why Are Some People Healthy and Others Not? The Determinants of Health of Populations* (Evans, Barer, and Marmor, 1994). The most recent volume from the CIAR group is *Developmental Health and the Wealth of Nations* (Keating and Hertzman, 1999), which considers how early childhood development influences population health.

In this chapter, health promotion is defined as a values-based approach to promoting health that has its genesis in World Health Organization (WHO) concepts of health. A concise statement of these principles and health promotion actions is contained within the Ottawa Charter for Health Promotion (World Health Organization, 1986). Health is seen as a resource for daily living and health promotion is the process of enabling people to increase control over, and to improve, their health. Health is promoted through building healthy public policy, creating supportive environments, strengthening community action, developing personal skills, and reorienting health services. Histories of the field are available (Pederson, O'Neill, M. and Rootman, 1994; Pan American Health Organization, 1998), as are recent overviews (Scriven and Orme, 1996; Jones and Sidell, 1997; Katz and Peberdy, 1997; Macdonald and Davies, 1998; Naidoo and Wills, 1998).

Population health, as defined by the CIAR, considers processes by which system-level variables influence the health of populations. It operates within the epidemiological tradition of illness prevention and identification of cause and effect relations under a claim of scientific objectivity. Research on how income inequality affects population health contains aspects of a population health approach (Chapter Seven; Kawachi, Kennedy, and Wilkinson, 1999; Ross et al., 2000), as does recent work on the impact of race on health status (Krieger, 1987, 2000; Krieger et al., 1993). These latter researchers think about system-level factors, however, in more complex ways than do many CIAR writers.

Population health as developed by the CIAR is challenging health promotion as the dominant approach to Canadian public health policy. Its increased influence is seen in the renaming of government branches and departments, the content of many federal and provincial health documents, and the establishment of a national population health research institute that is well funded by the federal government (Robertson, 1998; Raphael and Bryant, 2000).

Why the CIAR version of population health has garnered such acceptance by Canadian governments at the expense of health promotion concepts remains unclear (Wong, 1997; Legowski and McKay, 2000). Canada was an acknowledged leader in health promotion, introducing its key ideas of reducing health inequities, empowering individuals and communities, and building healthy cities and communities through civic engagement and support of social infrastructure (Epp, 1986; Hancock and Duhl, 1986).

U.S. policy makers are now examining the value of CIAR population health concepts. The National Committee on Vital and Health Statistics of the Centers for Disease Control and Prevention is considering the relevance of CIAR concepts (National Center for Health Statistics, 2000); the National Policy Association solicited a CIAR fellow for a contribution to a volume on income, socio-economic status and health (Hertzman, 2001); the state of Minnesota identified health determinants clearly drawn from the CIAR list (Minnesota Department of Health, 1998); and the Population Health Group at the University of Washington is drawing upon CIAR work to advance its agenda of identifying societal-level influences upon population health (International Health Program, 2001).

At first glance, population health's ascendence may be due to its raising of important issues. According to CIAR fellow John Frank (1995) its tenets are:

1. The major determinants of human health status are cultural, social and economic.

2. Societies in which there is a high level and relatively equitable distribution of wealth enjoy the highest health status.

3. One's immediate social environment and the way this environment interacts with one's psychological resources and coping skills have a strong relationship with health.

4. The early developmental environment is important for health.

5. Health policy should take a broad multi-sectoral view.

6. New insights into health are likely to come from interdisciplinary research collaborations.

Frank argues, "a broad population health perspective requires us to examine with a critical eye the conditions of life and work that damage the health of our communities and, in the view of this author, to work to change them" (p. 164). This is a compelling vision that challenges the public health emphasis upon lifestyle choices. An illustration of the power of a population health approach toward understanding and working to influence health determinants can be seen in the reawakened interest in income and social status as a health determinant in the United States (Auerbach and Krimgold, 2001). But interest in income, class and health has a long history in the United Kingdom and elsewhere that existed well prior to the CIAR work (Townsend, Davidson, and Whitehead, 1992; Davey Smith, Dorking, and Shaw, 2001).

HOW IS POPULATION HEALTH DIFFERENT FROM HEALTH PROMOTION?

Frank's views are consistent with health promotion theory and practice. It has been noted, however, that "Frank has a very progressive viewpoint that may contrast with others in the population health camp" (Wong, 1997, p. 13). It is the viewpoints of these others—especially some of the most influential—in the CIAR population health camp with whom issue is taken.

Canadian documents such as *Population Health Promotion: An Integrated Model of Population Health and Health Promotion* (Hamilton and Bhatti, 1996) and *Taking Action on Population Health: A Position Paper for Health Promotion and Programs Branch Staff* (Health Canada, 1998) draw upon population health and health promotion concepts. To illustrate this, the Health Canada commissioned document *Population Health: Putting Concepts into Action* (Zöllner and Lessof, 1998) briefly discusses, but dismisses, the differences between health promotion and population health. It then outlines a values-based health promotion approach based on European Health for All (HFA) documents. The emphasis upon values of equity, solidarity, participation, sustainability, ethics and accountability is interesting, considering that statements of values are absent in CIAR discussions of health or its determinants, a theme returned to later.

The bulk of *Population Health: Putting Concepts into Action* is concerned with strategies to enhance population health. These include providing leadership, building partnerships, engaging the private sector, putting public health to work, looking for evidence and monitoring success, making population health attractive, and raising the stakes toward accountability. None of this is based upon CIAR population health work. Indeed, these ideas are drawn from health promotion principles and practices developed by HFA committees. Why population health is entered into this discussion at all is puzzling.

The key aspect of the CIAR version of population health is that economic and social forces serve as determinants of health. The most explicit presentation of the CIAR population health programme is contained in their Web site:

> Since its inception, the program has systematically explored socio-economic status (SES) gradients and their relationship to health outcomes. It is now well-established that, on average, people with higher levels of income, education, and social position live longer and are healthier than those at lower levels. Moreover, societies with greater variations in income, education, or social position tend to have higher levels of mortality. Program members are now furthering studies in this area by examining the SES gradient at the individual, neighbourhood, and community levels (CIAR, 2001).

CIAR has outlined 10 health determinants that have achieved an orthodoxy within Canadian government documents on population health. These are income and social status, social support networks, education, employment and working conditions, physical environments, social environments, biology and genetic endowment, personal health practices and coping skills, healthy child development and health services (Health Canada, 1998). Health Canada sees population health as a plan of action as well as a means of understanding health determinants: "Population health is an approach to health that aims to improve the health of the entire population and to reduce health inequities among population groups. In order to reach these objectives, it looks at and acts upon the broad range of factors and conditions that determine health" (Health Canada, 1998, p. 1). Health Canada's definition of population health is much more than the CIAR version. It is (i) a conceptual framework for thinking about health; (ii) a method for making decisions based on evidence; (iii) a framework for taking action; and (iv) an approach requiring collaboration among sectors for effective action. It is also more than the CIAR version of population health as it sees health as a capacity and a resource for living, which is not the case for the CIAR (see below). Health Canada documents also support pluralism in data gathering by accepting the validity of both quantitative and qualitative methods in needs assessment and evaluation—an idea absent from CIAR thinking.

It is important to consider to what extent the Health Canada version of population health diverges from the CIAR version, as contradictions that arise between these versions may need to be reconciled. Such reconciliations should consider what may be serious shortcomings in the CIAR approach as a model of a new public health.

Our main concern with the CIAR vision is its reliance on epidemiological thought. "Epidemiology—particularly in its most modern forms—is a militantly quantitative, empiricist discipline" (Williams and Popay, 1997, p. 260). CIAR also emphasizes scientific understanding over action. Finally, its lack of a critical perspective on the role of societal structures limits the likelihood that population health findings will effect significant policy change. Many of these issues were raised at the Roundtable on Population Health and Health Promotion held in 1996 and are still unresolved (Wong, 1997).

Population Health Is Rooted in Epidemiological Thinking

The CIAR version of population health is epidemiological in its orientation and incorporates the basic tenets of the biomedical approach to research. It emphasizes observables, specifies exposures to environmental stimuli, cause and effect relationships, and natural science methods involving quantitative data collection and experimental research designs. Not surprisingly, CIAR does not use the WHO definition of health as a resource for daily living: "Our work proceeds from a particular notion of 'health' about which it is important to be clear at the outset. For the most part we simply assume that health is the absence of illness" (Evans, 1994, p. 24). Macdonald and Davies state the issue as follows:

> There is a growing realization that traditional logical positivist approaches to health promotion research and evaluation no longer provide the right questions (or indeed answers) for many health promotion interventions. These approaches tend to be firmly rooted in the biomedical model and the origins of disease, which although the mainstay of many early health promotion research programs, are now giving way to more pluralist, post-modernist approaches, based on the origins of health (Macdonald and Davies, 1998, p. 1).

Another criticism of epidemiological approaches is the lack of interest in, and inability to focus upon, the lived experience of people (Lincoln and Guba, 1985; Raphael, 2000a). To validly assess need and to identify causes of phenomena requires recognition that individuals' motivations involve complex patterns of interactions and situations that cannot easily be dealt with through traditional approaches (Blaxter, 1990; Lincoln, 1994; Raphael et al., 2001b).

Population Health Lacks an Explicit Values Base

Consistent with its positivist orientation, the CIAR version of population health eschews any statement of values. Tesh outlines how particular theories of illness causation are inextricably linked to values and political ideology (Tesh, 1988). Seedhouse concurs, stating that all health-related research and practice decisions involve aspects of values, opinions and prejudice (Seedhouse, 1997). This is not problematic. What is problematic is not making explicit the values base underlying these decisions (Collins, 1995). The CIAR values base is that of not having a values base. CIAR writings therefore ignore important community health issues of participation, equity, community, collaboration and social justice (Minkler, 1997).

One result of this emphasis is a reliance on expert knowledge dominated by the use of large-scale data collection approaches that ignore individuals and the community within which they live. In essence, the population is taken out of population health. The CIAR version is also remarkably non-reflexive, the importance of which is described by Tesh: "The reality that truth is only dis-coverable by human beings, in all their humanness, does not mean that we must abandon the hope of finding it. We just have to hold facts lightly, contin-ually testing them against experience and logic, recognizing their connections to the rules and contexts within which they appear, and more important, never ceasing to scrutinize the values that necessarily permeate them" (Tesh, 1988, p. 177).

Population Health Neglects Political and Socio-Economic Forces

CIAR offers no theory of society (Coburn and Poland, 1996). Lack of a theory of society leads to a neglect of how the current state of health determinants come to be and the potent forces that either support or oppose the status quo. Population health has a troubling blind spot (as does health promotion at times) to work in the political economy area that sheds lights on the forces that drive health determinants.

To illustrate this, the work of North American Vicente Navarro, one of the most important contributors to the political economy of health literature and editor of the volume *The Political Economy of Social Inequalities: Consequences for Health and Quality of Life* (Navarro, 2001), is not mentioned in any CIAR work. Similarly, there is no place for consideration of the role of neoliberal ide-ology (Chapter Fourteen) or changing tax structures plays in population health (Raphael, 2001) because CIAR thinking is firmly rooted within biomedical con-cepts of health. It lacks a critical perspective that could consider the role of structural forces, specifically power, in the organization of societies and the effects these structures have on health determinants.

British population health workers have long maintained a critical approach that allowed consideration of societal organization and how it influences health (Gordon et al., 1999; Shaw et al., 1999a, 1999b; Pantazis and Gordon, 2000). It should not be surprising, then, that U.K. researchers have contributed to think-ing about social exclusion as a process by which health inequalities come about (Shaw et al., 1999a; Percy-Smith, 2000). U.S. researchers have also begun to evoke such a critical perspective in their population health work. Inquiries have been carried out into how racism (Krieger, 1987, 2000; Krieger et al., 1993), class relations (Muntaner and Lynch, 1999; Muntaner, Lynch, and Oates, 1999), the market economy (Navarro, 1998, 1999a, 1999b, 2000), and government ide-ology (Terris, 1999; Kaplan, 2001) affect the health of the U.S. population. This work shows how even within the epidemiological tradition, developments from political economy can illuminate the factors that affect health. Notwithstanding the importance of a critical perspective in population health work, there are still some intrinsic aspects of population health research methodology that bear scrutiny.

Population Health Leads to Context Stripping

Context stripping refers to research approaches that consider the health of individuals removed from the community and societal structures within which they live (Lincoln and Guba, 1985). It results from use of positivist models of understanding that seek to identify general laws of cause and effect or, in the case of health research, general risk and protective factors. Within the health field, context stripping manifests itself through large-scale studies that attempt to identify the general determinants of health for the entire population. Even though contextual variables can be introduced into study designs, these approaches are a pale version of the rich insights that can be gathered through ethnographic approaches.

In these approaches, the individual—his or her perceptions, behaviours and health status—becomes removed from the rich and complex environments, including communities, to which they are linked. The data that result from these studies cannot consider individuals' health in relation to local societal structures, nor do they consider the forces that influence how these societal structures are organized.

In the CIAR version of population health, analyses of how societal structures come to influence individuals' sense of control and well-being give way to study of personal coping devices and the biological mechanisms by which personal stressors become translated into illness and disease. Such individual-level analyses are important, but inquiry is directed away from critical analysis of societies toward studies focused on individual-level variables. Such context stripping within a population health framework is not inevitable, as shown by recent U.S. and Canadian analyses of health determinants (Frankish, Veenstra, and Moulton, 1999; Kaplan, 2001).

Population Health Provides a Model of Research, Not Change

The CIAR version of population health does not provide a model of change, and writings suggest that there is little interest among some CIAR adherents in instituting change. In *Why Are Some People Healthy and Others Not?* Evans wrote, "We cannot offer a detailed prescription of what is to be done" (1994, p. 24), a sentiment he repeated five years later at a population health conference (Evans, 1999). Additionally, there is a disturbing tendency among CIAR writings to ignore the problem of poverty—its causes, consequences, and solutions—a sentiment that, not surprisingly, was enthusiastically taken up by high-level government health bureaucrats who provided key note addresses at this same population health conference. In *Why Are Some People Healthy and Others Not?* Evans, after discussing the health differences that occurred among British civil servants in the Whitehall studies, states, "A common interpretation of the correlation between socioeconomic status and health—that the poor are deprived of some of the material conditions of good health and suffer from poor diet, bad housing, exposure to violence, environmental pollutants, crowding, and infection—cannot explain these observations. Indeed, a focus on poverty can block progress in understanding, because it can be dismissive of further questions" (1994, p. 5).

Besides the problem of using research about people not living in poverty to state conclusions about those who are, Evans's sentiments—which he repeated at the population health conference—should be especially welcome to government officials faced with high levels of family and child poverty. From any vantage point, poverty is clearly one of the strongest determinants of health (Reutter, 1995; Lessard, 1997; Canadian Institute on Children's Health, 2000), but from the CIAR perspective, focusing on poverty, and perhaps working to alleviate it, distracts us from asking "further questions." While pursuing further questions is a worthy goal, using research to improve the lives of the large number of citizens living in poverty should be one of the highest priorities among public health researchers.

Population Health Has a Top-Down Emphasis on Expert Knowledge

The CIAR framework emphasizes identification of risk conditions and behaviours that influence illness. These studies are important and serve to illuminate how, for example, the structure of economic inequality influences the health status of the population. What is disturbing, however, is the CIAR denial of the validity of alternate forms of knowledge such as lay knowledge, the importance of community participation, and the value of enabling and empowering people. These shortcomings have been ignored in the rush to incorporate "population health" principles into Canadian government health documents. It must not be forgotten that traditional biomedical and epidemiological approaches to health research can potentially work against health. This argument against biomedical and epidemiological approaches to health research is best stated by Davies and Macdonald: "Its underlying ideology is expert-driven, authoritarian and disempowering, seeking evidence through narrow clinically based methods and short-term quantitative outcome measures" (Davies and Macdonald, 1998, p. 209). One interesting illustration of this is an examination of the extent to which community members' perceptions of the determinants of health are consistent with those outlined by CIAR. The authors examined older persons' perceptions of the CIAR-identified determinants of health. In these projects, seniors did not find these concepts to be particularly meaningful, nor were these determinants consistent with their experiences of what determines health (Raphael et al., 2001a).

CIAR research projects involve large-scale quantitative data surveys that should certainly be part of any population health strategy. However, sole reliance on these methods can lead to context stripping, denigrating of lay knowledge, disempowering community members, and limiting focus and analysis to individual level processes.

AN ALTERNATE VISION: PUTTING THE POPULATION INTO POPULATION HEALTH

Problems associated with the CIAR version of population health have been outlined. Some considerations that should inform a new public health include the validity of lay knowledge, explicit statements of values, use of methods that identify the complexity of health determinants, acknowledging the political dimension in health research, and providing information for change. Many components of this vision are based on modern health promotion principles and practices.

Importance of Lay and Critical Knowledge

Park outlines three forms of knowledge (Park, 1993). *Instrumental knowledge* is also known as traditional, scientific, positivist, quantitative or experimental knowledge, and is the dominant paradigm in health research and in the CIAR version of population health. *Lay* or *interactive knowledge* is derived from lived experience. Also known as constructivist, naturalistic, ethnographic or qualitative knowledge, its focus is on meanings and interpretations individuals provide to events. *Critical knowledge* is reflective knowledge and is concerned with the role that societal structures and power relations play in promoting inequalities and disenabling people.

The increasing focus on lay and critical knowledge comes from three sources. The first is that lay and critical knowledge may more accurately reflect the kinds of information about health, health status and health determinants that are necessary to understand and improve health. The second source is a belief that to effect positive change, knowledge not only has to be derived from individuals but should be done in a manner that respects them and supports their autonomy and empowerment. The third is that traditional approaches, by limiting health research focus to variables that can be isolated and measured, are incapable of providing useful models of health and its determinants.

If public health research is to develop more robust and holistic explanations for patterns of health and illness in contemporary society and contribute to more appropriate and effective policies, then the key is to utilize and build on lay knowledge—the knowledge that lay people have about illness, health, risk, disability and death (Williams and Popay, 1997, p. 267).

Making Values and Principles Explicit

Tesh argues that adherence to a particular theory may be based more on values than on the available objective evidence. The current health debates about the determinants of health are about the relative importance of genetic, personal lifestyle and structural factors in determining health. Health promotion research and action have been informed by principles of equity, collaboration, participation and capacity building. These principles shape the forms and focus of health promotion research and action. The lack of an explicit set of principles by CIAR-oriented population health researchers does not mean that population health research does not have a set of principles but rather that these principles are hidden. And, it has been argued, these principles are not particularly oriented towards changing the status quo.

Recognizing the Complexity of Health Determinants

There is increasing focus upon political and social structures and how these influence health (Chapter Fourteen). CIAR-inspired health research, however, remains focused on individuals as a means of assessing broad health determinants. There is need to recognize the role that community structures play in mediating the effects of system level factors on individual health and well-being (Raphael, 2000a). Williams and Popay describe this issue as follows: "Population health research in the future must reinstate a political dimension to intellectual enquiry and develop more sensitive measures for exploring and understanding the context of people's lives" (Williams and Popay, 1997, p. 262). The most important and relevant work that has been done in identifying the contextual factors that support health has been carried out within the framework of the healthy cities movement (Ashton, 1992; Davies and Kelly, 1993). The healthy cities approach is based on principles of equity, justice, participation and support for institutions that enhance health.

Making Explicit the Political Dimension in Health Research

Biomedical approaches, despite their protestations of objectivity and detachment from politics, actually reflect conservative values of preserving the status quo (Seedhouse, 1997). Similarly, Seedhouse sees community development approaches as representing values of egalitarianism and social democracy. That all health research decisions involve aspects of ideology is not in itself problematic. What is problematic is not making explicit the values base underlying health research decisions. Political ideology influences the focus of research and the recommended responses to the problems identified through the research. As argued by Williams and Popay, "The future of population health requires attention to the politics of public health issues, from the multiple causes of inequalities in health to the complex issues of global economics involved in environmental pollution, and doing so through exploration of the many discourses which may have a contribution to make" (Williams and Popay, 1997, p. 273).

Part of working toward health is developing means of incorporating these ideas into a model of policy change. The public policy change process is informed by various conceptions of knowledge and how different groups in society use knowledge to influence policy outcomes (Bryant, 2002). The field of political science has developed models to explain the input of ideas and knowledge into the public policy process (Hall, 1993; Sabatier, 1993). Most of these models focus on the knowledge contributions of professional social and health scientists and not on the contributions of lay political actors. To develop relevant and effective public health policy, it is necessary that contributions of lay actors, i.e. non-experts, be valued and solicited.

In the CIAR version of population health, knowledge creation resides solely in the realm of health and social scientists. Additionally, valid knowledge is restricted to forms that are positivist, quantitative and reductionist. In the past, there has always been room for the contributions of both groups of actors: scientists and lay people. The CIAR version of population health has room for the contribution of only one group: the professional scientists. Such a view will not, in the short or long-term, improve population health.

WHAT IS TO BE DONE?

The deficiencies of the CIAR vision are focused in two key areas: the lack of a critical perspective and the reliance on one form of knowledge. U.S. and U.K. public health researchers have demonstrated that findings from well designed epidemiological studies can be understood within frameworks based on critical theory and political economy.

However, it is important to remember that the "new public health" is about the values of participation, enablement, empowerment, equity and social justice (Minkler, 1997; Robertson, 1999). As attempts are made to address inequalities in health, such efforts must be rooted within the communities with which public health workers are concerned. There is an emerging literature showing that such action will be most effective when the participation and understandings of citizens are incorporated into such actions (Williams and Popay, 1997).

Such ideas have seen application in community-based Canadian efforts such as the Pathways to Building Healthy Communities project in eastern Nova Scotia (PATH Project, 1997) and the Community Quality of Life project in Toronto (Raphael et al., 1999, 2001b). There, community members identify and act upon social determinants of health by drawing upon their experiences and developing critical understandings of how societies operate. Armed with these understandings, they identify policy issues that become the basis of efforts to influence government actions.

At the municipal, regional and national levels, public health workers can support citizens in examination and discussions of the importance of the social determinants of health. It is in these sorts of undertakings that the traditions of public health can combine with those of civic involvement and participation to create effective action to improve the health of the population. These lay perceptions of the determinants of health are remarkably similar to those identified in large-scale surveys. The difference is that in these approaches the complexity of determinants and their interactions are not only acknowledged but revealed as integrally related to local contexts, including municipal, regional, provincial and national policy decisions. Additionally, information is collected and considered in manners consistent with the principles and values of participation and respect. Results are presented in a manner that is likely to lead to change.

We have argued that implementation of the CIAR version of population health will not by itself support a new public health. By lacking an explicit values base and a critical perspective on health, it fails to provide an alternate vision of society. Unfortunately, in many nations, the status quo is one of consistent or increasing inequalities in health. Additionally, the current policy atmosphere is one of weakening communities by removing supports such as social safety nets. Health promotion points out these developments; CIAR population health does not. Policy makers should consider the benefits of both approaches as they develop means of improving population health.

References

Ashton, J. *Healthy Cities.* Maidenhead, England: Open University Press, 1992.

Auerbach, J., and Krimgold, B. *Income, Socioeconomic Status, and Health: Exploring the Relationships.* Washington, D.C.: National Policy Association, 2001.

Blaxter, M. *Health and Lifestyles.* London: Routledge, 1990.

Bryant, T. "The Role of Knowledge in Public Health and Health Promotion Policy Change." *Health Promotion International,* 2002, *17,* 89–98.

Canadian Institute for Advanced Research. "Population Health Program." 2001. [http://www.ciar.ca].

Canadian Institute on Children's Health. *The Health of Canada's Children: A CICH Profile.* Ottawa: Canadian Institute on Children's Health, 2000.

Coburn, D., and Poland, B. "The CIAR Vision of the Determinants of Health: A Critique." *Canadian Journal of Public Health,* 1996, *87,* 308–310.

Collins, T. "Models of Health: Pervasive, Persuasive, and Politically Charged." *Health Promotion International,* 1995, *10,* 317–324.

Davey Smith, G., Dorking, D., and Shaw, M. *Poverty, Inequality, and Health in Britain, 1800–2000: A Reader*. Bristol, England: Policy Press, 2001.

Davies, J. K., and Kelly, M. P. *Healthy Cities: Research and Practice*. New York: Routledge, 1993.

Davies, J. K., and Macdonald, G. "Beyond Uncertainty: Leading Health Promotion into the Twenty-First Century." In J. K. Davies and G. Macdonald (eds.), *Quality, Evidence, and Effectiveness in Health Promotion: Striving for Certainties*. London: Routledge, 1998.

Epp, J. *Achieving Health for All: A Framework for Health Promotion*. Ottawa: Health and Welfare Canada, 1986. [http://www.hc-sc.gc.ca/english/care/achieving_health.html].

Evans, R. G. "Introduction." In R. G. Evans, M. Barer, and T. R. Marmor (eds.), *Why Are Some People Healthy and Others Not? The Determinants of Health of Populations*. Hawthorne, N.Y.: Aldine de Gruyter, 1994.

Evans, R. G. Keynote address presented at the conference Population Health Perspectives: Making Research Work, Winnipeg, Manitoba, Canada, Oct. 7, 1999.

Evans, R. G., and Stoddart, G. L. "Producing Health, Consuming Health Care." *Social Science and Medicine*, 1990, *31*, 1347–1363.

Evans, R. G., Barer, M., and Marmor, T. R. (eds.). Why *Are Some People Healthy and Others Not? The Determinants of Health of Populations*. Hawthorne, N.Y.: Aldine de Gruyter, 1994.

Frank, J. "Why Population Health?" *Canadian Journal of Public Health*, 1995, *86*, 162–164.

Frankish, C. J., Veenstra, G., and Moulton, G. (eds.). "Advancing the Population Health Agenda." *Canadian Journal of Public Health*, 1999, *90*(Suppl. 1), S1–S75.

Gordon, D., and others. *Inequalities in Health: The Evidence Presented to the Independent Inquiry into Inequalities in Health*. Bristol, England: Policy Press, 1999.

Hall, P. A. "Policy Paradigms, Social Learning and the State: The Case of Economic Policy Making in Britain." *Comparative Politics*, 1993, *25*, 275–296.

Hamilton, N., and Bhatti, T. *Population Health Promotion: An Integrated Model of Population Health and Health Promotion*. Ottawa: Health Promotion Development Division, Health Canada, 1996. [http://www.hc-sc.gc.ca/hppb/phdd/php/php.htm].

Hancock, T., and Duhl, L. *Healthy Cities: Promoting Health in the Urban Context*. Copenhagen: World Health Organization European Regional Office, 1986.

Health Canada. *Taking Action on Population Health: A Position Paper for Health Promotion and Programs Branch Staff*. Ottawa: Health Canada, 1998. [http://www.hc-sc.gc.ca/hppb/phdd/pdf/tad_e.pdf].

Hertzman, C. "Population Health and Child Development: A View from Canada." In J. Auerbach and B. Krimgold (eds.), *Income, Socioeconomic Status, and Health: Exploring the Relationships*. Washington, D.C.: National Policy Association, 2001.

International Health Program. *Equity and Health*. Seattle, Wash.: International Health Program, 2001. [http://depts.washington.edu/eqhlth].

Jones, L., and Sidell, M. (eds.). *The Challenge of Promoting Health: Exploration and Action*. London: Macmillan, 1997.

Kaplan, G. A. "Economic Policy Is Health Policy: Conclusions from the Study of Income Inequality, Socioeconomic Status, and Health." In J. Auerbach and B. Krimgold (eds.), *Income, Socioeconomic Status, and Health: Exploring the Relationships*. Washington, D.C.: National Policy Association, 2001.

Katz, J., and Peberdy, A. (eds.). *Promoting Health: Knowledge and Practice*. London: Macmillan, 1997.

Kawachi, I., Kennedy, B. P., and Wilkinson, R. G. (eds.). *The Society and Population Health Reader*, Vol. 1: *Income Inequality and Health*. New York: New Press, 1999.

Keating, D. P., and Hertzman, C. (eds.). *Developmental Health and the Wealth of Nations*. New York: Guilford Press, 1999.

Krieger, N. "Shades of Difference: Theoretical Underpinnings of the Medical Controversy on Black/White Differences in the United States, 1830–1870." *International Journal of Health Services*, 1987, *17*, 259–278.

Krieger, N. "Discrimination and Health." In L. Berkman and I. Kawachi (eds.), *Social Epidemiology*. Oxford: Oxford University Press, 2000.

Krieger, N., and others. "Racism, Sexism, and Social Class: Implications for Studies of Health, Disease, and Well-Being." *American Journal of Preventive Medicine*, 1993, *9*(Suppl.), 82–122.

Labonte, R. "Population Health and Health Promotion: What Do They Have to Say to Each Other?" *Canadian Journal of Public Health*, 1995, *86*, 165–168.

Labonte, R. "The Population Health/Health Promotion Debate in Canada: The Politics of Explanation, Economics, and Action." *Critical Public Health*, 1997, *7*, 7–27.

Legowski, B., and McKay, L. *Health Beyond Health Care: Twenty-Five Years of Federal Health Policy Development*. Ottawa: Canadian Policy Research Network, 2000. [http://www.cprn.ca/cprn.html].

Lessard, R. *Social Inequalities in Health: Annual Report of the Health of the Population*. Montreal: Direction de la Santé, 1997.

Lincoln, Y. S. "Sympathetic Connections Between Qualitative Methods and Health Research." *Qualitative Health Research*, 1994, *2*, 375–391.

Lincoln, Y. S., and Guba, E. G. *Naturalistic Inquiry*. Thousand Oaks, Calif.: Sage, 1985.

Macdonald, G., and Davies, J. K. "Reflection and Vision: Proving and Improving the Promotion of Health." In J. K. Davies and G. Macdonald (eds.), *Quality, Evidence, and Effectiveness in Health Promotion: Striving for Certainties*. London: Routledge, 1998.

Minkler, M. *Community Organizing and Community Building for Health*. New Brunswick, N.J.: Rutgers University Press, 1997.

Minnesota Department of Health. *Healthy Minnesotans: Public Health Improvement Goals, 2004*. St. Paul: Minnesota Department of Health, 1998.

Muntaner, C., and Lynch, J. W. "Income Inequality, Social Cohesion, and Class Relations: A Critique of Wilkinson's Neo-Durkheimian Research Program." *International Journal of Health Services*, 1999, *29*, 59–81.

Muntaner, C., Lynch, J. W., and Oates, G. L. "The Social Class Determinants of Income Inequality and Social Cohesion." *International Journal of Health Services,* 1999, *29,* 699–732.

Naidoo, J., and Wills, J. *Practising Health Promotion: Dilemmas and Challenges.* London: Balliere-Tindall, 1998.

National Center for Health Statistics. *21st-Century Vision for Health Statistics.* Hyattsville, Md.: National Center for Health Statistics, 2000.

Navarro, V. "Neo-Liberalism, 'Globalization,' Unemployment, Inequalities, and the Welfare State." *International Journal of Health Services,* 1998, *28,* 607–682.

Navarro, V. "Health and Equity in the World in the Era of 'Globalization.'" *International Journal of Health Services,* 1999a, *29,* 215–226.

Navarro, V. "The Political Economy of the Welfare State in Developed Capitalist Countries." *International Journal of Health Services,* 1999b, *29,* 1–50.

Navarro, V. "Are Pro-Welfare State and Full-Employment Policies Possible in the Era of Globalization?" *International Journal of Health Services,* 2000, *30,* 231–251.

Navarro, V. (ed.). *The Political Economy of Social Inequalities: Consequences for Health and Quality of Life.* Amityville, N.Y.: Baywood Press, 2001.

Pan American Health Organization. *Health Promotion: An Anthology.* New York: Pan American Health Organization, 1998.

Pantazis, C., and Gordon, D. (eds.). *Tackling Inequalities: Where Are We Now and What Can Be Done?* Bristol, England: Policy Press, 2000.

Park, P. "What Is Participatory Research? A Theoretical and Methodological Perspective." In P. Park and others (eds.), *Voices of Change: Participatory Research in the United States and Canada.* Toronto: Greenwood, 1993.

PATH Project. *Pathways to Building Healthy Communities in Eastern Nova Scotia: The PATH Project Resource.* Antigonish, Nova Scotia, Canada: People Assessing Their Health, 1997.

Pederson, A., O'Neill, M., and Rootman, I. *Health Promotion in Canada: Provincial, National, and International Perspectives.* Toronto: Saunders, 1994.

Percy-Smith, J. *Policy Responses to Social Exclusion: Towards Inclusion?* Maidenhead, England: Open University Press, 2000.

Poland, B., and others. "Wealth, Equity, and Health Care: A Critique of a Population Health Perspective on the Determinants of Health." *Social Science and Medicine,* 1998, *46,* 785–798.

Raphael, D. "Health Inequalities in Canada: Current Discourses and Implications for Public Health Action." *Critical Public Health,* 2000a, *10,* 193–216.

Raphael, D. "The Question of Evidence in Health Promotion." *Health Promotion International,* 2000b, *15,* 355–367.

Raphael, D. "From Increasing Poverty to Societal Disintegration: How Economic Inequality Affects the Health of Individuals and Communities." In H. Armstrong, R. Armstrong, and D. Coburn (eds.), *Unhealthy Times: The Political Economy of Health and Health Care in Canada.* Toronto: Oxford University Press, 2001.

Raphael, D., and Bryant, T. "Putting the Population into Population Health." *Canadian Journal of Public Health,* 2000, *91,* 9–12.

Raphael, D., and others. "The Community Quality of Life Project: A Health Promotion Approach to Understanding Communities." *Health Promotion International,* 1999, *14,* 197–207.

Raphael, D., and others. "How Government Policy Decisions Affect Seniors' Quality of Life: Findings from a Participatory Policy Study Carried Out in Toronto, Canada." *Canadian Journal of Public Health,* 2001a, *92,* 190–195.

Raphael, D., and others. "Making the Links Between Community Structure and Individual Well-Being: Community Quality of Life in Riverdale, Toronto, Canada." *Health and Place,* 2001b, *7*(3), 17–34.

Reutter, L. "Poverty and Health: Implications for Public Health." *Canadian Journal of Public Health,* 1995, *86,* 149–151.

Robertson, A. "Shifting Discourses on Health in Canada: From Health Promotion to Population Health." *Health Promotion International,* 1998, *13,* 155–166.

Robertson, A. "Health Promotion and the Common Good: Theoretical Considerations." *Critical Public Health,* 1999, *9,* 117–133.

Ross, N., and others. "Income Inequality and Mortality in Canada and the United States." *British Medical Journal,* 2000, *320,* 898–902.

Sabatier, P. A. "Policy Change over a Decade or More." In P. A. Sabatier and H. C. Jenkins-Smith (eds.), *Policy Change and Learning: An Advocacy Coalition Approach.* Boulder, Colo.: Westview Press, 1993.

Scriven, A., and Orme, J. (eds.). *Health Promotion: Professional Perspectives.* London: Macmillan, 1996.

Seedhouse, D. *Health Promotion: Philosophy, Prejudice, and Practice.* New York: Wiley, 1997.

Shaw, M., and others. "Poverty, Social Exclusion, and Minorities." In M. G. Marmot and R. G. Wilkinson (eds.), *Social Determinants of Health.* Oxford: Oxford University Press, 1999a.

Shaw, M., and others. *The Widening Gap: Health Inequalities and Policy in Britain.* Bristol, England: Policy Press, 1999b.

Terris, M. "The Neoliberal Triad of Anti-Health Reforms. Government Budget Cutting, Deregulation, and Privatization." *Journal of Public Health* Policy, 1999, *20,* 149–167.

Tesh, S. N. *Hidden Arguments: Political Ideology and Disease Prevention Policy.* New Brunswick, N.J.: Rutgers University Press, 1988.

Townsend, P., Davidson, N., and Whitehead, M. (eds.). *Inequalities in Health: The Black Report and the Health Divide.* New York, Penguin, 1992.

Williams, G., and Popay, J. "Social Science and the Future of Population Health." In L. Jones and M. Sidell (eds.), *The Challenge of Promoting Health: Exploration and Action.* London: Macmillan, 1997.

Wong, D. *Paradigms Lost: Examining the Impact of a Shift from Health Promotion to Population Health on HIV/AIDS Policy and Program in Canada.* Ottawa: Canadian AIDS Society, 1997.

World Health Organization. *Ottawa Charter on Health Promotion.* Geneva: World Health Organization, 1986.

Zöllner, H., and Lessof, S. "Population Health: Putting Concepts into Action." Copenhagen: World Health Organization European Regional Office. 1998. [http://www.hc-sc.gc.ca/hppb/phdd/pube/report.html].

CHAPTER NINETEEN

Theories for Social Epidemiology in the Twenty-First Century

An Ecosocial Perspective

Nancy Krieger

Both thinking and facts are changeable,
if only because changes in thinking manifest themselves in changed facts.
Conversely, fundamentally new facts can be discovered only through new thinking.
—Ludwick Fleck, 1935, pp. 50–51

Once we recognize the state of the art is a social product,
we are freer to look critically at the agenda of our science,
its conceptual framework, and accepted methodologies,
and to make conscious research choices.
—Richard Levins and Richard Lewontin, 1987, p. 286

In social epidemiology, to speak of theory is simultaneously to speak of society and biology. It is, I will argue, to speak of embodiment. At issue is how we literally incorporate, biologically, the world around us, a world in which we simultaneously are but one biological species among many—and one whose labour and ideas literally have transformed the face of this earth. To conceptualize and elucidate the myriad social and biological processes resulting in embodiment and its manifestation in populations' epidemiological profiles, we need theory. This is because theory helps us structure our ideas, so as to explain

This chapter was originally prepared as a paper for Theory and Action, a series of meetings to link research and practice, London, England, 27–29 March 2000. Sponsored by World Health Organization, Centers for Disease Control and Prevention, and United Kingdom Health Development Agency. It was originally published in the *International Journal of Epidemiology* 2001; 30:668–677.

Thanks to Sofia Gruskin, Mary Basset, George Davey Smith, and also to two anonymous reviewers for their helpful comments. No funds from any grant supported this project. A small honorarium, however, was paid by the organizers of the Theory and Action conference at which a preliminary version of this chapter was first presented.

causal connections between specified phenomena within and across specified domains by using interrelated sets of ideas whose plausibility can be tested by human action and thought (Fleck, 1935; Levins and Lewontin, 1987; Ziman, 1984). Grappling with notions of causation, in turn, raises not only complex philosophical issues but also, in the case of social epidemiology, issues of accountability and agency: simply invoking abstract notions of "society" and disembodied "genes" will not suffice. Instead, the central question becomes: who and what are responsible for population patterns of health, disease, and well-being, as manifested in present, past and changing social inequalities in health?

Not surprisingly, theorizing about social inequalities in health runs deep. One reason is that it is fairly obvious that population patterns of good and bad health mirror population distributions of deprivation and privilege. Comments to this effect can be found in the Hippocratic corpus and in early texts of ancient Chinese medicine (Lloyd, 1983; Veith, 1966). Shared observations of disparities in health, however, do not necessarily translate to common understandings of cause; it is for this reason theory is key. Consider only centuries of debate in the United States over the poor health of black Americans. In the 1830s and 1840s, contrary schools of thought asked: is it because blacks are intrinsically inferior to whites?—the majority view, or because they are enslaved?—as argued by Dr. James McCune Smith (1811–1865) and Dr. James S. Rock (1825–1866), two of the country's first credentialled African American physicians (Krieger, 1987). In contemporary parlance, the questions become: do the causes lie in bad genes? bad behaviours? or accumulations of bad living and working conditions born of egregious social policies, past and present? (Krieger, 2000a; Williams, 1999). The fundamental tension, then and now, is between theories that seek causes of social inequalities in health in innate versus imposed, or individual versus societal, characteristics.

Yet despite the key role of theory explicit or implicit, in shaping what it is we see—or do not see, what we deem knowable—or irrelevant, and what we consider feasible—or insoluble, literature articulating the theoretical frameworks informing research and debates in social epidemiology—and epidemiology more broadly—is sparse (Stallones, 1980; Krieger, 1994; Krieger and Zierler, 1995; Schwartz, Susser, and Susser, 1999). In this chapter, I accordingly note the emergence of self-designated social epidemiology in the mid-20th century, review key theories invoked by contemporary social epidemiologists, and highlight the need for advancing theories useful for the 21st century.

SOCIAL EPIDEMIOLOGY GAINS A NAME

Building on holistic models of health developed between World War I and World War II and on the "social medicine" framework forged during the 1940s (Lawrence and Weisz, 1998; Galdston, 1947; Ryle, 1948; Porter 1997), it is in the mid-20th century that "social epidemiology" gains its name-as-such. The term apparently first appears in the title of an article published by Alfred Yankauer in the *American Sociological Review* in 1950: "The Relationship of Fetal and Infant Mortality to Residential Segregation: An Inquiry into Social Epidemiology," (Yankauer, 1950), a topic as timely now as it was then; Yankauer later becomes editor of the *American Journal of Public Health*. The term then reappears in the introduction to one of the first books pulling together the behavioural and medical sciences, edited by E. Gartly Jaco, published in 1958, *Patients, Physicians, and Illness: Sourcebook in Behavioral Science and Medicine* (Jaco, 1958), and is included in the title of Jaco's next book, *The Social Epidemiology of Mental Disorders: A Psychiatric Survey of Texas* (Jaco, 1960), published in 1960. By 1969, enough familiarity with the field exists that Leo G. Reeder presents a major address to the American Sociological Association called "Social Epidemiology: An Appraisal." Defining social epidemiology as the "study of the role of social factors in the aetiology of disease, he asserts that "social epidemiology . . . seeks to extend the scope of investigation to include variables and concepts drawn from a theory" (1972, p. 97)—in effect, calling for a marriage of sociological frameworks to epidemiological inquiry.

Soon thereafter, the phrase "social epidemiology" catches on in the epidemiological literature. Articles appear with such titles as "Contributions of Social Epidemiology to the Study of Medical Care Systems" (Syme, 1971) and "Social Epidemiology and the Prevention of Cancer" (Graham and Schneiderman, 1972). By the end of the century, the first textbook is published with the title *Social Epidemiology,* co-edited by Lisa Berkman and Ichiro Kawachi (2000). Despite these gains, it is nevertheless sobering to realize that among the slightly over 432,000 articles indexed in Medline by the keyword *epidemiology* between 1966 and 2000, only 4% also employ the keyword *social,* and—as Reeder surely would be sorry to learn—fewer than 0.1 % are additionally indexed by the term *theory.* Clearly, there is room for improvement—and reflection.

CURRENT THEORETICAL TRENDS IN SOCIAL EPIDEMIOLOGY

Contemporary social epidemiology, however, is not without its theories. The three main theories explicitly invoked by practising social epidemiologists are: (1) psychosocial, (2) social production of disease and/or political economy of health, and (3) ecosocial theory and related multi-level frameworks. All seek to elucidate principles capable of explaining social inequalities in health, and all represent what I would term theories of *disease distribution* (Krieger, 2000b), which presume but cannot be reduced to mechanism-oriented theories of *disease causation.* Where they differ is in their respective emphasis on different aspects of social and biological conditions in shaping population health, how they integrate social and biological explanations, and thus their recommendations for action.

PSYCHOSOCIAL THEORY

First, psychosocial theory. As is typically the case with scientific theories (Fleck, 1935; Levins and Lewontin, 1987; Ziman, 1984), its genesis can be traced to problems that prior paradigms could not explain, in this case, why it is that not all people exposed to germs become infected and not all infected people develop disease (Greenwood, 1935; Dubos, 1959). One response, first articulated in the 1920s (Frost, [1928] 1976; Lawrence and Weisz, 1998) and refined in the 1950s as epidemiologists increasingly study cancer and cardiovascular disease, is to expand the aetiological framework from simply "agent" to "host-agent-environment" (Gordon, 1953; Galdston, 1954). Despite conceptual expansion, several restrictive assumptions still pervade the new framework's very language (Krieger, 1994). "Agency," for example, remains located in the "agent"—typically an exogenous entity that acts upon a designated "host"; terminology alone renders it inhospitable to conceive of the host having agency! "Environment," moreover, serves as a catch-all category with no distinctions offered between the natural world, of which we humans are a part and can transform, and social institutions and practices which we, as humans, create and for which we can hold each other accountable. Gaining complexity without an explicit accounting of social agency, the model becomes increasingly diffuse and, by 1960, the spiderless "web of causation" is born (Krieger, 1994).

The importance of the "host-agent-environment" model for psychosocial epidemiology is evidenced by the title of one of the field's still-defining papers: John Cassel's (1921–1976) final opus, "The Contribution of the Social Environment to Host Resistance." Published in the *American Journal of Epidemiology* in 1976, the year of Cassel's death, this article expands upon frameworks elaborated in the 1940s and 1950s linking vulnerability to disease to both physical and psychological stress (Gordon, 1953; Galdston, 1954; Lawrence and Weisz, 1998). Positing that in "modern" societies exposure to pathogenic agents is ubiquitous, Cassel argues that to explain disease distribution we must therefore investigate factors affecting susceptibility: "The question facing epidemiological inquiry then is, are there categories or classes of environmental factors that are capable of changing human resistance in important ways and making subsets of people more or less susceptible to these ubiquitous agents in our environment?" (1976, p. 108).

To Cassel, in prosperous nations, relevant modifying factors are unlikely to include "nutritional status, fatigue, overwork, or the like" (1976, p. 108). More promising candidates lie in what he calls the "social environment," comprised of psychosocial factors generated by human interaction.

Cassel's central hypothesis is that the social environment alters host susceptibility by affecting neuroendocrine function. His list of relevant psychosocial factors includes: dominance hierarchies; social disorganization and rapid social change; marginal status in society, including social isolation; bereavement; and, acting as a buffer to all of the above, the "psychosocial asset" of "social support." In Cassel's view, these psychosocial factors, considered together, explain the puzzle of why particular social groups are disproportionately burdened by otherwise markedly distinct diseases, e.g., tuberculosis, schizophrenia and suicide. Shifting attention from "specific aetiology" to "generalized susceptibility"—while acknowledging that what disease a person gets is dependent on prior exposures—Cassel ultimately concludes that, in his own words, the most "feasible" and promising interventions to reduce disease will be "to improve and strengthen the social supports rather than reduce the exposure to stressors" (1976, p. 121).

Following Cassel's article, research in psychosocial epidemiology blossoms. Between 1966 and 1974, the keywords *psychosocial* and *epidemiology* together index only 40 articles in Medline; between 1995 and 1999 alone, the number jumps to nearly 1,200. Indicating new ideas are in the air, new polysyllabic terms emerge—such as *psychoneuroendocrinology* (Smythies, 1976), *psychoneuroimmunology* (Masek and others, 2000), and *biopsychosocial* (Engel, 1978)—whose proliferating prefixes hint that some important concepts have yet to be tabbed down. Fortunately, newer additions gaining currency are appreciably shorter. One is *allostasis,* introduced as an alternative to *homeostasis* in 1988 by Peter Sterling and Joseph Eyer to describe systems that achieve balance through change. Its successor, *allostatic load,* is then introduced by Bruce McEwen to describe "wear-and-tear from chronic overactivity or underactivity" of systems "that protect the body by responding to internal and external stress," including "the autonomic nervous system, the hypothalamic-pituitary-adrenal (HPA) axis, and cardiovascular, metabolic, and immune systems" (1998, p. 171). One new implication is that psychosocial stressors can be directly pathogenic, rather than alter only susceptibility. And consonant with the emerging lifecourse perspective—which holds that health status at any given age reflects not only contemporary conditions but prior living circumstances, in utero onwards (Kuh and Ben-Shlomo, 1997)—*allostatic load* draws attention to long-term effects of both chronic and acute stressors. Other new work extends Cassel's insights to focus on "social capital" and "social cohesion," which—although defined differently by diverse schools (Portes, 1998)—are construed (and contested) as population-level psychosocial assets which shape population health by influencing norms and strengthening bonds of "civil society" (Kawachi and Berkman, 2000; Wilkinson, 1996; Lynch and others, 2000; Baum, 1999).

In summary, then, a psychosocial framework directs attention to endogenous biological responses to human interactions. Its focus is on responses to stress and on stressed people in need of psychosocial resources. Comparatively less attention, theoretically and empirically, is accorded to: (1) who and what generate psychosocial insults and buffers, and (2) how their distribution—along with that of ubiquitous or non-ubiquitous pathogenic physical, chemical, or biological agents—is shaped by social, political and economic policies. Time also takes a back seat, in that except for reference to periods of rapid social change, the question of whether changing levels of stress are sufficient to explain secular trends in disease and death receives little attention. It is as if, paraphrasing Aaron Antonovsky's (1923–1994) penultimate lament (1987), the study of why some people swim well and others drown when tossed into a river displaces study of who is tossing whom into the current—and what else might be in the water. To ask the latter questions, however, brings us to other schools of thought.

SOCIAL PRODUCTION OF DISEASE/ POLITICAL ECONOMY OF HEALTH

A second theoretical framework accordingly introduces agency to the "upstream-downstream" metaphors increasingly invoked in social epidemiology today (McKinlay and Marceau, 2000; Susser, 1999; McMichael, 1999). Hearkening back to social analyses of health of the 1830s and 1840s, as well as 1930s and 1940s, this school of thought—emerging in the politically turbulent 1960s and 1970s—focuses on what it terms the "social production of disease" and/or "political economy of health" (Doyal, 1979; Breilh, 1979; Conrad and Kern, 1981a). Articles appear with such titles as: "A Case for Refocusing Upstream: The Political Economy of Illness" (McKinlay, 1979), "The Social Production of Disease and Illness" (Conrad and Kern, 1981b), and—recalling the trend's Marxist origins and its advocacy of "materialist" analyses of health, even: "Hypertension in American Society: An Introduction to Historical Materialist Epidemiology" (Schnall and Kern, 1981). These and kindred papers are published, however, in journals unlikely to be on the regular browsing list of most epidemiologists—for example, the *International Journal of Health Services,* founded in 1971 by Vincente Navarro (Navarro, 1971), and *Review of Radical Political Economics* (Eyer and Sterling, 1977). By 1979, the trend's broad theoretical contours are encapsulated in two books: *The Political Economy of Health* by Lesley Doyal (Doyal, 1979), a British health policy analyst, and *Epidemiología Economía Medicina y Política,* by Jamie Breilh, an Ecuadorian epidemiologist (Breilh, 1979).

Arising in part as critique of proliferating blame-the-victim "lifestyle" theories, which emphasize individuals' responsibility to "choose" so-called healthy lifestyles and to cope better with stress (Doyal, 1979; Crawford, 1977; Navarro, 1986; Tesh, 1988), these new analyses explicitly address economic and political determinants of health and disease, including structural barriers to people living healthy lives (Doyal, 1979; Breilh, 1979; Conrad and Kern, 1981a; Eyer and

Sterling, 1977; Crawford, 1977; Navarro, 1986; Sanders, 1985; Tesh, 1988; Turshen, 1989). At issue are priorities of capital accumulation and their enforcement by the state, so that the few can stay rich (or become richer) while the many are poor (Townsend, 1986)—whether referring to nations or to classes within a specified country. Recast in this manner, determinants of health are analysed in relation to who benefits from specific policies and practices, at whose cost. Core questions include: how does prioritizing capital accumulation over human need affect health, as evinced through injurious work-place organization and exposure to occupational hazards, inadequate pay scales, profligate pollution, and rampant commodification of virtually every human activity, need, and desire? What, too, is the public health impact of state policies enforcing these priorities?—whether by regulation or de-regulation of corporations, the real estate industry, and interest rates; or by enactment or repeal (or enforcement or neglect) of tax codes, trade agreements, labour laws, and environmental laws; or by absolute and relative levels of spending on social programmes versus prisons and the military; or by diplomatic relations with, economic domination of, and even invasion of countries abroad? The underlying hypothesis is that economic and political institutions and decisions that create, enforce, and perpetuate economic and social privilege and inequality are root—or "fundamental"—causes of social inequalities in health. Revisiting issues of agency and accountability, theoretical analyses examine interdependence of institutional and interpersonal manifestations of unjust power relations; resources to counter these adverse conditions are reframed, no longer "buffers" but rather strategies for community (not just individual) "empowerment" and social change (Tesh, 1988).

Within this trend, initial conceptual and empirical analyses chiefly focus on class inequalities in health within and between countries (Kitagawa and Hauser, 1973; Black and others, 1982; Navarro, 1986). Related contemporary questions include: what are the health impacts of rising income inequality, of structural adjustment programmes imposed by the International Monetary Fund and the World Bank, of neoliberal economic policies favouring dismantling of the welfare state, or of free-trade agreements imposed by the World Trade Organization? (Wilkinson, 1996; Kim and others, 2000; Bijlmakers, Bassett, and Sanders, 1996; Wise, Chavkin, and Romero, 1999; O'Campo and Rojas-Smith, 1998; Scott-Samuel, 1998). Other analyses address social inequalities involving race/ethnicity, gender and sexuality, as they play out within and across socioeconomic position, within and across diverse societies. Relevant questions include: what are the health consequences of experiencing economic and non-economic forms of racial discrimination? (Krieger, 2000a; Williams, 1999)—or of men dominating and abusing women? (Doyal, 1995; Fee and Krieger, 1994; Ruzek, Olesen, and Clarke, 1997)—or of civilians and soldiers verbally or physically queer-bashing lesbian, gay, and transgendered people? (Solarz, 1999; American Medical Association, 1996; Krieger and Sidney, 1997; Meyer, 1995;

Becker, 2000). Recently emerging environmental justice movements likewise bring critical attention to corporate decisions and government complicity in transferring toxic waste to poor countries and to poor regions within wealthy countries, especially poor communities of colour (Kim and others, 2000; Committee on Environmental Justice, 1999). The call for action premised on this framework is thus, minimally, for "healthy public policies," especially redistributive polices to reduce poverty and income inequality (Shaw and others, 1999; Whitehead, Scott-Samuel, and Dahlgren, 1998), if not for "wider campaigns for sustainable development, political freedom, and economic and social justice" (Doyal, 1995, p. 232).

Four implications for action accordingly flow from a social production of disease/political economy of health perspective. One is that strategies for improving population health require a vision of social justice, backed up by active organizing to change unjust social and economic policies and norms (Kim and others, 2000; Doyal, 1995; Krieger and Birn, 1998). Another is that absent concerns about social equity, economic growth and public health interventions may end up aggravating, not ameliorating, social inequalities in health if the economic growth exacerbates economic inequality and if the public health interventions are more accessible and acceptable to affluent individuals (Szreter, 1997; Link and Phelan, 1996). A third is that greater familiarity with the emerging field of health and human rights—supplemented by analyses of who gains from neglecting or violating these rights—is likely to improve the real-world efficacy of social epidemiologists' work, by providing a systematic framework for delineating governmental accountability to promote and protect health, premised, in the first instance, upon the 1948 Universal Declaration of Human Rights and its recognition of the indivisibility and interdependence of civil, political, economic, social and cultural rights (Mann and others, 1999). And fourth, social epidemiologists must be key actors in ensuring viability of the vital public health activity of monitoring social inequalities in health, for without such work—which is our particular job to do—it is impossible to gauge progress and setbacks in reducing social inequalities in health (Kitagawa and Hauser, 1973; Black and others, 1982; Shaw and others, 1999; Whitehead, Scott-Samuel, and Dahlgren, 1998; Krieger, Chen, and Ebel, 1997).

Yet despite its invaluable contributions to identifying social determinants of population health, a social production of disease/political economy of health perspective affords few principles for investigating *what* these determinants are determining (Krieger, 1994). Biology is opaque. Focusing on relative risks across specified social groups, these analyses rely chiefly on critical appraisals of population distributions of known risk and protective factors, most of which ironically are individual-level characteristics identified by conventional epidemiological research. In the case of breast cancer, for example, analyses might focus on social determinants of a variety of reproductive risk factors (e.g., age at menarche, use of oral contraceptives, age at and number of pregnancies), but would be as constrained as conventional analyses in explaining the portion of cases not attributable to these factors (Kelsey and Bernstein, 1996; Krieger, 1989). Nor does an emphasis on "fundamental social causes" (Link and Phelan, 1996) offer principles for thinking through, systematically, *whether*—and if so, *which*—specific public health and policy interventions are needed to curtail social inequalities in health, above and beyond securing adequate living standards and reducing economic inequality. In the background is Thomas McKeown's (1914–1988) famous argument (1976, 1988) that 19th century declines in infectious disease mortality in the United Kingdom and United States are due chiefly to improved nutrition, not medical interventions. Yet as Simon Szreter (1988) and other public health historians (Fairchild and Oppenheimer, 1998; Porter, 1999) have convincingly demonstrated, McKeown is only half right: although medical care per se can claim little credit for declines in incidence or mortality before World War II, economic growth alone did not improve health. Rather, specific public health policies, e.g., those aimed at cleaning the water and eliminating bovine tuberculosis, were also of fundamental importance. Stated another way, both improved living standards and noneconomic interventions (albeit with economic costs and consequences) matter. Moving from an "either/or" to a "both/and" logic requires multi-level frameworks integrating social and biological reasoning and history, and it is to such new theoretical efforts in social epidemiology—building on prior ideas infused into "social medicine" in the 1940s (Galdston, 1947; Ryle, 1948; Porter, 1997) that I now turn.

ECOSOCIAL THEORY AND RELATED MULTI-LEVEL DYNAMIC PERSPECTIVES

Perhaps one sign of the ferment in contemporary social epidemiological thought is the fact that pictorial depictions of newer frameworks to explain current and shifting patterns of disease distribution refuse to stay in a single plane. Instead, unlike prior images—whether of a triangle connecting host, agent and environment (Gordon, 1953) or a "chain of causes" (Duncan and others, 1988) arrayed along a scale of biological organization, from "society" to "molecular and submolecular particles" (Stallones, 1980) or a spiderless two-dimensional "web of causation," (MacMahon, Pugh, and Ipsen, 1960) or a "causal pie" sans cook (Rothman, 1986)—the new mental pictures are both multidimensional and dynamic (Krieger, 1994; McMichael, 1999; Susser and Susser, 1996). The terminology, too, is changed, as each invokes literal—and not just metaphorical—notions of ecology, situating humans as one notable species among many co-habiting, evolving on, and altering our dynamic planet. I refer especially to three explicitly named frameworks:

1. *Ecosocial theory,* a term I introduced in 1994, with its visual fractal metaphor of an evolving bush of life intertwined at every scale, micro to macro, with the scaffolding of society that different core social groups daily reinforce or seek to alter (Krieger, 1994);

2. *Eco-epidemiology,* proposed by Mervyn and Ezra Susser in 1996, with its image of Chinese boxes, referring to nested "interactive systems," each with its localized structures and relationships (Susser and Susser, 1996); and

3. The *social-ecological systems perspective* invoked by Anthony McMichael in 1999, depicting a cube, representing the "present/past," whose three axes extend from individual-to-population, proximate-to-distal, static/modular to life course and which is projected forward, to "future" (McMichael, 1999)

Their goal is not a totalizing theory to explain everything (and therefore nothing), but rather to generate a set of integral (and testable) principles useful for guiding specific inquiry and action, much as evolutionary theory (broadly writ, with contending interpretations) guides biological disciplines ranging from paleontology to molecular biology (Levins and Lewontin, 1987; Lewontin, 2000; Mayr and Provine, 1980; Sober, 2000). And specifically in the case of ecosocial theory, its fractal image deliberately fosters analysis of current and changing population patterns of health, disease and well-being in relation to *each* level of biological, ecological and social organization (e.g., cell, organ, organism/individual, family, community, population, society, ecosystem) as manifested at *each* and every scale, whether relatively small and fast (e.g., enzyme catalysis) or relatively large and slow (e.g., infection and renewal of the pool of susceptibles for a specified infectious disease).

That each of these frameworks explicitly incorporates the prefix *eco-* or term *ecological* in its name is revealing. Ecology, after all, is a science devoted to study of evolving interactions between living organisms and inanimate matter and energy over time and space (Roughgarden, 1998; Peterson and Parker, 1998). Core to an ecological approach are concerns with:

1. *Scale:* referring to quantifiable dimensions of observed spatio-temporal phenomenon, whether measured in nanoseconds or millennia, microns or kilometres

2. *Level of organization:* theorized and inferred, in relation to specified nested hierarchies, from individual to population to ecosystem

3. *Dynamic states:* reflecting combined interplay of specified animate and inanimate inputs and outputs, with recognition that operative processes and phenomena may be scale-dependent (e.g., factors relevant to self-regulation of an organism's body temperature differ from those involved in self-regulation of the earth's global temperature)

4. *Mathematical modeling:* employed to illuminate how groupings of organisms and processes work together, using both idealized minimal and detailed synthetic models—both to render complexity intelligible and because large-scale experiments are rarely feasible

5. *Understanding unique phenomena in relation to general processes:* in the case of populations, for example, no two forests are ever identical, yet share important features and processes in common relevant to understanding their genesis, longevity, and degradation or decline

Recognizing, however, the importance of social, political, and economic processes in shaping epidemiological profiles, two of the frameworks—ecosocial and social-ecological systems perspective—additionally explicitly indicate in their very names that ecological analysis is not intended to be a substitute or metaphor for social analysis. Rather, they distinguish ecological theory from the diverse social theories upon which they and the other social epidemiological frameworks rely. In doing so, these frameworks part company with other theoretical perspectives that invoke ecology as a metaphor, e.g., social ecology and human ecology, and which employ organic analogies that obscure accountability for social divisions and processes by reinterpreting them as "natural" phenomena (e.g., migration of populations to cities and gentrification recast as analogous to plant succession; Alihan, 1938; Honari and Boleyn, 1999).

Nascent, these emerging ecologically inclined multi-level social epidemiological frameworks remain rather sketchy, the bare beginnings of a mental map. Much more elaboration is required; calling the question can perhaps spur the needed work. Concomitantly, explicit applications to aetiologic inquiry and to interventions are only just underway. From an ecosocial perspective, however, it is possible to formulate several constructs that can begin to serve as a mental checklist for epidemiological research. Focused on the guiding question of who and what drives current and changing patterns of social inequalities in health, the ecosocial approach (but not necessarily the other multi-level frameworks) fully embraces a social production of disease perspective while aiming to bring in a comparably rich biological and ecological analysis. Relevant ecosocial constructs thus minimally include (Krieger, 1994; Krieger, 2000a):

1. *Embodiment,* a concept referring to how we literally incorporate, biologically, the material and social world in which we live, from conception to death; a corollary is that no aspect of our biology can be

understood absent knowledge of history and individual and societal ways of living

2. *Pathways of embodiment,* structured simultaneously by: (a) societal arrangements of power and property and contingent patterns of production, consumption, and reproduction and (b) constraints and possibilities of our biology, as shaped by our species' evolutionary history, our ecological context, and individual histories, that is, trajectories of biological and social development

3. *Cumulative interplay* between exposure, susceptibility and resistance, expressed in pathways of embodiment, with each factor and its distribution conceptualized at multiple levels (individual, neighbourhood, regional or political jurisdiction, national, inter- or supra-national) and in multiple domains (e.g., home, work, school, other public settings), in relation to relevant ecological niches, and manifested in processes at multiple scales of time and space

4. *Accountability and agency,* expressed in pathways of and knowledge about embodiment, in relation to institutions (government, business and public sector), households and individuals, and also to accountability and agency of epidemiologists and other scientists for theories used and ignored to explain social inequalities in health; a corollary is that, given likely complementary causal explanations at different scales and levels, epidemiological studies should explicitly name and consider the benefits and limitations of their particular scale and level of analysis

With these constructs at hand, we can begin to elucidate population patterns of health, disease and well-being as biological expressions of social relations, and can likewise begin to see how social relations influence our most basic understandings of biology (Fleck, 1935; Levins and Lewontin, 1987; Krieger, 2000a, 2000c) and our social constructions of disease (Fleck, 1935; Rosenberg and Golden, 1992)—thereby potentially generating new knowledge and new grounds for action.

Consider, as one example, the phenomenon of pregnancy in relation to risk of cancer. Let us start with breast cancer. As is well known, pregnancy decreases risk of breast cancer over the lifetime if it occurs early, but thereafter increases risk, especially after age 35. This phenomenon is often invoked to explain, in part, why incidence of breast cancer increases with affluence and why the rate has climbed during the 20th century (over and above increases due to earlier age at menarche), since more educated women tend to have children later in life and educational level of women, especially in industrialized societies, has generally been on the rise (Kelsey and Bernstein, 1996; Krieger, 1989). Notably, all three social epidemiological frameworks—psychosocial, social production of disease, and ecosocial—would highlight how social conditions, including women's social status, available birth control technology and access to abortion, affect age at first pregnancy (Krieger, 1989; dos Santos Silva and Beral, 1997). An ecosocial approach, however, would raise questions beyond social determinants of age at first pregnancy to inquire how pregnancy itself is conceptualized in relation to risk of breast cancer (Krieger, 1989). Constructs of "embodiment," "pathways of embodiment," and the "dynamic and cumulative interplay between exposure, susceptibility and resistance" would require analysing pregnancy in relation to developmental biology of the breast (especially maturation of lobules and ducts and also altered rates of apoptosis) as well as its effects on the endocrine system (synthesis of hormones within the breast plus alteration in magnitude and frequency of hormonal fluctuations) and cardiovascular system (increased vascularization of the breast) (Krieger, 1989; Russo and Russo, 1997). A concern with accountability and agency, as well as scale and level, would additionally challenge gender-biased views positing reproductive hormones as primary determinants of women's health (Doyal, 1995; Fee and Krieger, 1994; Ruzek, Olesen, and Clarke, 1997; Oudshoorn, 1994). The net result would be to reconceptualize pregnancy not simply as an "exposure" but also as a biological process capable of altering susceptibility to exogenous carcinogens (Krieger, 1989; Russo and Russo, 1997; Davis and others, 1997). This is the thinking, in part, behind new aetiologic research on environmental pollution and breast cancer; although answers are not yet in as to causal relationships, at least the question is posed (Krieger and others, 1994; Wolff and Toniolo, 1995; Davis and others, 1997).

Similar fresh and integrative thinking motivates a recent novel study including men and women which asks if relationships between parity and cancer incidence are due to the biology of pregnancy or to other social factors "that are influenced by or are influencing family size" (Kravdal, 1995, p. 477). Tellingly, parity is *equally* associated among women and men with risk of three types of cancer: oral and pharyngeal (reflecting greater use of tobacco and alcohol by childless men and women, a topic itself meriting investigation) and malignant melanoma—for which the parity/risk association had been previously interpreted only in hormonal terms and only for women. For two sites, however, thyroid and Hodgkin's disease, parity is associated with incidence only among women. One implication of these findings is not to presume parity exerts effects solely by pregnancy-related biological processes; the other is to consider the social meaning of parity even when the biology of pregnancy is relevant. Simplistic divisions of the social and biological will not suffice.

Consider, too, how an ecosocial perspective can contribute to unravelling the unexplained excess risk of hypertension among African Americans (Krieger, 2000a). Moving beyond eclectic, purely psychological, or purely economic sets of risk factors, the four ecosocial constructs can systematically be used to propose six discrete—yet entangled—multi-level pathways linking expressions of racial discrimination and their biological embodiment across the lifecourse (Krieger and others, 1993; Krieger, 2000a). These are:

1. *Economic and social deprivation:* for example, residential and occupational segregation lead to greater economic deprivation among African Americans and increased likelihood of living in neighbourhoods without good supermarkets; risk of hypertension is increased by cheap, high fat, high salt and low vegetable diets; also, economic deprivation increases risk of being born preterm, thereby harming development of kidneys and increasing likelihood of chronic salt retention (Krieger, 2000a; Krieger and others, 1993; Williams, 1999; Anderson and others, 1989; Lopes and Port, 1995).

2. *Toxic substances and hazardous conditions:* residential segregation increases risk of exposure to lead paint in older houses and to soil contaminated by lead from car exhaust (due to closer proximity of residences to streets or freeways); lead damages renal physiology, increasing risk of hypertension (Krieger, 2000a; Krieger and others, 1993; Williams, 1999; Sorel and others, 1991; Lanphear, Weitzman, and Eberly, 1996).

3. *Socially inflicted trauma:* perceiving, recalling or anticipating interpersonal racial discrimination provokes fear and anger, triggering the "flight-or-fight" response; chronic triggering of this pathway increases allostatic load, leading to sustained hypertension (Krieger, 2000a; Krieger and Sidney, 1996; Krieger and others, 1993; Williams, 1999; Sterling and Eyer, 1988; McEwen, 1998; Anderson and others, 1989; Clark and others, 1999).

4. *Targeted marketing of commodities:* targeted marketing of high-alcohol content beverages to black communities increases likelihood of harmful use of alcohol to reduce feelings of distress; excess alcohol consumption elevates risk of hypertension (Lopes and Port, 1995; Moore, Williams, and Qualls, 1996).

5. *Inadequate health care:* poorer detection and clinical management of hypertension among African Americans increases risk of untreated and uncontrolled hypertension (Lopes and Port, 1995; Svetkey and others, 1996).

6. *Resistance to racial oppression:* individual and community resources and social movements to counter racism and to enhance dignity, along with enactment and implementation of legislation to outlaw racial discrimination, reduces risk of hypertension among African Americans (Cooper and others, 1981; Krieger, 2000a; Krieger and others, 1993; Williams, 1999).

Embracing social determinants ignored by biomedical approaches, the ecosocial approach thus recasts alleged racial differences in biology (e.g., kidney function, blood pressure) as mutable and embodied biological expressions of racism (Krieger, 2000c). Emphasizing accountability, it extends beyond psychosocial explanations focused on anger and hostility (Gentry, 1985; Brosschot and Thayer, 1998) to the social phenomena—in this case, interpersonal and institutional discrimination—eliciting these responses, as mediated by material pathways. Highlighting dynamic and cumulative interplay between exposure, susceptibility and resistance, it advances beyond social production of disease analyses typically focused on racial/ethnic disparities in socioeconomic position among adults (Schnall and Kern, 1981), to highlight discrimination within class strata plus ongoing biological impact of economic deprivation in early life (Krieger, 2000a; Krieger and others, 1993; Kuh and Ben-Shlomo, 1997; Williams, 1999). Urging conceptual integration, it advocates coordinated research and action cognizant of the specified multiple pathways and geared to explaining current and changing rates of hypertension, premised on the view that our common humanity demands no less if we are to understand and rectify social inequalities in health (Mann and others, 1999; Krieger and Davey Smith, 2000). Thus, more than simply adding "biology" to "social" analyses, or "social factors" to "biological" analyses, the ecosocial framework begins to envision a more systematic integrated approach capable of generating new hypotheses, rather than simply reinterpreting factors identified by one approach (e.g., biological) in terms of another (e.g., social). Suggesting much work remains to be done, however, few of the proposed pathways have been extensively studied and, to date, fewer than 25 epidemiological studies have explicitly investigated somatic consequences of racial discrimination—a mere 0.06% of the nearly 40,000 articles indexed by the keyword *race* in Medline since 1966.

CONCLUSION: THEORY MATTERS

In conclusion, theory matters: both to define social epidemiology and to distinguish among trends within this field. These diverse frameworks encourage us to think critically and systematically about intimate and integral connections between our social and biological existence—and, especially in the case of social production of disease and ecosocial theory, to name explicitly who benefits from and is accountable for social inequalities in health. By focusing attention on under-theorized and under-researched conjoint social and biological determinants of disease distribution, these theories, even in nascent form, can potentially give new grounds for action—and underscore that theory, absent action, is an empty promise.

Ultimately, it remains to be seen whether any of the three theoretical frameworks discussed in this article—psychosocial, social production of disease/political economy of health, and emerging ecosocial and other multi-level frameworks—is best suited for guiding social epidemiological research in the 21st century. If not these theories, however, other frameworks will need to be elaborated to enhance social epidemiologists' ability to analyse and provide evidence useful for addressing the myriad ways we both embody and transform the co-mingled social and biological world in which we live, love, work, play, fight, ail and die. To generate the data required to test and refine our theoretical frameworks, priority must thus be accorded to: (1) enhanced monitoring of social inequalities of health, so that data are available—cross-stratified—by class, gender, and race/ethnicity and any other social groups subject to economic and social deprivation and discrimination, to gauge progress and setbacks in reducing social inequalities in health, (2) funding interdisciplinary aetiologic research to identify conjoint social and biological determinants of disease at appropriate spatiotemporal scales and levels of organization, and (3) funding interventions based on the findings of this research—with the content of all three priority areas determined by coalitions including sectors of society most burdened by social inequalities in health.

If social epidemiologists are to gain clarity on causes of and barriers to reducing social inequalities in health, adequate theory is a necessity, not a luxury. The old adage still stands: "If you don't ask, you don't know, and if you don't know, you can't act" (Krieger, 1992, p. 412). Ultimately, it is theory which inspires our questions, which enables us to envision a far healthier world than the one in which we live, and which gives us the insight, responsibility, and accountability to translate this vision to a reality. Who shall create this theory? The task is ours.

References

Alihan, M. A. *Social Ecology: A Critical Analysis.* New York: Columbia University Press, 1938.

American Medical Association, Council on Scientific Affairs. "Health Care Needs of Gay Men and Lesbians in the United States." *Journal of the American Medical Association,* 1996, *275,* 1354–1359.

Anderson, N.B., and others. "Hypertension in Blacks: Psychosocial and Biological Perspectives." *Journal of Hypertension,* 1989, *7,* 161–172.

Antonovsky, A. *Unraveling the Mystery of Health: How People Manage Stress and Stay Well.* San Francisco: Jossey-Bass, 1987, 90–91.

Baum, F. "Social Capital: Is It Good for Your Health? Issues for a Public Health Agenda." *Journal of Epidemiology and Community Health,* 1999, *53,* 195–196.

Becker, E. "Harassment in the Military Is Said to Rise: More Gays Abused, Legal Groups Report." *New York Times,* Mar. 10, 2000, p. A15.

Berkman, L. F., and Kawachi, I (eds.). *Social Epidemiology.* New York: Oxford University Press, 2000.

Bijlmakers, L. A., Bassett, M. T., and Sanders, D. M. *Health and Structural Adjustment in Rural and Urban Zimbabwe.* Uppsala, Sweden: Nordiska Afrikainstitutet, 1996.

Black, D., and others. *Report of the Working Group on Inequalities in Health.* Harmondsworth, England: Penguin, 1982.

Breilh, J. *Epidemiología Economía Medicina y Política.* Quito: Universidad Central del Ecuador, 1979.

Brosschot, J. E., and Thayer, J. F. "Anger Inhibition, Cardiovascular Recovery, and Vagal Function: A Model of the Link Between Hostility and Cardiovascular Disease." *Annals of Behavioral Medicine,* 1998, *20,* 326–332.

Cassel, J. "The Contribution of the Social Environment to Host Resistance." *American Journal of Epidemiology,* 1976, *104,* 107–123.

Clark, R., and others. "Racism as a Stressor for African Americans. A Biopsychosocial Model." *American Psychologist,* 1999, *54,* 805–816.

Committee on Environmental Justice, Health Sciences Policy Program, Health Sciences Section, Institute of Medicine. *Toward Environmental Justice: Research, Education, and Health Policy Needs.* Washington, D.C.: National Academy Press, 1999.

Conrad, P., and Kern, R. (eds.). *The Sociology of Health and Illness: Critical Perspectives.* New York: St. Martin's Press, 1981a.

Conrad, P., and Kern, R. "The Social Production of Disease and Illness." In P. Conrad and R. Kern (eds.), *The Sociology of Health and Illness: Critical Perspectives.* New York: St. Martin's Press, 1981b;9–11.

Cooper, R., and others. "Racism, Society, and Disease: An Exploration of the Social and Biological Mechanisms of Differential Mortality." *International Journal of Health Services,* 1981, *11,* 389–414.

Crawford, R. "You Are Dangerous to Your Health: The Ideology and Politics of Victim Blaming." *International Journal of Health Services,* 1977, *7,* 663–680.

Davis, D. L., and others. "Avoidable Causes of Breast Cancer: The Known, the Unknown, and the Suspected." *Annals of the New York Academy of Science,* 1997, *833,* 112–128.

dos Santos Silva, I., and Beral, V. "Socioeconomic Differences in Reproductive Behavior." *IARC Scientific Publications,* 1997, *138,* 285–308.

Doyal, L. *What Makes Women Sick? Gender and the Political Economy of Health.* New Brunswick, N.J.: Rutgers University Press, 1995.

Doyal, L. *The Political Economy of Health.* London: Pluto Press, 1979.

Dubos, R. J. *Mirage of Health: Utopias, Progress, and Biological Change.* New York: Doubleday, 1959.

Duncan, D. F., and others. *Epidemiology: Basis for Disease Prevention and Health Promotion.* New York: Macmillan, 1988.

Engel, G. L. "The Biopsychosocial Model and the Education of Health Professionals." *Annals of the New York Academy of Science,* 1978, *310,* 169–187.

Eyer, J., and Sterling, P. "Stress-Related Mortality and Social Organization." *Review of Radical Political Economics,* 1977, *9,* 1–44.

Fairchild, A. L., and Oppenheimer, G. M. "Public Health Nihilism vs. Pragmatism: History, Politics, and the Control of Tuberculosis." *American Journal of Public Health,* 1998, *88,* 1105–1117.

Fee, E., and Krieger, N. *Women's Health, Politics, and Power: Essays on Sex/Gender, Medicine, and Public Policy.* Amityville, N.Y.: Baywood, 1994.

Fleck, L. *Genesis and Development of a Scientific Fact.* Chicago: University of Chicago Press, 1935.

Frost, W. H. "Some Conceptions of Epidemics in General." *American Journal of Epidemiology,* 1976, *103,* 141–151. (Originally published 1928)

Galdston, I. (ed.). *Social Medicine: Its Derivations and Objectives.* New York: Commonwealth Fund, 1947.

Galdston, I. (ed.). *Beyond the Germ Theory: The Roles of Deprivation and Stress in Health and Disease.* New York: Health Education Council, New York Academy of Medicine, 1954.

Gentry, W. D. "Relationship of Anger-Coping Styles and Blood Pressure Among Black Americans." In M. A. Chesney and R. H. Rosenman (eds.), *Anger and Hostility in Cardiovascular and Behavioral Disorders.* Washington, D.C.: Hemísphere, 1985, 139–147.

Gordon, J. E. "The World, the Flesh, and the Devil as Environment, Host, and Agent of Disease." In I. Galdston (ed.), *The Epidemiology of Health.* New York: Health Education Council, 1953, 60–73.

Graham, S., and Schneiderman, M. "Social Epidemiology and the Prevention of Cancer." *Preventive Medicine,* 1972, *1,* 371–380.

Greenwood, M. *Epidemics and Crowd-Diseases: An Introduction to the Study of Epidemiology.* London: Williams & Norgate, 1935.

Honari, M., and Boleyn, T. (eds.). *Health Ecology: Health, Culture, and Human-Environment Interaction.* London: Routledge, 1999.

Jaco, E. G. "Introduction: Medicine and Behavioral Science." In E. G. Jaco (ed.), *Patients, Physicians, and Illness: Sourcebook in Behavioral Science and Medicine.* New York: Free Press, 1958, 3–8.

Jaco, E. G. *The Social Epidemiology of Mental Disorders: A Psychiatric Survey of Texas.* New York: Russell Sage Foundation, 1960.

Kawachi, I., and Berkman, L. F. "Social Cohesion, Social Capital, and Health." In L. F. Berkman and I. Kawachi (eds.), *Social Epidemiology.* New York: Oxford University Press, 2000, 174–190.

Kelsey, J. L, and Bernstein, L. "Epidemiology and Prevention of Breast Cancer." *Annual Review of Public Health,* 1996, *17,* 47–67.

Kim, J.-Y., and others. *Dying for Growth: Global Inequality and the Health of the Poor.* Monroe, Maine: Common Courage Press, 2000.

Kitagawa, E., and Hauser, P. *Differential Mortality in the United States: A Study in Socio-Economic Epidemiology.* Cambridge, Mass.: Harvard University Press, 1973.

Kravdal, O. "Is the Relationship Between Childbearing and Cancer Incidence Due to Biology or Lifestyle? Examples of the Importance of Using Data on Men." *International Journal of Epidemiology,* 1995, *24,* 477–484.

Krieger, N. "Shades of Difference: Theoretical Underpinnings of the Medical Controversy on Black-White Differences, 1830–1870." *International Journal of Health Services,* 1987, *7,* 258–279.

Krieger, N. "Exposure, Susceptibility, and Breast Cancer Risk: A Hypothesis Regarding Exogenous Carcinogens, Breast Tissue Development, and Social Gradients, Including Black/White Differences, in Breast Cancer Incidence." *Breast Cancer Research and Treatment,* 1989, *13,* 205–223.

Krieger, N. "The Making of Public Health Data: Paradigms, Politics, and Policy." *Journal of Public Health Policy,* 1992, *13,* 412–427.

Krieger, N. "Epidemiology and the Web of Causation: Has Anyone Seen the Spider?" *Social Science and Medicine,* 1994, *39,* 887–903.

Krieger, N. "Discrimination and Health." In L. F. Berkman and I. Kawachi (eds.), *Social Epidemiology.* New York: Oxford University Press, 2000a, 36–75.

Krieger, N. "Epidemiology and Social Sciences: Toward a Critical Reengagement in the 21st Century." *Epidemiologic Reviews,* 2000b, *11,* 155–163.

Krieger, N. "Refiguring 'Race': Epidemiology, Racialized Biology, and Biological Expressions of Race Relations." *International Journal of Health Services,* 2000c, *30,* 211–216.

Krieger, N., and Birn, A. E. "A Vision of Social Justice as the Foundation of Public Health: Commemorating 150 Years of the Spirit of 1848." *American Journal of Public Health,* 1998, *88,* 1603–1606.

Krieger, N., Chen, J. T., and Ebel, G. "Can We Monitor Socioeconomic Inequalities in Health? A Survey of U.S. Health Departments' Data Collection and Reporting Practices." *Public Health Reports,* 1997, *112,* 481–491.

Krieger, N., and Davey Smith, G. "Re: 'Seeking Causal Explanations in Social Epidemiology.'" Letter to the editor. *American Journal of Epidemiology,* 2000, *151,* 831–832.

Krieger, N., and Sidney, S. "Racial Discrimination and Blood Pressure: The CARDIA Study of Young Black and White Adults." *American Journal of Public Health,* 1996, *86,* 1370–1378.

Krieger, N., and Sidney, S. "Prevalence and Health Implications of Anti-Gay Discrimination: A Study of Black and White Women and Men in the CARDIA Cohort: Coronary Artery Risk Development in Young Adults. *International Journal of Health Services,* 1997, *27,* 157–176.

Krieger, N., and Zierler, S. "What Explains the Public's Health? A Call for Epidemiologic Theory." *Epidemiology*, 1995, *7*, 107–109.

Krieger, N., and others. "Racism, Sexism, and Social Class: Implications for Studies of Health, Disease, and Well-Being." *American Journal of Preventive Medicine*, 1993, *9*(Suppl.), 82–122.

Krieger, N., and others. "Breast Cancer and Serum Organochlorines: A Prospective Study Among White, Black, and Asian Women." *Journal of the National Cancer Institute*, 1994, *86*, 589–599.

Kuh, D., and Ben-Shlomo, Y. (eds.). *A Life Course Approach to Chronic Disease Epidemiology.* Oxford: Oxford University Press, 1997.

Lanphear, B. P., Weitzman, M., and Eberly, S. "Racial Differences in Urban Children's Environmental Exposures to Lead." *American Journal of Public Health*, 1996, *86*, 1460–1463.

Lawrence, C., and Weisz, G. (eds.). *Greater Than the Parts: Holism in Biomedicine, 1920–1950.* New York: Oxford University Press, 1998.

Levins, R., and Lewontin, R. C. *The Dialectical Biologist.* Cambridge, Mass.: Harvard University Press, 1987.

Lewontin, R. C. *The Triple Helix: Gene, Organism, and Environment.* Cambridge, Mass.: Harvard University Press, 2000.

Link, B. G., and Phelan, J. C. "Understanding Sociodemographic Differences in Health: The Role of Fundamental Social Causes." *American Journal of Public Health*, 1996, *86*, 471–473.

Lloyd, G.E.R. (ed.), *Hippocratic Writings.* Harmondsworth, England: Penguin, 1983.

Lopes, A. A., and Port, F. K. "The Low-Birthweight Hypothesis as a Plausible Explanation for the Black/White Differences in Hypertension, Non-Insulin-Dependent Diabetes, and End-Stage Renal Disease." *American Journal of Kidney Disease*, 1995, *25*, 350–356.

Lynch, J. W., and others. "Income Inequality and Mortality: Importance to Health of Individual Incomes, Psychological Environment or Material Conditions." *British Medical Journal*, 2000, *320*, 1200–1204.

MacMahon, B., Pugh, T. F., and Ipsen, J. *Epidemiologic Methods.* New York: Little, Brown, 1960, 18–22.

Mann, J. M., and others (eds.). *Health and Human Rights.* New York: Routledge, 1999.

Masek, K., and others. "Past, Present and Future of Psychoneuroimmunology." *Toxicology*, 2000, *142*, 179–188.

Mayr, E., and Provine, B. (eds.). *The Evolutionary Synthesis: Perspectives on the Unification of Biology.* Cambridge, Mass.: Harvard University Press, 1980.

McEwen, B. S. "Protective and Damaging Effects of Stress Mediators: Allostasis and Allostatic Load." *New England Journal of Medicine*, 1998, *338*, 171–179.

McKeown, T. *The Role of Medicine: Dream, Mirage or Nemesis.* London: Nuffield Provincial Hospital Trust, 1976.

McKeown, T. *The Origins of Human Disease.* Oxford: Blackwell, 1988.

McKinlay, J. B. "A Case for Refocussing Upstream: The Political Economy of Illness." In *Applying Behavioral Science to Cardiovascular Risk,* proceedings of the American Heart Association conference in Seattle, June 17–19, 1974, pp. 7–17. Republished in Jaco, E.G. (ed.), *Patients, Physicians, and Illness: A Sourcebook in Behavioral Science and Health.* New York: Free Press, 1979, 9–25.

McKinlay, J. B., and Marceau, L. D. "To Boldly Go . . ." *American Journal of Public Health,* 2000, *90,* 25–33.

McMichael, A. J. "Prisoners of the Proximate: Loosening the Constraints on Epidemiology in an Age of Change." *American Journal of Epidemiology,* 1999, *149,* 887–897.

Meyer, I. H. "Minority Stress and Mental Health in Gay Men." *Journal of Health and Social Behavior,* 1995, *36,* 38–56.

Moore, D. J., Williams, J. D., and Qualls, W. J. "Target Marketing of Tobacco and Alcohol-Related Products to Ethnic Minority Groups in the United States." *Ethnicity and Disease,* 1996, *6,* 83–98.

Navarro, V. "Editorial: A Beginning." *International Journal of Health Services,* 1971, *1,* 1–2.

Navarro, V. *Crisis, Health, and Medicine: A Social Critique.* New York: Tavistock, 1986.

O'Campo, P., and Rojas-Smith, L. "Welfare Reform and Women's Health: Review of the Literature and Implications for State Policy." *Journal of Public Health Policy,* 1998, *19,* 420–446.

Oudshoorn, N. *Beyond the Natural Body: An Archaeology of Sex Hormones.* New York: Routledge, 1994.

Peterson, D. L., and Parker, V. T. (eds.). *Ecological Scale: Theory and Application.* New York: Columbia University Press, 1998.

Porter, D. "The Decline of Social Medicine in Britain in the 1960s." In D. Porter (ed.), *Social Medicine and Medical Sociology in the Twentieth Century.* Atlanta: Rodopi, 1997, 97–119.

Porter, D. *Health, Civilization, and the State: A History of Public Health from Ancient to Modern Times.* London: Routledge, 1999.

Portes, A. "Social Capital: Its Origins and Applications in Modern Sociology." *Annual Review of Sociology,* 1998, *24,* 1–24.

Reeder, L. G. "Social Epidemiology: An Appraisal." In E. G. Jaco (ed.), *Patients, Physicians, and Illness: A Sourcebook in Behavioral Science and Health.* (2nd ed.) New York: Free Press, 1972, 97–101.

Rosenberg, C. E., and Golden, J. *Framing Disease: Studies in Cultural History.* New Brunswick, N.J.: Rutgers University Press, 1992.

Rothman, K. J. *Modern Epidemiology.* New York: Little, Brown, 1986.

Roughgarden, J. *Primer of Ecological Theory.* Upper Saddle River, N.J.: Prentice Hall, 1998.

Russo, J., and Russo, I. H. "Toward a Unified Concept of Mammary Carcinogenesis." *Progress in Clinical Biology Research,* 1997, *396,* 1–16.

Ruzek, S. B., Olesen, V. L., and Clarke, A. E. (eds.). *Women's Health: Complexities and Differences.* Columbus: Ohio State University Press, 1997.

Ryle, J. A. *Changing Disciplines: Lectures on the History, Method and Motives of Social Pathology.* Oxford: Oxford University Press, 1948.

Sanders, D. *The Struggle for Health: Medicine and the Politics of Underdevelopment.* London: Macmillan, 1985.

Schnall, P. L., and Kern, R. "Hypertension in American Society: An Introduction to Historical Materialist Epidemiology." In P. Conrad and R. Kern (eds.), *The Sociology of Health and Illness: Critical Perspectives.* New York: St. Martin's Press, 1981.

Schwartz, S., Susser, E., and Susser, M. "A Future for Epidemiology?" *Annual Review of Public Health,* 1999, *20,* 15–33.

Scott-Samuel, A. "Health Impact Assessment: Theory into Practice." *Journal of Epidemiology and Community Health,* 1998, *52,* 704–705.

Shaw, M., and others. *The Widening Gap: Health Inequalities and Policy in Britain.* Bristol, England: Policy Press, 1999.

Smythies, J. R. "Perspectives in Psychoneuroendocrinology." *Psychoneuroendocrinology,* 1976, *1,* 317–319.

Sober, E. *Philosophy of Biology.* (2nd ed.) Boulder, Colo.: Westview Press, 2000.

Solarz, A. L. (ed.). *Lesbian Health: Current Assessment and Directions for the Future.* Washington, D.C.: National Academy Press, 1999.

Sorel, J. E., and others. "Black-White Differences in Blood Pressure Among Participants in NHANES II: The Contribution of Blood Lead." *Epidemiology,* 1991, *2,* 348–352.

Stallones, R. A. "To Advance Epidemiology." *Annual Review of Public Health,* 1980, *1,* 69–82.

Sterling, P., and Eyer, J. "Allostasis: A New Paradigm to Explain Arousal Pathology." In J. Fisher and J. Reason (eds.). *Handbook of Life Stress, Cognition, and Health.* New York: Wiley, 1988.

Susser, M. "Should the Epidemiologist Be a Social Scientist or a Molecular Biologist?" *International Journal of Epidemiology,* 1999, *28,* 1019–1022.

Susser, M., and Susser, E. "Choosing a Future for Epidemiology: II. From Black Boxes to Chinese Boxes and Eco-Epidemiology." *American Journal of Public Health,* 1996, *86,* 674–677.

Svetkey, L. P., and others. "Effects of Gender and Ethnic Group on Blood Pressure Control in the Elderly." *American Journal of Hypertension,* 1996, *9,* 529–535.

Syme, S. L. "Contributions of Social Epidemiology to the Study of Medical Care Systems: The Need for Cross-Cultural Research." *Medical Care,* 1971, *9,* 203–213.

Szreter, S. "The Importance of Social Intervention in Britain's Mortality Decline, c.1850–1914: A Reinterpretation of the Role of Public Health." *Social History of Medicine,* 1988, *1,* 1–37.

Szreter, S. "Economic Growth, Disruption, Deprivation, Disease, and Death: On the Importance of the Politics of Public Health for Development." *Popular Development Review,* 1997, *23,* 693–728.

Tesh, S. N. *Hidden Arguments: Political Ideology and Disease Prevention Policy.* New Brunswick, N.J.: Rutgers University Press, 1988.

Townsend, P. "Why Are the Many Poor?" *International Journal of Health Services,* 1986, *16,* 1–32.

Turshen, M. *The Politics of Public Health.* New Brunswick, N.J.: Rutgers University Press, 1989.

Veith, L. (trans.). *The Yellow Emperor's Classic of Internal Medicine* [Huang Ti Ne Ching So Wen]. Berkeley: University of California Press, 1966.

Whitehead, M., Scott-Samuel, A., and Dahlgren, G. "Setting Targets to Address Inequalities in Health." *Lancet,* 1998, *351,* 1279–1282.

Wilkinson, R. G. *Unhealthy Societies: The Afflictions of Inequality.* New York: Routledge, 1996.

Williams, D. R. "Race, Socioeconomic Status, and Health. The Added Effects of Racism and Discrimination." *Annals of the New York Academy of Science,* 1999, *896,* 173–188.

Wise, P., Chavkin, W., and Romero, D. "Assessing the Effects of Welfare Reform Policies on Reproductive and Infant Health." *American Journal of Public Health,* 1999, *89,* 1514–1521.

Wolff, M. S., and Toniolo, P. G. "Environmental Organochlorine Exposure as a Potential Etiologic Factor in Breast Cancer." *Environmental Health Perspectives,* 1995, *103*(Suppl. 7), 141–145.

Yankauer, A. "The Relationship of Fetal and Infant Mortality to Residential Segregation: An Inquiry into Social Epidemiology." *American Social Review,* 1950, *15,* 644–648.

Ziman, J. *An Introduction to Science Studies: The Philosophical and Social Aspects of Science and Technology.* Cambridge: Cambridge University Press, 1984.

PART THREE

STRATEGIES: PERSPECTIVES ON SOCIAL POLICY AND PRACTICE

As many contributors to this volume suggest, particularly in Part Three, research findings indicate that making major improvements in the health of vulnerable populations and anticipating future increases in health inequities depend on a coordinated agenda aimed at structural and institutional change. Cures, treatments, and individual interventions will not be enough. Although behavior clearly influences premature mortality and health, more basic socioeconomic conditions that continue over time play a larger role in determining behavior. Therefore, attention must focus on the foundations of health: the social roots of suffering, premature death, and disability within and among population groups. Contributors in Part Three consider a variety of policy menus and options, along with actions to strengthen communities.

Dennis Raphael briefly summarizes a variety of policy options for the United States, based on approaches taken in Britain, Finland, Sweden, and Canada that might influence the structural social determinants of health. He reviews the ideas of political economists, the World Health Organization, and the Healthy Cities Movement.

Given mounting evidence of the negative impact of global trade and neoliberal policies on public health, Ronald Labonte presents a case for appending global trade agreements to ensure that they are socially just and environmentally sustainable. He proposes the creation of a strong public health lobby, nationally and internationally, to work with NGOs in creating these social clauses.

Nancy Moss suggests action strategies to place public health priorities on the policy agenda, drawn from the European experience in reducing socioeconomic disparities in morbidity and mortality. The author argues for the necessity of creating a climate of unacceptability for socioeconomic disparities in health and dissemination to broad audiences. She also suggests the need for the formation of state and community task forces, attention to social justice issues, creative use of media, and attraction of new funders.

Hilary Graham presents the case for bringing scientific knowledge to bear on policy to eliminate health inequities. This means more than description and evaluation; she feels that we must examine how inequalities in health result from inequalities in socioeconomic status and how they are produced and maintained. Such an analysis will require consideration of how the socioeconomic structure influences individual circumstances in order to intervene in the disadvantaged pathways that increase exposure to health risks.

Observing changes in African American neighborhoods in impoverished urban areas, Arline T. Geronimus describes the need to tackle poverty, socioeconomic disadvantages, and other structural forces—such as housing, transportation, employment, and investment policies—in order to reverse continuing inequities in health. She also focuses on the importance of developing race-conscious policies that deal with institutional discrimination and racism. Calling for research that examines differences within population groups, she, like Jennie Popay in Part Two, suggests providing the links between personal experience and structural barriers to improved health and well-being.

From the perspective of someone working within a local public health agency, Rajiv Bhatia describes the options and challenges to serving marginalized communities in their efforts to achieving greater democratic and community control over social and economic decisions that affect people's health. He explores three case studies related to environmental health, the development of the Health Impact Assessment, and attempts to enact a living wage law.

At the state level, Gavin Kearney analyzes the process and outcomes of a group of organizations and government agencies in Minnesota to address the social and economic conditions associated with health inequalities. Describing the story of the Social Conditions and Health Action Team, working under the Minnesota Department of Health, he summarizes the findings of the group's research, recommendations, and strategies and offers a critique of accomplishments to date.

Lawrence Wallack argues that mass media approaches to improving the public's health need to be rethought in light of recent developments in social epidemiology, political science, sociology, and mass communications. Traditional behavior-oriented media campaigns have been limited in improving health status. This is because they fail to adequately address fundamental public health values related to social justice, participation, and social change—values made more important by the increasing research on the relationship between social inequality and health inequality. Future media approaches must focus on skill development for participation in the social change process rather than primarily on information for personal change.

CHAPTER TWENTY

Toward the Future

Policy and Community Actions to
Promote Population Health

Dennis Raphael

My chapter in Part One of this volume described the forces driving the deterioration of a variety of social determinants of health in the United States. Overall, they included the economic globalization and the concentration of wealth and power supported by a neoliberal public discourse. The chapter analyzed how these social determinants of health were affecting population health in the United States. The U.S. public policy and public health communities must begin to address the structural sources of increasing income and wealth inequality and the deterioration of other social determinants of population health.

This chapter presents an overview of policy recommendations that can begin to improve population health by addressing structural sources of health inequities. The underlying concepts owe much to political economists who argue for a basic reorganization of the creation and distribution of societal resources. Practical ideas for action, however, are drawn primarily from developments in the field of health promotion as outlined by the World Health Organization (WHO). The WHO concept of health promotion is very different from its meaning in the United States, where it is usually restricted to lifestyle approaches associated with behavioral change (Raphael and Farrell, 2002b).

The WHO's Ottawa Charter for Health Promotion (1986) contains the concepts necessary for a multisectoral, multilevel approached to improving population health. These concepts have been applied in numerous health promotion approaches at the national, state or provincial, municipal, and community levels around the world. With some notable exceptions, these ideas have not penetrated into public policy and public health practice in the United States (Raphael, 2000).

TARGETS FOR ACTION:
THE POLITICAL ECONOMY PERSPECTIVE

The concentration of wealth and power in a nation leads to growing inequality in terms of income and wealth among the population, along with a weakening of social infrastructure and processes associated with civil society (see Chapter Fourteen). The United States and other nations have experienced periods in which wealth and power had become concentrated to the point that the public pressured the government to enact legislation to control their influence (Phillips, 2002). Kevin Phillips's comprehensive historical review of the U.S. experience provides two good examples: Progressive Era antitrust legislation, enacted in reaction to the excesses of the Gilded Age of the late 1800s, and New Deal legislation, enacted as a reaction to the stock market crash and resultant depression of the 1930s. Such a period of profound reorganization, on an international scale, may now be a necessary response to the current excesses and health-threatening processes of economic globalization.

Gary Teeple (2000) pessimistically argues that citizens can do little to resist deteriorating political, economic, social, and health conditions under the circumstances of contemporary globalization. He contends that governments generally find it impossible to resist the power of multinational corporations and hence have little choice but to become complicit in these processes. Yet the effects of economic globalization have not been identical in all nations, and some have resisted the forces that heighten economic inequality and threaten population health (Mishra, 1990; Coburn, 2001).

Michael Zweig (2000) argues for greater equity in political power and the possibility of achieving it. He calls for restoration of programs and services that have been reduced and the reintroduction of more progressive income tax rates. Independent unions are a necessity, as is legislation that strengthens the ability of workers to organize. Reregulating many industries would serve to reverse current trends toward the concentration of power and wealth. Internationally, the development and enforcement of agreements to provide adequate working and living standards would support and promote health and well-being across national barriers is essential. The provision of a social wage—government-provided services that people need to live and develop their ability to work—is a way to help restore the social infrastructure that has been so weakened in the United States, along with resistance to the privatization of public services needs.

BACK TO THE BASICS: THE OTTAWA CHARTER FOR HEALTH PROMOTION

Although many of the issues discussed in this volume are best addressed in the political sphere rather than through population and public health initiatives, strong links exist between political economy and population health issues (Navarro, 2002). But as important an intrinsic concern as health is among Americans, the public remains focused on medical and lifestyle issues. It is time to raise these population health issues, recognizing that the structural sources of power, wealth, and health differences among citizens play an important role in determining the success of attempts to influence social determinants of health.

The Ottawa Charter for Health Promotion defines health promotion as the process of enabling people to increase control over their health and to improve their health (World Health Organization, 1986). In line with its predominantly structural approach to promoting health, the Charter identifies the basic prerequisites for health as peace, shelter, education, food, income, a stable ecosystem, sustainable resources, social justice, and equity. It further outlines five pillars of action: building healthy public policy, creating supportive environments, strengthening community action, developing personal skills, and reorienting health services. *[handwritten margin note: all these must things be working together]*

Social justice and equity are the core values driving this approach, themes usually absent from discussions of population health (see Chapter Eighteen). Nations that have seriously implemented health promotion approaches consistent with the Charter offer clear commitments to these principles (Mackenbach and Bakker, 2002).

American attitudes toward having governments provide full employment, ensure decent standards of living for the unemployed, and guarantee a basic income are profoundly more conservative than among citizens of the United Kingdom, Germany, the Netherlands, or Italy (Kawachi and Kennedy, 2002). Indeed, low-income Americans are less likely than the wealthy in these other nations to believe that the unemployed should be provided with a basic income and a decent standard of living. The same is true regarding the belief that governments should work to reduce the income gap between rich and poor and should tax the rich to help the poor. Clearly, any efforts to redress the issues identified in this volume face an uphill battle in the United States.

WORKING FROM THE TOP: NATIONAL POLICY OPTIONS TO PROMOTE HEALTH

Two examples of nations with commitments to improving the health of citizens through progressive public policy are Sweden (Burstrom and others, 2002) and Finland (Lahelma, Keskimaki, Rahkonen, 2002). Both have a tradition of incorporating equity in governmental policies. The new National Swedish Health Policy outlines six policy recommendations to improve population health of which five are focused on structural issues. (Agren and Hedin, 2002). These activities are the responsibility of the National Institute of Public Health. These strategies are as follows:

- *To increase social capital in Swedish society.* This includes efforts to decrease social inequality, counteract discrimination of minority groups, and promote local democracy.

- *To promote better working conditions.* The most important issues are to decrease long-term negative stress, increase employees' influence at work, and achieve more flexible working hours.

- *To improve conditions for children and young people.* The intent is to improve social support for families with children and for health-promoting schools.

- *To improve the physical environment.* This involves coordinating the work for a sustainable environment with the struggle for improved health.

- *To provide good structural conditions for public health work at all levels of society.* This entails support and coordination of research and education in public health science.

The Finnish government's commitment is to preventive public policy with the following elements: supporting growth and development of children and young people, preventing exclusion, supporting personal initiative and involvement among the unemployed, and promoting basic security in housing (Ministry of Social Affairs and Health, 2001). The means of achieving these goals clearly recognize the social determinants of health; they include

- Improving efficiency and cooperation among primary, specialized, and occupational health care providers

- Providing support for the general functional capacity of people of differing ages

- Promoting lifelong learning

- Promoting well-being at work

- Increasing gender equality and social protection, which provides an incentive to work
- Giving priority to preventive policy, early intervention, and actions to interrupt long-term unemployment
- Reducing regional welfare gaps
- Promoting multiculturalism
- Controlling substance abuse
- Promoting active participation in international policymaking
- Providing adequate income security as the key to building social cohesion

RECENT POLICY REPORTS FROM THE UNITED KINGDOM AND CANADA

Britain has one of the longest traditions of considering health inequalities, their causes, and means of alleviating the differences (Davey Smith, Dorling, and Shaw, 2001). Canada, too, has been a world leader in developing concepts of health promotion and population health (Health Canada, 2001).

The United Kingdom

British researchers have recommended strong government action to close the widening health gap between the rich and poor, thereby improving population health. The authors of *The Widening Gap* (Shaw and others, 1999) make two main points in relation to reducing the health gap:

> The key policy that will reduce inequalities in health is the alleviation of poverty through the reduction of inequalities in income and wealth.
> Poverty can be reduced by raising the standards of living of poor people through increasing their incomes "in cash or in kind." The costs would be borne by the rich and would reduce inequalities overall—simultaneously reducing inequalities in health [p. 169].

Acheson's *Independent Inquiry into Inequalities in Health* (1998) reached a similar conclusion concerning the importance of income and wealth distribution in Britain. Its key recommendations focus on the need for health impact assessment of public policies and more equitable distribution of income and other societal resources:

- We recommend that as part of health impact assessment, all policies likely to have a direct or indirect impact on health should be evaluated in terms of their impact on health inequalities and should be formulated in such a way that by favouring the less well off they will, wherever possible, reduce such inequalities [p. 31].

- We recommend that further reductions in poverty of women of child-bearing age, expectant mothers, young children and older people should be made by increasing benefits in cash or in kind to them [p. 36].

Other recommendations address numerous social determinants of health, such as education, employment, housing and environment, mobility, transportation, pollution policy, nutrition and agricultural policy, and the provision of health care.

Canada

Three recent Canadian reports concerning the future of health care (Kirby, 2002; Mazankowski, 2001; Romanow, 2002) all identified the importance of the social determinants of population health and the need to address population health from a public policy perspective. Compared to the United States, Canada is more equal in its distribution of income and wealth, is stronger in the quality of many of its social determinants of health, and presents a more positive population health profile (Dunn, Hargreaves, and Alex, 2002). A recent publication by the National Policy Association (Auerbach and Krimgold, 2001) praised the Canadian social policy tradition of transfer payments, strong services, and other policies that promote equalization of income as a model for improving the health of citizens. Yet these Canada-specific policies are under threat in the current Canadian policy environment (Raphael, 2003).

Drawing on various U.K. and Canadian documents, I outlined three general policy areas to reduce health inequalities and to improve the population health of Canadians (Raphael, 2002b). These concern the incidence of low income, reducing social exclusion, and restoring the social infrastructure—all social determinants of health identified as influencing health inequalities and population health. Many of these recommendations certainly apply to the United States.

Policies to Reduce the Incidence of Low Income. The incidence of low income has been increasing in Canada, as have income and wealth inequalities. The following steps would serve to reduce the number of Canadians living with low incomes, reduce economic inequality, and improve population health.

- *Raise the minimum wage to a living wage.* Canadians working full time at current Canadian minimum-wage levels do not even come close to the current Statistics Canada low-income cutoff levels. Furthermore, in many provinces, minimum wages have not been adjusted for increased living costs or the impact of inflation for some time.
- *Improve pay equity.* Low income is becoming concentrated more and more among Canadian women. Single mothers are especially disadvantaged, with associated health consequences for both themselves and their children. Traditional women's occupations continue to pay only a

fraction of those of men. Reducing the salary differentials between these occupations would go a long way toward assuring the health of many at-risk Canadian families.

- *Restore and improve income supports for individuals unable to gain employment.* Social assistance rates do not come close to allowing many recipients to meet basic needs and participate in Canadian society. In Ontario, profound reductions in social assistance benefits has led to an alarming increase in homelessness and the use of food banks. And most users of food banks are families whose children are especially at risk for poor health outcomes. Other provinces have not reduced benefits to such a drastic extent as in Ontario, yet few have raised them to levels that come close to lifting people out of dire life circumstances.

- *Provide a guaranteed minimum income.* Since the health effects of low income are well documented, it may be more cost-effective to provide Canadians with a basic minimum income in order to reduce the overall incidence of disease as well as various other social ills such as crime and poor school performance. A variety of possible schemes exist, and recent analyses of the benefits of such programs are available (Van Parijs, 2000; Lerner, Clark, and Needham, 2000).

Policies to Reduce Social Exclusion. Numerous analyses have considered how social exclusion occurs and the role it plays in threatening population health (Atlantic Centre of Excellence, 2000; Shaw, Dorling, and Davey Smith, 1999). The following steps—in addition to reducing low income—would reduce social exclusion in Canada.

- *Enforce legislation that protects the rights of minority groups,* particularly concerning employment rights and antidiscrimination. New immigrants to Canada and visible minorities are especially at risk for low income and social exclusion.

- *Ensure that families have sufficient income to provide their children with the means of attaining healthy development.* The provision of these resources will reduce the proportion of children born into and living in poverty, which will have short-term as well as long-term effects on health.

- *Reduce inequalities in income and wealth within the population through pro-gressive taxation of income and inherited wealth.* Canada is one of the few industrialized nations with no inheritance tax. (The United States has such a tax but is considering eliminating it.) In addition, the income tax rates for the very wealthy are lower than in many other industrialized nations.

- *Ensure access to educational, training, and employment opportunities,* especially for individuals such as the long-term unemployed.

- *Remove barriers to health and social services;* this requires learning where and why such barriers exist.

- *Provide adequate follow-up support for individuals leaving institutional care.*
- *Establish housing policies that provide enough affordable housing of a reasonable standard.*
- *Institute employment policies that preserve and create jobs.*
- *Direct attention to the health needs of immigrants* and to the unfavorable socioeconomic position of many groups, including the particular difficulties many New Canadians face in accessing health and other care services.

Policies to Restore and Enhance Canada's Social Infrastructure. Canadian federal program spending as a percentage of gross domestic product has been decreasing since 1987 such that current federal spending is at 1950s levels (Raphael, 2002a). These decreases have occurred in tandem with decreases in tax revenues resulting from modifications to the tax structure that favor the well-off. The concept of universality is an important cornerstone of policies designed to promote social inclusion. Programs that apply to all are more likely to garner political support from the public. The federal and provincial governments should do all of the following:

- *Restore health and service program spending to the average level of the OECD nations.* Federal spending on programs as a percentage of GDP is among the lowest of Organization for Economic Cooperation and Development nations. As noted earlier, such spending is now at 1950s levels (Raphael, 2002a).
- *Develop a national housing strategy and allocate an additional 1 percent of federal spending for affordable housing.*
- *Provide a national day care program.* Such a program—long promised by the federal government—would help many women enter the workforce and reduce the stress associated with carrying out both homemaking and working responsibilities.
- *Provide a national pharmacare program.* Such a program would ensure that individuals with low incomes and on social assistance would have access to needed medication. In addition, such a program would actually reduce health care and drug costs as it improved the health of Canadians (Lexchin, 2001).
- *Restore eligibility and employment benefits to previous levels.*
- *Require that provincial social assistance programs be accessible and be funded at levels to ensure health.*
- *Ensure that supports are available to support Canadians through critical life transitions.*

WORKING FROM THE MIDDLE:
MUNICIPAL ACTION TO PROMOTE HEALTH

The most developed program addressing health and its determinants at the municipal level is that of the Healthy Cities movement (Ashton, 1992; Davies and Kelly, 1993). The movement originated in Toronto, Canada, but it was the European Office of the WHO that turned it into a major political force. Though not explicitly focused on structural issues of power and the concentration of wealth, it provides means by which citizens can leverage local governments to strengthen the social determinants of health and resist the forces that threaten their health and well-being. A WHO Collaborating Center for Healthy Cities has been established at Indiana University.

The Healthy Cities movement has historical roots in public health, considerable consensus on principles, and a core group of theoreticians and researchers (Ashton, 1992; Davies and Kelly, 1993). Healthy Cities is rooted in WHO concepts of health, health promotion, and notions of justice and equity. In practice, Healthy Cities work emphasizes developing healthy municipal public policy. Acting on economic, social, and environmental forces is key in producing a community's health, as is an emphasis on community involvement (Hancock and Duhl, 1986).

Healthy Cities projects are committed to promoting health by influencing local social structures and environments. The movement has a strong values base and considers health in a manner consistent with Canadian and European ways of thinking about a nation's social responsibilities toward its citizens. There are six key elements to the approach (World Health Organization, 1997):

- *Commitment to health.* Projects are based on a commitment to and definition of health as involving the interaction of physical, mental, social, and spiritual dimensions.

- *Political decision making for health.* Since housing, environment, education, social services, and other city programs have a major effect on health in cities, strengthening these is important.

- *Intersectoral action.* Healthy Cities requires creating organizational mechanisms by which city departments and community members come together to contribute to health.

- *Community participation.* Projects promote active roles for people so that they can have a direct influence on project decisions, the activities of city departments, and local life.

- *Innovation.* Projects recognize that promoting health and preventing disease require a constant search for innovative ideas and methods and support for their implementation.

- *Healthy public policy.* Projects achieve their goals by working to create policies that lead to healthier homes, schools, workplaces, and other parts of the urban environment.

The WHO Healthy Cities office in Copenhagen has developed numerous guides for developing healthy cities projects. These provide syntheses of work in the area and are valuable resources. Its strong value of participation reminds health workers of the need to focus on community members' input in identifying community issues. The Healthy Cities center at Indiana University can also be a resource at the local level for anyone addressing the societal issues identified in this chapter.

WORKING FROM THE BOTTOM: COMMUNITY ACTION TO PROMOTE HEALTH

The Ottawa Charter for Health Promotion identifies creating supportive environments and strengthening community action as key areas for health promotion action. A multitude of local efforts across the United States involve attempts by community workers to promote local health and well-being. Frequently, decisions made at the municipal, state, and federal levels damage the quality of the social determinants of health and handicap these efforts. If identifying and influencing governmental and other institutional decisions that threaten health are identified as areas of appropriate activity, these efforts can promote health by engaging local community members in these kinds of analyses (Minkler, 1997; Minkler, Wallerstein, and Hall, 2002).

The health promotion literature identifies numerous means to carry out these efforts. To date, however, the overwhelming proportion of community-based health promotion activities in the United States focus on health behaviors such as diet, physical activity, and tobacco use (Raphael and Farrell, 2002a). Narrow and expert-driven, they are unlikely to consider societal factors that influence health. These efforts are also unlikely to acknowledge and respond to issues that community members themselves may indicate as being important to their health and well-being (Raphael, Steinmetz, and Renwick, 1999).

As it turns out, studies that allow community members to identify their own health needs find that these concerns are remarkably consistent with the view that societal factors are the primary ones that affect their health and the health of those around them (Raphael and others, 2001a, 2001b). Such approaches allow for the integration of the best aspects of health promotion by allowing individuals and communities to increase control over the determinants of their health through strengthening communities and advocating for healthy public policy. They provide a direction for community-based health workers consistent with the main arguments concerning the social determinants of health covered in this volume (Popay and Williams, 1994; Williams and Popay, 1997).

These community-based health promotion activities should be based on the following principles (Raphael, 2002b):

1. The most important determinants of health in Western societies such as the United States are related to how societal and community institutions are organized and resources are distributed. This assumption is in stark contrast to current medical and public health preoccupations with the provision of health care services and altering "healthy lifestyle" behaviors.

2. The lay knowledge that community members possess about their health and its determinants, accumulated from their life experiences, are as valid, if not more so, than knowledge collected by experts through traditional scientific procedures such as indicator analyses and health surveys.

3. Identifying and responding to community health needs involves the commitment to a set of principles guided by the best values of health promotion: empowerment, participation, holistic emphasis, intersectoral action, equity, sustainability, and use of multiple strategies.

These three assumptions are common to the best community-based health promotion work. They also guided the planning and implementation of two community quality-of-life studies in Toronto than can serve as examples of the directions community-based health promotion can take (Raphael, 2001a, 2001b).

The community quality-of-life projects increased understanding about the aspects of community and society that community members believe affect their health and well-being. When asked, "What is it about your neighborhood or community that makes life good for you and the people you care about?" and "What is it about your neighborhood and community that does not make life good for you and the people you care about?" community members identified access to community agencies and services, crime and safety, housing, low income and poverty, municipal support of community infrastructure, and public transportation as key issues. Service providers offered insights concerning agency funding and mandates, and elected representatives discussed the current political environment at the municipal, provincial, and national levels. These concerns are remarkably similar to those identified in the social determinants of health literature.

In addition, community members explored the political dimensions associated with the issues that affected their health and well-being. They made connections between political, economic, and social policies and their effects on both community and individual health.

At local levels, health workers can support citizens in examining and discussing the importance of the social determinants of health. Results can be fed back and used as the basis for concerted community action. These actions can address issues at the local, state, or national levels. Undertakings of this sort, combining the traditions of public health with those of civic involvement and participation, lead to effective actions to improve the health of the population (Fischer, 2000).

CONCLUSION

Teeple (2000) and Laxer (1998) argue that the powerful forces associated with economic globalization and the internationalization of capital are systematically dismantling the welfare state, with health consequences for the majority of the world's people. Developments in Europe indicate that concerted public health and community efforts can profoundly influence the development of policies that determine the extent of health inequalities and the overall state of population health in a nation. The policy directions being undertaken by nations such as Sweden and Finland are two such examples. Similarly, the success of the WHO Healthy Cities initiative demonstrates the power of cities and communities to influence health policy. The Canadian example shows that concerted public pressure can lead to positive policy change.

The United States may present a different situation. American public opinion opposes significant elements of policy associated with reducing income and wealth inequalities and strengthening population health. Much of this is a result of the dominant neoliberal discourse that is promoted by the media and the weakening of unions, public advocacy organizations, and women's groups opposed to such developments. But there are a few bright spots.

In the United States and elsewhere, many efforts are under way to address issues of societal health and well-being. Much of this activity occurs outside the health sector by social welfare, social justice, antipoverty, and other organizations who work to promote community well-being. For example, many organizations such as United for a Fair Economy have raised the issues of income and wealth inequality (Collins, Hartman, and Sklar, 1999; Collins, Leondar-Wright, and Sklar, 1999). The Living Wage movement has scored many notable victories across the nation (Association of Community Organizations for Reform, 2003). The Association of Community Organizations for Reform explains, "Living wage campaigns seek to pass local ordinances requiring private businesses that benefit from public money to pay their workers a living wage. Commonly, the ordinances cover employers who hold large city or county service contracts or receive substantial financial assistance from the city in the form of grants, loans, bond financing, tax abatements, or other economic development subsidies."

In the United States, a series of policy-oriented volumes have addressed the economic inequality issue with little emphasis on health-related aspects (Auerbach and Belous, 1998; Galbraith, 1998; Wolff, 1995). For example, Karoly (1998) discusses the potential benefits of narrowing the income gap and protecting the bottom ranks of Americans from economic shocks. The report *Shifting Fortunes: The Perils of the Growing American Wealth Gap* (Collins, Leondar-Wright, and Sklar, 1999) proposes asset-building policies (broadening employee ownership; establishing individual development accounts), ensuring a living wage and full employment, expanding the earned income credit and raising the no-tax threshold, creating dedicated tax-exempt savings programs, providing affordable housing, and policies addressing the overconcentration of wealth (an income equity law, taxing capital gains like wages, maintaining strong estate and inheritance taxes and wealth taxation).

Finally, the state of Minnesota is one of the few that has moved to highlight the social determinants of health and the role they play in health inequalities in the population (Minnesota Department of Health, 2001; see also Chapter Twenty-Six). Its report *Populations of Color in Minnesota: Health Status Report* (Minnesota Department of Health, 1997) explicitly recognizes the role that poverty plays as a health determinant.

The Minnesota Health Improvement Goals (Minnesota Department of Health, 1998) foster understanding and promotion of social conditions that support health. In addition, they call for promotion of a philosophy of shared responsibility for addressing the social conditions that affect health and collaboration with community efforts to improve social conditions that affect health.

Americans' conservative opinions persist even as the living conditions of many Americans either stagnate or deteriorate. Moving U.S. public opinion and public policy discourse even to the point of approaching the developments seen in Europe may seem impossible. Seriously addressing health inequities in the United States will require some radical rethinking of priorities in social and economic policy. It will also take a great deal of organized political effort and will. Whether that happens in the coming years, without a shift in values supportive of social and economic equality and a belief that everyone deserves good health and well-being, is an open question.

References

Acheson, D. *Independent Inquiry into Inequalities In Health.* London: Stationery Office, 1998.

Agren, G., and Hedin, A. *The New Swedish Public Health Policy.* Stockholm: National Institute of Public Health, 2002.

Ashton, J. *Healthy Cities.* New York: Routledge, 1992.

Association of Community Organizations for Reform. "Living Wage." 2003. [http://www.acorn.org].

Atlantic Centre of Excellence for Women's Health. *Social and Economic Inclusion in Atlantic Canada.* Halifax, Nova Scotia, Canada: Atlantic Centre of Excellence for Women's Health, 2000.

Auerbach, J. A., and Belous, R. (eds.). *The Inequality Paradox: Growth of Income Disparity.* Washington, D.C.: National Policy Association, 1998.

Auerbach, J. A., and Krimgold, B. (eds.). *Income, Socioeconomic Status, and Health: Exploring the Relationships.* Washington, D.C.: National Policy Association, 2001.

Burstrom, B., and others (eds.). *Reducing Inequalities in Health: A European Perspective.* London: Routledge, 2002.

Coburn, D. "Health, Health Care, and Neo-Liberalism." In H. Armstrong, P. Armstrong, and D. Coburn (eds.), *Unhealthy Times: The Political Economy of Health and Care in Canada.* Toronto: Oxford University Press, 2001.

Collins, C., Hartman, C., and Sklar, H. *Divided Decade: Economic Disparity at the Century's Turn.* Boston: United for a Fair Economy, 1999.

Collins, C., Leondar-Wright, B., and Sklar, H. *Shifting Fortunes: The Perils of the Growing American Wealth Gap.* Boston: United for a Fair Economy, 1999.

Davey Smith, G., Dorling, D., and Shaw, M. (eds.). *Poverty, Inequality and Health in Britain, 1800–2000: A Reader.* Bristol, England: Policy Press, 2001.

Davies, J. K., and Kelly, M. P. (eds.). *Healthy Cities: Research and Practice.* New York: Routledge, 1993.

Dunn, J., Hargreaves, S., and Alex, J. S. "Are Widening Income Inequalities Making Canada Less Healthy?" In Ontario Public Health Association, *The Health Determinants Partnership–Making Connections Project.* Toronto: Ontario Public Health Association, 2002.

Fischer, F. *Citizens, Experts, and the Environment: The Politics of Local Knowledge.* Durham, N.C.: Duke University Press, 2000.

Galbraith, J. *The Crisis in American Pay.* New York: Free Press, 1998.

Hancock, T., and Duhl, L. *Healthy Cities: Promoting Health in the Urban Context.* Copenhagen: World Health Organization Regional Office for Europe, 1986.

Health Canada. *The Population Health Template: Key Elements and Actions That Define a Population Health Approach.* Ottawa: Strategic Policy Directorate, Population and Public Health Branch, Health Canada, 2001.

Karoly, L. A. "Growing Economic Disparity in the U.S.: Assessing the Problem and the Policy Options." In J. A. Auerbach and R. Belous (eds.), *The Inequality Paradox: Growth of Income Disparity.* Washington, D.C.: National Policy Association, 1998.

Kawachi, I., and Kennedy. B. P. *The Health of Nations: Why Inequality Is Harmful to Your Health.* New York: New Press, 2002.

Kirby, M. J. *The Health of Canadians: The Federal Role.* Ottawa, Ontario, Canada: Standing Senate Committee on Social Affairs, Science and Technology, 2002.

Lahelma, E., Keskimaki, I., and Rahkonen, O. "Income Maintenance Policies: The Example of Finland." In J. Mackenbach and M. Bakker (eds.), *Reducing Inequalities in Health: A European Perspective.* London: Routledge, 2002.

Laxer, J. *The Undeclared War: Class Conflict in the Age of Cybercapitalism.* Toronto: Viking, 1998.

Lerner, S., Clark, C., and Needham, W. *Basic Income: Economic Security for All Canadians.* Toronto: Between the Lines Press, 2000.

Lexchin, J. *A National Pharmacare Plan: Combining Efficiency and Equity.* Ottawa: Canadian Centre for Policy Alternatives, 2001.

Mackenbach, J., and Bakker, M. (eds.). *Reducing Inequalities in Health: A European Perspective.* London: Routledge, 2002.

Mazankowski, D. *A Framework for Reform: Report of the Premier's Advisory Council on Health.* Edmonton: Government of Alberta, 2001.

Ministry of Social Affairs and Health. *Government Resolution on the Health 2015 Public Health Program.* Helsinki, Finland: Ministry of Social Affairs and Health, 2001.

Minkler, M. (ed.). *Community Organizing and Community Building for Health.* New Brunswick, N.J.: Rutgers University Press, 1997.

Minkler, M., Wallerstein, N., and Hall, B. *Community Based Participatory Research for Health.* San Francisco: Jossey-Bass, 2002.

Minnesota Department of Health. *Populations of Color in Minnesota: Health Status Report.* St. Paul: Minnesota Department of Health, 1997.

Minnesota Department of Health. *Healthy Minnesotans: Public Health Improvement Goals, 2004.* St. Paul: Minnesota Department of Health, 1998.

Minnesota Department of Health. *A Call to Action: Advancing Health for All Through Social and Economic Change.* St. Paul: Minnesota Department of Health, 2001.

Mishra, R. *The Welfare State in Capitalist Society.* Toronto: University of Toronto Press, 1990.

Navarro, V. (ed.). *The Political Economy of Social Inequalities: Consequences for Health and Quality of Life.* Amityville, N.Y.: Baywood Press, 2002.

Phillips, K. *Wealth and Democracy.* New York: Broadway Books, 2002.

Popay, J., and Williams, G. H. (eds.). *Researching the People's Health.* London: Routledge, 1994.

Raphael, D. "Health Inequities in the United States: Prospects and Solutions." *Journal of Public Health Policy,* 2000, *21,* 392–425.

Raphael, D. *Poverty, Income Inequality and Health in Canada.* Toronto: Foundation for Research and Education, Centre for Social Justice, 2002a.

Raphael, D. *Social Justice Is Good for Our Hearts: Why Societal Factors—Not Lifestyles—Are Major Causes of Heart Disease in Canada and Elsewhere.* Toronto: Foundation for Research and Education, Centre for Social Justice, 2002b.

Raphael, D. "When Social Policy Is Health Policy: Why Increasing Poverty and Low Income Threaten Canadians' Health and Health Care System." *Canadian Review of Social Policy,* 2003, *51,* 9–28.

Raphael, D., and Farrell, E. S. "Addressing Cardiovascular Disease in North America: Shifting the Paradigm." *Harvard Health Policy Review,* 2002a, *3,* 18–29.

Raphael, D., and Farrell, E. S. "Beyond Medicine and Lifestyle: Addressing the Societal Determinants of Cardiovascular Disease in North America." *Leadership in Health Services,* 2002b, *15,* 1–5.

Raphael, D., Steinmetz, B., and Renwick, R. "The Community Quality of Life Project: A Health Promotion Approach to Understanding Communities." *Health Promotion International,* 1999, *14,* 197–210.

Raphael, D., and others. "Community Quality of Life in Low-Income Urban Neighbourhoods: Findings from Two Contrasting Communities in Toronto, Canada." *Journal of the Community Development Society,* 2001a, *32,* 310–333.

Raphael, D., and others. "Making the Links Between Community Structure and Individual Well-Being: Community Quality of Life in Riverdale, Toronto, Canada." *Health and Place,* 2001b, *7*(3), 17–34.

Romanow, R. J. *Building on Values: The Future of Health Care in Canada.* Saskatoon, Saskatchewan: Commission on the Future of Health Care in Canada, 2002.

Shaw, M., Dorling, D., and Davey Smith, G. "Poverty, Social Exclusion, and Minorities." In M. G. Marmot and R. G. Wilkinson (eds.), *Social Determinants of Health.* Oxford: Oxford University Press, 1999.

Shaw, M., and others. *The Widening Gap: Health Inequalities and Policy in Britain.* Bristol, England: Policy Press, 1999.

Teeple, G. *Globalization and the Decline of Social Reform.* Aurora, Ontario: Garamond Press, 2000.

Van Parijs, V., and others. "Delivering a Basic Income." *Boston Review,* Oct.-Nov. 2000, pp. 4–8.

Williams, G. H., and Popay, J. "Social Science and the Future of Population Health." In L. Jones and M. Sidell (eds.), *The Challenge of Promoting Health.* Maidenhead, England: Open University Press, 1997.

Wolff, E. N. *Top Heavy: The Increasing Inequality of Wealth in America and What Can Be Done About It.* New York: New Press, 1995.

World Health Organization. *Ottawa Charter for Health Promotion.* Geneva: World Health Organization, 1986.

World Health Organization. *Twenty Steps for Developing a Healthy Cities Project.* Copenhagen: World Health Organization Regional Office for Europe, 1997.

Zweig, M. *The Working-Class Majority: America's Best-Kept Secret.* Ithaca, N.Y.: Cornell University Press, 2000.

CHAPTER TWENTY-ONE

Globalization, Trade, and Health

Unpacking the Links and
Defining the Public Policy Options

Ronald Labonte

Globalization describes a process by which nations, businesses, and people are becoming more connected and interdependent across the globe through increased economic integration and communication exchange, cultural diffusion (especially of Western culture), and travel. It is not a new phenomenon. One might actually call it a basic human drive. Jared Diamond, in *Guns, Germs, and Steel* (1997), recounts how the history of humankind has been one of pushing against borders, exploring, expanding, conquering, and assimilating. In ancient Western times, "global" simply meant throughout the Middle East, once a Garden of Eden that, despoiled by overuse, became an eroding desert that drove people eastward to what is now China and westward to the Mediterranean and continental Europe. In Western medieval times, "global" referred to the exploration, colonization, and exploitation of the "New World" of the Americas. As Eduardo Galeano showed in the brilliant *Open Veins of Latin America* ([1973] 1998), only the wealth of the exploited colonies—their resources, their peoples—allowed Western capitalism to depose feudalism. Today's globalization, some argue, is simply capitalism's attempt to complete this global colonization process.

Globalization is not something that we should necessarily fear or protest against. Thirty years ago, many members of the public health community were passionate globalizers, concerned over international inequalities and the unjust burden of environmentally and socially induced diseases borne by many of the world's poor. We wanted to share our wealth, our democracies, and the empowering lessons of our own progressive social movements. We wanted to learn from and to support the emancipating people's movements that arose in the wake of postcolonial struggles in Africa, Asia, and Latin America. We wanted to travel and meet people from other cultures. We wanted a global village. That is the kind of globalization we can still embrace. Our populist protests over contemporary globalization have erroneously adopted the media moniker of "antiglobalization." We are not antiglobalizers; we are democratic and just globalizers. Therein lies the rub of globalization's critics, for what we have today is not a global village so much as a global marketplace where the dictates of capital and economic self-interest have made our earlier discourses of dignity and justice seem somehow obscene or archaic.

This chapter provides novice democratic globalizers with a map of the territory. It defines how today's globalization differs from previous eras and outlines, from a health perspective, key proglobalization arguments and the response of the skeptics. It provides a framework for how we might assess globalization's impacts on health and assesses two key health-determining pathways: inequalities of poverty and income and environmental sustainability. These necessarily broad strokes lead to a more focused discussion of the World Trade Organization and the known or potential effects of specific trade agreements on national governments' abilities to regulate for human health. The chapter concludes with a discussion of several health public policy options that can be— and are being—pursued by health activists, organizations, and professional groups in national and international forums to aid in creating a system of global governance based on human need rather than human greed.

CONTEMPORARY GLOBALIZATION

Contemporary globalization, abetted by innovations in communications technologies, is characterized by increasing liberalization in the cross-border flow of finance capital and trade in goods and services. It differs from previous eras in several aspects:

- *The scale and speed of such movement, particularly of finance capital.*
  Over U.S.$1.5 trillion (perhaps as much as $2 trillion) in currency transactions occurs daily, more than double the total foreign exchange reserves

of all governments. Such transactions reduce the ability of governments to intervene in foreign exchange markets to stabilize their currencies, manage their economies, and maintain financial autonomy (United Nations Development Programme, 1999).

- *The establishment of binding rules, primarily through the World Trade Organization.* Trade agreements are increasingly establishing enforceable supranational obligations on nation-states. Countries have also entered into scores of other multilateral conventions and agreements on human rights and environmental protection, but few of these carry any penalties. This asymmetry between enforceable economic (market-based) rules and unenforceable social and environmental reciprocal obligations is the biggest governance challenge of the new millennium (Labonte, 1998; United Nations Development Programme, 1999; Kickbusch, 2000).

- *The size of transnational companies involved,* several of which are economically larger than many nations or world regions. Much of the global trade in goods is intrafirm, meaning that a company's subsidiary in one country sells parts or products to a subsidiary in another country (Reinicke, 1998). This allows companies to locate labor-intensive parts of the production chain in low-wage countries (often in exclusive export production zones) and to declare most of their profits in low-tax countries (leading to global tax competition and lower corporate tax revenues in all countries).

- *The apparent commitment of most countries to continue the project of global economic integration through increased market liberalization.* This commitment is built on two decades' dominance of neoliberal economic assumptions, reflected in the macroeconomic policies of most governments, the World Bank and International Monetary Fund, and most trade agreements (see Exhibit 21.1). It is somewhat tempered by the reluctance of many of the world's wealthiest nations to abide by these assumptions if the assumptions are not to their benefit, witnessed by the continued presence and even increase of trade-distorting domestic agricultural subsidies in the European Union, Japan, and the United States.

- *Social, economic, environmental, and health issues are becoming "inherently global"* rather than purely national or domestic (Labonte and Spiegel, 2001). Environmental impacts of human activities are planetary in scale and scope, disease pandemics and economic stagnation partly underpin state collapse and regional conflict (Price-Smith, 2002), and almost one-sixth of humanity is "on the move" to escape environmental or economic degradation and conflict, straining against the borders of other nations. The risk of a return to unilateralism by the more powerful nations is always present; the evidence of the need for multilateral (global) solutions is irrefutable.

Exhibit 21.1. Basic Neoliberal (Neoconservative) Economic Assumptions Driving Contemporary Globalization.

Policy Area	Assumption
Liberalization	Open markets work best for everyone.
Privatization	States should not own or operate productive or profitable sectors of the economy.
Private sector	States should not only sell off their assets but should also open their programs or services to private sector competition.
Deregulation	The fewer the restrictions on the private sector, the better.
State minimalism	To help pay their debts, balance their budgets, and promote the private sector, states should reduce their public spending and taxation rates and introduce cost-recovery programs.

THE PROGLOBALIZATION ARGUMENT

From a health vantage point, there are several compelling arguments in favor of globalization. The diffusion of new knowledge and technology through trade and investment, for example, can aid in disease surveillance, treatment, and prevention. There is also broad consensus on the positive effects of a globalization of gender rights and empowerment, though with the caveat that these rights are not simply an invention of the West but existed (often more strongly in pre-Western colonization times) in many countries that are presumably less emancipated today (Sen, 1999). In economic terms, the proglobalization argument posits that increased trade and foreign investment through liberalization can improve economic growth. Such growth can be used to sustain investment in necessary public goods, such as health care, education, and women's empowerment programs (Dollar, 2001; Dollar and Kraay, 2000). Such growth, particularly in poorer countries, also reduces poverty, which leads, in turn, to better health. Improved population health, particularly among the world's poorest countries, is increasingly associated with improved economic growth (Savedoff and Schultz, 2000; World Health Organization, 2001), and so the circle virtuously closes upon itself.

THE CRITICS' RESPONSE

Critics of the proglobalization thesis argue that globalization's virtuous circle can have a vicious undertow. This includes the more rapid spread of infectious diseases, some of which are becoming resistant to treatment; and the increased adoption of unhealthy lifestyle habits by larger numbers of people (Lee, 2001). The more significant challenge is that liberalization does not always or inevitably lead to increased trade, foreign investment, or economic growth and that when it does, it does not inevitably reduce poverty (Cornia, 2001; Weisbrot et al, 2001; United Nations Development Programme and others, 2000). Much depends on preexisting social, economic, and environmental conditions in countries and on specific national programs and policies that enhance the capacities of citizens, such as health, education, and social welfare programs (United Nations Development Programme, 1999; United Nations Development Programme and others, 2000). China, Korea, Thailand, Malaysia, Indonesia, and Vietnam did dramatically increase their role as global traders, but this was primarily in terms of their exports. They retained tariff and nontariff barriers that shielded important sectors of their economy from competitive imports and public ownership of large segments of banking and placed restrictions on foreign capital flows—which is precisely how wealthier European and North American economies developed historically (Rodriguez and Rodrik, 2000; Rodrik, 1999). World Trade Organization rules now largely prohibit poorer countries from doing the same, with only modest provisions for "special and differential treatment" (trade agreement exemptions) that are being actively opposed by many of the world's richest economies. Weaker economies with fewer domestic protections, largely removed through earlier World Bank and International Monetary Fund (IMF) "structural adjustment" loan policies, have fared poorly under liberalization, notably those in Africa and Latin America. The net effect for these countries has been suppressed domestic economic activity, depressed wages and tax revenues, and a worsened balance of payments. Mexico, Uruguay, Zimbabwe, Kenya, India, and the Philippines all witnessed serious declines in income and corresponding increases in poverty and poor health among its rural farming population following liberalization (Hilary, 2001).

A FRAMEWORK FOR UNDERSTANDING GLOBALIZATION'S IMPACTS ON HEALTH

Globalization may improve people's health in some circumstances but damage it in others, especially when liberalization has been rapid and without government support to affected sectors and populations (United Nations Development Programme, 1999; Ben-David, Nordstrom, and Winters, 1999; Cornia, 2001). Liberalized trade in agricultural products may provide short-term economic benefit to less developed countries. This can improve people's health, depending on how equitably those benefits are allocated among all citizens. But food exports in poorer countries can also increase fossil-fuel-based transportation, creating short-term and longer-term health- and environment-damaging effects, and commodity-led exports produce lower long-term economic growth than manufactured ("value-added") exports (Kim and others, 2000). Protectionist policies, including subsidies, may preserve rural life and livelihoods, arguments frequently advanced by the European Union and Japan (Labonte, 2000). This benefits the health and quality of life of rural people. But such policies can also support ecologically unsustainable forms of production and increase oligopolistic corporate control over global food production. Trade openness might increase women's share of paid employment, which is an important element of gender empowerment (United Nations Development Programme, 1999). Yet much of women's employment remains low-paid, unhealthy, and insecure in "free trade" export zones that often prohibit any form of labor organization and employ only single women. Public support for young children has been declining in many trade-opened countries, portending future health inequalities. There is also evidence of a global "hierarchy of care." Women from developing nations employed as domestic workers in wealthy countries send much valued currency back home to their families, some of which is used to employ poorer rural women in the home country to look after the children they have left behind. These rural women, in turn, leave their eldest daughter (often still quite young and ill educated) to care for the family they left behind in the village (Hochschild, 2000).

What is the gain? What is the loss? Or perhaps more poignantly expressed, who gains and who loses? Tracing the impacts of globalization on health to answer such questions can be a daunting and complex task, but it is one in which public health activists need to engage if they are to become credible advocates for global healthy public policies. Figure 21.1, based on a more extensive study (Labonte and Torgerson, 2002), provides a simplified framework for understanding how contemporary globalization can affect health. The key points conveyed by this figure, in descending order of scale, are as follows:

- How contemporary globalization affects health depends on the historical context of particular countries—specifically, their political, social, and economic traditions (democratic, oligarchic, patriarchal, theocratic, dictatorial, and so on) and their stock of preexisting endowments (level of economic development, environmental resources, human capital development, and the like).

- Globally, the major vehicles through which contemporary globalization operates are imposed macroeconomic policies (notably the structural adjustment programs of the World Bank and International Monetary Fund, which are the precursors of today's "free trade" agenda); enforceable trade agreements (notably the World Trade Organization) and associated transborder flows in goods, capital, and services; official development assistance as a form of wealth transfer for public infrastructure development in poorer nations; and "intermediary global public goods," the numerous yet largely unenforceable multilateral agreements we have on human rights, environmental protection, women's rights, children's rights, and similar matters.

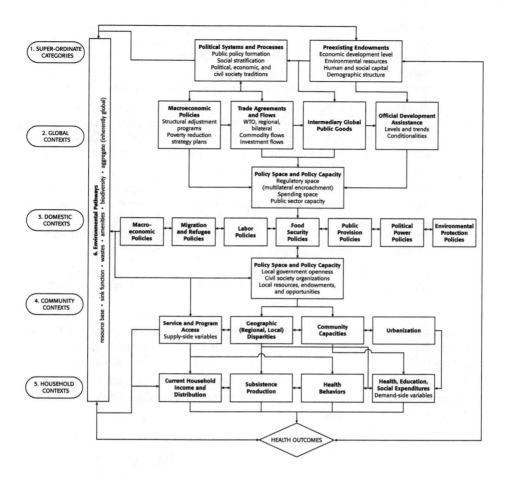

Figure 21.1. Globalization and Health: Selected Pathways and Elements.

- These vehicles have both positive and negative health effects on domestic policy by increasing or decreasing public sector capacity or resources and regulatory authority. Key domestic policies that condition health outcomes include universal access to education and health care, legislated human and labor rights, restrictions on health-damaging products such as tobacco or exposure to hazardous waste, and environmental protection. Liberalization, whether through trade agreements or through structural adjustment programs, lowers tariffs on imported goods. This has been particularly hard on developing countries, which derive much of their national tax revenue from tariffs and lack alternative revenue-generating sources. This affects their ability to provide the public health, education, and water and sanitation services essential both to health and to economic development. Global and regional trade agreements, in turn, are increasingly circumscribing the social and environmental regulatory options of national governments. *It is the impacts of globalization at this level of national policy and regulatory authority that cause health activists the greatest concern, for it can preclude governments from enacting policies that lead to health and equity at the local levels "where people live, work, and play."*

- National policies and resource transfers affect the abilities of regional or local governments to regulate their immediate environment, provide equitable access to health-promoting services, enhance generic community capacities (community empowerment), and cope with increased and usually increasingly rapid urbanization.

- At the household level, all of the foregoing factors in large measure determine family income and distribution (for example, under conditions of poverty, when women control household income, children's health tends to be better), health behaviors, and household expenditures (in time and in money) for health, education, and social programs.

- Each level affects, and is affected by, environmental pathways, chief among these being depletion of resources (water, land, forests), biodiversity loss, and pollution.

Although much remains to be understood about how globalization phenomena can be harnessed to improve global health outcomes, we have now lived through two decades of increased market integration and a decade of enforceable trade rules. With respect to trends in two fundamental health-determining pathways (poverty or inequality and environmental sustainability), the impacts have been largely negative.

POVERTY AND INCOME INEQUALITY

Globally, the past decade has seen a reduction in poverty rates at the $1-a-day level but a worsening in such rates at the $2-a-day level (Ben-David, Nordstrom, and Winters, 1999). This allows us to infer somewhat cynically that our recent era of globalization has successfully transferred income from the extremely poor to the absolutely destitute—a conclusion bolstered by more recent evidence that poverty rates at the $1-a-day level are once again increasing. Some counter that this is because poor countries have insufficiently globalized. If they liberalized more, they would benefit more. A 1999 United Nations Development Programme study of forty developing and least developed nations challenges this assumption. It found that trade openness (liberalization) increased poverty and inequality. The countries liberalizing the most rapidly fared the worst (Rao, 1999).

Although there is still some controversy over whether trade liberalization will succeed in poverty reduction—poverty being one of health's greatest threats—there is much less dispute that trade liberalization is increasing inequality.

Whether income inequality is the root of disease inequality remains a disputed topic among population health researchers (Deaton, 2001). Poverty, which is more widespread in high-income-inequality countries, may the bigger problem. But the greater the income inequality, the harder it becomes for the economic growth *presumed* to follow trade liberalization to actually lift people out of poverty. Moreover, inequalities *are* associated with declines in social cohesion, social solidarity, and support for states with strong redistributive income, health, and education policies that have been shown to buffer liberalization's unequalizing effects (Deaton, 2001; Global Social Policy Forum, 2001; Gough, 2001).

The evidence that trade and investment liberalization is leading to growing income inequality is compelling. Rodas-Martini (1999) discusses a review of 313 structural adjustment programs (SAPs) from 1968 to 1994, which increased liberalization and privatization of public services, found that inequality measures worsened dramatically in the first three years following such programs. Although there was some improvement in these measures by the fifth year, none recovered to their pre-SAP levels. David Dollar (2001) of the World Bank, however, argues that there is no consistent pattern between liberalization and income inequalities and that on average, incomes in the bottom percentiles rise at the same rate as those in highest percentiles as economic growth proceeds. Yet the same 10 percent rise on $1,000 and $100,000 nonetheless creates a larger absolute difference in wealth and the various health-enhancing capacities and privileges such wealth is able to purchase. Moreover, the very countries cited as evidence of the liberalization–growth–poverty reduction relationship (such as China, Vietnam, and India) are the outliers in terms of income distribution. The market-liberalizing developing countries experiencing the greatest growth are also the ones experiencing the sharpest increases in income inequalities.

From a health perspective, what remains contentious is where (or if) a trade-off should be made between economic growth that reduces poverty but increases income inequality (see Figure 21.2). Poverty reduction should lead to short-term health gains, but what are the longer-term risks of increased health inequalities associated with longer-term income inequalities? Many economists now argue that market-based economic growth may reduce income inequalities in the short term, but invariably increase them in the long term in the absence of government redistribution policies.

THE ENVIRONMENT AND SUSTAINABLE DEVELOPMENT

The two primary pathways linking globalization to the environment are the liberalization-induced effects of growth on resource depletion and pollution and increased transportation-based fossil fuel emissions. (What is it that moves all those goods from one part of the planet to another?) Ecological limits to growth

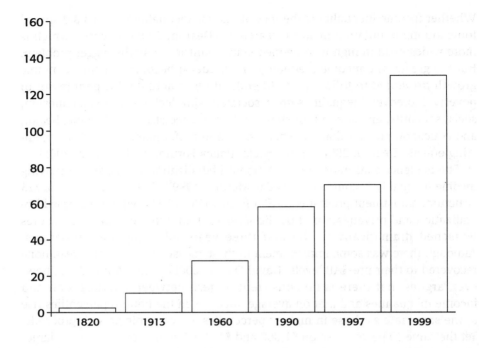

Figure 21.2. Rising Global Income Inequalities: Ratio of the Income of the Top and Bottom 20 Percent of the World's Population, 1820–1999.

Source: UNDP, 1999

and consumption are rarely considered in economic models, yet if all countries "developed" to the same consumption patterns found in the United States, our species would require four more planets to exploit. This estimate comes from the *Footprints of the Planet* report (no date) that calculates the hectares of biologically productive land per capita consumed by different nations. The United States consumed 10.3 hectares per capita in 1993, compared to 4.3 hectares in Japan, 2.5 hectares in Costa Rica, and 0.5 hectare in Bangladesh. Worldwide, current consumption outstrips capacity by 35 percent. There are also numerous instances of trade and investment liberalization having increased the pace of environmental despoliation:

- The combined effects of deregulation, privatization, and weak governmental controls on the Indonesian logging industry, implemented to increase economic growth through increased trade, have led to the loss of more than 1 million hectares of forest per year through logging in Indonesia. Health effects range from short-term and widespread respiratory disorders associated with extensive burning to long-term ecosystem disturbances and potential climatic change (Walt, 2000).

- In Uganda, trade liberalization in the form of industrial privatization and tariff reduction on fishing technology contributed to overfishing of the Nile perch in Lake Victoria and a degradation of the lake ecosystem and water quality (United Nations Environment Programme, 2001).

- Mauritania, a poor West African country, has sold fishing rights to factory ships from Europe, Japan, and China to earn the foreign currency it needs to pay back foreign loans made necessary by liberalization. Meanwhile, fish, the staple protein for the country's poor, has largely disappeared from local markets (Brown, 2002).

- In India, tariff reduction and liberalization of foreign investment in the automotive sector helped increase automobile production by 136 percent, which contributed to a doubling of air pollution levels between 1991 and 1997 (United Nations Environment Programme, 2001).

- In Argentina, trade liberalization and promotion of fisheries exports led to a quintupling of fish catches between 1985 and 1995. Fishing companies gained an estimated U.S.$1.6 billion from this growth, but depletion of fish stocks and environmental degradation have resulted in a net cost of U.S.$500 million (United Nations Environment Programme, 2001).

There are also potential indirect climate change effects due to deregulation of foreign investment. An example of this was the Brazilian currency crisis of 1998, precipitated by the greatest inflow and outflow of speculative capital ever experienced by a developing country (United Nations Development Programme, 1999; de Paula and Alves, 2000). The government lacked sufficient foreign reserves to stabilize its currency and was forced to borrow from the International Monetary Fund. The rescue package included the requirement for drastic public spending cuts, including a two-thirds reduction in Brazil's environmental protection spending. This led to the collapse of a multinationally funded project that would have begun satellite mapping of the Amazon rain forest as a first step in stemming its destruction. This destruction, in turn, may have a profound effect on climate change, with long-term and potentially severe health implications for much of the world's populations (Labonte, 1999). The commitment of the Brazilian government at the 2002 World Summit on Sustainable Development to set aside large tracts of the remaining Amazon rain forest partly obviates the bleak assessment made in 1999 (Mitchell, 2002). It also indicates how actions in one pathway category (in this case, a government's commitment to an intermediary global public good at the 2002 summit) can mitigate the effects of actions in another (capital market liberalization).

Most empirically based projections on the environmental impacts of trade liberalization show severe ecological damage (Labonte and Torgerson, 2002).

The only exceptions are trade agreement requirements to reduce trade-distorting agricultural and fisheries production subsidies. These subsidies go primarily to wealthy producers in wealthy countries, wreak havoc on local production in poorer countries by flooding the market with below-cost commodities, and severely damage the environment. World Trade Organization member nations in November 2001 committed themselves to "reductions, with a view to phasing out, all forms of [agricultural] export subsidies; and substantial reductions in trade-distorting domestic support" (World Trade Organization, 2001a). The European Union and Japan, which heavily subsidize their domestic farmers, have been slow to comply, and the Bush administration in the United States in 2002, despite the Doha agreement, signed into law the largest increase in domestic farm subsidies in American history.[1]

WORLD TRADE ORGANIZATION AGREEMENTS AND HEALTH-DETERMINING PATHWAYS

This brings the discussion to the narrower focus of trade agreements, specifically those of the World Trade Organization (WTO), and their impacts on globalization's health-determining pathways. The WTO was formed in 1995 out of the Uruguay Round of talks on the General Agreement on Tariffs and Trade (GATT). The GATT was a nonenforceable multilateral agreement aimed at decreasing import tariffs and export or production subsidies that impeded global trade in goods. The WTO is the only multilateral (supranational) organization with enforcement powers, in the form of fines or monetized trade concessions. It administers twenty-nine different trade, investment, and "trade-related" agreements, including the former GATT, and several new agreements, such as the General Agreement on Trade in Services (GATS), the Agreement on Trade-Related Aspects of Intellectual Property Rights (TRIPS), the Agreement on Agriculture (AoA), the Agreement on Trade-Related Investment Measures (TRIMS), and the Agreement on the Application of Sanitary and Phytosanitary Measures (SPS). Any of the 145 member countries (as of December 2002) can launch a complaint against other members they think are not fulfilling their WTO commitments. Key principles underpinning all WTO agreements are "national treatment" (in which foreign goods, investment, or services are regulated the same as domestic ones), and "most favored nation" (whatever special preferences might be given to one trading partner must be given to all member nations; social regulations a country adopts domestically that might fall within the scope of WTO agreements must be those that least impede global trade).

Several WTO agreements have specific bearing on these broad economic, social, and environmental pathways linking globalization and health. Indeed, the scope of these agreements, particularly their constraints on governments' domestic legal and regulatory capacities for social and environmental protection, is what has galvanized much of the opposition to the WTO.

TRIMS (Agreement on Trade-Related Aspects of Investment Measures)

There is growing consensus that various forms of social investment and worker protections are needed in the transition from a closed to an open economy. But it is these very protections that may be eroded through the new trade and investment regime. The TRIMS agreement, for example, prevents countries from placing "performance requirements" on foreign investment. Such requirements have been used to benefit corrupt political leaders, government officials, and their families. But such requirements have also proved useful in the development of viable national economies. Their removal benefits investors from developed countries much more than it does people living in developing countries (Greenfield, 2001). Many developing countries are requesting exemptions to this TRIMS requirement in order to retain some control over the direction of their local economic development. This may prove difficult, since a WTO dispute panel several years ago ruled against the use of import protections by developing nations for the purpose of improving poor living standards. "Development [or pro-poor] policy," the ruling concluded, is not the same as "macro-economic policy." Where there is a WTO dispute, the latter shall prevail (Raghavan, 1999). Moreover, exemptions from TRIMS for developing countries is opposed by the so-called Quad of rich countries—the United States, the European Union, Japan, and Canada (*BRIDGES Weekly Trade News Digest*, May 28, 2002).

TBT (Agreement on Technical Barriers to Trade)

The TBT agreement intends to make any "technical" barrier to trade minimally restrictive of trade. A technical barrier is a domestic regulation that has nothing to do with tariffs (the taxes governments impose on imports) or export subsidies (the assistance they give to exports). The TBT encourages use of international standards and allows domestic regulations to be higher only if they can be justified. Article XX(b) of the GATT permits exception to the general GATT rules, including the TBT, "necessary to protect human, animal or plant life or health." On the surface, this seems a reasonable health protection. But in only one instance has this exception been successful in a trade dispute. Part of the reason for this is that countries wishing to deviate from trade rules under this exception are responsible for proving that the measure is not really protectionism in disguise. Many health nongovernmental organizations (NGOs) argue that a reverse onus should apply: the complaining country should prove that the exception was *not* invoked to protect human, animal, or plant life or health. Given that most WTO disputes emanate from developed nations, with over half from the United States alone (Barlow, 2001), there are also suggestions that costs associated with filing a complaint should be borne by the wealthier disputant.

The one successful Article XX(b) exception is the Canadian asbestos case. In April 2001, the WTO rejected Canada's appeal against a French decree banning the importation of asbestos. Canada argued that its asbestos products were "like" the glass fiber products that France did permit; therefore, the asbestos ban was a technical barrier to trade. (Another element of WTO trade rules is that even if an imported product is not the same as any domestic product, if it is sufficiently "like" a domestic product, it cannot be subject to any special regulations.) The WTO dispute panel agreed with Canada that asbestos was "like" glass fibers and that the French ban did violate the TBT. The panel also considered the large body of research establishing asbestos as a proven human carcinogen, which made it "unlike" glass fibers. Therefore, the French ban qualified under the Article XX(b) exception (World Trade Organization, 2000). Such scientific certainty rarely applies to most human health risks, especially those mediated through the environment. There is also a price to be paid for WTO disputes, one that is often disproportionately borne by poorer countries (see Box 21.1).

Box 21.1. Regulatory Chill and the High Price of WTO Compliance.

The WTO regime can lead to a "regulatory chill" effect even before disputes go to a panel for settlement. Guatemala, for example, was threatened by the United States with trade sanctions after Gerber Foods argued that Guatemalan legislation to enact the WHO breast-milk substitutes code violated the TRIPS agreement. The code prohibits visual images that "idealize the use of bottle feeding," such as Gerber's "pudgy baby" logos. According to Gerber, Guatemala's legislation was a de facto expropriation of the company's trademark. The WTO never ruled on this because Guatemala, lacking the resources to fight such a challenge, buckled under pressure and rewrote its legislation to exempt imported baby food products (Wallach and Sforza, 1999). Developing nations need more resources to help shape the interpretation (and ultimately the promised global distributive justice) of these agreements. Small amounts of funding assistance for developing country participation at the WTO do exist, including the Geneva-based Advisory Centre on WTO Law, to which least developed countries have preferential access, and the new Global Trust Fund to assist developing countries in post-Doha negotiations, which has been established by the WTO with about U.S.$20 million in total funding (World Trade Organization, 2001, 2002).

But these rather meager assistance levels do not deal with domestic costs associated with trade agreement compliance. One recent study (Finger and Schuler, 2001) found that to comply with WTO obligations on the SPS agreement alone, Argentina spent over $80 million and Hungary over $40 million. Mexico spent over $30 million to upgrade intellectual property laws and enforcement. "The figures, for just three of the six Uruguay Round Agreements that involve restructuring of domestic regulations, come to $150 million . . . [and could] be higher in the least developed countries. . . .

One hundred and fifty million dollars is more than the annual development budget for eight of the twelve least developed countries for which we could find a figure for that part of the budget" (p. 129).

The current and future costs of WTO compliance seriously jeopardize the already weakened health, education, and human rights infrastructure in many of these countries; "for most of the developing and transition economies—some 100 countries—money spent to implement the WTO rules . . . would be money unproductively invested" (p. 129).

SPS (Agreement on the Application of Sanitary and Phytosanitary Measures)

Scientific uncertainty was the premise behind establishment of the precautionary principle that if evidence is suggestive but not conclusive, the benefit of the doubt should go to protecting human and environmental health. This principle has been weakened by the SPS agreement, which mandates a scientific risk assessment on all regulatory standards. Risk assessment, admittedly an important tool in understanding human threats to the environment and, in turn, environmental threats to humans, cannot deal with the multiple, cumulative impacts that now typify risk management issues. Indeed, risk assessment methods were first introduced in the United States specifically to slow down the rapid pace of environmental regulation during the 1970s (Ward, 1999). The risk assessment requirement invariably favors producers and exporting countries over citizens and importing countries, since there is no cost to the producers if their product eventually proves harmful. The higher order of scientific certainty under the SPS than that governing GATT Article XX(b) is thought to be one reason why the European Union lost to the United States and Canada on its attempt to ban imports of hormone-treated beef. The WTO dispute panel (which did not include any scientists as members) rejected as inadequate the scientific arguments presented to them by the EU, including evidence of possible, though not definitive, human carcinogenicity provided by the independent International Agency for Research on Cancer (Sullivan and Shainblum, 2001; Charnovitz, 2000). There is also concern that the SPS agreement conflicts with how the precautionary principle is enshrined in many multilateral environmental agreements, including the Cartagena Protocol on Biosafety to the Convention on Biodiversity. The SPS puts the burden of proof on the importer while the Cartagena Protocol, more in keeping with the precautionary principle, puts the burden of proof on the exporter.

Both the TBT and the SPS constitute what some call "trade creep," whereby trade rules limit how national governments can regulate their domestic health and environment affairs even if they treat products from other countries no differently than their own—that is, even if they honor trade liberalization's over-arching principle of "national treatment" (Drache and others, 2002).

TRIPS (Agreement on Trade-Related Intellectual Property Rights)

Unlike other WTO agreements, TRIPS does not ensure "free" trade but is "protectionist" of trade by protecting intellectual property rights, almost all of which are held by companies or individuals in developed countries. The TRIPS agreement requires WTO member nations to legislate patent protection for twenty years, although the least developed countries do not have to implement such legislation until 2016. Debate over the TRIPS agreement, particularly regarding access to antiretroviral drugs, has been extensive and highly public. Few developing countries had any patent protection legislation prior to joining the WTO. One effect of the TRIPS agreement has been to sharply increase drug costs in most countries. This decreases the amount of public funding available for primary health care or other public programs (including environmental protection) in First World countries, where 75 percent of prescription drug costs are publicly or privately insured. But it is particularly hard on persons living in poor countries where the health portion spent on drugs is already much higher and often a direct personal cost.

Current TRIPS clauses do allow countries, in the event of public health emergencies, to issue compulsory licenses to generic drug manufacturers. These provisions were affirmed by the WTO Declaration on the TRIPS Agreement and Public Health (World Trade Organization, 2001b), essentially shutting down so-called TRIPS-plus bilateral agreements the United States had been negotiating with developing countries that limited their abilities to use these clauses.[2] While lauded as a major public health breakthrough and a victory by developing countries (particularly the group of African countries) at the WTO, the Doha Declaration fails to deal with substantive problems with TRIPS: With respect to drugs, how will countries lacking generic production capacity obtain their drugs at lower cost when faced with public health emergencies? The United States, Canada, Japan, and Switzerland are reportedly blocking efforts to seek a resolve to this in the TRIPS Council of the WTO (*BRIDGES Weekly Trade News Digest*, May 22, 2002). Presently, the United States is the only government not to agree with the final summary report of the TRIPS Council chair, which, in keeping with the "Declaration on the TRIPS Agreement and Public Health" allows developing countries the right to declare what constitutes a public health emergency within their borders.

GATS (General Agreement on Trade in Services)

The GATS is a "framework agreement" introduced at the conclusion of the Uruguay Round of the GATT. The contribution of services to economic growth and wealth has increased rapidly in comparison to the production of goods.

Its actual and potential contribution to trade has also grown (Sinclair, 2000). The GATS was conceived and continues to be defended primarily as a vehicle for the expansion of business opportunities for transnational service corporations (Hilary, 2001). The key concern is that the GATS will ineluctably lead to increased privatization of such essential public services as health care, education, and water and sanitation (see Box 21.2). Globally, roughly 30 percent of all economic activity lies in government-provided (public) services. Most of these services are essential, meaning that there is a guaranteed market for them, at least among citizens able to pay for them privately. When a crisis of overproduction occurs (too many goods for too few purchasers) or a volatile stock market collapses after years of excessive speculation, one might expect corporations with capital to look to formerly provided public services as a safe private investment. There is some evidence that this may be occurring; services account for 60 percent of foreign direct investment, "much of which is connected with privatization of state entities" (Corner House, 2001, p. 3).

Box 21.2. Globalization, Privatization, and Health Care.

Globalization and free trade agreements are not the cause of public service privatization, although both share the same source, namely, neoliberal economic theory and its five basic tenets. When we consider privatization in health care, we need to draw a distinction between public financing and private delivery (which most countries have to some degree and which can have degrees of progressivism depending on tax structures and on the extent of public regulation of private providers) and private financing and private delivery (which is regressive and excludes all but the wealthy).

Privatization of both forms is increasing worldwide. Between 1990 and 1995, the share of private health expenditure rose in fifteen of twenty-two Latin American countries (Brugha and Zwi, 2002). It has also risen in both Canada (Canadian Centre for Policy Alternatives, 2002) and the United States. The scope for private health care in Latin America is considered so large that in 1999, *The Economist* launched a new quarterly, *Healthcare Latin America*. The same year *The Economist* ran a feature on the "shift toward private health care," which quoted the president of American Association of Health Plans, who noted that "450 million Latin Americans constitute a health-care market of $120 billion a year—of which only 15% is spent on private insurance" (Lewis, 1999). By inference, 85 percent of the market is ripe for privatization. There is some evidence that governments are moving in this direction, often with World Bank or IMF prodding. Peru, in 1998, committed itself to IMF policies of increased privatization of public services, including concessions to private companies taking over public services and increased foreign investment in health and education. Bolivia, with World Bank, IMF, and USAID funding, is promoting a private, self-financed primary health care model (PROSALUD). "Regardless of the type of intervention, most [World Bank and International Development Bank] initiatives have favored the private financing and provision of health care over the former public financing and provision that predominated in most Latin American countries" (Armada, Muntaner, and Navarro, 2001, p. 735).

There are evocative examples of how such privatization creates inequalities in access. Between 1974 and 1989, total private health care expenditures in Chile rose substantially while public health care expenditures declined (Collins and Lear, 1995). Large segments of the poor population were left with underfunded, low-quality public health care. Although public health expenditures since the return of democratic regimes in 1990 have been increasing, growth in private health care expenditures in Chile still outstrips that for public health care (Leon, 2002), and foreign companies now provide 60 percent of Chile's health insurance (Wasserman and Cornejo, 2002). In Brazil, private health care provides 120,000 physicians and 370,000 hospital beds to the richest 25 percent of the population, while the public system has just 70,000 physicians and 565,000 hospital beds for the remaining 75 percent (Zarrilli, 2002a). Recent multilevel studies of structural (macroeconomic) adjustment programs in eight low- and middle-income countries similarly found that privatization of health, education, and other services leads to declining access by the poor via financial impediments, user fees, geographical location, and so on (Haddad and Mohindra, 2001). The situation has been especially bad in Africa, where World Bank structural adjustment policies resulted in user fees in 75 percent of all health, nutrition, and population projects in sub-Saharan countries, with disastrous consequences (Corner House, 2001).

Another effect of this trend, in all countries, is a decline in support for universal public programs by higher-income earners in favor of private insurance and health care systems. In some countries, this is actively supported by tax incentives to higher-income earners to purchase private health care coverage or education.

Private provision of health care (and of education and other essential public goods) is less efficient, often less effective, and always more inequitable than the public, risk-pooling programs that mark the greatest, most democratic, and most humane political system we have so far managed to create: the modern welfare state.

To understand how the GATS might affect health care and other health-promoting public services, one has to examine its "bottom-up" provisions. The GATS agreement has several "top-down" provisions binding on all members, including "national treatment" (foreign services are treated identically to domestic services), "most favored nation" (the foreign services of all WTO members must be treated equally), and "progressive liberalization" (commitments to liberalize services can only increase and cannot decrease without penalty). But its most important health impacts lie in its bottom-up provisions, in which countries specify which services they commit to liberalize, under which of four different modes, and with what, if any, restrictions, referred to in the GATS as commitments that are "bound." The four modes of service liberalization are as follows:

1. Cross-border delivery of trade (such as shipment of laboratory samples or provision of telehealth services)

2. Consumption of health services abroad (called "health tourism," whereby people from one country are treated by health services in another)

3. Commercial presence (foreign private investors provide private hospitals, clinics, treatment centers, or insurance or have management contracts for such facilities, whether they are public or private)

4. Movement of natural persons (the temporary movement of health professionals from one country to another)

As with globalization and trade liberalization generally, there are many arguments made in favor of liberalization in health services. For example, it is argued that GATS liberalization can lead to new private resources to support the public system, can introduce new techniques to health professionals in developing countries, can provide such professionals with advanced training and credentials, and can introduce new and more efficient management techniques (Zarrilli, 2002b). Several developing countries, such as Cuba and India, are specializing in liberalizing health services under modes 2 (health tourism) and 4 (export of health professionals), which earn these countries valuable foreign currency. But there are powerful counterarguments to each of these points. Private resources, whether from health tourism, foreign investment, or remittances from professionals working abroad, benefit the wealthy and increase the regressive privatization of health systems. There is a global crisis in the "brain drain" of trained health professionals from developing to developed countries, from poorer to richer developed countries, and from poorer to richer regions of developed countries. Developing countries are estimated to lose over U.S.$500 million in training costs of doctors and nurses who migrate each year to wealthier nations (Frommel, 2002). The problem is most acute for African countries but is also a problem for many Caribbean countries (International Development Research Centre, 2002) and could be worsened by the GATS. New management techniques are drawn primarily from private providers, the majority of which are from the United States, a country that has the most inefficient and most inequitable health care system of all economically advanced nations.

There is one country where liberalized trade in health services does work very well: Cuba. Years ago, Cuba set out to become a "world medical power." It is one of the few nations in the world producing far more health professionals, particularly physicians, than it needs. It has also developed surplus health care facility capacity. Cuban health professionals work abroad, both as agents of international solidarity and as a means of obtaining foreign exchange through remittances. Cuba's high-quality health care facilities are "value-adding" to its tourism industry. But Cuba is also unique in having surplus capacity, a fully universal public health care system for all of its citizens, and a commercialized health industry that is fully within the public sector. As recounted in Box 21.2, liberalization in health services, to the extent that it increases privatization, will increase inequalities in access.

To date, fifty-four WTO members have made commitments to liberalize some health services under the GATS (Adlung and Carzaniga, 2002). Many of these are developing countries. The number of health-liberalized countries grows to seventy-eight if one includes private health insurance. The GATS has a built-in requirement for "progressive liberalization," meaning that countries can only liberalize more, not less. Once a service sector has been liberalized under the GATS, there is no cost-free way of reversing it (Canadian Centre for Policy Alternatives, 2002). Canada, for example, has opened up private health insurance under the GATS. Should Canada ever wish to extend its public system into areas that are privately insured and so reverse the current trend away from privatization, its GATS commitments would trigger trade penalties. The same would apply to any developing country wishing to reverse its present-day commitments to health services liberalization. Imagine a poorer country where most of its former public services are now privately provided, partly as a result of earlier structural adjustment programs. Imagine that trade liberalization does eventually promote long-term economic growth and that the country is able to tax such growth so that it has sufficient revenue to increase its provision of public health, education, and sanitary services. If it provided any of these services under the GATS, it would have to pay some compensatory damages (in trade concessions, perhaps even as fines) should its public programs force private foreign providers out of the domestic market.

The GATS agreement does offer an exception for a government service that "is supplied neither on a commercial basis, nor in competition with one or more service suppliers" (Article 1:3b). This is often cited as evidence that concern over privatization is misplaced. This clause, however, may collapse under an eventual challenge, since most countries allow some commercial or competitive provision of virtually all public services (Sinclair, 2000; Pollock and Price, 2000). And, while concern over the impact of GATS on access to health care is important, there is also fear that GATS could limit access to such key health determinants as water (see Box 21.3) and education.

Box 21.3. Water Privatization and the GATS.

Water privatization in many poorer countries arose as a condition of structural adjustment programs, which promoted privatization even when the costs would be beyond the reach of most families. A review of IMF loan agreements in forty countries during 2000 found that privatization or full-cost recovery was a condition of twelve of them (Henning, 2001). Such programs in Nouakchott, the capital of Mauritania, led to water costs consuming more than one-fifth of total average household budgets for low-income families (World Bank, 2000) and to thousands of households being cut off from privatized water delivery systems in South Africa (Bond, 2002). Latin American water privatization schemes have been tried, and have failed, in Puerto Rico (1995–1999), Trinidad (1994–1998), Argentina (1995–1998), and several other countries. In each case, rates skyrocketed, service was sporadic or inefficient, huge deficits were created, and in most instances, the contracts were not renewed or the providers simply walked away (Shaffer, Brenner, and Yamin, 2002).

There is considerable concern that the GATS could be used to open up private trade in and increased privatization of water. If this were to occur, the reversal of the hugely unpopular water privatization scheme in Cochabamba, Bolivia, following popular riots, could not have been undertaken without massive compensation paid to foreign water supply companies. To date, forty countries have committed to liberalize environmental services under the GATS, including twenty-six developing and least developed countries. Such liberalization could lead to increased privatization in the provision of water.

SUMMARY: HEALTH PUBLIC POLICY OPTIONS

Globalization is not new, but it is assuming new forms. Specifically, liberalized trade in goods, services, and capital are now governed by enforceable trade rules. The dominant discourse on globalization is that of a "tide raising all boats." This has not been empirically demonstrated except in a few countries, where trade liberalization has lifted all boats but has also made the large ones much larger and the small ones much smaller. Environmentally, the seas supporting the boats, the air filling their sails, and the land on which they dock are all experiencing more severe stress.

How globalization more precisely determines people's health is affected by a complex set of preexisting political conditions and natural endowments, national policy capacities and resources, and publicly provided programs, such as health, education, labor rights, and environmental protection. The abilities of national governments to self-determine these regulatory policies continue to be constrained by the neoliberal economic prescriptions of the World Bank and the International Monetary Fund and are being increasingly compromised by World Trade Organization agreements with their "trade creep" behind the border.

Commercial interests in education, health care, and other public goods can rise and fall. Public provision of such programs can also experience periods of retrenchment and expansion. Trade agreements, however, are limiting national governments and national peoples' abilities to expand public provision, once private financing or services, particularly foreign provision, are allowed into the market. The GATS agreement will almost certainly penalize countries that have committed their health services to liberalization that then change their mind or whose people change governments. NAFTA already does so for its three member nations, which could extend to the hemisphere under the Free Trade Area of the Americas agreement, particularly if that agreement concludes its negotiations with its investor suit provisions still intact (see Box 21.4). Tinkering around the edges of these agreements, by putting in more "bounded" regulatory restrictions, is insufficient. Like Venezuela, which recently revoked a 1998 law committed to privatization of health and social services and declared in a new political constitution that health and social security are universal rights best guaranteed by the state (Armada, Muntaner, and Navarro, 2001), Canadian social and trade policy activists are urging the government to declare a full "carve-out" of health and other essential social programs from current and future trade agreements. In all future trade negotiations, including the Free Trade Area of the Americas agreement, our countries should not rely exclusively on country-specific exceptions for health, which have significant shortcomings and should only be regarded as stopgap measures. Instead, we should pursue generally agreed exceptions or safeguards—permanent features of treaties that are far more likely to endure over time.

Box 21.4. NAFTA and the FTAA.

The WTO is not the only free trade regime with implications for government regulatory capacity or provision of essential public services. The North American Free Trade Agreement (NAFTA) and the Free Trade Area of the Americas Agreement (FTAA, still in negotiation) also have potentially profound effects on the pathways linking globalization to health. NAFTA contains a particularly problematic section, Chapter 11, which permits private *foreign* companies to deny democratically elected governments the ability to regulate in the public health interests of their citizens. I provide some uniquely Canadian examples.

The Canadian government let its legislation for plain packaging of tobacco products die after representatives of Phillip Morris International and R. J. Reynolds Tobacco International argued that it constituted an expropriation of assets, violating NAFTA investment and intellectual property obligations. The Canadian government similarly repealed its ban on the gasoline additive MMT, a known neurotoxin, and paid U.S.$13 million in compensation after Ethyl Corporation argued, again on the strength of NAFTA Chapter 11, that the ban had the effect of expropriating its assets even if there was no "taking" in the classic understanding of expropriation. Both these NAFTA challenges achieved their goal of overturning a public health measure, although neither went to a dispute panel. More recently, a U.S.-based water company used NAFTA to sue the Canadian province of British Columbia for U.S.$220 million over restrictions on bulk water exports legislated by the government. The declared intent of Canadian federal and provincial governments to prohibit international trade in water (primarily to the United States) may be in violation of NAFTA (Shrybman, 1999). The CEO of the U.S. water company was quoted as saying, "Because of NAFTA, we are now stakeholders in the national water policy of Canada" (Barlow, 1999). U.S. states bordering the Great Lakes are currently drafting legislation to permit commercial diversion of water from the basin despite Canada's opposition, arguing that NAFTA gives them the right to do so. Of course, Chapter 11 can be used by Canadian companies to challenge U.S. regulations. Methanex Corporation, a Canadian-based producer of the gasoline additive MTBE, a suspect carcinogen, is suing for U.S.$970 million because California banned its use in 1999.

With respect to health care, NAFTA provides that governments can expropriate foreign-owned investments only for a public purpose *and* if they provide compensation. This opens the door to NAFTA claims that measures to expand public health insurance in Canada (where prescription drugs, home care, and dental care are currently privately insured) or to restrict private for-profit provision of health care services amount to expropriation and that compensation must be paid to American or Mexican investors who are adversely affected.

From a health vantage point, NAFTA's Chapter 11 should be rescinded. Article 15 of the FTAA chapter on investment, which similarly allows investor state suits, should be deleted. (It is currently bracketed text, meaning that there is as yet no agreement among the nations negotiating the FTAA on its content.)

Such a stance begins to build a fence around trade agreements to prevent their incursion into areas of important public domestic policy. There are other trade policy options health activists need to promote:

- Extend "special and differential" trade agreement exemptions for developing countries until their domestic economies are sufficiently developed to be able to compete more fairly in open global markets. This is a double standard. It contradicts neoliberalism's ideological commitment to "equality of opportunity"—one set of rules for everyone and let the chips fall where they may. But if our goal is to move toward equality of outcome, the social justice norm most consistent with health promotion and public health, we require inequalities of opportunity to overcome historically created inequalities in power (Labonte, 2000).

- Ban patenting of life forms, exempt patent protection legislation for poor countries indefinitely, decrease the patent protection period, and permit parallel importing under the TRIPS agreement. These are all positions variously argued by developing and least developed countries, as well as by health, environmental, and development NGOs and many United Nations agencies.

- Reverse the burden of proof in health and environmental protection cases argued under the exemptions in GATT Article XX(b) and under the SPS agreement. Countries claiming that another nation's domestic standards are unnecessarily restrictive of trade need to prove that they were *not* imposed for health reasons and that changing the standard would *not* create a health risk.

- Institute fines tied to gross domestic product rather than trade sanctions as penalties, since trade sanctions invariably hurt poor countries more than wealthy ones. The WTO has the option to levy fines instead of trade sanctions but rarely does. Apportion part of the fines to global funds for health, education, and social development, allowing the dozens of countries now lagging behind in reaching the international development goals for infant and child health, maternal health, gender empowerment and universal education to start catching up.

- Impose a "Tobin tax" on currency exchange. Such a tax, named after the Nobel Prize–winning economist who first proposed the idea, would impose a small tax each time foreign currencies were exchanged. This would dampen tremendously damaging speculation and would raise about U.S. $150 billion annually (based on 1995 data). Such a tax could be split three ways, with a third going to each national government whose currencies were being traded and the remainder to an international development fund.

- Strengthen the "special and differential" exemptions to the liberalization requirements in the Agreement on Agriculture. Sometimes referred to as a "development box," this would allow poorer countries to impose import tariffs and restrict foreign investment or ownership in order to protect domestic markets and ensure food security. Developing countries, under Article 6.2 of the AoA, already have the option to retain domestic support programs for local agriculture when (and if) developed countries finally get around to reducing their extremely generous production subsidies. But they do not have the same abilities to retain or reinstate tariffs for the purposes of food security, rural development, poverty alleviation, or rural employment.

- Negotiate an overarching and enforceable rule in all trade agreements to the effect that when there is any conflict, multilateral environmental agreements and human rights agreements (including the right to health) shall trump trade agreements. Some 109 countries recognize a right to health in some form in their constitution, and all but a few countries (including the United States) have ratified human rights conventions that include the right to health (Blouin, Foster, and Labonte, 2002).

Several health NGOs have been urging national governments with an interest in health to create a "like-minded group" to pursue negotiation of such an overarching rule within the scope of the WTO.

In addition to these reforms to trade agreements, the WTO itself needs some overhauling. The WTO dispute settlement process is one of its least transparent or democratic practices. Such panels should be opened to greater participation from civil society groups, whether in the form of amicus curiae ("friends of the court") briefs or actual representation. All proceedings of the panel should be public in the form of Web postings, except for information that may be legally sensitive or confidential. Such panels should also become "joint panels" involving other specialized multilateral or UN organizations (such as the United Nations Environment Programme, the World Health Organization, and the International Labor Organization) when a trade dispute has obvious cross-cutting effects on human health, human rights, and the environment. Panel members must always include representatives from developing countries (this is optional rather than mandatory at the moment) and should be drawn from experts in disciplines other than simply trade law.

In fairness, the WTO has gone some distance in being more open about its trade negotiating agendas, initiating more meetings with civil society groups, and convening discussions with UN agencies such as those just noted. These agencies, however, are still excluded from many of the negotiating sessions of the WTO and lack any official observer status. The WTO, for example, has the Committee on Trade and Environment. The Doha Declaration mandated this committee to reconcile conflicts between WTO agreements and multilateral environmental agreements, such as the Convention on Biodiversity and the Convention on International Trade in Endangered Species, both of which require trade restrictions against offending countries. But even observer status at the WTO Committee on Trade and Environment by the secretariats responsible for these environmental agreements is still not allowed.

Developing countries are much better organized and more vocal in WTO negotiations than they were in earlier years. At the same time, the United Nations Development Programme, in its 2002 report, chided the WTO (and the World Bank and the International Monetary Fund) for failing to adequately represent the interests of developing countries. Although developing and least developed countries are a majority at the WTO, their abilities to influence the WTO agenda and decision-making process remains constrained. Nearly half of least developed country members of the WTO have no representation in Geneva, compared to the presence of over 250 full-time negotiators from the United States alone (with more flown in for particular meetings or issues). Many developing countries have only one representative, who lacks the time and expertise to attend all of the different weekly meetings scheduled by the WTO. The push for expanding existing agreements and introducing new issues for negotiation will only further WTO bias toward the economic interests of developed nations.

Several NGOs argue that "WTO processes should be designed to suit the capacity of the least powerful members" and that "this aim should override concerns about the speed of decision-making"(ActionAid and others, 2001). Among other requirements, this means direct financial assistance from developed to developing countries for WTO participation (see Box 21.1), reductions in the number of trade-related issues for negotiation at the WTO, fewer meetings, and no use of executive body or other subdividing of decision making away from the General Council. Within negotiating rounds themselves, the practice of elite caucusing and negotiations (referred to as the "green room" process) that partly led to the collapse of the 1999 Seattle WTO ministerial meetings must be prevented.

WTO legitimacy as a democratic global institution extends to its engagement with civil society. Presently, private sector corporations dominate NGO involvement at the WTO. The extent of this influence is not fully known, but a study by Corporate European Observer (cited in ActionAid and others, 2001) found that a committee of thirteen major companies, including General Motors and Monsanto, introduced intellectual property rights into the Uruguay Round. The U.S. delegation participating in subsequent negotiations leading to the TRIPS agreement had 111 members, 96 of whom were from the private sector. In the lead-up to the failed Seattle meetings, U.S. organizers offered businesses special access to key negotiators in exchange for donations to subsidize the costs of the round (ActionAid and others, 2001). Although the WTO has made efforts at greater openness, there is a risk that these will be partial and tokenistic or will favor those NGOs with the resources required to participate. Special efforts to engage NGOs from developing countries must be made, and means to support their engagement in discussions must be created. Capacity building for NGOs from developing and least developed countries is no less important than capacity building for official delegates from those countries. Precedents and models for funding NGO participation in public policy reviews exist in several developed countries and could be emulated by the WTO.

Finally, existing agreements must continue to be analyzed for their impacts on internationally agreed basic rights, human development, and health and environmental sustainability goals, with changes made when WTO agreements conflict in any way with their accomplishment. More important, the WTO as an institution should be judged for how it contributes to the accomplishment of these goals, rather than simply on the degree to which it succeeds in trade and investment liberalization.

CONCLUSION

We live in perhaps the most important historical moment of our species. Our planet is dying amid excessive affluence and poverty. Once far-away conflicts and diseases imperiled global health and security. At the same time, activists are struggling toward some system of global governance for our common good.

In Western countries, a similar national struggle took place in the nineteenth century. The first laws and regulatory systems in such countries protected the interests of the capitalist class at the expense of the workers, women, the poor, and the environment. But such laws became the platform around which progressive social struggles constructed reciprocal responsibilities for both state and market, giving rise to the twentieth-century welfare state.

A similar struggle is being enacted globally today. Trade agreements are the first truly enforceable international laws we have created. They benefit the capitalist class. They have also become the focus of worldwide progressive social movements demanding that governments similarly abide by their agreements to protect the environment, promote human rights, achieve health for all, and redistribute wealth through universal education and social support systems. The WTO originally served the rich countries' benefit, as much of this chapter laid out. Its enforceable rules constraining the domestic regulatory space of national governments risk environmental deregulation. Its "level playing field"—one set of rules for all nations with only limited special treatment for poor countries—is pushing many of these countries into deeper health-compromising poverty. Its negotiations to open public services to trade will hasten their privatization, with loss of access for the poor. But the WTO is also increasingly under siege by developing countries, UN agencies, and nongovernmental organizations, collectively attempting to harness the first global rules with penalties attached to the goal of human development and ecological sustainability. Some democratic globalizers urge the WTO's abolition. This would be a mistake, for we have no other vehicle capable of enforcing an improvement in the unequal balance of global economic power. Civil society and developing country struggles to wrest reforms in the WTO are giving rise to a new system of global governance for the common good.

We cannot say whether these struggles will succeed. But we know the global policy options that will work to promote health. We know where these must be advocated—with our national governments, our fellow citizens, our global institutions.

Notes

1. The U.S. trade representative, Robert Zoellick, subsequently proposed global reductions in such subsidies, including those in the United States (*BRIDGES Weekly Trade News Digest,* Nov. 7, 2002). This is a common ploy by wealthier countries in the World Trade Organization. Before agreeing to reduce trade-distorting tariffs or subsidies in sectors important to their own economies, they first dramatically raise them.

2. The United States, however, is seeking to write such TRIPS-plus restrictions into the intellectual property rights chapter of the Free Trade Area of the Americas agreement, now in negotiation, in clear violation of its signing of the Doha Declaration (Human Rights Watch, 2002). It is also entering into free trade talks with the Southern African Customs Union—Lesotho, Botswana, South Africa, Namibia, and Swaziland—which includes agreements on "intellectual property rights," something that NGO observers believe could be another TRIPS-plus effort (*BRIDGES Trade Weekly Digest,* Nov. 14, 2002).

References

ActionAid and others. "Recommendations for Ways Forward on Institutional Reform of the World Trade Organization." Unpublished document (mimeo). 2001.

Adlung, R., and Carzaniga, A. "Health Services Under the General Agreement on Trade Services." In C. Vieira and N. Drager (eds.). *Trade in Health Services: Global, Regional, and Country Perspectives.* Washington, D.C.: Pan American Health Organization, 2002.

Armada, F., Muntaner, C., and Navarro, V. "Health and Social Security Reform in Latin America: The Convergence of the World Health Organization, the World Bank and Transnational Corporations." *International Journal of Health Services,* 2001, *31,* 729–768.

Barlow, M. "Global Rules Could Paralyze Us." *National Post,* Aug. 31, 1999.

Barlow, M. "The Free Trade Area of the Americas and the Threat to Social Programs, Environmental Sustainability and Social Justice in Canada and the Americas." Council of Canadians, 2001. [http://www.canadians.org/documents/campaigns-ftaa-threat-barlow.pdf].

Ben-David, D., Nordstrom, H., and Winters, L. A. *Trade, Income, Disparity and Poverty.* Geneva: World Trade Organization, 1999.

Blouin, C., Foster, J. and Labonte, R. *Canada's Foreign Policy on Health: Towards Coherence.* Commissioned research paper to the Commission on the Future of Health Care in Canada. Ottawa: Canadian Centre for Policy Alternatives, 2002.

Bond, P. (ed.). *Fanon's Warning: A Civil Society Reader on the New Partnership for Africa's Development.* Trenton, N.J.: Africa World Press, 2002.

Brown, P. "Europe's Catch-All Clause." *Guardian Weekly,* Mar. 29–Apr. 3, 2002, p. 26.

Brugha, R., and Zwi, A. "Global Approaches to Private Sector Provision: Where Is the Evidence?" In K. Lee, K. Buse, and S. Fustukian (eds.), *Health Policy in a Globalizing World*. Cambridge: Cambridge University Press, 2002.

Canadian Centre for Policy Alternatives. "Putting Health First: Canadian Health Care Reform, Trade Treaties and Foreign Policy." 2002. [http://www.healthcarecommission.ca].

Charnovitz, S. "The Supervision of Health and Biosafety Regulation by World Trade Rules." 2000. [http://www.netamericas.net/Researchpapers/Documents/Charnovitz/Charnovitz4.doc].

Collins, J., and Lear, J. *Chile's Free Market Miracle: A Second Look*. Oakland: Food First Books, 1995.

Corner House. *Trading Health Care Away? GATS, Public Services and Privatisation*. Sturminster Newton, England: Corner House, 2001.

Cornia, G. A. "Globalization and Health: Results and Options." *Bulletin of the World Health Organization*, 2001, *79*, 834–841.

Deaton, A. *Health, Inequality and Economic Development*. Geneva: Commission on Macroeconomics and Health, World Health Organization, 2001.

de Paula, L.F.R., and Alves, A. J., Jr. *External Financial Stability and the 1998–99 Brazilian Currency Crisis*. Rio de Janeiro, Brazil: Fundação Konrad Adenauer no Brasil, 2000.

Diamond, J. *Guns, Germs, and Steel: The Fates of Human Societies*. New York: Norton, 1997.

Dollar, D. "Is Globalization Good for Your Health?" *Bulletin of the World Health Organization*, 2001, 79, 827–833.

Dollar, D., and Kraay, A. *Growth Is Good for the Poor*. Washington, D.C.: World Bank, 2000.

Drache, D., and others. *One World, One System? The Diversity Deficits in Standard-Setting, Development and Sovereignty at the WTO*. Toronto: Robarts Centre for Canadian Studies, York University, 2002.

Finger, J. M., and Schuler, P. "Implementation of Uruguay Round Commitments: The Development Challenge." In B. Hoekman and W. Martin (eds.), *Developing Countries and the WTO: A Proactive Agenda*. Oxford: Blackwell, 2001.

Footprints of the Planet Report (n.d.) [http://www.iclei.org/iclei/ecofoot.htm]. Accessed September 15, 2001.

Frommel, D. "Global Market in Medical Workers." *Le Monde Diplomatique*, May 2002, pp. 28–29.

Galeano, E. H. *Open Veins of Latin America: Five Centuries of the Pillage of a Continent* (C. Belfrage, trans.). New York: Monthly Review Press, 1998. (Originally published 1973)

Global Social Policy Forum. "A North-South Dialogue on the Prospects for a Socially Progressive Globalization." *Global Social Policy*, 2001, *1*, 147–162.

Gough, I. "Globalization and Regional Welfare Regimes: The East Asian Case." *Global Social Policy*, 2001, *1*, 163–190.

Greenfield, G. "The WTO Agreement on Trade-Related Investment Measures." Ottawa: Canadian Centre for Policy Alternatives Briefing Paper Series: Trade and Investment, 2001, *2*(1).

Haddad, S., and Mohindra, K. *Macroeconomic Adjustment Policies, Health Sector Reform, and Access, Utilisation and Quality of Health Care: Studying the Macro-Micro Links.* Montreal: International Development Research Centre, University of Montreal, 2001.

Hennig, R. C. "IMF Forces African Countries to Privatise Water." [www.afrol.com]. Feb. 8, 2001.

Hilary, J. *The Wrong Model: GATS, Trade Liberalisation and Children's Right to Health.* London: Save the Children, 2001.

Hochschild, A. R. "Global Care Chains and Emotional Surplus Value." In W. Hutton and A. Giddens (eds.), *Global Capitalism.* New York: New Press, 2000.

Human Rights Watch. "The FTAA, Access to HIV/AIDS Treatment and Human Rights." Briefing paper. New York: Human Rights Watch, Oct. 29, 2002.

International Development Research Centre. *Trade in Health Services: Research Priorities to Address Emerging Policy Challenges in Latin America and the Caribbean.* Ottawa: International Development Research Centre, 2002.

Kickbusch, I. "The Development of International Health Policies: Accountability Intact?" *Social Science and Medicine*, 2000, *51*, 979–989.

Kim, J.-Y., and others (eds.). *Dying for Growth: Global Inequality and the Health of the Poor.* Monroe, Maine: Common Courage Press, 2000.

Labonte, R. "Healthy Public Policy and the World Trade Organization: A Proposal for an International Health Presence in Future World Trade/Investment Talks." *Health Promotion International*, 1998, *13*(3), 245–256.

Labonte, R. "Globalism and Health: Threats and Opportunities." *Health Promotion Journal of Australia*, 1999, *9*, 126–132.

Labonte, R. "Health Promotion and the Common Good: Toward a Politics of Practice." In D. Callahan (ed.), *Promoting Healthy Behavior: How Much Freedom? Whose Responsibility?* Washington, D.C.: Georgetown University Press, 2000.

Labonte, R., and Spiegel, J. *Health, Globalization and Research Priorities: A Briefing Paper Prepared for the Institute on Population and Public Health.* [http://www.spheru.ca]. 2001.

Labonte, R., Torgerson, R. *Frameworks for Analyzing the Links Between Globalization and Health,* SPHERU—University of Saskatchewan (mimeo, draft report to World Health Organization, Geneva). 2002. http://www.spheru.ca (accessed December 14, 2002).

Lee, K. "Globalization: A New Agenda for Health?" In M. McKee, P. Garner, and R. Scott (eds.), *International Cooperation in Health.* Oxford: Oxford University Press, 2001.

Leon, F. "The Case of the Chilean Health System, 1983–2000." In C. Vieira and N. Drager (eds.), *Trade in Health Services: Global, Regional, and Country Perspectives.* Washington, D.C.: Pan American Health Organization, 2002.

Lewis, J. "The Americas Shift Towards Private Health Care." *Economist,* May 8, 1999, pp. 27–29.

Mitchell, A. "Brazil to Conserve Tract of Rain Forest." *Globe and Mail,* Sept. 7, 2002, p. A14.

Pollock, A., and Price, D. "Re-Writing the Regulations: How the World Trade Organisation Could Accelerate Privatisation in Health-Care Systems." *Lancet,* 2000, *356,* 1995–2000.

Price-Smith, A. *The Health of Nations: Infectious Disease, Environmental Change, and Their Effects on National Security and Development.* Cambridge, Mass.: MIT Press, 2002.

Raghavan, C. "WTO Members Awaiting New Draft Text for Seattle." Third World Network, Oct. 17, 1999. [http://www.twnside.org.sg/title/newdraft-cn.htm].

Rao, J. M. "Openness, Poverty and Inequality." In United National Development Programme, *Background Papers, Human Development Report, 1999.* New York: United Nations Development Programme, 1999.

Reinicke, W. *Global Public Policy: Governing Without Government?* Washington, D.C.: Brookings Institution, 1998.

Rodas-Martini, P. "Income Inequality Between and Within Countries: Main Issues in the Literature." In United National Development Programme, *Background Papers, Human Development Report, 1999.* New York: United Nations Development Programme, 1999.

Rodriguez, F., and Rodrik, D. *Trade Policy and Economic Growth: A Skeptic's Guide to the Cross-National Evidence.* London: Centre for Economic Policy and Research, 2000.

Rodrik, D. *The New Global Economy and Developing Countries: Making Openness Work.* Washington, D.C.: Overseas Development Council, 1999.

Savedoff, W., and Schultz, T. P. (eds.). *Wealth from Health: Linking Social Investments to Earnings in Latin America.* Washington, D.C.: Inter-American Development Bank, 2000.

Sen, A. *Development as Freedom.* New York: Knopf, 1999.

Shaffer, E., Brenner, J., and Yamin, A. *Comments Regarding the Free Trade Area of the Americas Negotiations: Effects on Universal Access to Health Care and Water Services.* San Francisco: Center for Policy Analysis on Trade and Health, 2002.

Shyrbman, S. "A Legal Opinion Concerning Water Export Controls and Canadian Obligations under NAFTA and the WTO." [http://www.wcel.org/wcelpub/1999/12926.html]. 1999.

Sinclair, S. *GATS: How the World Trade Organization's New "Services" Negotiations Threaten Democracy.* Ottawa: Canadian Centre for Policy Alternatives, 2000.

Sullivan, T., and Shainblum, E. "Trading in Health: The World Trade Organization (WTO) and the International Regulation of Health and Safety." *Health Law in Canada,* Nov. 2001.

United Nations Development Programme. *Human Development Report, 1999*. New York: Oxford University Press, 1999.

United Nations Development Programme. *Human Development Report, 2002*. New York: Oxford University Press, 2002.

United Nations Development Programme and others. *World Resources, 2000–2001*. Washington, D.C.: World Resources Institute, 2000.

United Nations Environment Programme. *Trade Agreements Must Consider Environmental Issues*. Information Note 01/18. New York: United National Environment Programme, 2001.

Wallach, L., and Sforza, M. *Whose Trade Organization?* Washington, D.C.: Public Citizen, 1999.

Walt, G. "Globalisation of International Health." *Lancet*, 2000, *351*, 434–444.

Ward, H. "Science and Precaution in the Trading System." International Institute for Sustainable Development and the Royal Institute of International Affairs. [http://iisd1.iisd.ca/trade/wto/wto_pubs.htm]. 1999.

Wasserman, E., and Cornejo, S. "Trade in Health Services in the Region of the Americas." In C. Vieira and N. Drager (eds.), *Trade in Health Services: Global, Regional, and Country Perspectives*. Washington, D.C.: Pan American Health Organization, 2002.

Weisbrot, I., and others. "The Scorecard on Globalization, 1980–2000: Twenty Years of Diminished Progress." Center for Economic and Policy Research, 2001. [http://www.cepr.net/globalization/scorecard_on_globalization.htm].

World Bank. *World Development Indicators, 2000*. Washington, D.C.: World Bank, 2000.

World Health Organization. "Health in PRSPs: WHO Submission to World Bank/IMF Review of PRSPs." Department of Health and Development, World Health Organization, Dec. 2001. [http://www.worldbank.org/poverty/strategies/review/who1.pdf].

World Trade Organization. *European Communities—Measures Affecting Asbestos and Asbestos Containing Products: Report of the Panel*, WT/DS/135/R (accessed May 27, 2003). [http://www.wto.org]. 2000.

World Trade Organization. *Ministerial Declaration*, WT/MIN(01)/DEC/1. Geneva: Nov. 20 (accessed May 27, 2003). [http://www.wto.int/english/thewto_e/minist_e/min01_e/mindecl_e.htm]. 2001a.

World Trade Organization. *Declaration on the TRIPs Agreement and Public Health*, WT/MIN(01)/DEC/2. Geneva, Nov. 20 (accessed Sept. 18, 2002). [http://www.wto.org/english/thewto_e/minist_e/min01_e/mindecl_trips_e.htm]. 2001b.

Zarrilli, S. "The Case of Brazil." In C. Vieira and N. Drager (eds.), *Trade in Health Services: Global, Regional, and Country Perspectives*. Washington, D.C.: Pan American Health Organization, 2002a.

Zarrilli, S. "Identifying a Trade-Negotiating Agenda." In C. Vieira and N. Drager (eds.), *Trade in Health Services: Global, Regional, and Country Perspectives*. Washington, D.C.: Pan American Health Organization, 2002b.

CHAPTER TWENTY-TWO

Socioeconomic Disparities in Health in the United States

An Agenda for Action

Nancy E. Moss

The very earliest documents from the founding of the U.S. Republic make equality a governing principle for policy-making. In the eighteenth century, equality was about political power rather than social norms and was extended neither to women nor to slaves. Nevertheless, the ideal of equality has governed constitutional change and significant aspects of public policy-making for generations. The most recent of these was the wave of legislation that culminated in the Johnson administration's War on Poverty during the 1960s when the issues of racial, gender and economic equality of opportunity rose to the fore. The past decade has seen a resurgence of interest in inequality, motivated by concern with results attained rather than opportunity. In this chapter I examine recent trends in economic inequality in the United States; the relationship of economic inequality to variations in health; recent actions in the United States to draw attention to health inequalities; the creation of health inequalities as a public policy issue in the United States and Europe; and, based on these experiences, next steps that could be taken.

This chapter is based on a paper presented at the forum "Inequalities in Health and Health Care," held at the University of Utah, July 12, 1996. The assistance of all participants and especially Dr. Norman Waitzman is gratefully acknowledged.

INEQUALITY OF INCOME AND WEALTH IN THE UNITED STATES

The period of economic and social expansion that began in the post–World War II era ended in the early 1970s when income gains made by Americans during the 1950s and 1960s began to erode, leading to increasing income inequality between those at the top and those at the bottom of the nation's social hierarchy. During the 1980s, political and economic trends towards deregulation of financial markets, the globalization of capital, and social conservatism drove interest in socioeconomic equality and the consequences of poverty off of the public agenda. The demise of the Soviet Union as an external threat coincided with a reopening of internal debates about economic inequality within the United States, as issues which had been marginalized during the late 1970s and the 1980s moved back to center stage. Nonetheless, this change has occurred primarily among the media and academic elites, not in the public-at-large.

Despite the rhetoric of constitutional ideology and the recent rediscovery by the media of inequality of income and wealth, it is nothing new in the United States. The extent of inequality has risen and fallen periodically during the past 300 years (Williamson and Lindert, 1980). During the colonial and post-colonial periods inequality was relatively constrained, but it increased during the nineteenth century with the erosion of the frontier, urbanization and the technological development that made access to an educated workforce and financial capital more important and reinforced urban social hierarchies dominated by capitalist elites. After brief leveling during World War I, inequality of wealth and income rose during the 1920s to retreat during the years of the Great Depression and World War II.

During the post–World War II period, income inequality declined 7.4% (as measured by the Gini index),[1] a trend that reversed in 1968 (Williamson & Lindert, 1980; Weinberg, 1996). By 1982, income inequality equaled and then surpassed its post-war level, a trend that has continued, albeit somewhat less dramatically than during the 1980s (Figure 22.1). Since 1968 the share of total income received by the top 5% of households has grown from 16.6 to 21.2% in 1994, more than eight times as much as households at the 20th percentile or bottom of the income distribution (Weinberg, 1996). Accounting for non-cash income such as government transfers somewhat modifies but does not alter this picture. Only recently has there been some stabilization of the long-term growth in income inequality in the United States (Weinberg, 1997).

The recent rise in inequality of income and wealth in the United States is mirrored by trends in other industrialized countries (Atkinson, Rainwater and Smeeding, 1995a); data from the Luxembourg Income Study show that by 1987 income inequality was greater in the United States than in comparable industrialized nations (see Figure 22.2) (Atkinson, Rainwater and Smeeding, 1995b).

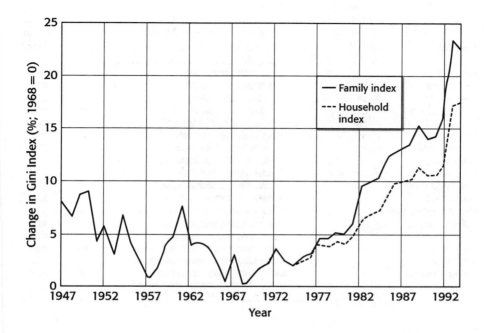

Figure 22.1. Change in Income Inequality in the United States, 1947–1992.
Source: Weinberg, 1996.

Explanations proposed to account for the recent rise in income inequality in the United States include the inflow of baby-boom age workers during the 1970s competing with lower-skilled, older workers, the decline of manufacturing and the erosion of good jobs for less-educated workers, globalization of labor and capital markets, the growth of the lower-wage service sector, changes in technology's demands on labor, and the decline of labor unions that could press for higher wages (Larin and McNichol, 1997). Changes in social welfare programs eroded the cash value of benefits (Danziger and Gottschalk, 1995). Income inequality for white households during this period would probably be even worse were it not for increased contributions of women's earnings to the household (Cancian, Danziger and Gottschalk, 1993), although there are signs that the moderating effect of women's wage work may be leveling off.

Inequalities in wealth, while less often studied than inequalities in income, present a similarly dismal picture. The share of marketable net worth held by the top 1% of wealth holders declined (unevenly) from 1930 until the mid-1970s when it began a steep and unabated rise back to pre–World War II levels (see Figure 22.3). In the United States, nearly 40% of total household wealth belongs to 1% of the population (Wolff, 1995).

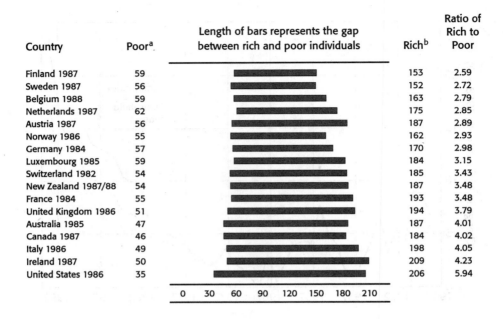

Country	Poor[a]	Length of bars represents the gap between rich and poor individuals	Rich[b]	Ratio of Rich to Poor
Finland 1987	59		153	2.59
Sweden 1987	56		152	2.72
Belgium 1988	59		163	2.79
Netherlands 1987	62		175	2.85
Austria 1987	56		187	2.89
Norway 1986	55		162	2.93
Germany 1984	57		170	2.98
Luxembourg 1985	59		184	3.15
Switzerland 1982	54		185	3.43
New Zealand 1987/88	54		187	3.48
France 1984	55		193	3.48
United Kingdom 1986	51		194	3.79
Australia 1985	47		187	4.01
Canada 1987	46		184	4.02
Italy 1986	49		198	4.05
Ireland 1987	50		209	4.23
United States 1986	35		206	5.94

```
0   30   60   90   120  150  180  210
```

Figure 22.2. Gap Between the Incomes of Rich and Poor Individuals in Various Countries (Percentage of Median in Each Country).

Source: Atkinson, Rainwater and Smeeding, 1995a.

[a]Relative income for individuals who are poorer than 90 percent of the individuals in the country and more affluent than 10 percent of the individuals, as a percentage of the national median.

[b]Relative income for individuals who are more affluent than 90 percent of the individuals in the country and poorer than 10 percent of the individuals, as a percentage of the national median.

Until recently, poverty rather than inequality was the focal point among U.S. policy makers and scholars trying to understand how social class differences affect people's well-being. While World War II had served as a leveler after the Great Depression, by the early 1960s the claims of poor whites and poor blacks left behind in the 1950s march towards affluence helped to make the War on Poverty the focus of social policy. The institutionalization of the "poverty line," an average subsistence income threshold adjusted by the annual Consumer Price Index and weighted by family size (U.S. Department of Commerce, 1993), made it possible to monitor health and social trends among the poor and non-poor (Citro and Michael, 1995). Trends such as the increasing concentration of income and wealth among a small percentage of Americans, and declines in wage growth for middle class households, have stimulated renewed attention to inequality and its consequences for health and well-being (Duncan, 1996; Duncan, Smeeding and Rodgers, 1993).[2]

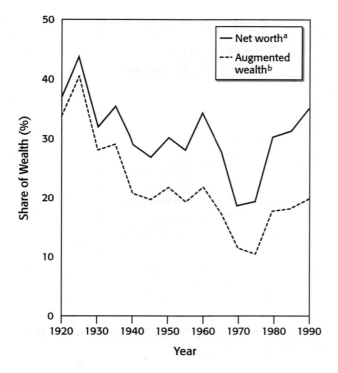

Figure 22.3. Share of Wealth Owned by the Top 1% of Households in the United States, 1922–1989.

Source: Wolff, 1995.

[a]Net worth is the difference between assets and liabilities (mortgage, consumer and other debt).

[b]Augmented wealth includes Social Security and pensions in addition to assets such as cash, money market accounts, bonds, cash value of life insurance, stocks, real estate and consumer durables.

INEQUALITY AND HEALTH

Variations in educational attainment, wealth, income and occupational position as markers of socioeconomic inequality have long been associated with variations in health and mortality risk (Antonovsky, 1967; Pappas, Queen, Hadden and Fisher, 1993; Adler et al., 1994; Amick, Levine, Tarlov and Walsh, 1995; Wilkinson, 1996; Kaplan et al., 1996; Kennedy, Kawachi and Prothrow-Stith, 1996). While the impact of socioeconomic inequality varies by gender, age and ethnicity (and by choice of independent and dependent measures), the overall message is consistent: socioeconomic inequalities affect health (Figure 22.4).

Not all inequalities in health or in health care are due to socioeconomic antecedents. Given the same socioeconomic profile and the same environmental

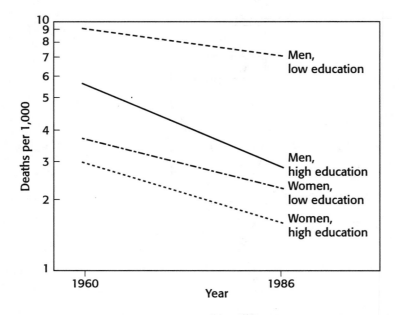

Figure 22.4. Death Rates in 1960 and 1986 Among Whites Between 25 and 64 Years of Age, by Sex and Educational Level.

Source: Pappas and others, 1993.

constraints, two individuals may differ in genetic heritage as well as behavioral choices, and the result may well be different sequelae of disease or disability. The effects of socioeconomic variation are likely to be intergenerational, and differences in fetal and early life environments combined with subsequent socioeconomic conditions across the lifecourse may contribute to the risk of adult morbidity and mortality (Elo and Preston, 1992; Lynch et al., 1994; Kuh and Ben-Shlomo, 1997; Barker, 1998). Whether socioeconomic inequality always leads to inequalities in health is an empirical question. This paper's purpose is to explore the relationship of socioeconomic inequality to health in the context of policy in the United States but not to suggest that inequalities in health will always be modified by socioeconomic equity.

The pathways by which socioeconomic inequality affects health are complex (Williams and Collins, 1995; Williams, 1997b). Macroeconomic events and policy—translated into investments—shape the occupations and industries of employment, which in turn determine labor-market opportunities and workplace conditions. In differing ways a number of the body's organs and systems are affected by expressions of inequality which influence the endpoints of disease, disability and death. Inequality shapes health through intergenerational genetic and socioeconomic heritage; neighborhood and environmental quality; household patterns, including gender and economic equity; and personal behaviors (Elo and Preston, 1992; Kaplan, 1996; Wilkinson, 1996; Williams, 1997b; Guest and Almgren, 1998). Access to goods and services, including health care, can be a consequence or modifier of inequality.

With an idea in mind of how inequality's effects shape health, we return to our major question: are there steps that policy makers can take to reduce the impact of inequality on health? How can data be used to make policy action possible?

ATTENTION TO INEQUALITIES IN HEALTH IN THE POLICY SPHERE

The relationship of socioeconomic inequality and health is an old—not a new—area of concern for public health policy (Amick et al., 1995). The public health community in the United States, like that in the United Kingdom, has a longstanding interest in socioeconomic differences in health, with advocates promoting and performing much of the work of monitoring and investigating these relationships (Krieger and Fee, 1996). Many public health researchers over the years have attempted to highlight the differences among Americans in health using a variety of socioeconomic measures (Krieger, Williams and Moss, 1997).

For the first time in 1998, the U.S. Department of Health and Human Services (HHS) issued its annual report, *Health, United States, 1998*, as a chartbook on socioeconomic status and health (Pamuk, Makuc, Heck, Reuben and Lochner, 1998).[3] Unlike the United Kingdom and many European countries, the United States has not routinely reported public health and vital registry data by occupational class or socioeconomic position (Krieger, Chen and Ebel, 1997; Krieger, Williams and Moss, 1997); instead, the emphasis has been on health differences by "race," color or ethnicity, with the choice of term depending upon the era. Yet the volume which sets decennial public health goals for the nation, *Healthy People 2000*, contains a surprising number of references to income disparities, albeit under the heading "Special Populations" (U.S. Department of Health and Human Services, 1991). As has been typical in the United States, particularly since the 1960s, the focus is on low-income populations—the "poor"—rather than on the effects of social gradients or social class.

Healthy People 2000 states, "Health disparities between poor people and those with higher incomes are almost universal for all dimensions of health. Those disparities may be summarized by the finding that people with low income have death rates that are twice the rates for people with incomes above the poverty level" (p. 29).

The section concludes with an interesting paragraph which highlights some of the contradictions in the government's approach:

> For the coming decade, perhaps no challenge is more compelling than that of equity. The disparities experienced by people who are born and live their lives at the lowest income levels define the dimensions of that challenge. The relationships between poverty and health are complex and cannot be reduced to a simple one-to-one relationship between dollars available and levels of health. Low income may, in fact, be a product of poor health, just as poor health may be caused by environmental exposures, material deficiencies and lack of access to health services that adequate income might correct or improve. While, from a public health perspective, the leverage available to effect improvements is limited largely to the availability and quality of health services, improvements in education, job training and other social services are necessary to erase the health effects of current income disparities [p. 31].

This excerpt from *Healthy People 2000* explicitly identifies equity as a public health objective. It brings the United States into line with the World Health Organization's European Region, where equity is "target 1" for reducing differences in health (Vagero, 1995; Whitehead, 1998). Subscribing to the goal of equity is an important rationale for the systematic collection and distribution of information and for public health and social policy (Whitehead, 1998).

There are some drawbacks to the approach of *Healthy People 2000*. Its emphasis is primarily on the poor versus the non-poor. It views poverty as affecting health through environmental effects, material deprivation and lack of access to health services; *Healthy People 2000* ignores the research showing that social and occupational hierarchies create conditions of control and subordination that differ all along the socioeconomic gradient and that there are health effects throughout (Karasek and Theorell, 1990; Marmot, Bobak and Davey Smith, 1995).[4] *Healthy People 2000* targets health policies and programs as the consequences of socioeconomic disparities; their existence is taken as a given. The text cited above highlights the "drift hypothesis," which views poverty as a product of poor health. Evidence supporting the drift hypothesis (Smith and Kington, 1997a, 1997b) is limited relative to evidence that supports the effects of poverty, social class and inequality on health. On the positive side, *Healthy People 2000* recognizes that improvement in health disparities attributable to income differentials will not come solely from improving access to medical care and recognizes the importance of cooperation with other sectors, such as education, job training and social services.

ACTIONS TO REDUCE SOCIOECONOMIC DISPARITIES IN HEALTH

During the past 25 years, U.S. government intervention to improve health has come almost entirely through initiatives aimed at changing individual behavior; the public has been urged to eliminate cigarette smoking, eat more fruits and vegetables, reduce fat consumption, modify alcohol intake and use seat belts (Marmor, Barer and Evans, 1994). The Clinton administration has moved only recently towards more regulatory action by limiting the tobacco companies' marketing efforts and by regulations aimed at improving food safety. The agencies charged with regulatory action, including the Food and Drug Administration, the Environmental Protection Agency and the Occupational Safety and Health Administration, are sometimes successful in socially-directed initiatives, although more often embattled. Individual behaviors are, to a large extent, shaped by social class position and the material environment (Kaplan, 1996). Yet there is increasing evidence that societal inequality reduces life expectancy independent of behavior (Kaplan et al., 1996; Kennedy, Kawachi and Prothrow-Stith, 1996; Williams, 1997b). And, at the micro-level, the work of Michael Marmot and his colleagues shows that, independent of individual health habits and access to health services, hierarchical position predicts morbidity, disability and mortality (e.g., Marmot, Bobak and Davey Smith, 1995; Hemingway et al., 1997).

Recognizing that increasing inequalities in wealth and income during the past 25 years have resulted in disparities in mortality and other health indicators, and cognizant of the power of the Black Report and *The Health Divide* in the United Kingdom to serve as rallying points for research and policy change (Townsend, Davidson and Whitehead, 1992), a number of scientists inside and outside the U.S. government have begun to search for ways to improve the monitoring of inequalities in health and to find new ways to report to the public on socioeconomic inequalities in health. Activities include:

- The publication in recent years of widely-cited papers drawing attention to the worsening consequences of socioeconomic inequalities for health (Pappas et al., 1993; Adler et al., 1994; Kaplan et al., 1996; Kennedy, Kawachi and Prothrow-Stith, 1996).

- The publication in 1994 of the revised National Institutes of Health (NIH) Guidelines on the Inclusion of Women and Minorities in Clinical Research explicitly encouraging researchers to take into consideration socioeconomic gradients among study populations.

- A workshop conducted at the National Institute of Child Health and Human Development in October 1993 on data and measurement issues relating to social class and health followed by a conference in Annapolis the following fall on the same topic (Moss and Krieger, 1995; Krieger and Moss, 1996); these meetings brought together federal officials and non-governmental researchers, including epidemiologists, economists, sociologists and advocates from the United States and Europe. A portion of the conference focused on the implications for health of macroeconomic changes such as globalization of labor and capital as well as trends in income and wealth inequality. With its unique, cross-disciplinary focus the meeting also drew attention to the conceptual issues underlying the selection of different measures. The Annapolis meeting resulted in recommendations to add and/or improve socioeconomic measures in vital statistics, government and nongovernment health surveys and disease registries to better monitor social inequalities in health and for research ("Recommendations," 1996).

- Support by Annapolis participants for what was to have been called the "Lee Report on Social Inequalities in Health in the United States," inspired by the United Kingdom's Black Report (Townsend, Davidson and Whitehead, 1992). The plan was for the Lee Report to be prepared at the National Center for Health Statistics (NCHS) under the auspices of then-Assistant Secretary for Health and head of the U.S. Public Health Service, Dr. Philip R. Lee. An expert panel convened in March 1995 at the National Institutes of Health (NIH) reviewed a draft plan for the report. The report became a highly contentious activity partly because of concerns raised by results of the 1994 congressional elections, which had resulted in a conservative Republican majority and the imminent 1996 presidential election. By the winter of 1995–1996, the Lee Report had been replaced by two distinct activities: the planned submission to a leading public health journal of a set of analytic papers, mostly by federal researchers; and a chart book similar in format to the annual *Health, United States* report, which was to use a variety of government health data sets to present descriptive tables on health differences by age, race, sex and education or income. By the end of 1997 there had been numerous changes of leadership at the NCHS and in the HHS. The articles planned for the single journal submission dispersed and appeared individually in a variety of places. *Health, United States, 1998* focused on ethnic and socioeconomic differences in health (Pamuk et al., 1998). Several of its authors were originally slated to participate in the Lee Report.

- The 1995 hiring of Norman Anderson, a social psychologist, as the first associate director of the Office of Behavioral and Social Science

Research, NIH. Anderson's major scientific work has been on the impact of race on hypertension; his conceptual model is explicitly focussed on the broader dimension of social inequality (Anderson, 1997).

- The 1995 conference on "Socioeconomic Status and Cardiovascular Health and Disease," organized by the National Heart, Lung and Blood Institute.

- Research initiatives of the Centers for Disease Control and Prevention addressing social class and racial differences in health (e.g., Rowley and Tosteson, 1993).

- A series of regional workshops in 1999 sponsored by the National Institute of Environmental Health Sciences on "Decreasing the Gap: Developing a Research Agenda on Socioeconomic Status, Environmental Exposures and Health Disparities."

At the same time, there has been a strong resurgence of interest in the topic of inequalities in health in the private sector. The John D. and Catherine T. MacArthur Foundation's support of a working group to explore how social inequality and specifically social hierarchies "get into the body" led to the creation of a research network (Adler et al., 1994). The 1999 meeting of the New York Academy of Sciences at the National Institutes of Health, "Socioeconomic Status and Health in Industrial Nations: Social, Psychological and Biological Pathways," was an important outgrowth of this network. Advocacy groups have joined forces with public health researchers to highlight health inequalities at meetings sponsored by organizations like the American Public Health Association and through groups like the Poverty and Race Research Action Council.

Despite the resurgence of economic productivity and full employment in the United States during the mid- and late 1990s, inequalities of income and wealth, if not their consequences for health, have enjoyed full play in the *New York Times* and the *Washington Post* (e.g., Bradsher, 1995; Rich, 1995; Pérez-Peña, 1995). Much thinking and communication about the issue of inequality and its consequences for Americans' well-being has been directed at elite audiences, but more attention needs to be directed at the public-at-large.

How can socioeconomic inequality and its consequences for health become a compelling issue for policy-makers and the public as it has in the United Kingdom, where The Black Report and *The Health Divide* (Townsend, Davidson and Whitehead, 1992) have received widespread attention? It also has been possible to put health inequalities on the health policy agendas of the Netherlands, Sweden and Spain, as well as the European Union (Whitehead, 1998). These efforts have partially counterbalanced the privatization of national insurance, dismantling of social safety nets and widening income disparities in European nations (Atkinson, Rainwater and Smeeding, 1995a, 1995b).

CREATING A PUBLIC POLICY ISSUE:
LESSONS FROM EUROPEAN COLLEAGUES

While member countries have varied in how health inequalities were identified as a policy issue, the European Union has identified related research as a priority area (Whitehead, 1998). Public debate on inequality in Europe is part of a long tradition supported by powerful political parties. The United States has neither the collective support of a supranational body nor a major political party that is comfortable addressing inequality. There are two other major differences between the United States and Europe:

- *Deteriorating social conditions.* The evidence from the United States is mixed. While inequalities in income and wealth as well as in health have increased during the past 25 years, the mid-to-late-1990s has been a time of prosperity, with decreasing unemployment and real income gains for some—though not all—population groups (Weinberg, 1997). The United States has lacked the visible crises and political and economic deterioration experienced in some areas of Western and Eastern Europe and the former Yugoslavia.
- *Population aging.* While both North America and Europe are experiencing population aging, public concern in the United States centers not around the vulnerability of the elderly but around the impact of the costs of services for the aging baby boom cohort. On the other hand, the United States shares with Europe a widening gap in health status between those better and worse off socioeconomically (Pappas et al., 1993).

Public action in European countries has depended on different country-specific strategies. The Dutch found, for example, that including a broad spectrum of governmental and non-governmental policy makers was as important as the language used to frame policy debate. In the Netherlands, politicians were more eager to act when debate centered "on the wasted potential attributable to the excess morbidity and mortality of the more disadvantaged social groups" than when the discussion concerned social justice or equity (Whitehead, 1998, p. 480).

The atmosphere around health policy in the United Kingdom was contentious following the release of the Black Report and continuing throughout the Thatcher period (Whitehead, 1997). The United Kingdom lacked the widespread agreement of a broad spectrum of advocacy organizations or politicians that health inequalities constituted a major public policy issue (U.K. Department of Health, 1996; Whitehead, 1998). Nonetheless, organizations like the King's Fund and civil servants in the Department of Health were able to reverse this dismal situation over time, working through European Union activities and within the United Kingdom by compromising, e.g., changing terminology from "inequalities in health" to "variations in health," keeping up a steady stream of pressure in elite publications such as the *British Medical Journal* and *Lancet* (e.g., Whitehead and Dahlgren, 1991; Davey Smith and Egger, 1993; Wilkinson, 1995; Haines and Smith, 1997; Whitehead, Scott-Samuel and Dahlgren, 1998) and making sure that the effect of poverty on well-being was highlighted in the media. The Black Report and its successor, *The Black Report and The Health Divide,* have received widespread attention (Townsend, Davidson and Whitehead, 1992), and there have been a number of reports on socioeconomic variations in health (e.g., U.K. Department of Health, 1996). A recent report in the United Kingdom, sponsored by the private King's Fund, has taken the next step of preparing a comprehensive program of policy initiatives and activities to reduce health inequalities (Benzeval, Judge and Whitehead, 1995). Its recommendations provide guidelines for U.S. policymakers (see Exhibit 22.1).

Exhibit 22.1. Recommendations on Inequalities in Health in the United Kingdom Pertinent to the United States: Levels of Policy Initiatives and Examples.

Strengthen individuals[a]
- Behavioral changes and supports (for example, stress management)
- Smoking cessation clinics
- Nutrition interventions
- Counseling services

Strengthen communities[a]
- Increase opportunities for healthy social interaction and networking
- Facilitate community development
- Strengthen community groups

Improve access to essential facilities and services[b]
- Ensure adequate and secure housing
- Build on and extend public health initiatives to improve infrastructure, reduce pollution
- Legislate for public health and safety (smoking, seat belts, and so on)
- Provide universal comprehensive health and social insurance

Encourage macroeconomic and cultural change[b]
- Provide income maintenance policies for broad adequate support
- Improve education and training policies shown to reduce long-term poverty
- Ensure equitable compensation, taxation, and income distribution policies
- Create new sources of access to investment capital to spur entrepreneurial activity

Source: Adapted from Benzeval, Judge and Whitehead, 1995.

[a]Some evidence for effects; treat symptoms, not causes; usually limited in place, scope, time.

[b]Strong evidence for effects; wide-ranging in scope.

Success in putting health inequalities on the public agenda in Europe has depended upon some of the same strategies that have been successful in getting public health issues like adolescent pregnancy and infant mortality on the policy agenda in the United States (Nathanson, 1991; Luker, 1996):

- Bringing research evidence to the attention of decision-makers by using elite publications including academic journals and national press; special reports that are visible and highly readable; and popular media that help to fan public attention.

- Reframing the categories and attending to language in ways that obtain and encourage consensus among divergent factions and agencies. Focusing on equity, disparities and variations in health proved more palatable than talking about inequality.

- Keeping action steps firmly in view of policy makers and advocates. These include policy alternatives as well as recommendations on measuring and monitoring.

- Communicating across a wide variety of settings and constituencies, using different media.

- Playing on public and political concern about international ranking.

- Linking common goals and action targets across agencies.

- Developing a research program supported by elite foundations, scientific agencies and other shapers of the policy agenda.

- Encouraging advocates, including authoritative medical and scientific organizations, to design realistic policy alternatives.

- Creating networks among public and private agencies and advocates to evaluate and disseminate policy options.

WHAT ELSE SHOULD THE UNITED STATES DO TO TAKE ACTION ON INEQUALITIES IN HEALTH?

The foregoing suggests that strategies can be grouped into three categories: those that raise the awareness level among the general public and policy makers as well as among scientists and advocates; those that address the policies at the federal, state and local levels that shape inequality; and the development of interventions that target the mediators and consequences of socioeconomic disparities in health. A first step in the United States is to create a climate of unacceptability for socioeconomic differentials in health. How can this be done? I recommend activities following from strategies that have been successful in Europe as well as the United States:

- Improve measures and data sources at local, state and national levels, and in the public and private sectors (Krieger, Chen and Ebel, 1997; Berkman and Macintyre, 1996). Local health and hospital systems can improve their socioeconomic data as, for example, a working group at Kaiser Permanente, the oldest and largest health maintenance organization in the United States, has attempted to implement in the 1990s in order to better monitor the health of its own patient populations. Core national health data sets should have the most succinct, best-validated socioeconomic measures (Williams, 1997a).

- Use the data which are available. Many socioeconomic measures are available in state and local health data systems, but too often the will or the resources to analyze them are not available (Krieger, Chen and Ebel, 1997). State and local advocacy groups can draw renewed attention to the availability of these data and pressure for increased funds for analysis, reporting and dissemination.

- In addition to identifying relevant scientific issues, research networks should make sure that findings are disseminated to popular as well as to scholarly audiences. The growth of the Internet, the development of geographic information systems and other new technologies are available to assist in this process.

- U.S. researchers and public officials should build on already existing initiatives that have some credibility, e.g., through WHO/SIDA (Braveman, 1996), *Healthy People* and the Healthy Cities program, and they should interweave attention to socioeconomic variations in health into behavior and disease-based initiatives.

- Partnerships could be created between public health advocates and officials with colleagues and agencies in education, labor and justice; these agencies have a stake in the consequences of increased socioeconomic disparities in the United States and maintain their own research and policy staffs. The Dutch example cited by Whitehead (1998) suggests that shared goals and moderate language facilitate intersectoral and cross-party alliances.

- State, county and city health departments could take the lead in forming task forces to monitor, report on and design interventions to tackle socioeconomic differences in health. Task forces have mobilized communities around adolescent pregnancy, infant mortality and AIDS. While the health of the poor, vulnerable and "special" populations is a natural focus at the community level, it will be important to educate the public about relationships that transcend all gradations in social hierarchies.

- It would be helpful to move away from the concept of the dependent poor and bring the issue into political debate in a way that highlights the human potential presented by reducing socioeconomic disparities in health. These include a more productive workforce, the lessening of social and interpersonal violence, diminished costs of health care and other economic and equity rationales (Miller, 1995).

- There are many opportunities to use media creatively. In 1996 Channel 4 (ITV) in the United Kingdom broadcast a series on poverty created by a small commission that included Peter Townsend among its members (Channel 4 Commission on Poverty, 1996). The series attracted significant media attention.

- Groups concerned with equity in health should try to attract new funders. Foundation assets have grown significantly during the 1990s, and a number of foundations are experiencing changes in leadership that open up new opportunities for individuals concerned about socioeconomic disparities in health. Academics and advocates have a role to play in shaping funders' priorities, and foundations often help to form the vanguard of public opinion. Conservatives have learned this lesson well by successfully using institutions like the Heritage Foundation and the Manhattan Institute to shape public discourse.

- Using *Healthy People* as a base, the federal government should establish quantitative targets for reducing socioeconomic disparities in health. Targets have been successfully established in both European Union and in-country documents. In the United States, *Healthy People* sets public health goals for the nation. It would be helpful to focus on socioeconomic gradients affecting the middle and upper classes as well as the poor. Targets should not be limited to "special populations"; they should cut across many, if not most, public health goals and activities. *Healthy People* should move from framing health goals for poor and non-poor populations to targeting health disparities across the socioeconomic spectrum while still recognizing the disproportionate disadvantage borne by vulnerable populations including the poor.

CONCLUSION

The renewed interest in socioeconomic disparities in health, sparked by growing inequality in an era of unprecedented prosperity, suggests that it is time to bring new thinking to this area. Although data from the United Kingdom and other Western European countries suggest that universal health care does not dissolve inequalities in outcomes, they provide instructive examples of how with will, imagination and energy, health inequalities can be tackled at local and national levels. Recent general prosperity in the US and the beginning of a new century provide an opportune moment for conveying the discussion of socioeconomic inequalities in health from academic to popular and policy discourse and action.

Notes

1. The Gini index is a statistical method for calculating the relative inequality of an income distribution. It ranges from 0, if every family or household had the same income, to 1, if one family or income had all of the income (Weinberg, 1996).

2. By contrast, public attention to racial/ethnic and gender inequality has been more pervasive, widespread and popularized. In the United States, the interactions of race/ethnicity and gender affect the shape and distribution of personal and household income and wealth. For a detailed discussion, see Massey and Denton (1993), Wilson (1987, 1996) and Smith and Kington (1997a).

3. *Health, United States, 1998* relies on data routinely collected by the National Center for Health Statistics via birth and death certificates and the National Health Interview Survey (Pamuk et al., 1998). Family income and education are the predominant socioeconomic measures. Diseases for which socioeconomic data are not routinely collected (e.g., cancer, AIDS and other sexually-transmitted diseases) were not included.

4. The 1999 New York Academy of Sciences conference, "Socioeconomic Status and Health in Industrial Nations: Social, Psychological and Biological Pathways," had as an explicit goal to investigate the relationship between social ordering and health and the policy implications of the socioeconomic gradient.

References

Adler, N. E., and others. "Socioeconomic Status and Health: The Challenge of the Gradient." *American Psychologist*, 1994, *49*, 15–24.

Amick, B. C., III, and others (eds.). *Society and Health.* New York: Oxford University Press, 1995.

Anderson, N. "Psychosocial, Behavioral, and Educational Factors That Affect Population Differences in Health Among Women." Paper presented at the workshop "Beyond Hunt Valley: Research on Women's Health for the 21st Century," Office of Research on Women's Health, National Institutes of Health, Santa Fe, N.M., 1997.

Antonovsky, A. "Social Class, Life Expectancy, and Overall Mortality." *Milbank Quarterly,* 1967, *45*, 31–73.

Atkinson, A. B., Rainwater, L., and Smeeding, T. M. *Income Distribution in Advanced Economies: Evidence from the Luxembourg Income Study.* Paris: Organization for Economic Cooperation and Development, 1995a.

Atkinson, A. B., Rainwater, L., and Smeeding, T. M. *Income Distribution in OECD Countries.* Paris: Organization for Economic Cooperation and Development, 1995b.

Barker, D.J.P. *Mothers, Babies and Health in Later Life.* Edinburgh, Scotland: Churchill Livingstone, 1998.

Benzeval, M., Judge, K., and Whitehead, M. *Tackling Inequalities in Health: An Agenda for Action.* London: King's Fund, 1995.

Berkman, L. F., and Macintyre, S. "The Measurement of Social Class in Health Studies: Old Measures and New Formulations." In M. Kogevinas and others, *Social Inequalities and Cancer.* Lyons: International Agency for Research on Cancer, 1996.

Bradsher, K. "Gap in Wealth in U.S. Called Widest in West." *New York Times,* Apr. 17, 1995, pp. A1, D4.

Braveman, P. *Equity in Health and Health Care: A WHO/SIDA Initiative.* Geneva: World Health Organization, 1996.

Cancian, M., Danziger, S., and Gottschalk, P. "The Changing Contributions of Men and Women to the Level and Distribution of Family Income, 1968–88." In G. Papadimitriou and E. Wolff (eds.), *Poverty and Prosperity in the Late Twentieth Century.* New York: Macmillan, 1993.

Channel 4 Commission on Poverty. *The Great, the Good and the Dispossessed.* London: Channel 4 Television, 1996.

Citro, C. F., and Michael, R. T. *Measuring Poverty: A New Approach.* Washington, D.C.: National Academy Press, 1995.

Danziger, S., and Gottschalk, P. *America Unequal.* Cambridge, Mass.: Harvard University Press, 1995.

Davey Smith, G., and Egger, M. "Socioeconomic Differentials in Wealth and Health: Widening Inequalities in Health—The Legacy of the Thatcher Years." *British Medical Journal,* 1993, *307,* 1085–1086.

Duncan, G. J. "Income Dynamics and Health." *International Journal of Health Services,* 1996, *16,* 419–444.

Duncan, G. J., Smeeding, T. M., and Rodgers, W. "W(h)ither the Middle Class? A Dynamic View." In G. Papadimitriou and E. Wolff (eds.), *Poverty and Prosperity in the Late Twentieth Century.* New York: Macmillan, 1993.

Elo, I. T., and Preston, S. N. "Effects of Early Life Conditions on Adult Mortality: A Review." *Population Index,* 1992, *58,* 186–212.

Guest, A. M., and Almgren, G.J.M. "The Ecology of Race and Socioeconomic Distress: Infant and Working-Age Mortality in Chicago." *Demography,* 1998, *35,* 23–34.

Haines, A., and Smith, R. "Working Together to Reduce Poverty's Damage: Doctors Fought Nuclear Weapons, Now They Can Fight Poverty." *British Medical Journal,* 1997, *314,* 529–530.

Hemingway, H., and others. "The Impact of Socioeconomic Status on Health Functioning as Assessed by the SF-36 Questionnaire: The Whitehall II Study." *American Journal of Public Health,* 1997, *87,* 1484–1490.

Kaplan, G. A. "People and Places: Contrasting Perspectives on the Association Between Social Class and Health." *International Journal of Health Services,* 1996, *26,* 507–519.

Kaplan, G. A., and others. "Inequality in Income and Mortality in the United States: Analysis of Mortality and Potential Pathways." *British Medical Journal,* 1996, *312,* 999–1003.

Karasek, R., and Theorell, T. *Health Work: Stress, Productivity, and the Reconstruction of Working Life.* New York: Basic Books, 1990.

Kennedy, B. P., Kawachi, I., and Prothrow-Stith, D. "Income Distribution and Mortality: Cross-Sectional Ecological Study of the Robin Hood Index in the United States." *British Medical Journal,* 1996, *311,* 1004–1007.

Krieger, N., Chen, J. T., and Ebel, G. "Can We Monitor Socioeconomic Inequalities in Health? A Survey of U.S. Health Departments' Data Collection and Reporting Practices." *Public Health Reports,* 1997, *112,* 481–494.

Krieger, N., and Fee, E. "Measuring Social Inequalities in Health in the United States: A Historical Review, 1900–1950." *International Journal of Health Services,* 1996, *26,* 391–418.

Krieger, N., and Moss, N. E. "Accounting for the Public's Health: An Introduction to Selected Papers from a U.S. Conference on Measuring Social Inequalities in Health." *International Journal of Health Services,* 1996, *26,* 383–390.

Krieger, N., Williams, D. R., and Moss, N. E. "Measuring Social Class in U.S. Public Health Research: Concepts, Methodologies, and Guidelines." *Annual Review of Public Health,* 1997, *18,* 341–378.

Kuh, D., and Ben-Shlomo, Y. (eds.). *A Lifecourse Approach to Chronic Disease Epidemiology: Tracing the Origins of Ill-Health from Early to Adult Life.* Oxford: Oxford University Press, 1997.

Larin, K., and McNichol, E. *Pulling Apart: A State-by-State Analysis of Income Trends.* Washington, D.C.: Center on Budget and Policy Priorities, 1997.

Luker, K. *Dubious Conceptions: The Politics of Teenage Pregnancy.* Berkeley: University of California Press, 1996.

Lynch, J. W., and others. "Childhood and Adult Socioeconomic Status as Predictors of Mortality in Finland." *Lancet,* 1994, *343,* 524–527.

Marmor, T. R., Barer, M. L., and Evans, R. G. "The Determinants of a Population's Health." In R. G. Evans, M. L. Barer, and T. R. Marmor (eds.), *Why Are Some People Healthy and Others Not? The Determinants of Health of Populations.* Hawthorne, N.Y.: Aldine de Gruyter, 1994.

Marmot, M. G., Bobak, M., and Davey Smith, G. "Explanations for Social Inequalities in Health." In B. C. Amick III and others (eds.), *Society and Health.* New York: Oxford University Press, 1995.

Massey, D. S., and Denton, N. A. *American Apartheid and the Making of the Underclass.* Cambridge, Mass.: Harvard University Press, 1993.

Miller, S. M. "Thinking Strategically About Society and Health." In B. C. Amick III and others (eds.), *Society and Health.* New York: Oxford University Press, 1995.

Moss, N. E., and Krieger, N. "Measuring Social Inequalities in Health." *Public Health Reports,* 1995, *110,* 302–305.

Nathanson, C. *Dangerous Passage: The Social Control of Sexuality in Women's Adolescence.* Philadelphia: Temple University Press, 1991.

National Commission to Prevent Infant Mortality. *Death Before Life: The Tragedy of Infant Mortality.* Washington, D.C.: U.S. Government Printing Office, 1988.

Pamuk, E., and others. *Socioeconomic Status and Health Chartbook: Health, United States, 1998.* Hyattsville, Md.: National Center for Health Statistics, 1998.

Pappas, G., and others. "The Increasing Disparity Between Socioeconomic Groups in the United States, 1960 and 1986." *New England Journal of Medicine,* 1993, *329,* 103–109.

Pérez-Peña, R. "New York's Income Gap Largest in Nation." *New York Times,* Dec. 19, 1995, p. A25.

"Recommendations of the Conference 'Measuring Social Inequalities in Health.'" *International Journal of Health Services,* 1996, *26,* 521–527.

Rich, S. "Study Finds Nest Eggs Vary Greatly." *Washington Post,* July 25, 1995, p. A11.

Rowley, D., and Tosteson, H. "Racial Differences in Preterm Delivery: Developing a New Research Paradigm" (special issue). *American Journal of Preventive Medicine,* 1993, *9*(Suppl.).

Smith, J. P., and Kington, R. S. "Demographic and Economic Correlates of Health in Old Age." *Demography,* 1997a, *34,* 159–170.

Smith, J. P., and Kington, R. S. "Race, Socioeconomic Status, and Health in Later Life." In L. G. Martin and B. J. Soldo (eds.), *Racial and Ethnic Differences in the Health of Older Americans.* Washington, D.C.: National Academy Press, 1997b.

Townsend, P., Davidson, N., and Whitehead, M. *Inequalities in Health: The Black Report and The Health Divide.* Harmondsworth, England: Penguin, 1992.

U.K. Department of Health. "Variations Sub-Group of the Chief Medical Officers Health of the Nation Working Group." In *The Health of the Nation: Variations in Health: What Can the Department of Health and the NHS Do?* London: Department of Health., 1996.

U.S. Department of Commerce and Bureau of the Census. "Current Population Reports, Series P60–185." In *Poverty in the United States, 1992.* Washington, D.C.: U.S. Government Printing Office, 1993.

U.S. Department of Health and Human Services, Public Health Service. *Healthy People 2000: National Health Promotion and Disease Prevention Objectives.* Washington, D.C.: Department of Health and Human Services, 1991.

Vagero, D. "Health Inequalities as Policy Issues: Reflections on Ethics, Policy, and Public Health." *Sociology of Health and Illness,* 1995, *17,* 1–19.

Weinberg, D. *A Brief Look at Postwar U.S. Income Inequality.* Washington, D.C.: U.S. Department of Commerce, Bureau of the Census, 1996.

Weinberg, D. *Money Income in the United States, 1996.* Washington, D.C.: U.S. Department of Commerce, Bureau of the Census, 1997.

Whitehead, M. *Bridging the Gap: Working Towards Equity in Health and Health Care.* Sundyberg, Sweden: Karolinska Institutet, 1997.

Whitehead, M. "Diffusion of Ideas on Social Inequalities in Health: A European Perspective." *Milbank Quarterly,* 1998, *76,* 469–492.

Whitehead, M., and Dahlgren, G. "What Can Be Done About Inequalities in Health?" *Lancet,* 1991, *338,* 1059–1063.

Whitehead, M., Scott-Samuel, A., and Dahlgren, G. "Setting Targets to Address Inequalities in Health." *Lancet,* 1998, *351,* 1279–1282.

Wilkinson, R. G. "'Variations in health': The Costs of Government Timidity." *British Medical Journal,* 1995, *311,* 1177–1178.

Wilkinson, R. G. *Unhealthy Societies: The Afflictions of Inequality.* New York: Routledge, 1996.

Williams, D. R. "Missed Opportunities in Monitoring Socioeconomic Status." *Public Health Reports,* 1997a, *112,* 492–494.

Williams, D. R. "Race and Health: Basic Questions, Emerging Directions." *Annals of Epidemiology,* 1997b, *7,* 322–333.

Williams, D. R., and Collins, C. "U.S. Socioeconomic and Racial Differences in Health: Patterns and Explanations." *Annual Review of Sociology,* 1995, *21,* 49–86.

Williamson, G., and Lindert, P. H. *American Inequality: A Macroeconomic History.* San Diego, Calif.: Academic Press, 1980.

Wilson, W. J. *The Truly Disadvantaged: The Inner City, the Underclass, and Public Policy.* Chicago: University of Chicago Press, 1987.

Wilson, W. J. *When Work Disappears: The World of the New Urban Poor.* New York: Knopf, 1996.

Wolff, E. N. *Top Heavy: The Increasing Inequality of Wealth in America and What Can Be Done About It.* New York: New Press, 1995.

CHAPTER TWENTY-THREE

From Science to Policy

Options for Reducing Health Inequalities

Hilary Graham

Tackling health inequalities is moving up the public health agenda, at both international and national levels. In the international arena, the declaration of the 1998 World Health Assembly confirmed that a reduction in socio-economic inequalities in health is a priority for all countries. In Europe, the European Union's Action Programme on Public Health is giving priority to improving the health of disadvantaged groups. Alongside this, the World Health Organization (WHO) has launched its new health strategy for Europe, *Health 21* (1998). Improving health and promoting equity are again the organising principles around which the health strategy is built. Underlying this two-track strategy is the recognition that reducing health inequalities is an essential pre-requisite for wider gains in public health. In other words, improved health turns on greater equity in health.

This two-track strategy is evident, too, in national public health policies. As one recent example, the U.K. government has launched new public health strategies in England, Northern Ireland, Scotland, and Wales built around the twin goals of reducing health inequalities and improving population health. As in the UK, governments elsewhere are recognising that achieving these goals requires a broader and more radical vision of public health policy. It is one that

The author thanks Sharon Matthews, Institute of Child Health, for unpublished data from the National Child Development Study, and Tanya Richardson for help with typing the chapter.

not only targets individuals and their risk behaviours, but also tackles the inequalities in life chances and living standards which shape people's lifestyles. Tackling health inequalities requires a comprehensive strategy which, in the words of the New Zealand report on health inequalities, "addresses the fundamental socio-economic determinants of health" (New Zealand National Advisory Committee, 1998, p. 14). Or as the Public Health Strategy for England put it, "Tackling inequalities generally is the best way of tackling health inequalities in particular" (Great Britain Department of Health, 1998, p. 12).

Tackling inequalities generally is clearly an ambitious policy objective, particularly at a time of rapid social and economic change. People's working and domestic lives are being transformed by the growth of the global economy, by increasing job insecurity and unemployment, and by a shift away from lifelong marriage. These changes are fuelling a wider process of social polarization in many societies, marked by a widening gap in living standards between work-rich, two-earner households and work-poor, no-earner households. This process of polarization is being played out on the international stage, with rich economies based on capital-intensive industries gaining at the expense of poor countries dependent on labour-intensive industries (United Nations Development Programme, 1996).

Social change and social polarization provide the backdrop against which the international community and national governments are seeking to reduce inequalities in health. And they are turning to the scientific community for advice on how to do so. Governments are looking, in the words of the WHO's strategy for Europe, for "a scientific framework for decision makers" and "a science-based guide to better health development" (1998, pp. 11–12). Research programmes and evidence-based reviews are being launched to furnish these science-based guides in the Netherlands, Finland, Sweden, New Zealand, and elsewhere (Mackenbach et al., 1994; Kunst, 1997; Arve-Pares, 1998; New Zealand National Advisory Committee, 1998). The Independent Inquiry into Inequalities in Health (1998), established by the U.K. government, is the latest example of this international trend. The Inquiry's terms of reference were to review the scientific evidence on health inequalities in order to identify policies with the potential to reduce them—in other words, to bring the science of health inequalities to bear on the process of policy development.

But what is the science of health inequalities? It clearly includes epidemiological studies which, since the nineteenth century have mapped the persistent association between individual socio-economic status and individual health. It includes, too, the more recent and smaller seam of experimental research which has sought to evaluate the effectiveness of interventions designed to narrow socio-economic differentials in health. I will discuss these fields of research briefly below.

But the science of health inequalities potentially covers a much larger canvas, one which moves beyond description and evaluation to explanation. This broader science is concerned with how inequalities in health result from inequalities in socio-economic status and how inequalities in socio-economic status are produced and maintained. It is a science concerned with what the socio-economic structure is doing to individual socio-economic circumstances as well as what individual socio-economic circumstances are doing to health. This dual scientific focus, structural and individual, upstream and downstream, is particularly important at times of social transformation, when the occupational structure is changing and income inequalities are widening. The central sections of the chapter broaden the base of health inequalities research to include these processes of change, moving beyond the disciplines of social epidemiology and public health to the social science disciplines of sociology, social policy, and welfare economics.

THE SCIENCE OF HEALTH INEQUALITIES: DESCRIBING HEALTH INEQUALITIES

At the core of health inequalities research is the long tradition of collecting data on the health and socio-economic status of individuals. In the nineteenth century, it was these data which brought the fact and scale of health inequalities to the attention of policy makers, prompting major investment in environmental health and sanitation. It is this descriptive science which revealed how socio-economic inequalities in childhood health had all but disappeared in Sweden by the 1960s (Whitehead and Diderichsen, 1997). And it is this descriptive science which is pointing to widening inequalities in morality in a number of countries, including the United Kingdom (Drever and Whitehead, 1997). Recording and publicising these trends has been an important catalyst in the policy process, ensuring that health inequalities remain on and move up the political agenda (Haines and Smith, 1997).

These descriptive studies also convey a simple and compelling policy message. Health inequalities are dynamic: their scale, and the causes of ill-health which underlie them, vary over time and between countries. The fact that health inequalities are not fixed and immutable provides evidence that they can be reduced.

THE SCIENCE OF HEALTH INEQUALITIES: INTERVENTION STUDIES

The evaluative studies are concerned with identifying interventions with the potential to reduce health inequalities. They represent, as is widely acknowledged, a small and underdeveloped field, and one where the research designs of the randomized control trial are ill-suited to assessing the impact of macro-trends and policies. As a result, evaluative research on health inequalities is disproportionately weighted towards the evaluation of interventions targeted at individuals rather than at the circumstances in which they live. Systematic reviews have found a predominance of interventions designed to reduce risk-related behaviours, like cigarette smoking, through providing individuals with information and support (National Health Service, 1995; Gepkins and Gunning-Schepers, 1996). There is little evidence that these behavioural interventions have either a positive effect on those in lower socio-economic groups or one that is differentially beneficial for these groups. As the Scottish public health green paper put it (Scottish Office, 1998, p. 33; underlining and italics in the original):

> *Simply addressing disease and lifestyle cannot deliver what is needed. The first part* of a cohesive strategy for a healthier, more equitable Scotland must be to counter the *life circumstances* which can give rise to poor health, and foster those which generate good health. These include a job, a home, a good education and an attractive environment.

There are few evaluated interventions designed to counter adverse life circumstances. The few, however, point to the potential impact that interventions targeted at life circumstances could have on health inequalities.

One example is of an intervention designed to achieve health gain by increasing financial resources to low-income families. In a randomized control trial conducted in the early 1970s in Indiana, the intervention group of low-income mothers received an expanded income support plan which guaranteed them a minimum income. Mothers at high risk of adverse pregnancy outcomes who were in the intervention group had heavier babies than control-group mothers (Kehrer and Wolin, 1979). Another example is the introduction of measures to reduce traffic accidents, a major cause of injury and death to children which displays a sharp socio-economic gradient. The introduction of 20-mph zones is associated with, on average, a 60% drop in pedestrian casualties and a 70% reduction in child pedestrian and cycling casualties (Great Britain Department of Environment, 1997).

A third and more developed field of intervention is the provision of out-of-home day care to improve the current and future life circumstances of disadvantaged children. Evidence from randomized control trials indicates that such interventions have positive effects on children's well-being and, through their impact on cognitive development and school performance, on future socio-economic status (Zoritch, Roberts, and Oakley, 1998).

While providing a guide to policy, the range of intervention studies is currently too limited to provide the evidence base on which a comprehensive strategy to reduce health inequalities could be built. In its place, scientists and policy makers are looking to a third area of health inequalities research, where evidence is derived from the analysis of causal pathways and not the effectiveness of interventions. As the New Zealand report on health inequalities put it (New Zealand National Advisory Committee, 1998, p. 70; emphasis in original), "Even if there is no specific evidence on the health outcomes of interventions, if there is evidence for a strong and consistent association between a particular socio-economic factor and health *and* there is good evidence that the association is causal, *then* specific initiatives, including policies that show a positive effect on that factor, are highly likely to lead to improved health."

THE SCIENCE OF HEALTH INEQUALITIES: EXPLANATORY STUDIES

This third area, concerned with consistent associations and causal pathways, has been traditionally resourced by social epidemiology. The dominant epidemiological model tracks the socio-economic patterning of individual health back through a series of intermediate factors to individual socio-economic status. As Figure 23.1 indicates, the causal chain is short and links up a range of individual-level influences on health. Some epidemiological models lengthen the causal chain to include the social structure as the upstream, independent variable (e.g., International Centre for Health and Society, 1998; Diderichsen, 1998). However, the social structure features as an unanalysed variable placed within but not incorporated into these extended models.

We need to look beyond social epidemiology to other disciplines, and to sociology and social policy in particular, for analyses which track macro-level influences on individual socio-economic status. And the evidence from these disciplines suggests that the socio-economic structure of many societies is undergoing a process of rapid change and fracturing in ways which are widening inequalities in living standards and life chances. This suggests that the science of health inequalities needs, to coin a well-used U.K. phrase, to be a "joined up" one. It should include both epidemiological research on individual health and sociological research on social inequality. Although these fields of research have developed separately, there is considerable potential for synergy. As one example, longitudinal studies of the socio-economic patterning of health

Individual SES ⟶ Intermediate factors ⟶ Health problems

Figure 23.1. An Individual-Level Model of Health Inequalities.
Source: Mackenbach, 1998, fig. 1.

over the life course could be integrated into sociological analyses of social polarization. Such an integration highlights a set of interlocking links in the chains which run from the social structure to individual health. Together, these two seams of research are uncovering how health is fashioned by risk exposures across the life course, within pathways of disadvantage, shaped by broader changes in the socio-economic structure.

As a case study—and I would emphasise that it is only one example—the sections below look in more detail at this joined-up science of health inequalities and at the policy framework it provides.

JOINED-UP EXAMPLE 1: CUMULATIVE EXPOSURE TO DISADVANTAGE

As Figure 23.1 indicates, social epidemiology has identified a cluster of individual-level factors which link individuals' socio-economic circumstances and their health. These include material factors, like poor housing and poor living standards, and psycho-social factors, like life events and chronic difficulties and the social networks and relationships which support people through them. These intermediate factors also include behavioural influences, like cigarette smoking and a diet with a limited nutrient base.

An important seam of research has described how these proximate influences cluster together. These studies have demonstrated that an individual exposed to material disadvantage is more likely to be disadvantaged with respect to their psychosocial environment and their health behaviour, while an individual protected from material hazards is more likely to have a protective psycho-social environment and to engage in health-promoting behaviours (Marmot and Davey Smith, 1997). These factors can also interact. For example, low levels of social support have been found to have a more negative effect on the psychological health of those living in poverty, and poverty has its most substantial effects on the psychological well-being of those who had limited access to social support (Whelan, 1993).

However, longitudinal studies are now tracking how these risks and resources not only cluster together but accumulate over the life course (Power et al., 1996; van de Mheen, 1998). The British 1958 birth cohort study provides a powerful and chilling insight into this process of cumulative disadvantage. It has followed children born in one week in 1958 through their childhood up to the age of 33 (Power and Matthews, 1997). And it is revealing how girls and boys born into families at the bottom of the class hierarchy (based on father's occupation) are much more likely to be exposed to material, psycho-social, and behavioural risks in the process of growing up than those in higher social classes. For example, they are more likely to live in overcrowded homes, to experience such life events as the divorce of their parents, and to be exposed to parental smoking.

JOINED-UP EXAMPLE 2: PATHWAYS OF DISADVANTAGE

Longitudinal studies are not only uncovering the socio-economic patterning of health risks—material, psycho-social, and behavioural—across the life course. They are also uncovering the socio-economic trajectories of which these exposures are part. In other words, they are beginning to move beyond individual socio-economic status to the social structure, identifying the pathways through which the occupational structure shapes the lives and life chances of individuals (Figure 23.2). Again, the 1958 National Child Development Survey provides an instructive example. Analyses of the 1958 cohort to the age of 33 indicate that those born and brought up on the lower rungs of the class ladder are more likely than their more advantaged peers to follow disadvantaged pathways across their adult lives. Their employment pathways are more likely to be characterized by low educational qualifications, unemployment, layoffs, and receipt of public assistance (income benefits provided through the welfare system).

Figure 23.3 maps the employment trajectories of young adults by social class at birth (Power and Matthews, 1997). The proportion of young people entering the labour market without educational qualifications, facing layoffs, and being in receipt of public assistance increases in line with declining social class, with working-class men particularly exposed to the risk of layoff. Ethnicity mediates the employment pathways young people follow into and through the labour market. U.K. studies point to an "ethnic penalty" paid by young people from minority ethnic groups in which they do less well with respect to employment and job level than similarly qualified whites. African Caribbean and Bangladeshi/Pakistani groups, in particular, face higher rates of unemployment and of employment in low-skilled jobs than their white peers (Modood, 1997).

Socio-economic status also structures young people's domestic pathways, with low SES linked to pathways which run through early parenthood, and for women, lone parenthood. As Figure 23.4 indicates, there is a sharp socio-economic gradient in the proportion of young people becoming parents by their

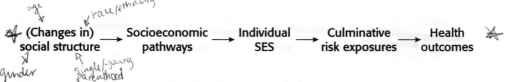

Figure 23.2. A Society-Level Model of Health Inequalities.

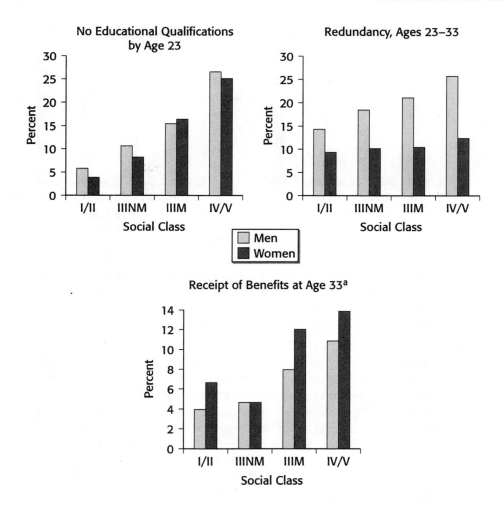

Figure 23.3. Socio-Economic Pathways by Social Class at Birth, According to the National Child Development Study ($p < .001$).

Source: Power and Matthews, 1997.

[a]Includes some support or supplementary unemployment benefits for participant or partner.

early twenties. Among men in the highest social class at the age of 23, less than 1 in 10 are fathers by that age; among women in the lowest social class, more than 6 in 10 are mothers. Single parenthood shows even more pronounced gender and class differences. Few men are lone fathers by the age of 33 and it is not patterned by their socio-economic status. The chances are significantly higher

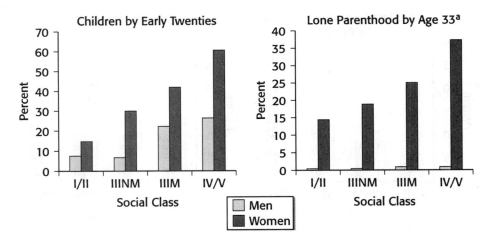

Figure 23.4. Domestic Pathways by Social Class at Age 23, According to the National Child Development Study (p < .001).

Source: Sharon Matthews, Institute of Child Health.

[a]Includes all who have ever been a lone parent for a period of more than one month.

for women and are closely related to occupational circumstances in early adulthood. The domestic pathways which run through early and lone parenthood bring additional layers of disadvantage, restricting opportunities to gain the skills and work experience necessary to move out of unemployment and low-paid work and into the better-paid and more secure sectors of the labour market. The result is a high level of dependence on income benefits provided through the welfare system, with living standards significantly below those taken for granted by the majority of the population (Bradshaw, 1993; Burstrom et al., 1999).

As Figures 23.3 and 23.4 suggest, longitudinal studies are broadening the scientific framework of health inequalities research, introducing a temporal as well as a spatial dimension to socio-economic status. It is not simply where an individual is in the socio-economic hierarchy which matters; it is how this position shapes exposure to health-damaging influences across their lives which is crucial.

The life-course perspectives provided by longitudinal studies have moved the science of health inequalities closer to the social structure, enabling it to measure the effects of disadvantage on the paths which individuals follow across their lives. But their individual-level focus means that the structural-level forces which shape these pathways remain hidden from view. Leaving out structural-level processes is particularly problematic during periods in which the social structure is undergoing rapid change. These are periods when the size and composition of the occupational categories which underpin the class structure are changing, and with them the socio-economic trajectories that individuals can expect to follow across their lives.

JOINED-UP EXAMPLE 3: CHANGES IN
THE SOCIO-ECONOMIC STRUCTURE

The science of health inequalities needs to include society-level as well as individual-level analyses, because the pathways that people track through their lives are framed by the wider socio-economic structure—by how life chances and living standards are distributed through the labour market, and by the tax and welfare system. The international pattern, repeated across Europe, the United States, and in the emergent economies of Africa, Asia, and South America, is of rising unemployment linked to a collapse in demand for low-skilled manual workers. However, the effect of these labour market changes on the distribution of income, and on the class structure more broadly, varies between countries. The United Kingdom provides an instructive example of a society in which the process of social polarization is well advanced.

From the mid-1970s to the mid-1990s, inequalities in living standards in the United Kingdom increased at a pace and on a scale unmatched in Europe (Goodman, Johnson, and Webb, 1997). While better-off households enjoyed rising living standards, the proportion of the population living in poverty rose sharply. Figure 23.5 plots the proportion of the U.K. population living in

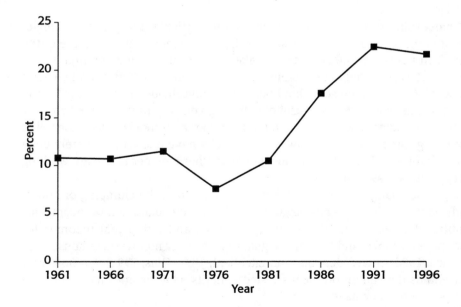

Figure 23.5. Proportion of the Population Below 50% of Average Income After Subtraction of Housing Costs, United Kingdom, 1961–1996.

Sources: Goodman and Webb, 1994; Great Britain Department of Social Security, 1998.

households below the European Community poverty line, represented by a household income below half of national average income. As the figure indicates, 7% of Britons were in poverty in the mid-1970s; by the mid-1990s, nearly a quarter (24%) of the population was living in households with incomes less than half the national average (after housing costs) (Endean, 1998).

Rising unemployment and widening income inequalities have been associated with a wider process of social polarization. Underlying this process have been changes in the structure of the labour market and, in particular, a rapid decline in manual and low-skilled work. As a result, unemployment rates for those in unskilled manual socio-economic groups have doubled, reaching 30% among white men and over 60% among African Caribbean men by the early 1990s (Office for National Statistics, 1998). Rising unemployment at the bottom of the class hierarchy has been matched by rising earnings among high-paid workers.

As elsewhere in Europe and in the United States, changes in the structure of the labour market and in the dispersal of earnings have been associated with a more far-reaching change. They have fuelled a redistribution of employment between households. Across the last two decades, there has been a rapid shift away from households containing a mix of employed and non-employed adults and a corresponding increase in two-earner and no-earner households (Gregg and Wadsworth, 1996). The proportion of no-earner households has doubled since the late 1970s, from less than 1 in 10 households in 1979 to more than 1 in 5 in 1995.

Changes in household composition, and in particular the growth in single-parent households and childless single-adult households, explains some of the growth in no-earner households. To take account of this demographic trend, Figure 23.6 is restricted to the dominant household form. It focuses on two-adult households, which represent about 60% of all households in Britain. As the figure indicates, male-earner households have given way to two-earner and no-earner households. The upward trend in no-earner households reflects the toll of increasing unemployment. However, new jobs have disproportionately been taken by those living in households where another member is already working (Gregg and Wadsworth, 1996).

With the changing household distribution of work, the clumping of households on middle incomes has begun to break up. In its place, a new income distribution has emerged, characterized by high and rising real incomes for working households and low and stagnant incomes for non-working households (Jenkins, 1996; Cowell, Jenkins, and Litchfield, 1997; Hills, 1998). For no-earner households dependent on means-tested benefits, real incomes have not even been stagnant; they have declined.

These trends suggest that the U.K. class structure no longer consists of a hierarchy of unequal but relatively stable positions. Increasingly, it is a structure composed of unequal and diverging socio-economic trajectories. Those in secure

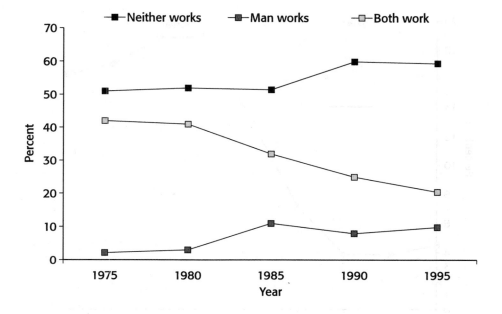

Figure 23.6. Employment in Two-Adult Households, Britain, 1975–1993.
Source: Gregg and Wadsworth, 1996.

and well-paid jobs can expect to increase their command over the material, psycho-social, and behavioural resources associated with good health: enjoying, for example, high living standards, high control at work, and high nutrient intake. Those in disadvantaged positions face the prospect of downward socio-economic trajectories. Low and declining living standards are likely to restrict opportunities to avoid the health risks which come with a poor material and psycho-social environment or to break health-damaging patterns of behaviour.

In examining the effects of macro socio-economic change on individual socio-economic trajectories, it is instructive to compare the United Kingdom with countries where labour market changes have been associated with less pronounced changes in the distribution of living standards and life chances. Finland provides an illuminating example. There the rapid economic growth which marked the 1970s and 1980s gave way to deep recession at the beginning of the 1990s. The economic reversal was rapid and profound: unemployment climbed from less than 4% in 1990 to over 18% in 1993 (Figure 23.7).

As in the United Kingdom, earnings differentials between higher-paid white collar workers and lower-paid blue collar workers widened and, with them, income inequalities increased. But the widening of income inequalities has been relatively small in comparison with the United Kingdom (Keskimaki et al., 1999).

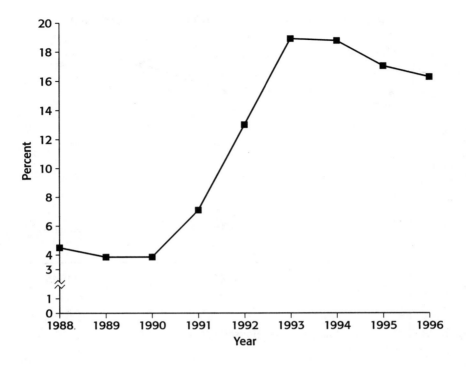

Figure 23.7. Unemployment Rate in Finland, 1988–1996.

Source: Keskimaki and others, 1999.

This is because fiscal and welfare policies have moderated the effects of rising unemployment. Tax rate increases have contained the rise in real incomes of those in better-paid jobs while, despite cuts, the public assistance system has protected the living standards of the increasing proportion of the population dependent on them for their economic survival. As a result, the cost of recession has been redistributed and shared. By 1996, real incomes for most income groups were below their pre-recession level. Only the higher-income decile have seen a rise in real incomes. As Keskimaki et al. (1999) note, the Finnish fiscal and welfare systems have been relatively successful in maintaining an equitable distribution of income in the face of forces which, in the United Kingdom, resulted in a rapid widening of income inequalities.

POLICY OPTIONS FOR REDUCING HEALTH INEQUALITIES

In the sections above, I have drawn selectively on health inequalities research, particularly on epidemiological research on life-course influences and sociological research on socio-economic inequality, to illustrate how, in the words of the

WHO *Health 21* strategy, research can yield "a scientific framework for decision makers" (1998, p. 12). The framework highlights a set of interlocking processes in the production of the socio-economic gradient in health and in particular the *cumulative exposure to risks along disadvantaged pathways* framed by *wider structures of inequality.* In so doing, it reveals multiple points where policy leverage can be exerted, as scientific and policy reviews have made clear (Great Britain Independent Inquiry, 1998; New Zealand National Advisory Committee, 1998). Two are highlighted below.

Pathways of Disadvantage

The evidence that exposure to health risks—material, psycho-social, and behavioural—is patterned by the socio-economic pathways individuals follow across their lives has a clear policy message. It argues for policies which intervene in the disadvantaged pathways which increase exposure to health risks. One policy option is to target points and periods in the life course when individuals are making changes likely to have long-term effects on their future socio-economic status. These critical life transitions include entering pre-school care and education, moving from primary and secondary school, (early) school, leaving and entering the labour market, being laid off, becoming a (lone) parent and, particularly for women, moving through separation and divorce. Recognizing these critical life transitions, and especially those relating to childhood and adolescence, offers a number of advantages.

Firstly, governments are already involved in helping and directing individuals through the key transitions which mark out childhood and adulthood: for example, entry into pre-school and compulsory education, into and off welfare, through pregnancy and into parenthood are all life events which are closely regulated by state agencies. Secondly, targeting these transitions goes with the grain of welfare policy. It is a principle and practice already integrated into welfare programmes and expenditure plans. There are many examples of programmes which aim to improve the educational levels and outcomes for children from disadvantaged communities and to promote education and training for low-skilled young people.

Informed by evaluations of established programmes, particularly those in the United States, early childhood programmes are being developed in the United Kingdom, New Zealand, and elsewhere with the aim of lifting disadvantaged children onto more advantaged socio-economic trajectories. The Sure Start programme in England is a targeted programme providing child care and primary health care services in 250 areas, reaching about 5% of the national population of 0–3 year olds. While a programme from which important research and policy messages will flow, its targeted focus means that its broader population impact will be limited.

Like the early childhood programmes, New Deal and Welfare-to-Work programmes are designed to break into disadvantaged socio-economic pathways by providing targeted groups with a springboard onto more advantaged trajectories. In the United States and the United Kingdom, these programmes are part of a wider set of policies aimed to help move key claimant groups off public assistance and into paid work by offering access to training and education and to subsidised jobs. In the United Kingdom, the largest recipient group for the Welfare-to-Work Programme are young adults aged 18 to 24 who have been claiming unemployment benefits (job seekers allowance) for 6 months or more.

Enhancing the skills of unemployed people is what economists call a supply side approach to tackling unemployment and reducing poverty. The aim is to increase the skills and employment chances of unemployed people, who are considerably less skilled than those in paid work. However, evaluated New Deal schemes have produced disappointing results. Employment rates among those recruited to the schemes are only fractionally above rates among welfare recipients excluded from them (Solow, 1998). This suggests that the schemes require parallel demand-side initiatives to improve the availability of the low-skilled jobs sought by unemployed people. Further, providing gateways out of unemployment for some groups offers little to those who remain on means-tested benefits (Graham, Benzeval, and Whitehead, 1999). To address these structural dimensions of disadvantage requires policies which generate low-skilled jobs and which improve the living standards of those unable to earn their living.

Structures of Inequality

In the United Kingdom, life chances and living standards polarized across two decades in which inequality was off the political agenda. From 1979 to 1997, the country was led by a Conservative government which adopted a free market approach to economic, social, and fiscal policy. As a result, inequalities resulting from labour market restructuring and the emergence of new patterns of family life were magnified rather than moderated.

As the example of the United Kingdom suggests, national policies play an important part in mediating the effects of social and socio-economic change. Change—whether at the level of the transitional corporation and the global labour market or in our patterns of cohabitation and parenthood—is not inevitably linked to widening inequalities in health and opportunity. Whether and how far social and economic change results in widening inequalities depends on national policies: social, economic, and fiscal (Bradshaw, 1996; Breen and Rothman, 1998; Black et al., 1999).

The role of social policy in tempering social inequality is underlined in a recent analysis by Richard Breen and David Rothman (1998). They analysed the occupational structure and extent of class inequality and mobility in countries occupying core positions in the global labour market (Australia, Belgium, France, Italy, Japan, the United States, Germany, Norway, and Sweden) and peripheral locations (Philippines and Malaysia). They concluded that national policies shape class structures and buffer the effects of low social class on life chances and living standards:

> Welfare and other state policies enacted and implemented in diverse ways at the level of the national state shape class structures and the consequences of class membership. The specifics of such policies are important vehicles linking class position and life chances As a result, national states that occupy a similar niche within the world [economic] system present us with diverse class structures, degrees of openness (as manifest in social mobility) and degree of class inequality [p.14].

As their analysis indicates, national state policies form an integral part of a public health strategy to reduce health inequalities. Attention has been drawn, in particular, to employment, income, and the provision of services like public housing, health care, and transport as mechanisms through which to temper inequalities in the labour market and improve the living standards of those groups whose earning power is low (for example, Great Britain Independent Inquiry, 1998; New Zealand National Advisory Committee, 1998; Black et al., 1999). In these policy domains, governments exercise a high degree of direct control, providing considerable opportunity for leverage and impact.

Participation in paid employment is the major determinant of living standards, with poverty concentrated among households outside the labour market. The sharp socio-economic differentials in the opportunities for paid work are widely recognised by governments, with welfare-to-work programmes seeking to reduce unemployment among low-skilled workers. However, analyses suggest that the demand for low-skilled labour in an increasing number of societies is falling short of the supply, even when the quality of that supply is enhanced through welfare-to-work programmes. Increasing the availability of low-skilled jobs in the public sector is an important policy option (Solow, 1998).

A second option is to act directly on the distribution of income. The tax and public assistance systems are redistributive systems through which governments can influence the scale of income inequality and can protect the living standards of the poorest groups. As evidence from Finland and Sweden indicates, progressive tax structures narrow differentials in (post-tax) incomes, while the introduction of a more regressive tax structure in the United Kingdom widened inequalities in income (Hills, 1998; Burstrom and Diderichsen, 1999; Keskimaki et al., 1999). The simplest way of protecting the living standards of households dependent on welfare benefits is to peg benefit levels to average earnings. This maintains their relative value and avoids the downward drift in living standards experienced by welfare recipients in the United Kingdom (Hills, 1998).

A third potential lever on inequalities is provided by publicly-funded welfare state services. These include health care and education, subsidised housing, personal social services (social work and social care), subsidised public transport, and local amenities (parks, playgrounds, leisure centres) open to and free for the whole community. Evidence from the United Kingdom suggests that poorer households derive significantly greater benefit than richer households from these services (Sefton, 1998). As a result, universally-provided welfare services are an important mechanism for raising the living standards of the poor, for moderating the impact of income inequalities and for redistributing wealth. Services which are targeted at, and disproportionately used by, those in need, like subsidised rented housing, personal social services, and subsidised bus networks, have the most pronounced redistributive effects. Investment in these elements of the welfare state therefore offers an effective strategy for targeting groups and areas in which disadvantage is concentrated.

CONCLUSION

My review of the science/policy interface has been necessarily selective. I have looked briefly at descriptive and evaluative studies and in more depth at the scientific contribution of longitudinal studies of individuals and of time-series analyses of societies. In this narrow focus, key areas have been omitted. I have not, for example, discussed how areas and communities exert their own and independent effects on the class gradient in health and how gender and ethnicity mediate the effects of class disadvantage. Nonetheless, I hope my selective approach has uncovered the long interface that runs between science and policy.

I have highlighted how socio-economic inequalities are at least in part the outcome of risks accumulated along disadvantaged life-course pathways, which in turn are fashioned by wider structures of inequality. I have pointed to how science can inform and intersect with policy, underlying the importance of policies which intervene in disadvantaged pathways and temper socio-economic inequality.

My selective focus also has a broader policy message. Because health inequalities are multi-determined, policies need to exert leverage at multiple points. As the Acheson report concludes, a broad-front approach is required. I give my final word to the report (Great Britain Independent Inquiry, 1998, p.7):

> A broad front approach reflects scientific evidence that health inequalities are the outcome of causal chains which run back into and from the basic structure of society. Such an approach is necessary because many of the factors are interrelated. It is likely to be less effective to focus solely on one point if complementary action is not in place which influences a linked factor in another policy area.

References

Arve-Pares, B. (ed.). *Promoting Research on Inequality in Health.* Stockholm: Swedish Council for Social Research, 1998.

Black, D., and others. "Better Benefits for Health: Plan to Implement the Central Recommendation of the Acheson Report." *British Medical Journal,* 1999, *318,* 724–727.

Bradshaw, J. *Household Budgets and Living Standards.* York, England: Joseph Rowntree Foundation, 1993.

Bradshaw, J. *The Employment of Lone Parents: A Comparison of Policy in 20 Countries.* London: Family Policy Studies Centre, 1996.

Breen, R., and Rothman, D. B. "Is the National State the Appropriate Geographical Unit for Class Analysis?" *Sociology,* 1998, *32,* 1–22.

Burstrom, B., and Diderichsen, F. "Income-Related Policies in Sweden, 1990–98." In J. P. Mackenbach and M. Droomers (eds.), *Interventions and Policies to Reduce Socio-Economic Inequalities in Health.* Rotterdam: Erasmus University, 1999.

Burstrom, B., and others. "Lone Mothers in Sweden: Trends in Health and Socio-Economic Circumstances, 1979–1995." *Journal of Epidemiology and Community Health,* 1999, *53,* 750–756.

Cowell, F. A., Jenkins, S. P., and Litchfield, J. A. "The Changing Shape of the UK Income Distribution: Kernal Density Estimates." In J. Hills (ed.), *New Inequalities: The Changing Distribution of Income and Wealth in the United Kingdom.* Cambridge: Cambridge University Press, 1997.

Diderichsen, F. "Understanding Health Equity in Populations: Some Theoretical and Methodological Considerations." In B. Arve-Pares (ed.), *Promoting Research on Inequality in Health.* Stockholm: Swedish Council for Social Research, 1998.

Drever, F., and Whitehead, M. (eds.). *Health Inequalities: Decennial Supplement.* London: Stationery Office, 1997.

Endean, R. (ed.). *Households Below Average Income, 1979 to 1996/97.* Leeds, England: Department of Social Security, 1998.

Gepkins, A., and Gunning-Schepers, L. J. "Interventions to Reduce Socio-Economic Health Differences." *European Journal of Public Health,* 1996, *6,* 218–226.

Goodman, A., Johnson, P., and Webb, S. *Inequality in the UK.* Oxford: Oxford University Press, 1997.

Goodman, A., and Webb, S. *For Richer, for Poorer. The Changing Distribution of Income in the United Kingdom.* London: Institute for Fiscal Studies, 1994.

Graham, H., Benzeval, M., and Whitehead, M. "Social and Economic Policies in the UK with a Potential Impact on Health Inequalities." In J. P. Mackenbach and M. Droomers (eds.), *Interventions and Policies to Reduce Socio-Economic Inequalities in Health.* Rotterdam: Erasmus University, 1999.

Great Britain Department of Environment, Transport and the Regions. *Road Safety: Current Problems and Future Solutions.* London: Great Britain Department of Environment, Transport and the Regions, 1997.

Great Britain Department of Health. *Our Healthier Nation.* London: Stationery Office, 1998.

Great Britain Department of Social Security. *Social Security Statistics, 1997.* London: Stationery Office, 1998.

Great Britain Independent Inquiry into Inequalities in Health. *Report of the Independent Inquiry into Inequalities in Health.* London: Stationery Office, 1998.

Gregg, P., and Wadsworth, J. "More Work in Fewer Households." In J. Hills (ed.), *New Inequalities: The Changing Distribution of Income and Wealth in the United Kingdom.* Cambridge: Cambridge University Press, 1996.

Haines, A., and Smith, R. "Working Together to Reduce Poverty's Damage." *British Medical Journal,* 1997, *314,* 529–530.

Hills, J. *Income and Wealth: The Latest Evidence.* York, England: Joseph Rowntree Foundation, 1998.

International Centre for Health and Society. "Socio-Economic Circumstances and Health Outcomes." In Great Britain Independent Inquiry into Inequalities in Health, *Report of the Independent Inquiry into Inequalities in Health.* London: Stationery Office, 1998.

Jenkins, S. "Recent Trends in the UK Income Distribution: What Happened and Why?" *Oxford Review of Economic Policy,* 1996, *12,* 29–46.

Kehrer, B., and Wolin, V. "Impact of Income Maintenance or Low Birth Weight: Evidence from the Gary Experiment." *Journal of Human Resources,* 1979, *14,* 434–462.

Keskimaki, I., and others. "Policy Changes Related to Income Distribution and Income Differences in Health in Finland in the 1990s." In J. P. Mackenbach and M. Droomers (eds.), *Interventions and Policies to Reduce Socio-Economic Inequalities in Health.* Rotterdam: Erasmus University, 1999.

Kunst, A. E. *Cross-National Comparisons of Socio-Economic Differences in Mortality.* Rotterdam: Erasmus University, 1997.

Mackenbach, J. P. "The Dutch Experience with Promoting Research on Inequality in Health." In B. Arve-Pares (ed.), *Promoting Research on Inequality in Health.* Stockholm: Swedish Council for Social Research, 1998.

Mackenbach, J. P., and others. "Socio-Economic Inequalities in Morbidity and Mortality in Western Europe." *Lancet,* 1994, *349,* 1655–1659.

Marmot, M. G., and Davey Smith, G. "Socio-Economic Differentials in Health." *Journal of Health Psychology,* 1997, *2,* 283–296.

Modood, J. "Employment." In J. Modood and R. Berthoud (eds.), *Ethnic Minorities in Britain: Diversity and Disadvantage.* London: Policy Studies Institute, 1997.

National Health Service Centre for Reviews and Dissemination. *Review of the Research on the Effectiveness of Health Service Interventions to Reduce Variations in Health.* York, England: National Health Service Centre for Reviews and Dissemination, University of York, 1995.

New Zealand National Advisory Committee on Health and Disability. *The Social, Cultural and Economic Determinants of Health in New Zealand: Action to Improve Health.* Wellington, New Zealand: National Health Committee, 1998.

Office for National Statistics. *Living in Britain: Results from the 1996 General Household Survey.* London: Stationery Office, 1998.

Power, C., and Matthews, S. "Origins of Health Inequalities in a National Population Sample." *Lancet,* 1997, *350,* 1584–1585.

Power, C., and others. "Transmission of Social and Biological Risk Across the Life Course." In D. Blane, E. Brunner, and R. G. Wilkinson (eds.), *Health and Social Organization: Toward a Health Policy for the 21st Century.* London: Routledge, 1996.

Scottish Office. *Working Together for a Healthier Scotland.* Edinburgh, Scotland: Stationery Office, 1998.

Sefton, T. *The Changing Distribution of the Social Wage.* London: London School of Economics, 1998.

Solow, R. M. *Work and Welfare.* Princeton, N.J.: Princeton University Press, 1998.

United Nations Development Programme. *Human Development Report, 1996.* New York: Oxford University Press, 1996.

van de Mheen, D. *Inequalities in Health: To Be Continued? A Lifecourse Perspective on Socio-Economic Inequalities in Health.* Rotterdam: Erasmus University, 1998.

Whelan, C. T. "The Role of Social Support in Mediating the Psychological Consequences of Economic Stress." *Sociology of Health and Illness,* 1993, *15,* 86–101.

Whitehead, M., and Diderichsen, F. "International Evidence on Social Inequalities in Health." In F. Drever and M. Whitehead (eds.), *Health Inequalities: Decennial Supplement.* London: Stationery Office, 1997.

World Health Organization Regional Office for Europe. *Health 21: Health for All in the 21st Century.* Copenhagen: World Health Organization Regional Office for Europe, 1998.

Zoritch, B., Roberts, I., and Oakley, A. "The Health and Welfare Effects of Day-Care: A Systematic Review of Randomised Controlled Trials." *Social Science and Medicine,* 1998, *47,* 317–327.

CHAPTER TWENTY-FOUR

Addressing Structural Influences on the Health of Urban Populations

Arline T. Geronimus

A compounding series of changes in the urban socioeconomic and demographic landscape since World War II have resulted in staggering and growing rates of excess mortality in urban areas of concentrated poverty (McCord and Freeman, 1990; Geronimus, Bound, and Waidmann, 1999; Geronimus and others, 1996). By 1990, African American youth in some urban areas faced lower probabilities of survival to age 45 than white youth nationwide faced of survival to 65 years. Popularized images emphasize the role of homicide among urban youth, although chronic diseases in young and middle adulthood are key contributors to these health inequalities and to their growth. For example, among young and middle-aged men in Harlem, the number of excess deaths attributed to homicide per 100,000 persons remained stable between 1980 and 1990 and then began to decline. In contrast, throughout the 1980s, excess deaths attributed to circulatory disease or cancer each *doubled* among young and middle-aged Harlem men (Geronimus, Bound, and Waidmann, 1999).

In developing these ideas, I benefitted tremendously from exchanges with J. Philip Thompson. I am also grateful to Sherman James, Sylvia Tesh, and Adam Becker for commenting on earlier drafts and for the financial support provided by the William T. Grant Foundation and by a Robert Wood Johnson Foundation Investigator in Health Policy Research Award. The views expressed are my own.

Attempts to understand and to reverse these growing health inequalities will be partial without consideration of the socioeconomic factors and, even more critical, the historical and structural factors that have produced modern ghettos in central cities with predominantly minority populations. About 80% of the residents of high-poverty urban areas in the United States are minorities; the figure is over 90% in the largest metropolitan areas. African Americans alone account for 50% of residents of high-poverty urban areas nationally and between 80 and 90% of the population in some of the largest urban ghettos, such as in Detroit and Chicago (Jargowsky, 1997). A range of policies, some now old and all apparently disconnected from health considerations, have reaped dire consequences for the health of these urban residents. In the wake of these policies, unless public health professionals take poverty *and* race/ ethnicity into account, they risk exaggerating the returns that can be expected of narrow or conventional public health campaigns or overlooking important targets, approaches, and resources for mounting successful interventions.

POVERTY

Central city populations are characterized by extreme, persistent, and pervasive poverty that intensified in the late 20th century. There was a decline in the real value of working-class wages and government transfers and, by extension, of the material resources available through the pooling of income across kin networks; at the same time, the cost of living increased.

The association between health and poverty (or more broadly defined, socioeconomic position) is among the most robust findings of social epidemiology (Antonovsky, 1967; Kitagawa and Hauser, 1973; Adler and others, 1994; Williams and Collins, 1995; Backlund, Sorlie, and Johnson, 1996). Consider the list of social and psychosocial factors that have demonstrated associations with morbidity and mortality, and consider that those in poverty suffer increased exposure to most of them. These include material hardships, psychosocial conditions of acute and chronic stress or of overburdened or disrupted social supports, and toxic environmental exposures (Lantz and others, 1998; Marmot, Kogevinas, and Elston, 1987; Williams and House, 1991; Geronimus, 1992; Mohai and Bryant, 1992. Generally and persistently difficult psychosocial conditions contribute to the increased tendency of the poor to engage in some unhealthy behaviors, suffer depression, or engage in persistent high-effort coping, which in itself is a risk factor for stress-related diseases in low-income populations (Lantz and others, 1998; Marmot, Kogevinas, and Elston, 1987; Williams and House, 1991; Geronimus, 1992; James, 1994; James and others, 1987; Northridge and others, 1998). As Link et al. (1998) have outlined, those of a lower socioeconomic position also have less ability than others to gain access to information, services, or technologies that could protect them from or ameliorate risks. Further, there appears to be a "dose/response" relationship: long-term poverty is more devastating to health than short poverty spells, both for children and adults (Lynch, Kaplan, and Shema, 1997; Miller and Korenman, 1994). For impoverished African Americans, excess morbidity and mortality increase over the young and middle adult years, suggesting the *cumulative* health impact of persistent disadvantage (Geronimus, 1992).

While poverty has intensified in central city areas, it has also come to interact with characteristics of the urban environment to produce a particularly lethal combination. Several social and environmental factors are likely contributors to this phenomenon. First, economic restructuring away from a manufacturing to a service economy resulted in extraordinarily high levels of urban unemployment and the loss of well-paying unionized jobs. Those now employed in the service sector often face unreliable and shifting part-time hours and have little or no health or retirement benefits. Second, there is a lack of adequate housing in major urban areas: increased housing prices have been a formidable problem for those whose already low incomes have failed to keep pace. The scarcity of housing has been exacerbated by reductions in municipal services, including fire department closings, which, among other consequences, have resulted in large numbers of burned-out buildings and the deterioration of the remaining housing stock (Wallace and Wallace, 1990).

Third, massive reductions in outlays to maintain and supervise public parks in urban areas have led to the dramatic deterioration of these facilities and their use for illicit purposes (Kelly, 1997). One can imagine the cascade of events, as suggested by Wallace and Wallace (1990), triggered by reductions in city services in low-income minority neighborhoods in New York City: an upsurge in family homelessness; the profound disruption of social networks, as those network members who lose their homes and can avert homelessness do so by fleeing or doubling up with other families; and the movement of drug users and traffickers into burned-out buildings and dilapidated public play spaces. These service reductions allowed urban areas to become the staging ground for the violence we have come to associate with urban neighborhoods and for other severe public health problems, including the crack and HIV/AIDS epidemics and the re-emergence of tuberculosis. That stress-related diseases are on the increase hardly seems surprising. Meanwhile, the urban poor have confronted new challenges in gaining access to medical care (Fossett and Perloff, 1995; Fossett and others, 1990; Polednak, 1996; Schlesinger, 1987).

This description suggests that poverty and urban decay are among the causes of early health deterioration and excess mortality among residents of distressed urban areas. It also suggests several possible program and policy levers for improving the health of urban populations, among them, (1) implementing jobs programs and measures to raise family incomes, (2) improving the quality, quantity and affordability of housing, (3) improving municipal services, (4) redressing environmental inequities, and (5) expanding health insurance coverage and increasing the number of physicians in depressed urban areas. Each of these measures deserves serious attention. However, without addressing the question of how urban decay, with its attendant health problems, was allowed to happen and the role of race in this process, the promise of such policies may be limited. Socioeconomic characteristics of urban populations are unlikely to be transformed in isolation; they are not associated with an otherwise level playing field.

RACE/ETHNICITY

For this discussion of the role of race/ethnicity in understanding poverty and urban health, race will be conceptualized in two intertwined ways. One is as a set of social relationships *between* majority and minority populations that have been institutionalized over time (O'Connor, 1998), that privilege the majority population, and are *prior* to the poverty that is associated with race (Cooper and David, 1986; Thompson, 1998). The other is as a set of autonomous institutions *within* the minority population that are developed and maintained—even in the face of burdensome obligations or costs to individuals—because, on balance, they mitigate, resist, or undo the adverse effects imposed by institutionalized discrimination.

In terms of the first conceptualization, the current urban environment developed under the influence of race-conscious policies. A large-scale migration of African Americans from the South to northern urban locations began in the 1940s, initially in response to increased demand for labor to sustain the war effort. In northern urban destinations, European immigrant neighborhood groups, government officials, and developers worked to avoid the integration of African Americans with established immigrant neighborhoods, producing the outlines of urban black ghettoes (Halpern, 1995). Highway construction and public housing projects isolated black neighborhoods from other areas, while other policies prevented blacks from moving to emerging suburbs. Following World War II, African Americans were effectively frozen out of suburbs by racial covenants, discriminatory mortgage practices and racial steering. In contrast, whites were offered low-cost homes in suburbs and low-interest rates on government subsidized home mortgages, and they benefited from publicly funded transportation projects that linked their suburban homes to employment and cultural centers (Oliver and Shapiro, 1995; Massey and Denton, 1993).

Such housing and transportation policies promoted segregation and prevented many African Americans from escaping poverty as urban centers lost jobs (first as industry moved to the suburbs and later because of macroeconomic restructuring away from industrialized jobs). They also precluded blacks from enjoying the wealth associated with the vast appreciation of suburban housing values (Conley, 1999). Meanwhile, there has been little sustained investment—public or private—in central city areas. Race has consistently been an explicit factor in this circumstance (Halpern, 1995).

In terms of the second conceptualization of race/ethnicity, African Americans have historically participated in community networks of exchange and support in order to mitigate social and economic adversity (Stack, 1974; Stack and Burton, 1993). These networks are dynamic systems that help to shore up material resources among members and also serve to provide social support and identity-affirming cultural frameworks across generations. In 1919, W.E.B. Du Bois wrestled with the "curious paradox" that without the strength of conviction and cultural identity forged through vital *separate* ethnic organizations, the determination of African Americans to fight against being *segregated* into an "ill-lighted, unpaved, unsewered ghetto" might have been dilute rather than resolute (Weinberg, 1970, p. 268). More recently, James (1993) has speculated that members of minority groups find health-preserving protection in cultural frameworks that are alternatives to the dominant cultural framework in which they are marginalized. James proposes a model that can be interpreted to resolve the paradox Du Bois observed: As a minority group's economic strength diminishes, its ability to supply the protection conferred by social support and identity-affirming symbols may be especially critical to preserving the health of its members.

In a vexing double-whammy, policies and macroeconomic realities that gave rise to the ghettoization of poor African Americans in urban areas may have also dealt a series of hard blows to their critical social network systems, leaving such networks with fewer resources of any kind to meet the increasing needs of their members. Joblessness, homelessness, doubling-up in overcrowded, substandard housing, ill-health, and early death all undermine the efforts of kin to provide mutual aid or cultural affirmation. In addition, African Americans must vie with the dominant American culture to define urban black identity. The dominant culture often defines urban minorities in disconfirming, negative stereotypes or ones that are affirming only in a narrow, perverse and self-serving way—for example, in corporate images of urban athletes in high-priced athletic shoes. Kelly (1997) summarizes this restricted and confusing menu of images as "the circulation of the very representations of race that generate terror in all of us at the sight of young black men and yet compels most of America to want to wear their shoes" (p. 224).

Apart from this materialistic fantasy, few sincerely attempt to walk in the shoes of the urban African American poor. Instead, pervasive negative images inform policies with flawed logic. For example, the growing inability of community networks in poor urban areas to avert material hardship, violence, or disease is interpreted through the prism of the dominant cultural (pre)occupation with a perceived decline in personal responsibility and family values. Rather than consider the historical or structural precursors of urban decay, citizens and policy makers—liberal and conservative—identify the behavior of urban residents (and the disturbing values their behavior is thought to represent) as an important source of urban poverty and distress (Gans, 1995). One hard-hitting extension of this reasoning is the reduction of antipoverty policy into welfare policy institutionalized in the Personal Responsibility and Work Opportunity Reconciliation Act of 1996 (PRWORA; welfare reform), a bill misguided and demeaning in many of its fundamental premises about the goals and motivations of the poor (Geronimus, 1997).

IMPLICATIONS FOR PUBLIC HEALTH

HealthyPeople 2010 (U.S. Department of Health and Human Services, 2000) calls attention to socioeconomic disparities in health and, for the first time, boldly calls for the *elimination,* not simply the reduction, of racial/ethnic and socioeconomic disparities in health. The unfortunate truth is that descriptive documentation of these disparities is matched neither by well-tested explanations for them nor by evaluation research on *socioeconomic* interventions. Without progress in research, specific socioeconomic interventions cannot be confidently proposed. Yet the preceding "structural" analysis suggests some activities and leads to guiding principles for action and continued research.

First Do No (More) Harm
In a structural framework, policies that affect the context of urban poverty—such as the distribution of wealth, the built environment, segregation, and access to technologies, information or other resources—influence fundamental causes of health inequality. So, too, do policies that affect the integrity of the autonomous institutions—formal organizations, informal networks, ideologies, and cultural frameworks—that members of oppressed groups work to develop and maintain to mitigate, resist, or undo the structural constraints they face. Policies that are likely to erode income, housing, or neighborhood conditions; fragment or impose new obligations on already overburdened networks; or proliferate demeaning and demoralizing stereotypes affect the material and psychosocial conditions of life for the urban poor and thus their health. Public health professionals can describe the health impact of proposed policies by evaluating the likelihood that they will do any of the above and bring these considerations to the table.

For example, if such an analysis had been part of the deliberations on PRWORA, those concerned with its probable health impact would have noted not only its implications for Medicaid eligibility (which were considered) but also its likelihood of intensifying the material hardship, stress, and uncertainty faced by poor residents of urban areas (through, for example, its time-limits provisions) *and* its potential to impose further perturbations on the protective systems worked out by kin networks (through, for example, requiring all adult family members to work, no matter whether they then compete with each other for the same scarce low-wage jobs or whether this requirement depletes the reserve of kin members available to offer childcare to others). By intensifying their exposure to risks and undermining their autonomous protections, PRWORA could further erode the health of the urban poor.

Similarly, a press to revitalize urban areas now comes from environmentalists and upper- middle-class Americans who, ironically, now bemoan the sprawl wrought of increasing suburbanization and white flight. However, if plans to reverse sprawl and reclaim urban areas for the socio-economically advantaged have no equity component, they risk leading to the dispersion and fragmentation of poor, inner-city neighborhood residents as real estate prices increase. Already, evidence of this possibility is available in urban "success" sites such as downtown Atlanta, the South End of Boston, and San Francisco. On a more positive note, broad interest in reversing sprawl may offer opportunities for urban community leaders to build coalitions with environmentalists to galvanize interest in the revitalization of American cities.

Work to Alter Public Perspectives on Race

Negative stereotypical judgments of African Americans led to, and continue to reinforce, ghettoization; affect the treatment decisions of health providers (Chasnoff, Landress, and Barrett, 1990; Schulman and others, 1999); influence the hiring practices of potential employers (Wilson, 1996); fuel distrust of public health initiatives (Dalton, 1989); weaken public support for initiatives to improve the health of urban populations; and deny young, urban African Americans health promoting, identity-affirming symbols. In a structural framework, understanding what shapes public sentiment on race and how it might be influenced becomes a critical public health objective. Incorporating the historical underpinnings of ghettoization and the deterioration of urban areas into discussions of urban life and health may alter the ways people think about the minority poor and their health. To the extent that social epidemiologists elucidate the social conditions and contexts that trigger unhealthy behaviors among the urban poor, these should be described to broad audiences as a means to alter public understanding of these behaviors. For example, as King (1997) points out, high smoking rates in urban poor communities may in part be a response to pervasive psychosocial stress, and to the targeting of these communities by tobacco companies for advertising.

When social epidemiologists find evidence that in the face of formidable structural impediments to success, there is a physical price attached even to coping in socially approved ways, this information should also be disseminated. For example, James (1994; James and others, 1987) has suggested and found evidence of a culturally salient behavioral predisposition among African Americans to engage in persistent high-effort coping with social and economic adversity ("John Henryism"). In low-income African American populations, individuals who exhibit high levels of John Henryism are the ones most apt to be hypertensive. This evidence contradicts demeaning stereotypic notions that fatalism and indolence precipitate cardiovascular disease among low-income African Americans. Put another way, the empirical evidence on John Henryism suggests that low-income African Americans who work hard to mobilize their internal resources to cope with or surmount structural barriers to their achievement also express values and take actions that are in sync with the greater American ideological emphasis on self-control and a strong work ethic. However, these actions can exact a physical price, whether or not they are successful in producing social mobility.

Distinguish Between "Ameliorative" and "Fundamental" Approaches

Positing that many social conditions are "fundamental causes" of disease, Link and Phelan (1995, 1996; Link and others, 1998) describe the social patterning of health and disease as a potent force that may take new shape but persists undeterred by the identification and amelioration of the risk factors that express that patterning in a given time period. In the realm of intervention, this conceptual model implies a distinction between "ameliorative" and "fundamental" actions. Ameliorative approaches target the risk factors that link socioeconomic position to health in a particular context, but do not fundamentally alter the context (or underlying inequalities). Public health practitioners are often engaged in what can be seen, by this rubric, as ameliorative actions. A substantial literature assesses ameliorative interventions, including ones specific to the urban context (Freudenberg, 1998).

Continued implementation of and refinements in ameliorative approaches are necessary to avoid health disparities from widening uncontrollably. Certainly, it is wise to build on the accumulated base of knowledge on how best to implement health promotion initiatives or expand access to medical services; it is also wise to target and tailor them appropriately for urban and minority populations. Still, such initiatives and services alone will not result in the *elimination* of health disparities. As Link and Phelan (1995, 1996; Link and others, 1998) outline, energy put forth to address a specific risk factor will achieve limited success in improving the health of a disadvantaged population. The risk factor may be virtually inevitable in a given social context, or it may be only one of the many risk factors that follow from a set of social conditions. Even the eradication of specific risk factors may be followed by the emergence of new risks that, similar to the old risks, are more likely to be averted by a population in more favorable social circumstances than by the population one is trying to help. From this perspective, the only way to eliminate differentials in health is to address the underlying "social inequalities that so reliably produce them" (Link and Phelan, 1996, p. 472).

It is easiest to understand individual behavior change strategies or the expansion of access to (especially tertiary services) as falling under the rubric of ameliorative interventions. It is also important to recognize that community-based public health initiatives can also be ameliorative rather than fundamental. The value of community partners in research, the importance of community members on boards of local health care facilities, and the necessity of the participation and leadership of community members in social or policy change efforts is clear and has been well-described elsewhere (Schlesinger, 1987; Dalton, 1989; Thompson, 1998; Israel and others, 1998). In fact, aspects of the structural paradigm urge working in partnerships with communities, engaging in "bottom-up" approaches, and recognizing that historically important and effective social movements derive their moral, political, and practical force from the autonomous networks and institutions developed and kindled within minority communities.

However, the paradigm also suggests a caveat to over-reliance on community-centered approaches. As Halpern (1995) notes, one possible pitfall of over-reliance on such approaches is that "those who have the least role in making and the largest role in bearing the brunt of society's economic and social choices [are left] to deal with the effects of those choices" (p. 5). If social, political, and economic exclusion are among the distal causes of the disproportionate health burden absorbed by the urban minority poor, and if, as a result, community members own and control little, the prospects for local community initiatives to alter fundamental causes of morbidity and mortality may be modest. The comments of a community legal aid activist of the 1960s are cautionary: "We undoubtedly brought some solace and relief to many individual tenants. . . . Nevertheless in those same three years the housing situation in San Francisco became a great deal worse. . . . [It] might appear [that we made] the process a little more humane without having any effect on the underlying machinery" (Carlin, 1973, p. 146).

In addition to cautioning against having unrealistic expectations of what community-based public health approaches can be expected to achieve, this caveat also suggests broadening the set of community-based networks and organizations that can be enlisted to address structural barriers to include organizations with substantial economic leverage. For example, the largest and wealthiest minority organizations include labor unions. In some cities, minority-run public sector unions are a major force in city/state politics and policy. More generally, altering fundamental causes of health inequality requires working at multiple levels and making connections between levels. The scope and target of public health activity can move (as they have, to an extent) from the individual to the family to the community and also to encompass large societal institutions, pervasive and influential ideologies, inter-group relations, and macroeconomic policy.

Increase Attention to the Needs of Adults

Many public health activities target or favor the health and well-being of youths over those of adults, because youths are viewed a being either more deserving of our efforts or as more at risk. However, adults are critical to the vitality of families and communities, and research findings suggest the merit of stimulating increased attention to the needs of young and middle-aged adults in impoverished urban areas. As noted previously, social differentials in morbidity and mortality are most pronounced among adults of reproductive and working-age (Geronimus, 1992; House and others, 1994).

Adults of these ages play critical social roles as economic providers and caretakers. Improving adult health in impoverished urban areas would reap advantages for residents of all ages. Some examples are straightforward, such as the importance of maternal health to infant health. In addition, high levels of health-induced disability among working-age African American men and women contribute to their relatively low rates of participation in the labor force and thereby to their ability to support families economically (Bound, Schoenbaum, and Waidmann, 1996). Meanwhile, extensive and competing obligations to family and larger social networks as well as to paid jobs lead to stress-related disease, particularly among women (Geronimus, 1992; Le Clere, Rogers, and Peters, 1998). More speculatively, pervasive health uncertainty regarding young adult and middle-aged members of a community shapes the expectations of youths and may influence the timing of childbearing towards earlier ages (Geronimus, 1992, 1997) or the propensity of some youth to engage in risk-taking behaviors (Wilson and Daly, 1997).

CONTINUED RESEARCH

To inform efforts to reduce or eliminate urban health disadvantages, continued research should evaluate the impact of social and economic policies on the health of urban residents. In addition, evidence of important interactions of race, poverty, and local place in influencing health is growing (Davey Smith and others, 1998; Geronimus, Bound, and Waidmann, 1999), but social epidemiologists more often look at general patterns of the relationship between socioeconomic position and health (e.g., providing estimates based on national or statewide averages or averaging across all residents of major metropolitan areas). Stepping up research on variation among local poor populations may prove beneficial to those hoping to remedy the problems of urban life on health.

Indicators of personal experience with racism and racialized stress have been added to the set of studied influences on health (Williams and others, 1997), yet few investigators have systematically considered the health consequences of the manifestations of racism in the *structures* of society (Williams and Collins, 1995; Polednak, 1996). Conceptually, research in this area would benefit from the development of dynamic and contextualized understandings of the role of culture in health. This development would replace static constructions of culture as an imported set of behaviors, practices, or values that are subject to change only inasmuch as they are traded in for the dominant set.

As part of this activity, investigators should become more attuned to the *functioning* of autonomous social institutions within communities and less concerned with their *form*. For example, classifying mothers as married or unmarried provides more questionable information about children's well-being or local social organization than does understanding who, in a broader social network, is expected and available to participate in the care and support of children. Classifying mothers as married or unmarried also overlooks important questions such as why autonomous caretaking systems evolved and how they are maintained (Stack, 1974; Stack and Burton, 1993; Geronimus, 1997; Sharff, 1998). To this end, development and empirical testing of theories that draw from African American (or other urban ethnic) culture, history, and life experience to hypothesize links between structural barriers, personal and social coping mechanisms, and their physiological effects and health manifestations offer more promise than studies that draw from political theories abstracted from the lived experience of urban Americans.

A deeper understanding of how culture relates to inequalities in health will also require evaluation of the role the dominant cultural system plays in the maintenance of inequality. The history of race-based ghettoization suggests there is a cultural component to the perpetuation of poverty, and it comes, in the main, from the dominant culture, not from the poor. One interpretation is that the health of the African American poor has been sacrificed to maintain the core American myth that "some people are more equal than others." In this myth, the populace is divided into those who are responsible members of civil society, deserving of its full benefits, and those who are deemed a threat to civil society, who are to be segregated, marginalized, or even policed (Brodkin, 1998).

These comments have focused on African American residents of impoverished urban areas because both real and imagined threats to public health emanate from the long-term ghettoization of African Americans. Historical processes underpin this ghettoization, but there are also emerging racial/ethnic challenges and opportunities that affect the landscape and dynamics of urban centers. The 1990s witnessed the greatest influx of immigrants in 50 years, and many of these immigrants moved into high poverty urban areas. Whether they become long-term residents of ghettos or barrios or whether, like some immigrant populations before them, they are enabled to move through these areas, and into higher-income areas is an open question. Meanwhile, their needs and perspectives deserve articulation, and the influence of inter-group dynamics, coalitions, and tensions on health must also be examined and incorporated into programs and policies to improve the health of urban residents. In the spirit of this structural analysis, a key part of the process of examination is to discern the ways dominant American cultural ideologies and institutions shape, relieve, or reinforce the tensions between new immigrant groups and urban African Americans. Otherwise, a race-based culture of exclusivity will continue to draw its support by taxing the health of African Americans.

References

Adler, N. A., and others. "Socioeconomic Status and Health." *American Journal of Psychology*, 1994, *49*, 15–24.

Antonovsky, A. "Social Class, Life Expectancy, and Overall Mortality." *Milbank Quarterly*, 1967, *45*(2), 31–73.

Backlund, E., Sorlie, P. D., and Johnson, N. J. "The Shape of the Relationship Between Income and Mortality in the United States: Evidence from the National Longitudinal Mortality Study." *Annals of Epidemiology*, 1996, *6*, 12–20.

Bound, J., Schoenbaum, M., and Waidmann, T. A. "Race Differences in Labor Force Attachment and Disability Status." *Gerontologist*, 1996, *36*, 311–321.

Brodkin, K. *How Jews Became White Folks and What That Says About Race in America.* New Brunswick, N.J.: Rutgers University Press, 1998.

Carlin, J. "Storefront Lawyers in San Francisco." In M. Pilisuk and P. Pilisuk (eds.), *How We Lost the War on Poverty.* New Brunswick, N.J.: Transaction, 1973.

Chasnoff, I. J., Landress, H. J., and Barrett, M. E. "The Prevalence of Illicit-Drug or Alcohol Use During Pregnancy and Discrepancies in Mandatory Reporting in Pinellas County, Florida." *New England Journal of Medicine*, 1990, *322*, 1202–1206.

Conley, D. *Being Black, Living in the Red: Race, Wealth, and Social Policy in America.* Berkeley: University of California Press, 1999.

Cooper, R., and David, R. "The Biological Concept of Race and Its Application in Public Health and Epidemiology." *Journal of Health Politics, Policy and Law*, 1986, *11*, 97–116.

Dalton, H. "AIDS in Blackface." *Daedalus*, Summer 1989, pp. 205–223.

Davey Smith, G., and others. "Individual Social Class, Area-Based Deprivation, Cardio-vascular Disease Risk Factors, and Mortality: The Renfrew and Paisley Study." *Journal of Epidemiology and Community Health,* 1998, *52,* 399–405.

Fossett, J. W., and Perloff, J. D. "The 'New' Health Reform and Access to Care: The Problem of the Inner City." Report prepared for the Kaiser Commission on the Future of Medicaid, Dec. 1995.

Fossett, J. W., and others. "Medicaid in the Inner City: The Case of Maternity Care in Chicago." *Milbank Quarterly,* 1990, *68,* 111–141.

Freudenberg, N. "Community-Based Health Education for Urban Populations: An Overview." *Health Education and Behavior,* 1998, *25,* 11–23.

Gans, H. J. *The War Against the Poor.* New York: Basic Books, 1995.

Geronimus, A. T. "The Weathering Hypothesis and the Health of African American Women and Infants." *Ethnicity and Disease,* 1992, *2,* 207–221.

Geronimus, A. T. "Teenage Childbearing and Personal Responsibility: An Alternative View." *Political Science Quarterly,* 1997, *112,* 405–430.

Geronimus, A. T., Bound, J., and Waidmann, T. A. "Poverty, Time, and Place: Variation in Excess Mortality Across Selected U.S. Populations, 1980–1990." *Journal of Epidemiology and Community Health,* 1999, *53,* 325–334.

Geronimus, A. T., and others. "Excess Mortality Among Blacks and Whites in the United States." *New England Journal of Medicine,* 1996, *335,* 1552–1558.

Halpern, R. *Rebuilding the Inner City: A History of Neighborhood Initiatives to Address Poverty in the United States.* New York: Columbia University Press, 1995.

House, J. S., and others. "The Social Stratification of Aging and Health." *Journal of Health and Social Behavior,* 1994, *35,* 213–234.

Israel, B. A., and others. "Review of Community-Based Research: Assessing Partnership Approaches to Improve Public Health." *Annual Review of Public Health,* 1998, *19,* 173–202.

James, S. A. "Racial and Ethnic Differences in Infant Mortality and Low Birth Weight: A Psychosocial Critique." *Annals of Epidemiology,* 1993, *3,* 130–136.

James, S. A. "John Henryism and the Health of African-Americans." *Culture, Medicine and Psychiatry,* 1994, *18,* 163–182.

James, S. A., and others. "Socioeconomic Status, John Henryism, and Hypertension in Blacks and Whites." *American Journal of Epidemiology,* 1987, *126,* 664–673.

Jargowsky, P. A. *Poverty and Place: Ghettos, Barrios, and the American City.* New York: Russell Sage Foundation, 1997.

Kelly, R.D.G. "Playing for Keeps: Pleasure and Profit on the postindustrial playground." In W. Lubiano (ed.), *The House That Race Built.* New York: Pantheon, 1997.

King, G. "The 'Race' Concept in Smoking: A Review of Research on African Americans." *Social Science and Medicine,* 1997, *45,* 1075–1087.

Kitagawa, E. M., and Hauser, P. M. *Differential Mortality in the United States: A Study in Socioeconomic Epidemiology.* Cambridge, Mass.: Harvard University Press, 1973.

Lantz, P. M., and others. "Socioeconomic Factors, Health Behaviors, and Mortality." *Journal of the American Medical Association,* 1998, *279,* 1703–1708.

Le Clere, F. B., Rogers, R. G., and Peters, K. "Neighborhood Social Context and Racial Differences in Women's Heart Disease Mortality." *Journal of Health and Social Behavior,* 1998, *38,* 91–107.

Link, B. G, and Phelan, J. C. "Social Conditions as Fundamental Causes of Disease." *Journal of Health and Social Behavior,* 1995 (Special Issue), 80–94.

Link, B. G., and Phelan, J. C. "Understanding Sociodemographic Differences in Health: The Role of Fundamental Social Causes." *American Journal of Public Health,* 1996, *86,* 471–473.

Link, B. G., and others. "Social Epidemiology and the Fundamental Cause Concept: On the Structuring of Effective Cancer Screens by Socioeconomic Status." *Milbank Quarterly,* 1998, *76,* 375–402.

Lynch, J. W., Kaplan, G. A., and Shema, S. J. "Cumulative Impact of Sustained Economic Hardship on Physical, Cognitive, Psychological, and Social Functioning." *New England Journal of Medicine,* 1997, *337,* 1889–1895.

Marmot, M. G., Kogevinas, M., and Elston, M. A. "Socioeconomic Status and Disease." *Annual Review of Public Health,* 1987, *8,* 111–135.

Massey, D., and Denton, N. *American Apartheid: Segregation and the Making of the Underclass.* Cambridge, Mass.: Harvard University Press, 1993.

McCord, C., and Freeman, H. P. "Excess Mortality in Harlem." *New England Journal of Medicine,* 1990, *322,* 173–177.

Miller, J. E., and Korenman, S. "Poverty and Children's Nutritional Status in the United States." *American Journal of Epidemiology,* 1994, *140,* 233–243.

Mohai, P., and Bryant, B. "Environmental Injustice: Weighing Race and Class as Factors in the Distribution of Environmental Hazards." *University of California Law Review,* 1992, *63,* 921–932.

Northridge, M. E., and others. "Contribution of Smoking to Excess Mortality in Harlem." *American Journal of Epidemiology,* 1998, *147,* 250–258.

O'Connor, A. "Historical Perspectives on Race and community revitalization." Paper presented at the meeting of the Race and Community Revitalization project of the Aspen Institute Roundtable on Comprehensive Community Initiatives, Wye River Conference Center, Md., 1998.

Oliver, M. L., and Shapiro, T. M. *Black Wealth/White Wealth: A New Perspective on Racial Inequality.* New York: Routledge, 1995.

Polednak, A. P. "Segregation, Discrimination, and Mortality in U.S. Blacks." *Ethnicity and Disease,* 1996, *6,* 99–108.

Schlesinger, M. "Paying the Price: Medical Care, Minorities, and the Newly Competitive Health Care System." *Milbank Quarterly*, 1987, *65*(Suppl. 2), 270–296.

Schulman, K. A, and others. "The Effect of Race and Sex on Physicians' Recommendations for Cardiac Catheterization." *New England Journal of Medicine*, 1999, *340*, 618–626.

Sharff, J. W. *King Kong on 4th Street*. Boulder, Colo.: Westview Press, 1998.

Stack, C. B. *All Our Kin*. New York: HarperCollins, 1974.

Stack, C., and Burton, L. M. "Kinscripts." *Journal of Comparative Family Studies*, 1993, *24*, 157-170.

Thompson, J. P. "Universalism and Deconcentration: Why Race Still Matters in Poverty and Economic Development." *Politics and Society*, 1998, *26*, 181–219.

U.S. Department of Health and Human Services. *Healthy People 2010: Understanding and Improving Health*. Washington, D.C.: U.S. Government Printing Office, 2000.

Wallace, R., and Wallace, D. "Origins of Public Health Collapse in New York City: The Dynamics of Planned Shrinkage, Contagious Urban Decay, and Social Disintegration." *Bulletin of the New York Academy of Medicine*, 1990, *66*, 391–434.

Weinberg, M. (ed.). *W.E.B. Du Bois: A Reader*. New York: HarperCollins, 1970.

Williams, D. R., and Collins, C. "U.S. Socioeconomic and Racial Differences in Health: Patterns and Explanations." *Annual Review of Sociology*, 1995, *21*, 349–386.

Williams, D. R., and House, J. S. "Stress, Social Support, Control, and Coping: A Social Epidemiological View." *WHO Regional Publications, European Series*, 1991, *37*, 147–172.

Williams, D. R., and others. "Racial Differences in Physical and Mental Health: Socioeconomic Status, Stress and Discrimination." *Journal of Health and Psychology*, 1997, *2*, 335–351.

Wilson, M., and Daly, M. "Life Expectancy, Economic Inequality, Homicide, and Reproductive Timing in Chicago Neighbourhoods." *British Medical Journal*, 1997, *314*, 1271–1274.

Wilson, W. J. *When Work Disappears: The World of the New Urban Poor*. New York: Knopf, 1996.

CHAPTER TWENTY-FIVE

Swimming Upstream in a Swift Current

Public Health Institutions and Inequality

Rajiv Bhatia

We have sought too diligently to find the causes
of poverty among the poor and not in ourselves.
—Richard Titmuss

Health depends on meeting our common human needs (Max-Neef, Elizade, and Hopenhayn, 1989; Sen, 1995). It requires adequate food and shelter, a safe environment, and a secure livelihood along with the ability to acquire and use skills, exercise political freedom, and participate in the culture of the times. Societies do not ensure that needs are met equally for all their members. In many of the world's wealthiest countries, including the United States, economic inequality is increasing. In this context, inequalities in health outcomes are not unexpected.

Does identifying health inequalities advance the struggle for social equity? Health has a unique standing among human needs because it relates to conditions from which no one is immune. In contrast, many individuals living in societies of privilege may take the fulfillment of other human needs for granted. Because wealthy states have significant rhetorical commitments to ensuring the health of populations, examining the basis for health inequalities may have unique political currency to challenge inequity more broadly. Accordingly, some advocates for health promotion have called for examination and action on social structures, institutions, and policies that affect health and health equity (World Health Organization, 1986, 1998; Raphael, 2000).

Yet economic and social policymaking does not identify an explicit role for public health institutions. Traditionally, public health concerned itself with the control of adverse physical environmental conditions and communicable disease. Over time, these responses led to highly structured practices such as sanitation, environmental regulations, and communicable disease surveillance. New public institutions responsible for municipal water, waste disposal, occupational health, and building safety were also created for public health.

Today, public health activities, firmly anchored to preventing or treating disease, remain fragmented by disease category and risk factor. Strong disciplinary traditions and boundaries between disciplines limit action beyond institutional mandates (McKinlay and Marceau, 2000). Epidemiology and biomedical sciences, the dominant cognitive tools in public health, also discount experiential knowledge and reduce the understanding of the human ecology to an understanding of mechanisms and parts (Krieger, 2001). However, the relationship between social and economic circumstances and physical health eludes simple mechanistic explanations. More important, these tools do not question how social forces create and perpetuate unequal circumstances (Raphael and Bryant, 2002).

A critical demand of equity is equal political power, which requires the capacity of all people to "participate in, negotiate with, influence, control, and hold accountable the institutions that affect their lives" (Narayan, 2002, p. 11). Health promotion has been similarly defined as "the process of enabling people to increase control over, and to improve, their health" (World Health Organization, 1986, p. 1). In contrast, public health institutions are driven more by expertise and scientific analysis than by popular participation and community experience. Unfortunately, the paradigm of rational, linear, or evidence-based policymaking does not acknowledge the selective creation and use of evidence. Often evidence hides assumptions, worldviews, values, and contested political interests (Fischer, 2000; Keeley and Scoones, 1999; Campbell, 2002; Callicott, 2001).

In order to seize opportunities for public health to confront inequity, we must first examine critically how ideas and interests drive our practice and techniques. Institutional culture is both reproduced by internal forces and constrained by accountability to political, legal, and administrative structures. Institutional accountability is coherent with the social distribution of power and privilege, and increased institutional responsiveness to the socially excluded must support conditions for their self-representation. The participation of ordinary people requires that they have the capacity to meet basic needs, aspire, organize, deliberate, and choose. Equally, it demands guaranteeing that institutions make information available, be open to citizen voices, and limit the influence of powerful elites (Smulovitz and Walton, 2003). Initiatives in partnership with traditionally excluded populations have become more frequent in public health practice and represent movement toward equity.

This chapter describes the experience of an environmental health agency within a U.S. urban public health department seeking to support conditions for greater social equality. Our agency's primary mandate is to enforce state and local laws and regulations with regard to food safety, neighborhood sanitation, and chemical hazards. The first part of the chapter provides examples from and reflections on our agency's practice. These examples include the collaboration with community residents to address environmental hazards, the application of epidemiological research to policy analysis on a living wage law, and the development of a community health impact assessment. The experiences illustrate the evolution of our practice and the challenges to working for equity within a public institution. Our experiences with environmental justice struggles led to a greater understanding of how institutional partners might support social change, how public health research might legitimate issues, and how environmental health activities might advance from physical to social domains. Attempting to use public health research to influence economic policy also revealed the political context of evidence and demanded new structures to apply public health knowledge. Exploring health impact created a way to conduct policy analysis based on popular participation and influence.

The second part of the chapter discusses how we negotiated workplace culture and what acting in solidarity with socially excluded populations implies for public servants. It also projects future possibilities for public health practice to address inequity.

EVOLVING PRACTICE
Collaboration and Environmental Health

Community residents frequently ask public health agencies to respond to adverse environmental conditions such as chemical exposures from industries. Hazardous environmental conditions, more commonly found in low-income and predominantly minority neighborhoods, may reflect discriminatory land use decisions, population dynamics, or economic factors (Lee, 2002). They illustrate a direct pathway through which social disadvantage can lead to poorer health outcomes (Schulz and others, 2002). Action to change adverse environmental conditions is a common target of organizing efforts to mobilize community members.

Traditional public health responses to environmental justice claims include assessments of environmental exposure and health status. Regulatory agencies may also ensure the strict enforcement of existing laws. More recently, health agencies have developed partnerships with community organizations to address the conditions of environmental justice. Participatory research makes explicit the issues of agency and representation, questioning the privileged position of experts and demanding a greater role for lay citizens (Freire, [1970] 1999). Participatory research raises practical challenges for institutions. For example, what work skills does collaborative practice require? And how does the agency ensure that the individuals they work with represent the communities?

In 1994, our department began a community dialogue with members of a disadvantaged neighborhood in San Francisco on concerns about environmental health. Many community residents believed that a high rate of cancer existed in the neighborhood and attributed this to the presence of polluting industries and the legacy of a hazardous waste landfill. At the community's request, the department agreed to investigate environment-disease relationships in order to support actions toward environmental change.

The initiative centered on issues that had been voiced for several years. Until 1974, a federal naval shipyard had provided steady jobs for residents, including many African Americans fleeing racial and economic segregation in the South. The ceasing of military operations and the decline of urban manufacturing jobs damaged the community's livelihood. In 1989, the naval base was put on the national Superfund list due to significant soil and groundwater contamination. A few years later, an article in the local paper attributed an observed cluster of breast cancer to environmental contamination.

When concerned community members and environmental organizations requested that our agency investigate the health consequences of environment contamination, some employees were skeptical about a cause-and-effect relationship. They also raised more practical concerns about the methodological limits to demonstrating a relationship using epidemiological tools. Nevertheless, the agency's leaders chose to respond to the concerns, in part acknowledging their responsibility for the historic distrust between the community and government.

The department began meeting monthly with community members, advocacy organizations, and academic researchers. Our first actions involved the creation of a map of sites with hazardous materials uses and hazardous waste sites. We also conducted an analysis of common cancers, revealing an unusually high number of cases of breast cancer among young African American females. Although agency researchers considered the breast cancer findings speculative, the study validated long-standing community beliefs. Community organizations used the information on "toxic sites," emissions data, and the analysis of breast cancer to call for a moratorium on new power plants in the neighborhood. The department publicly supported the community position, arguing that the residents constituted a vulnerable population and bore a disproportionate burden of environmental exposures. These supportive efforts contributed to a relationship between our agency and community members. At the same time, the links between the community's poor health and environmental hazards became potent public and political facts.

In 1998, a new analysis of breast cancer data argued that the earlier findings represented a transient increase due to early detection. However, the new information had limited influence. At public meetings, key opinion leaders and environmental advocacy organizations challenged the new results despite similar sources of data and analytical approaches. Even after the new analysis, community members, political leaders, and some health officials continued to represent rates of cancer in this neighborhood as among the highest in the state.

Contested Evidence as Contested Power

Differences in interpretation of the epidemiological analyses underscore many of the well-recognized challenges to shared understanding between researchers and community members. Hidden values and assumptions contribute to these challenges (Brown, 1987). For example, epidemiologists seek objective truth about the causes of illness, while community residents want to solve problems. Trust is equally important. Community members frequently feel that expertise works against their interests, for example, when studying a problem means delaying action for change.

Our agency staff wanted to be effective advocates for this community, but they needed evidence to support their positions. If the findings of analyses did not validate community beliefs, researchers could be perceived as disinterested in health, threatening both the credibility of expert techniques and the trust of community members. Conversely, if researchers reinterpreted the findings to be consistent with the perceptions or interests of the community, they would be at odds with professional beliefs. Beyond the impacts on the agency-community relationships, some researchers believed that downplaying negative findings could increase insecurity among those members of the community looking for straightforward answers.

Through this dialogue we came to realize the enormous demands that contested policy contexts, such as the cleanup of contaminated properties, place on scientific research. The community expected scientific analysis to be understandable, reduce uncertainty, explain complexity, be trustworthy, and respond to the practical needs of decision makers and community members. But epidemiological methods did not produce certainty, and with interests competing to determine the fate of the shipyard, multiple interpretations of same scientific studies produced different meanings.

Despite the contested interpretations of research, policymakers, the Navy, advocates, and community members all relied on scientific studies. Environmental health research was alternatively supported and contested as a strategic lever to gain influence in a situation of otherwise limited power. By successfully engaging the agency in the study of environmental health, the community's concerns were given legitimacy, increasing political attention to the cleanup of the shipyard.

The community demands on our agency occurred in the broader context of the community residents' aspirations for a better future. The conflicts surrounding the reuse of the base transcended issues of health and safety and included the related issues of community power and economic development. Unfortunately, community members had little chance to address these issues together. For example, community involvement processes for cleanup and redevelopment activities had different goals, participants, and sponsoring institutions. Many participating community members were skeptical that cleanup and redevelopment efforts would ever meet the residents' needs. Residents questioned the assumptions guiding planning and the community assets and needs determined by nonresident consultants. Some argued that planned employment opportunities did not reflect the current skills, capacities, and ambitions of the residents, fueling fears around gentrification and displacement.

Though etiological issues with regard to health remained "unproven," community members still gained influence in land use planning and public resource allocation. Over the next few years, community organizations used neighborhood health statistics to secure funding for community organizing, a neighborhood environmental health resource center, and technical resources for oversight of the shipyard's cleanup. As issues of environmental health gained political currency, many community leaders developed influence in key decision-making processes. For example, city leaders asked advocates for environmental health to participate in the legal negotiation of the transfer of shipyard property, influencing the conditions under which the city would accept the property.

Beyond the Disciplinary Boundaries of Environmental Health

While supporting environmental justice struggles, our agency began to work on other adverse neighborhood conditions. In 2001, a community survey, assessing perceptions of environmental concerns, found that only 14 percent of residents rated chemical contamination and pollution as a major concern (Bayview–Hunter's Point Health and Environmental Assessment Task Force, 2001). Residents felt that addiction, crime, and unemployment were more important environmental issues. Upon revealing the survey's findings at a community forum, community residents identified corner food markets as a source of access to drugs and a cause of violence and poor nutrition. Some advocated for increased regulatory and criminal enforcement of corner stores, while others advocated for creating economic incentives for changes in business practices. However, at the time, neither approach attracted the support of our community partners.

The community survey did create an opportunity for our agency to attend to environmental issues other than pollution. We used a small amount of discretionary funding to collaborate with an urban gardening and agriculture organization to conduct research on neighborhood food access. The research led to the creation of a new seasonal farmer's market and the commitment by some small market owners to increase fresh food (Bhatia and Ona, 2002). Improving food quality subsequently became a demand of environmental justice in this neighborhood.

Next, our agency worked with elected leaders to request that other city departments also support the conditions for neighborhood health. A short series of interagency meetings with department leaders resulted in concrete outcomes and commitments. The local transit authority created a new daytime shuttle bus route between the neighborhood and larger retail food businesses. Commitments were made to public improvements such as street lighting and enhanced services such as recreational facilities. The redevelopment agency invited our department to play a role in neighborhood land use planning.

Our work on other issues of neighborhood disadvantage did not change popular perceptions of environmental health. Environmental contamination remained a prominent concern of opinion leaders, and protest activities frequently target our agency. Our agency has not tried to prove or to disprove an environment-disease relationship. As we have learned, good working relationships with community organizations alone can advance public health goals.

While studying environmental health concerns strengthened the claims of advocates, the realization of equity and participation remained uncertain. Advocacy for environmental health was not linked with other neighborhood priorities such as food security and violence. The neighborhood survey illustrated that concerns about environmental pollution were more limited than opinion makers and advocates claimed. Concerns about representation highlighted the need to examine whose voices were being heard and whose overlooked.

Applying Epidemiological Research to Economic Policy

In participatory research, participants develop and apply evidence for shared purposes and to develop capacity for social change. In the more traditional approach to knowledge translation, public health practitioners bring "objective" evidence to a question or problem already on the public policy agenda. The application of public health evidence depends on a legitimate claim on the policy being considered. For example, an abundance of evidence exists on the relationship between economic position and health, yet its influence on public policy has been limited.

Poverty is an established etiological factor for poor health. Local policies help determine labor market conditions, education, and wages and can thus affect poverty. Recently, our agency considered the effectiveness of applying epidemiological research on poverty to economic and social policy. A proposed local law requiring a "living wage" provided the catalyst for such an investigation.

Because the proposal was controversial, the legislature appointed a task force to study the ordinance and commissioned a local university to conduct an economic analysis. The official economic analysis identified the change in wages, the public and private monetary costs, and labor market effects due to the ordinance. No one mentioned the social benefits of increasing wages to workers, neighborhoods, and the city.

Several epidemiologists in our agency, familiar with the literature on income and health, believed that documenting the effects of increased wages on health could make the full costs and benefits of this proposal more transparent. A health-oriented analysis could potentially generate political support for the living wage. At the request of a legislator, we produced an analysis illustrating how the living wage decreased the risk of premature death for adults, increased completed education, and decreased the risk of early childbirth for offspring (Bhatia and Katz, 2001). The ordinance ultimately passed, although the legislated "living wage" was lower than originally proposed.

We conducted the analysis independent of community organizations advocating for the living wage. At the time, we did not have a working relationship with such organizations. In hindsight, conducting the analysis in partnership with such organizations might have given the findings a stronger voice in the political process. More recently, another legislator invited our agency to participate in discussions exploring a living wage requirement for all local employers. This discussion established the desirability of the consideration of social and health impacts in future city wage policy.

Although the analysis applied public health evidence to an economic policy, practical limits to this use of health research emerged. The living wage decision hinged primarily on economic factors. The legislators questioned us during public testimony about how the living wage could decrease the city's expenditures for safety net health services. In other words, these policymakers equated the health benefits of the wage increase only with economic savings to the city.

Evidence in a Context of Interests and Ideas

How does establishing an etiological role for poverty in health lead to the reduction of poverty? Our analysis of the living wage assumed the existence of an evidence-based culture that would use the analysis to inform the decision reached. Scientists typically value research only against standards for building knowledge within their own disciplines. In general, the efforts to describe health inequities do not address the translation of research into policy or practice (Raphael, 2000).

Linear or rational models of policymaking are prevalent, particularly in public health. A problem appears on the public agenda resulting in the identification of alternative courses of action followed by weighing the costs and benefits, making a decision, and ensuring its implementation (Sutton, 1999). Hidden in this scenario are three questionable assumptions: all options for change will be considered, scientific and analytical methods can be objective, and evidence will result in the selection of the best choice.

Values, interests, and ideas influence the use of evidence in policymaking. For example, values and beliefs holding the poor responsible for their own condition limit poverty interventions such as cash assistance programs and the living wage. Policymakers posed welfare reform as a response to the illegitimate transfer of income from working taxpayers to the undeserving (Campbell, 2002). Similarly, many people attribute health risk behaviors, though more prevalent in disadvantaged communities, to personal choices. The strength of values in policymaking can be stronger than the economic calculus. For example, society has not universally supported methadone maintenance, an effective and socially efficient intervention for treating injection drug use, in large part because of values holding individuals responsible for their addiction.

The failure to apply social resources to collective ends such as equal opportunities for education suggest that public health evidence alone has a limited impact on social and economic policymaking. Strategic efforts to use public health evidence to influence policy need to be coupled with efforts to challenge the way a problem is framed. Challenging the dominant problem frames around inequity can mean showing that beneficiaries of cash assistance policies have adequate work motivation but limited opportunities for work or illustrating that public programs subsidize employers who pay low wages. Historically, interventions for public health have required political struggles (Szreter, 2003).

Healthy Public Policy and Health Impact Assessment

Healthy public policy may be desirable; however, its accomplishment requires that policymakers agree on how collective actions affect health and, more important, that they are willing to change policies in the interest of health. As noted, these two needs, gaining knowledge and exerting influence, become intertwined in the political process. Methods for achieving healthy public policy need to be systematic and have institutional and political legitimacy.

Healthy public policy poses a number of challenges. Typically, reasons other than health motivate policies (Kemm, 2001). Furthermore, costs and benefits vary among different populations, challenging consensus. The diverse institutions whose decisions and actions determine social, economic, and environmental conditions plan and act independently. The working relationships required for interdisciplinary practice do not exist, and conventional public and political expectations currently reinforce boundaries. Public health evidence, created for institutionally specific needs, suggests the need for new methods to translate public health knowledge across disciplinary boundaries. Finally, public health practitioners need practical experience in the policy process.

Health impact assessment (HIA) has been defined as "any combination of procedures or methods by which a proposed policy or program may be judged as to the effect(s) it may have on the health of a population." (Frankish and others, 1996). HIA is not a new idea, but it seeks to integrate systematically diverse assessment methods using health promotion as a unifying lens or perspective.

Conceptually related to environmental impact assessment (EIA), HIA emphasizes social, economic, and environmental conditions that influence health (Kemm, 2001). EIA, developed to anticipate adverse consequences of human interaction with the environment, allows for the consideration of health effects; however, in practice, health effects considered under EIA are limited environmental exposures such as air pollution (Council on Environmental Quality, 1997a; Arquiaga, Canter, and Nelson, 1994; Davies and Sadler, 1997). HIA uses procedures similar to EIA but includes methods and evidence from public health and the social sciences (Ison, 2000; Kemm, 2001; Banken, 2001; Lehto and Ritsatakis, 1999). Health equity is a motivation, goal or value in most models of HIA (Parry and Stevens, 2001).

In the United States, public health rarely influences the development and practice of EIA, in part because agencies responsible for land use, transportation, and environmental resource management conduct them. Practices for more comprehensive HIA in the United States have only recently been proposed (Minnesota Health Improvement Partnership, 2001). Our agency believed that a more ecological approach to impact assessment could address equity by considering a broader range of health impacts and making transparent the relationships among impacts and their distribution in affected populations.

Our agency reviews the public health components of EIA reports on behalf of our city's planning agency. City planners in San Francisco acknowledge the limited consideration of health effects in traditional EIA; however, they assert that the state legislation that mandates EIA, the California Environmental Quality Act (CEQA), does not require the additional consideration of social effects. They are cautious about broadening the scope of the assessment, citing the lack of resources, the lack of analytical tools to predict social and health impacts, and the need for objective criteria against which to value significance.

The limited consideration of social effects under the CEQA coexists with a perception that social effects are more difficult to predict relative to physical environmental effects. State guidelines for community impact assessment describe how incorrect assumptions in EIA practice are propagated: "Many people in California, including some decisionmakers, harbor the general belief that CEQA addresses only purely 'environmental' issues, not social, demographic, or economic issues often raised by proposed projects. This is erroneous. The assumption, however, is understandable due to the complex linkage that must be demonstrated between the physical, social, and economic environment, and the determination of 'Significance'" (California Department of Transportation, 1997, p. 3).

Contrary to these assumptions, governmental guidelines provide adequate methods for assessing social effects (Interorganizational Committee, 1994). California's CEQA guidelines list several significance criteria relevant for equity, such as displacing people or housing and disrupting or dividing the physical arrangement of an established community. The national goal of eliminating health inequalities or achieving environmental justice may also serve as criteria to determine significance (U.S. Department of Health and Human Services, 2000; Council on Environmental Quality, 1997b).

Some have raised cautions about the lack of a standardized method and an evidence base to support HIA (Parry and Stevens, 2001). Realizing that precise pathways to health are not quantifiable may not limit the appeal of HIA (Lock, 2000). The significance of HIA arises from its attempt to join diverse disciplinary interests and practices and to value experiential and intuitive knowledge. This in itself changes the relationship of public health to public policy.

Exploring Impact Assessment as Participatory Research

Although a technical appraisal of the health impacts of social policies seemed feasible, we anticipated challenges to its support and legitimacy. Mindful of the challenges to public participation, we felt that conducting impact assessment as a collaborative activity provided an alternative. Existing relationships with community organizations represented a potential opportunity for exploring impact assessment. A participatory approach to impact assessment could result in the identification of relevant knowledge not considered by experts and could develop community capacity to influence policy and ensure its implementation. Demonstrating a successful alternative framework for assessment might also lead to political will for innovation within institutions.

In November 2001, our agency sponsored a workshop on health impact assessment for San Francisco–based community organizations. Hypothetically applied to two proposed land use projects in that city, the assessments let participants identify unanticipated project impacts and helped link those impacts to health. Some participants also changed their prior positions on the value of the proposed projects. Following this workshop, we offered to support these organizations in conducting a health impact assessment on a policy issue relevant to their organizational mission.

These exploratory assessments represented a first step in disseminating the concept of health impact assessment practice in our local communities. For these exploratory assessments, collaborating community organizations identified the policy target and recruited participants. The participants engaged in a structured dialogue that defined the policy question, brainstormed impacts, identified knowledge needs, and discussed opportunities for future actions. We conducted five workshops on a range of issues, including community food strategies, locally funded tenant subsidies, school ground improvements, and minimum wage policy. (Exhibit 25.1 describes one of these workshops.)

Exhibit 25.1. Health Impact Assessment Workshop on the San Francisco Dislocation Rent Assistance Ordinance.

Partner and Setting. The Quality Housing Work Responsibility Act (QHWRA), a federal law enacted in 1998, denies noncitizens and nonnaturalized legal immigrants federal subsidies for public housing. In 2001, the San Francisco Board of Supervisors proposed a QHWRA Dislocation Rent Assistance Ordinance that would provide a local rent subsidy in order to prevent displacement. At the request of Homeless Prenatal Advocates, the ordinance was examined using a rapid Health Impact Assessment method in February 2002. Participants were representatives of community organizations that supported the city subsidy, and the explicit purpose of assessment was to identify the breadth of the law's issues and impacts, as well as to identify evidence that may help document the value of the proposed law.

Findings. The primary impact of the proposed ordinance related to the *economic well-being* of tenants and their families. Without this ordinance, participants predicted the following impacts:
- Reduction in available income for other basic needs, such as education, food security, and health care
- Increased pressure for multiple jobs and multiple household members working
- Increased demands in the labor supply for the city and county due to the displacement of immigrant populations from San Francisco
- Erosion of existing family assets due to the loss of subsidy
- A decrease in the level of social interaction among family members
- Conditions conducive to child labor exploitation
- Conditions conducive to illegal economic activities

The passage of a city ordinance to create a subsidy would lead to benefits including:
- Increase in economic security and employment
- Employment continuity for affected immigrants with subsequent benefits on job training and career advancement
- Development of economic assets for immigrant families
- Effective use of public services by immigrants
- Time for parent-child interactions

Implications for Practice. Participants recommended repeating the assessment with a broader group of stakeholders that included people who were affected by the new law. The participants challenged us to demonstrate the usefulness of the method as a tool for change as opposed to an object of research. One participant concluded, "we already understand the impacts; the point is, how do we get the decision makers to understand the impacts?" They believed that summarizing the findings of an assessment in a report and disseminating it to city opinion leaders, including the San Francisco Health Commission and the Department of Public Health's community advisory bodies, may advance their policy interests. The participants further observed that if the ordinance were enacted, some of the effects identified in the HIA could be used prospectively to inform the evaluation of pilot programs.

Though constrained by time, these exploratory workshops allowed a broad look at the target proposal's impacts and suggested that a participatory version of impact assessment could be useful for policy evaluation and for capacity building. For a public health agency, the assessment provided an additional way to engage with community members on social and economic issues. If the assessments identified unrecognized links to health, public agencies could have greater legitimacy in weighing in on a policy debate. At the same time, participants raised important questions. For example, could a community-based impact assessment have credibility and voice in the political context? Participants appeared ready to use such tools if decision makers would be accountable to their findings.

Reflecting on our experience, our agency outlined a model for an interdisciplinary practice of health impact assessment. The proposed assessment, situated among other political and institutional processes for policy analysis and advocacy, allows stakeholders to take ownership of the assessment. It envisions that an oversight committee plans the assessment, identifies methods, and ultimately achieves consensus on recommendations. The model provides a starting point for local government agencies or community members to conduct health impact assessments and creates an alternative to compare to the existing practice of EIA. (See Exhibit 25.2 for some of the major elements of our model.)

Exhibit 25.2. Stages and Elements in a Model Health Impact Assessment Process.

Stage	Issues and Tasks
1. Context and goals	• Who are stakeholders and what values, resources, and interests are influencing decisions?
	• How are policies set and decisions made?
	• How could additional assessment influence policy?
2. Planning	• What questions will the assessment answer?
	• What tools or methods will be used?
	• How will stakeholders be represented in the assessment?
	• What resources are required to conduct the assessment?
3. Assessment	• Train researchers and participants
	• Conduct surveys, interviews, observations, workshops, and focus groups
	• Access existing data, documents, and published literature
4. Synthesis and consensus	• What policy alternative best reflects stakeholders' values and visions?
	• How can institutions be more responsive to needs?
	• What actions are required for successful policy implementation?
5. Communication	• Prepare report
	• Disseminate to community, decision makers, and media
	• Monitor policy process, decision, and implementation

Developing a New Practice of Impact Assessment

Our agency is using the model assessment process within a developing community-agency partnership to assess alternative neighborhood zoning plans. Community organizations have proposed a "people's plan," which will be considered along with alternative city-proposed plans. All alternatives require an environmental impact assessment, and our collaboration has been exploring the value of conducting a community-led impact assessment for the alternatives complementary to the required EIA. The proposed assessment would consider issues such as requirements for affordable housing in any new development and the siting of housing and industry from the perspective of current community residents.

The local planning agency initially expressed reluctance to consider the assessment of additional social effects in the EIA procedures, however, the omitted issues have been subsequently identified by other community members. The planning agency recently invited us to participate in developing an environmental impact assessment on transportation and health. A catalyst for this partnership was a controversial decision not to rebuild a damaged freeway. Community members in this neighborhood recognized that the existing environmental analysis might not provide a full accounting of the transport-related benefits of removing the freeway. The city's current transit impact assessment guidelines do not assess health impacts such as traffic accidents, physical activity, psychosocial effects, neighborhood economic development, and access to goods, services, and employment. These effects may disproportionately affect the disadvantaged. The planners believed that applying research from urban planning and public health might demonstrate the distribution of costs and benefits.

We believe that health impact assessment can be a tool both for political accountability and capacity development. Our attempts to work simultaneously with both community organizations and planning agencies may serve as a bridge toward a more inclusive and comprehensive practice of impact assessment within the planning agency. At the same time, this work may result in policy analysis tools for popular use, reflecting community values and needs.

BARRIERS AND OPPORTUNITIES IN CURRENT INSTITUTIONS

Acting in an Institutional Culture

At the beginning of my tenure at the department, the environmental health agency conducted an internal planning effort to identify how current staff could extend their traditional regulatory roles to other community health issues. However, employee-management relations and opportunities for career advancement dominated the discussions. Most employees were skeptical about approaches that relied on dialogue with community members. For example, according to one district inspector, the lack of demand explained a lack of access to nutritious food in disadvantaged neighborhoods. Some employees believed that improving food quality and reducing chemical use are inconsistent with the agency's regulatory roles. For others, less structured activities threatened employment security.

Reorienting an existing public health workforce toward new endeavors challenges habit and familiarity. Public health professionals are strongly committed to their work. Programs, especially those providing health services, develop motivated constituencies who will advocate for existing benefits and services. Although such commitments, internal and external to institutions, may limit change, the personal values of individuals are also a force for change. Many working in public health professions and institutions have strong personal commitments to social justice principles. Public health institutions, directly involved in providing health and social services to the disadvantaged, witness the lives and living conditions of the socially excluded, often strengthening these commitments.

The environment health agency had sufficient flexibility to initiate new practices so long as we met our legal mandates and maintained a high level of responsiveness to community concerns. Leadership supported employees to work on issues in disadvantaged communities. For example, an environmental health inspector worked with local day laborers to develop a health and safety training program that led to a commitment among the laborers, the department, and other institutions to work toward both safety and economic opportunities. In another example, employees participating in a research project on asthma and the home environment challenged their traditional enforcement roles, ultimately developing understanding of the barriers faced by low-income tenants to improving their housing conditions.

Reorganizing institutional resources is often necessary for change. For example, balancing the workload among employees enabled an environmental inspector to begin a program for reducing the use of toxic chemicals among city businesses. Reprioritizing activities also led to the creation of a new unit for health inequities within our agency. Now supported through a mix of grant and departmental funding, the unit develops its practice in collaboration with community organizations as well as through the support of community members as researchers.

Employees in this unit recognize that these opportunities are tenuous. Though the department's leadership supports us at present, new issues can emerge on the public agenda rapidly (bioterrorism is an example), and these issues change both the orientation and priorities of our agency.

Solidarity and Advocacy

Can employees in public health institutions support social justice agendas and their constituencies? Targets of social equity struggles lie outside institutional responsibilities, yet illustrating their relationship to health can support their legitimacy and visibility. Community organizing for environmental justice demonstrates that framing equity issues as public health problems can mobilize supporters and leverage resources for social change. Public health practitioners may have a unique and powerful position as advocates acting in solidarity with these organizations. They can bring both the symbolic values of public health and their own credibility as experts and health professionals.

Public health practitioners may be most useful in supporting roles. Community and grassroots organizations are already leaders for social change and have a long track record of policy advocacy, coalition building, and mobilizing constituencies. These organizations also have greater opportunities to hold institutions and elected officials accountable. The willingness to advocate on behalf of an organization also does not always mean that the issues of health will be at the forefront of a community struggle. Health is one of a constellation of issues on an organization's advocacy agenda.

Advocating for social change has practical limits for a local public health agency. The public expects responsive institutions but wants them accountable to elected leaders (Goetz and Gaventa, 2001). Disciplinary boundaries restrict the positions to which public health credibility can lend authority. For example, health policy's current orientation toward clinical service provision limited our argument for increasing the minimum wage. Unfortunately, public health practitioners may more legitimately advocate for service needs for individuals at a social disadvantage than it can against the conditions that sustain disadvantage.

If public health is able to support community advocacy, it also needs to look critically at how advocacy organizations claiming to represent the voice of the disadvantaged incorporate and articulate their interests (Goetz and Gaventa, 2001). As noted, the survey of community perceptions on environmental health issues highlighted differences of interest between opinion leaders and the community residents. Before entering into a coalition with an organization, practitioners must learn whom the organization claims to represent, how it listens to the voices of its constituency, and what principles govern its decisions.

Toward Capacity and Accountability

Fundamentally, inequity reflects unequal power. Inequities underscore both the limited capacities of the excluded and the lack of accountability of social institutions. State institutions not only fail to meet the needs of the socially excluded but also fail to ensure their capacity to influence the conditions of their lives.

Moreover, institutional activities can distance individuals from the exercise of their own power. Increasingly, people are aware that political institutions are accountable to the rich and their interests, creating a crisis of political apathy for those whose needs and aspirations are most marginalized by the political system (Narayan, 2000; Goetz and Gaventa, 2001).

Though collaborative efforts can advance health equity, they are often dependent on the individuals who occupy leadership roles. Increasing the capacity for participation and the opportunity for influence among the socially excluded must become working principles in public health practice. Agencies must acknowledge not only the enormous practical barriers for community members to participate as informed and equal participants but also that historic exclusion from policy influence has led to mistrust of experts and institutions. Public health practitioners can explore structures for more democratic institutional accountability, which may create models for other institutions. Conversely, models from outside public health can serve as examples to follow.

Opportunities for participation do not imply influence, and most efforts to incorporate community member voices fail to recognize the potential of citizens as shapers of policies and providers of needs (Cornwall and Gaventa, 2001; Arnstein, 1969). In most public participation processes led by state institutions, participants are simply listeners, informed or instructed about decisions, while others gather information through activities such as surveys, opinion polls, and focus groups. Substantial participation and more significant citizen power involve an open dialogue with opportunities to name problems and the range of solutions and determine how knowledge will be obtained and used. Full participation means that institutions and citizens are acting together towards shared goals.

Public health institutions already use a variety of means to increase responsiveness to clients. However, although community advisory bodies can function in the interest of better service delivery, they have less opportunity to prioritize needs or the mechanism for providing for these needs. Public health support of collaborative methods may allow for more meaningful community involvement with regard to defining, assessing, and solving problems and may lead to new lines of institutional accountability.

A number of approaches are demonstrating the feasibility of incorporating deliberations among laypeople to influence policy. In the Consensus Conference approach, the Danish Board of Technology recruits lay citizens to evaluate the evidence on a particular science or technology issue and provide political leaders with a consensus report of their findings and recommendations (Andersen and Jaeger, 1999). The approach allows ordinary residents to interact with experts to exchange knowledge and experience and develop common visions of the future. Both the Consensus Conference and the related Citizen Jury demonstrate the feasibility of involving ordinary people in technical decisions otherwise left to institutions and their experts (Pimbert and Wakeford, 2002).

Other international efforts illustrate more direct institutional accountability to citizens. For example, the city of Porto Alegre, Brazil, involves citizens directly in deliberative processes that inform and influence the annual municipal budget. The process, initiated and supported by a political party in power, relies on open community meetings, a citywide assembly, and an elected municipal budget council. The process, sustained in Porto Alegre and replicated in a number of large cities in South America, builds capacity for participation. It has increased neighborhood activism, improved participation skills among residents, and supported more collective perspectives (Goetz and Gaventa, 2001). Forest Protection Committees in West Bengal, India, provide an example of joint community-agency service provision. Villagers share the responsibility of forest management with the National Forest Department in exchange for a share of net forest income and the rights to responsible use of forest products (Joshi, 1998).

Recently, our agency began a community partnership premised on the need for more integrated approaches to food system issues such as food security, poor food quality, unhealthy food choices, and environmentally costly and unsustainable food production and distribution practices. The initiative, developed as a collective endeavor, includes institutions responsible for health, education, and social services; nonprofits responding to hunger and environmental degradation; academic experts; regional food producers and distributors; and local community members. Our agency provides core operating costs to build this network, create a physical home for the project, and conduct community research. The initiative provides an opportunity to create a new institution accountable to participants with a range of authority and expertise.

CONCLUSION

The Institute of Medicine's 1988 report, *The Future of Public Health,* implied that the mission of public health is to support social conditions in which we all can be healthy. However, while public health research helps identify what health requires, it fails to explain how to attain healthy social conditions. The key determinants of health are outside the domain of public health practice, and our sanctioned roles are coherent with those of other institutions. Accountability to political, administrative, and fiscal structures, as well as the internal work culture, maintains the status quo. In practice, the tight focus on disease limits the scope of public health. Disciplinary fragmentation, narrow mandates, and professional satisfaction all absolve public health from advancing the values and mission of health promotion.

We often use the idea of the "upstream" to describe the rationale for prevention in public health. It speaks to the narrow vision of contemporary public health practitioners, so busy pulling drowning people out of the water that they don't see them falling in farther upstream. Descriptions of the conditions causing health inequities help reveal what occurs upstream but do not tell us how to get upstream or what to do once we arrive.

Building on this idea, public health practitioners are not on the banks; they are also in the water, perhaps on a raft. The water, swollen by rapid global cultural and technological and economic change, is moving faster and pushing us farther downstream. Supporting the social conditions required for the health of *all of us* means not only challenging the current version of public health but also challenging the dominant views of human development.

The experiences described in this chapter have led to a conviction that health and social equity require sustained and representative social participation in the structures of government. The development of new institutional practices with the participation of ordinary people can lead toward more popular forms of institutional accountability. The success of new approaches depends on the breadth and quality of sustained social participation.

Social change requires working at the margins of culture; yet many individuals in public health remain attached to the status quo through familiarity and privilege. On the other hand, the motivation and commitment of individuals in public health who witness the needs of the socially excluded are powerful catalysts for change. Moving forward requires gaining confidence and recognizing our opportunities to think and work outside traditional boundaries. Viewing health from different disciplines and from the perspectives of the communities we serve can illustrate how public health is *part* of the landscape of inequities. Through reflection and communication, openness and solidarity, we may be able to create new meanings, practices, and institutions not recognized today.

References

Andersen, I. A., and Jaeger, B. "Scenario Workshops and Consensus Conferences: Toward More Democratic Decision Making." *Science and Public Policy,* 1999, *26,* 331–340.

Arnstein, S. "A Ladder of Citizen Participation." *Journal of the American Planning Association,* 1969, *35,* 216–224.

Arquiaga, M. C., Canter, L. W., and Nelson, D. I. "Integration of Health Impact Considerations in Environmental Impact Studies." *Impact Assessment,* 1994, *12,* 175–197.

Banken, R. *Strategies for Institutionalising HIA.* Brussels, Belgium: European Centre for Health Policy, 2001. [http://www.phel.gov.uk/hiadocs/19_echp_strategies_for_institutionalising_hia.pdf].

Bayview–Hunter's Point Health and Environmental Assessment Task Force. *Community Survey.* San Francisco, Apr. 2001.

Bhatia, R., and Katz, M. "Estimation of Health Benefits Accruing from a Living Wage Ordinance." *American Journal of Public Health,* 2001, *91,* 1398–1402.

Bhatia, R., and Ona, F. "Youth ENVISION: A Collaboration for Community Food Security." *Health Education and Behavior,* 2002, *29*(3), 284–286.

Brown, P. "Popular Epidemiology: Community Response to Toxic Waste–Induced Disease in Woburn, Massachusetts." *Science, Technology, and Human Values,* 1987, *12,* 78–85.

California Department of Transportation. *CalTrans Environmental Handbook.* Vol. 4. Sacramento, California: Cultural Studies Office, CalTrans Environmental Program, 1997.

Callicott, J. B. "Multicultural Environmental Ethics." *Journal of the American Academy of Arts and Sciences,* 2001, *130*(4), 77–97.

Campbell, J. L. "Ideas, Politics, and Public Policy." *Annual Review of Sociology,* 2002, *28,* 21–38.

Cornwall, A., and Gaventa, J. *From Users and Choosers to Makers and Shapers: Repositioning Participation in Social Policy.* Working Paper no. 127. Brighton, England: Institute of Development Studies. University of Sussex, 2001.

Council on Environmental Quality. *Environmental Justice: Guidance Under the National Environmental Health Policy Act.* Washington, D.C.: Executive Office of the President, 1997a.

Council on Environmental Quality. *The National Environmental Health Policy Act: A Study of Its Effectiveness After Twenty-Five Years.* Washington, D.C.: Executive Office of the President, 1997b.

Davies, K., and Sadler, B. *Environmental Assessment and Human Health: Perspectives, Approaches, and Future Directions.* Ottawa: Health Canada, 1997.

Fischer, F. *Citizens, Experts and the Environment: The Politics of Local Knowledge.* Durham, N.C.: Duke University Press, 2000.

Frankish, C. J., and others. *Health Impact Assessment as a Tool for Population Health Promotion and Public Policy: A Report Submitted to the Health Promotion Development Division of Health Canada.* Vancouver: Institute of Health Promotion Research, University of British Columbia, 1996. [http://www.hc-sc.gc.ca/main/hppb/healthpromotiondevelopment/pube/impact/impact.htm].

Freire, P. *Pedagogy of the Oppressed.* New York: Continuum, 1999. (Originally published 1970)

Goetz, A. M., and Gaventa, J. *Bringing Citizen Voice and Client Focus into Service Delivery.* Working Paper no. 138. Brighton, England: Institute of Development Studies, University of Sussex, 2001.

Institute of Medicine. *The Future of Public Health.* Washington, D.C.: National Academy Press, 1988.

Interorganizational Committee on Guidelines and Principles for Social Impact Assessment. *Guidelines and Principles for Social Impact Assessment.* Washington, D.C.: U.S. Department of Commerce, 1994.

Ison, E. "Resource for Health Impact Assessment." *London's Health,* Oct. 2000. [http://www.doh.gov.uk/pub/docs/doh/nletter08.pdf].

Joshi, A. *Progressive Bureaucracy: An Oxymoron? The Case of Joint Forest Management in India.* Rural Development Forestry Network Paper no. 24a. London: Overseas Development Institute, 1998.

Keeley, J., and Scoones, I. *Understanding Environmental Policy Processes: A Review.* Working Paper no. 89. Brighton, England: Institute of Development Studies, University of Sussex, 1999.

Kemm, J. "Health Impact Assessment: A Tool for Healthy Public Policy." *Health Promotion International,* 2001, *16,* 79–85.

Krieger, N. "Theories for Social Epidemiology in the 21st Century: An Ecosocial Perspective." *International Journal of Epidemiology,* 2001, *30,* 668–677.

Lee, C. "Environmental Justice: Building a Unified Vision of Health and the Environment." *Environmental Health Perspectives,* 2002, *110*(Suppl. 2), 141–144.

Lehto, J., and Ritsatakis, A. "Health Impact Assessment as a tool for Intersectoral Health Policy: From Theory to Practice." Paper presented at the European Centre for Health Policy Conference on Health Impact Assessment, Gothenburg, Sweden, Oct. 28–31, 1999.

Lock, K. "Health Impact Assessment." *British Medical Journal,* 2000, *320,* 1395–1398.

Max-Neef, M., Elizade, A., and Hopenhayn, M. "Human Scale Development: An Option for the Future." *Development Dialogue,* 1989, *1,* 7–80.

McKinlay, J. B., and Marceau, L. D. "To Boldly Go . . ." *American Journal of Public Health,* 2000, *90,* 25–33.

Minnesota Health Improvement Partnership. *A Call to Action: Advancing Health for All Through Social and Economic Change.* St. Paul: Minnesota Department of Health, 2001.

Narayan, D. *Voices of the Poor: Can Anyone Hear Us?* New York: Oxford University Press, 2000.

Narayan, D. *Empowerment and Poverty Reduction: A Sourcebook (draft).* Washington, D.C.: The World Bank, May 2002. [http://www.worldbank.org/poverty/empowerment/sourcebook/draft.pdf].

Parry, J., and Stevens, A. "Prospective Health Impact Assessment: Pitfalls, Problems, and Possible Ways Forward." *British Medical Journal,* 2001, *323,* 1177–1182.

Pimbert, M. P., and Wakeford, T. *Prajateerpu: A Citizen's Jury/Scenario Workshop on Food and Farming Futures for Andhra Pradesh, India.* London: International Institute for Environment and Development; and Brighton, England: Institute for Development Studies, University of Sussex, 2002.

Raphael, D. "Health Inequities in the United States: Prospects and Solutions." *Journal of Public Health Policy,* 2000, *21,* 394–427.

Raphael, D., and Bryant, T. "The Limitations of Population Health as a Model for a New Public Health." *Health Promotion International,* 2002, *17,* 189–199.

Schulz, A. J., and others. "Racial and Spatial Relations as Fundamental Determinants of Health in Detroit." *Milbank Quarterly,* 2002, *80,* 677–707.

Sen, A. *Inequality Reexamined.* Cambridge, Mass.: Harvard University Press, 1995.

Smulovitz, C., and Walton, M. "Evaluating Empowerment." Paper presented at the World Bank workshop "Measuring Empowerment: Cross-Disciplinary Perspectives," Washington, D.C., Feb. 4–5, 2003.

Sutton, R. "The Policy Process: An Overview." Working Paper no. 118. London: Overseas Development Institute, 1999.

Szreter, S. "The Population Health Approach in Historical Perspective." *American Journal of Public Health,* 2003, *93,* 421–431.

U.S. Department of Health and Human Services. *Healthy People 2010: Understanding and Improving Health.* (2nd ed.) Washington, D.C.: U.S. Government Printing Office, 2000.

World Health Organization. *Ottawa Charter for Health Promotion.* Geneva, Switzerland: World Health Organization, 1986.

World Health Organization. *Adelaide Recommendations on Healthy Public Policy.* Geneva, Switzerland: World Health Organization, 1998.

CHAPTER TWENTY-SIX

Minnesota's Call to Action

A Starting Point for Advancing Health Equity Through Social and Economic Change

Gavin Kearney

In 2001, organizations and individuals committed to understanding and addressing the effect of social and economic conditions on health in Minnesota published a report titled *A Call to Action: Advancing Health for All Through Social and Economic Change*. The group, the Social Conditions and Health Action Team, was born out of a larger effort in Minnesota's public health community to address public health needs and the large racial and ethnic health disparities that exist in Minnesota. Completed under the stewardship of the Minnesota Department of Health, this report strongly urges that Minnesota's public health community adapt to the growing understanding of the relationship between the health of individuals and communities and the social and economic environment in which they live. To an extent, this shift has already begun. The *Call to Action* and the efforts from which it arose have led to a number of positive developments in Minnesota. However, the ultimate goal of remedying health disparities and promoting health for all is necessarily a continuous effort.

This largely descriptive chapter tells the story of the *Call to Action*. It begins by discussing the developments that led to the formation of the action team and the production of the report. It then provides a summary review of the report, discussing key findings and highlighting recommendations and strategies. Next, it overviews the primary ways in which the report's approach and recommendations have been implemented in Minnesota. It concludes by critiquing our accomplishments thus far, analyzing in broad terms the challenges that lie ahead.[1]

A CALL TO ACTION IN CONTEXT

The *Call to Action* report and the shift in thinking that it embodies were driven by several developments affecting the public health community in Minnesota. For a time in the 1990s, universal health care appeared to be a real possibility for the United States. It was one of the most prominent (and contentious) political issues and for a time had the support of President Clinton. Its realization would have had significant implications for Minnesota's public health community.

Public health in Minnesota focused primarily on service delivery and filling the gaps of the health care system, roles that would be obviated significantly under a universal system. As a result, members of the community began to contemplate what public health in a society with universal health care would look like. From this contemplation arose the idea of creating a more effective and integrated public health system by ensuring that the various sectors within it—public, private, and nonprofit—functioned in concert. The Minnesota Health Improvement Partnership (MHIP) was created in 1997 to further this aim.

MHIP is composed of a variety of state, regional, and local health agencies in Minnesota, along with other public and private entities such as hospitals, community-based organizations, university-based researchers, and representatives of the business community. In addition, governmental actors from critical areas outside of the traditional health sector, such as planning, education, and human service agencies, are also members.[2] The purpose of MHIP is to "develop coordinated public, private, and nonprofit efforts to improve the health of Minnesota residents."[3] As one of its first actions, MHIP reviewed and updated a set of health improvement goals that the state had developed in 1995. Completed in 1998, a report titled *Healthy Minnesotans 2004* presented updated goals, along with a preliminary set of strategies for pursuing them.

A growing awareness that while Minnesota's population was generally among the healthiest in the country, the state possessed some of the country's largest racial and ethnic disparities in critical health areas affected the goal-setting process. In addition, research indicated that these disparities were in large part a function of the disparate socioeconomic conditions of different racial and ethnic groups in the state. In 1997, the Minnesota Department of Health (MDH) collaborated with the Urban Coalition, a nonprofit research and advocacy organization, to publish the *Populations of Color Health Status Report*. This report found that populations of color in Minnesota have significantly higher levels of risk than whites for a number of leading causes of death. The report also found that the overall mortality rates for African Americans, American Indians, and Hispanics was up to 3.5 times higher than that of whites in Minnesota.[4] Moreover, a growing body of research suggested that these disparities were not solely a product of behavioral differences and disparate access to health care. Clearly, phenomena beyond the de facto sphere of public health, such as education, housing, employment, and the environment, played large roles in generating these disparities.

MINNESOTA'S HEALTH IMPROVEMENT GOALS: HEALTHY MINNESOTANS 2004

In setting health goals for the state, MHIP sought to define goals and develop strategies that could be pursued and implemented at all levels of geography and by various public, private, and nonprofit actors.

"None of the public health goals or objectives contained in this publication," states *Healthy Minnesotans 2004*, "are intended to prompt new legislative mandates. Instead, each is intended to inspire voluntary action on issues that affect the health and well-being of people across the state, from reducing the number of tobacco users, to ensuring babies are born healthy, to helping the aged maintain their independence, to preventing or controlling the spread of infectious diseases such as tuberculosis, hepatitis and sexually transmitted diseases."[5]

Healthy Minnesotans identifies eighteen health improvement goals to be accomplished by 2004. Of these, seventeen are updated versions of goals originally articulated in 1995, and many of these target specific health risks or risk behaviors. The new goal, Goal 18, reflects the broadened understanding of health emerging at the time and is the goal that led to the *Call to Action* report. Generally stated, the goal is to "foster the understanding and promotion of social conditions that support health."[6] The report suggests that critical steps toward achieving this goal are raising awareness of the connections between health and social conditions and raising awareness of the need for critical actors within the state to establish "voluntary partnerships" across disciplines and sectors.

MHIP articulated the following objectives for the public health community and other key actors to achieve by 2004 in furtherance of Goal 18:

- Review and summarize existing studies and data sources that identify concrete linkages between social conditions and health.
- Stimulate and support efforts to develop the knowledge base to better characterize the multidimensional relationships between social conditions and health.
- Promote societal attitudes that include a philosophy of shared responsibility for addressing the social conditions that affect health.
- Discuss the impact of social conditions that contribute to poor health in terms of their organization's sphere of influence.
- Collaborate with community efforts to improve social conditions that affect health.

Subsequent to the adoption of these updated health goals, MHIP chose to make the pursuit of Goal 18 one of its priority areas and formed the Social Conditions and Health Action Team (SCHAT). The SCHAT's charge included developing strategies for the public, private, and nonprofit sectors to use to increase understanding of the ways in which social conditions affect health and to address the conditions underlying Minnesota's health outcomes. Funded through the Robert Wood Johnson Foundation's Turning Point program, the SCHAT was an interdisciplinary, intersectoral group that met from 1999 to 2001. Its work culminated in April 2001 with the submission of *A Call to Action* to the commissioner of health, Jan Malcolm.[7]

A CALL TO ACTION: ADVANCING HEALTH FOR ALL THROUGH SOCIAL AND ECONOMIC CHANGE

The *Call to Action* reviews the state of health in Minnesota and summarizes research findings about the relationship between social conditions and health. After discussing some of the implications and conclusions of these research findings, it culminates with recommendations and strategies for implementing a public health agenda responsive to the role that social conditions play in generating health outcomes and responsive to health needs in Minnesota. This section overviews the report, placing particular emphasis on the recommendations and strategies.

The report highlights several key aspects of the health status of Minnesota. First is the significant racial and ethnic disparities across key health indicators, despite Minnesota's relatively high overall level of health. The report also notes that Minnesota's rapidly growing foreign-born populations tend to have lower health status than most Minnesotans, in part due to barriers in accessing the health system as a result of such factors as language, culture, and religion. The report draws a direct link between social and economic factors and these disparities. It references the roles that discrimination, segregation, and unequal access to resources and opportunity in critical life areas such as education and housing play in generating health inequalities and notes the lesser role of behavior in explaining these outcomes.

The report then summarizes existing research on the relationship between health and social and economic conditions. It indicates that as with measures of health, Minnesota fares well in the aggregate on socioeconomic measures such as employment, income, and poverty, but these overall measures mask areas of concern. Minnesota has high child poverty rates, a growing portion of the job market that pays poverty-level wages, significant levels of racial and economic segregation, a significant lack of affordable housing, and growing income inequalities.

Moreover, the report finds that these socioeconomic concerns have important implications for health. Reviews of outside research established the following, among other things:

- Community and social support promote health; social exclusion generates negative health consequences.

- Housing plays a significant role in determining a family's well-being, depending on whether it is affordable, safe, and connected to resources such as transportation, education, and employment, and amenities such as quality grocery stores, cultural centers, and recreational facilities.

- Health is affected by various aspects of employment conditions, including wages, safety of the working environment, scheduling, and health and family policies.

- Macroeconomic trends, such as income distribution, employment rates, and other labor market trends, have important health consequences.

In sum, the SCHAT found that "more supportive social and economic conditions are needed to eliminate disparities and achieve Minnesota's overall health improvement goals." While the SCHAT suggested a need for more research "to understand precisely how these factors affect health and health disparities, and how to translate these findings into the most promising policies and programs," it found existing evidence compelling enough to recommend significant changes in the public health community. The *Call to Action* concluded that "the challenge is clear: public, private, and non-profit organizations in Minnesota need to act collectively on this deeper understanding of the social determinants of health, at the same time that we increase access to culturally competent health care, promote healthy behaviors, and strengthen the existing public health infrastructure." As a way of spurring future action, the SCHAT developed a series of recommendations and strategies for implementing the recommendations.

RECOMMENDATIONS AND STRATEGIES FOR IMPLEMENTATION
Identify and Advocate for Healthy Public Policies

Because public policy in multiple areas within and beyond the conventional health sector have significant effects on the health of Minnesotans, the SCHAT suggested that the public health community educate itself and the larger community on the types of policies that support or undermine health and to advocate accordingly. The SCHAT identified several specific strategies for accomplishing this goal.

First, the SCHAT asserted that MHIP should take actions necessary to develop and pilot health impact assessment (HIA) tools and methodologies in Minnesota. HIA was seen as a valuable method for explicitly injecting health objectives into the various areas of policymaking that have unacknowledged health consequences (for example, housing, transportation, and economic development). The SCHAT believed that by developing these tools, MHIP could do all of the following, among other things:

- Begin to model the health implications of programs and policies in other sectors
- Spur collaboration with related state and local agencies
- Assess and provide testimony on the health implications of pending legislation
- Identify political and organizational barriers to HIA and strategies for overcoming these barriers
- As a long-term goal, establish a foundation for requiring use of these tools in policymaking and propose appropriate legislative language for doing so

The SCHAT believed that a more general strategy for implementing this recommendation is to create opportunities to turn the growing body of knowledge around health and social conditions into action through policies and programs. Team members placed a strong emphasis on moving beyond a description of the determinants of health to pushing healthy public policy. Based on current evidence, the report lists several broad examples of the kinds of policies that are necessary to create a healthy environment and reduce health inequalities, including the following:

- Increasing opportunities for optimal early childhood development through affordable and high-quality child care, appropriate family support services, and employment practices that increase paid family leave
- Increasing opportunities for people to meet their basic needs by increasing the supply of affordable, accessible housing, boosting family income, and providing the support services that people need to obtain and retain employment
- Linking economic and community development policies and practices with health improvement goals as a way to foster sustainable development that makes planning in areas such as housing, transportation, and economic development mutually supportive and healthy
- Generating local policies and practices that serve broader regional interests and in doing so expand access to resources and opportunities for all communities

As initial first steps, the SCHAT recommended that MHIP and MDH work with appropriate partners to develop policy briefs that present evidence on the relationship between social conditions and health and articulate healthy policy approaches. They also recommended that these partnerships identify barriers to moving a broader agenda forward and strategies for overcoming these barriers.

Build and Use a Representative and Culturally Competent Workforce

As noted earlier, the SCHAT found that the health needs of communities of color and foreign-born populations in Minnesota are unmet, in part, because the health community is not prepared to address unique health needs that arise in areas such as language, culture, and religion. Consequently, team members decided that all sectors of Minnesota's health community should create and maintain a workforce that is both representative of the populations that it serves and able to understand and address the needs that arise from their characteristics. In order to accomplish this goal, the SCHAT asserted that MDH and MHIP member organizations will have to "establish and adhere to practices to recruit, retain, and promote personnel who reflect the cultural and ethnic diversity of the communities served."

The *Call to Action* includes several strategies designed to achieve these goals. First, health organizations and agencies need to create an environment that welcomes, accepts, and values all employees and community residents by making workforce diversity a core value and by explicitly demonstrating that harassment and discrimination are intolerable. Another strategy identified by the SCHAT is to ensure that organization functions are accessible to all employees through measures such as providing ongoing multicultural competency training for all employees and by assessing all policies and procedures to ensure equality of opportunity and cultural responsiveness. The SCHAT also indicated that organizations ought to take measures to create diverse applicant pools now and in the future through targeted recruitment, creation of internship and fellowship opportunities, and inclusive hiring processes and that organizations work to retain people of color who do enter the workforce through measures such as building support systems and networks and conducting retention surveys. Finally, the *Call to Action* recommends that organizations develop measures for assessing progress in achieving these goals and build these measures into assessments of organizational success and the success of supervisors and managers.

Increase Civic Engagement

A critical recommendation included creating public health models that engage the communities that they serve and increase the assets of these communities. Based on research in the area, the SCHAT believed that interventions that engage and build relationships with the communities they serve will better equip them to address the full range of conditions that affect health in a manner that is "comprehensive, flexible, responsive, and enduring." In doing so, they hoped to avoid past problems with fragmented services and programs and address underlying causes that drive multiple health outcomes.

The SCHAT recommended that the Department of Health convene a group "charged with identifying opportunities, as well as barriers, and solutions to broadly support the implementation of health improvement programs that use principles of community development, civic engagement, and participatory research and evaluation." It also suggested that this group develop recommendations for implementing such programs, coordinating health improvement activities with efforts and initiatives outside of the traditional health sector that favorably affect the social and economic environment, and transforming the health communities' systems and institutions to make them more accessible and responsive to community-based health improvement initiatives and to allow for mutually beneficial relationships between the two.

Reorient Funding

For public health programs to adapt to new understandings of the role of social and economic conditions in creating health outcomes, members of the SCHAT strongly believed that it is also necessary to rethink approaches to funding. Most grant programs at the federal and state levels have been disease- or issue-specific and competitive, based on the assumption that structuring funding in this manner makes it more effective and more efficient. Resulting programs have been similarly narrowly focused. In the aggregate, fragmented health programs often leave gaps in fulfilling health needs. Such funding structures impede the development of comprehensive health programs responsive to the relationships between health outcomes and the conditions that contribute to them. They also make it difficult to develop sustainable, community-based initiatives and to invest in building community assets. Moreover, although funding had been available to communities of color in the past, team members believed it necessary to increase funding targeted specifically for reducing health disparities.

The SCHAT recommended strategies for accomplishing this goal, including that MDH reorient its grant programs to involve people and organizations more broadly in proposal evaluation, ensure the inclusion of community of color–based organizations on funding notification lists, and make grant application processes accessible. They further supported building goals to eliminate health inequities into funding formulas and requiring prospective grantees to include organizations representing underserved communities in proposal planning and implementation.

To make funding more effective, they also recommended that health agencies build collaborations with institutions and agencies outside of the health sector as a way to focus on social and economic conditions by linking disparate funding streams to provide for more comprehensive programs and initiatives. The team also recommended that MDH, MHIP, and SCHAT members inform legislators of the shortcomings of categorical funding and seek to strengthen links with local and national foundations that address social and economic conditions or health.

Strengthen Assessment, Evaluation, and Research

Just as the SCHAT sought to modify and strengthen funding in order to address the social conditions that affect health more effectively, it also argued for modifying and strengthening the measurement of health and the evaluation of health activities. The team supported better use of population health data and development of measures and indicators that include the factors that affect health and the interrelationships among them.

Specific strategies recommended for accomplishing this goal include requiring that local public health agencies (community health service agencies) incorporate social and economic factors into the required community health assessment plans every four years. The SCHAT also recommended that these agencies conduct their assessments with significant involvement from all community members, including people of color, foreign-born populations, and low-income populations.

The report urged the commissioner of health to work with MHIP, MDH's Minority Health Advisory Committee, and MDH's Population Health Assessment Work Group to conduct a comprehensive baseline assessment of the social and economic factors that affect health and health disparities. The report further suggested that these groups also work to strengthen the capacity of state and local actors to link traditional health measures with measures such as income, education, and race/ethnicity and with research on the distribution of and access to resources and opportunities for Minnesota's various communities.

The report concludes a charge to MDH, MHIP, and the action team members to become responsible for communicating the findings of the report and championing its recommendations. Similarly, it urges these actors to create opportunities to engage individuals, organizations, and communities in dialogue around these findings and recommendations and to identify opportunities to mobilize and collaborate with individuals and groups outside the health community already committed to improving the social and economic conditions of all Minnesotans.

PUBLIC HEALTH EFFORTS AFTER THE *CALL TO ACTION*

Since submitting the *Call to Action* to the commissioner of health, several significant activities have occurred in Minnesota's public health community in direct response to its recommendations or consistent with and influenced by its analysis and findings. In particular, the Minnesota Health Improvement Partnership adopted "workplan objectives" for 2001–2002, two of which are specific recommendations found in the *Call to Action*. MHIP decided to "identify, pilot test, and disseminate civic engagement tools that can be used by communities in addressing disparities in health status" through the work of the Civic Engagement and Health Disparities Work Group and to "develop and pilot test health impact assessment methodology" through the work of the Health Impact Assessment Action Team.[8] In response to the efforts of Minnesota's health community, the Minnesota State Legislature also enacted legislation in 2001 to create and fund the Eliminating Health Disparities Initiative. Minnesota's public health planning framework has also been modified to encourage local agencies to incorporate social and economic conditions and an explicit focus on health disparities into their assessment of local health needs and planning to address them.

The Civic Engagement and Health Disparities Work Group

In 2001, MDH and MHIP convened the Civic Engagement and Health Disparities Work Group with a threefold charge: to explore models of civic engagement for engaging communities and institutions in addressing health disparities; to identify, pilot, and disseminate tools for increasing civic engagement and community involvement in addressing health disparities; and to recommend ways to integrate these approaches into state and local public health efforts.[9]

The work group defined civic engagement as a process involving the "participation of members of a community in assessing, planning, implementing, and evaluating solutions to problems that affect them." To be effective, the work group found that such engagement demands trust, two-way communication, and meaningful collaboration. To aid public health actors in Minnesota in efforts to address health disparities through civic engagement, the group placed a number of resources on the World Wide Web, including: an articulation of key principles for designing, implementing, and assessing civic engagement efforts; several models of engagement and participation, including asset-based community development (ABCD) and cultural complementarity; and lists of specific strategies and tips useful for increasing the engagement of communities in general and communities of color in particular.[10]

The Health Impact Assessment Action Team

Pursuant to the *Call to Action,* the Health Impact Assessment Action Team was created and charged with the following:

- To develop a shared understanding of HIA and its potential applications as a tool for developing healthy public policy and illuminating the potential effects of policy decisions on health disparities.

- To identify potential pilots for HIA in Minnesota and oversee their implementation.

- To describe the potential utility and feasibility of HIA in Minnesota based on findings from pilot projects.[11]

As discussed earlier, HIA was seen as a promising tool for ensuring that policymaking in areas traditionally viewed as beyond the health sector occur in a manner that acknowledges and accounts for health consequences in general and the need to remedy health disparities in particular.

Although the work of the HIA Action Team is ongoing, thus far the team has developed preliminary screening tools for assessing the potential utility of applying HIA to a given project or policy.[12] The team has also worked, with mixed results, to identify potential pilot projects and provide oversight and support for the implementation of HIA in these projects. While potential partners for these pilots have generally understood the value of considering the health implications of their policymaking or programming, efforts to pilot HIA have been hindered by the limited resources of the HIA Action Team and partner organizations, limited understanding of how to implement the assessment process, and difficulties in demonstrating the benefits of doing so in a given situation. The work of the action team should conclude by 2005 and will include an assessment of lessons learned from efforts to pilot HIA and the implications of these efforts for the long-term goal of broadly integrating health impact assessment into policymaking processes in Minnesota.

The Eliminating Health Disparities Initiative

As discussed earlier, members of the health community have become increasingly aware since the early 1990s of significant, and in some cases growing, racial and ethnic health disparities in Minnesota. Addressing them has been a priority of MDH and MHIP over the past several years, reflected in the focus of the *Call to Action* on the role of social and economic conditions in generating health disparities and methods of eliminating them. In response to the advocacy efforts of the health community and of communities of color around the issue of disparities (though not directly in response to the recommendations of the *Call to Action*), the Minnesota Legislature in 2001 created the Eliminating Health Disparities Initiative (EHDI) and provided it with $12.7 million to fund EHDI grant programs in the first two years of its existence.[13]

The legislature established the EHDI to decrease health inequities in infant mortality and immunization rates by 50 percent by 2010 and to narrow health disparities in breast and cervical cancer, HIV/AIDS and other sexually transmitted diseases, cardiovascular disease, diabetes, and accidental injury and violence during the same period. MDH is responsible for implementing the initiative, and the primary vehicle for achieving these goals is through Community and Tribal Grant programs that provide planning or implementation grants to organizations working to address disparities in these areas. Planning grants are short-term, designed to help communities assess their needs and assets and develop strategies for addressing these needs as they relate to the EHDI's target areas. To some extent, these grants have been used to help local public health organizations and communities of color develop stronger, sustainable relationships.

The legislation establishes several priorities for MDH to consider in awarding grants. Priority is to be given to applications and strategies supported by their target community that complement related activities within the community they will serve, have a positive effect on multiple priority areas, and embody racially and ethnically appropriate approaches or are to be implemented by organizations that reflect the race and ethnicity of the communities that they serve.

MDH is creating a comprehensive plan for evaluating the effectiveness of the EHDI. By means of a participatory research partnership with community-based organizations, community research experts, the University of Minnesota, and others, it will develop measurable outcomes for the initiative's overall goals and identify the types of intermediate outcomes that will affect the health of diverse individuals and communities in Minnesota.[14]

Public Health Planning at the Local Level

To receive some forms of state funding, local public health agencies in Minnesota must submit a community health services plan to the Minnesota Department of Health every four years.[15] In these plans, local agencies must conduct an assessment of public health in their community and develop a community health plan that details actions to be taken. MDH issued guidelines for the next round of planning (covering the period from 2004 to 2007), and although the mandated planning requirements have not changed, the guidelines recommend that local agencies adopt a number of the recommendations and strategies discussed in the *Call to Action* and developed by the Civic Engagement Work Group and HIA Action Team.

The new guidelines urge local agencies to engage their communities in the needs assessment process, in setting public health priorities, and in establishing public health plans. Although agencies are legally required to conduct public hearings, the guidelines consider these steps the bare minimum and urge that more significant efforts be undertaken to create more comprehensive, sustained community engagement.

The guidelines also acknowledge growing evidence that social and economic conditions affect health, and they reference "key aspects" of the social and economic environment that drive health outcomes, including income, education, housing, and employment conditions. The guidelines state generally that "these social and economic factors should be considered in the assessment and prioritization steps and incorporated into the plan." At the same time, the guidelines also identify twelve "categories of public health"—such as alcohol, tobacco, and other drug use; mental health; unintended pregnancy; and violence—that community assessment and planning should use to structure activities. Although planning to address social conditions and categorizing public health needs and objectives in this manner are not mutually exclusive, this method of categorization reflects some of the pitfalls of funding identified in the *Call to Action* and may impede efforts to get local agencies to focus on underlying conditions that drive multiple health outcomes.

FUTURE DIRECTIONS AND CHALLENGES

In a relatively short period of time, Minnesota's public health community has made significant advances in addressing the role that social and economic conditions play in generating health outcomes and health disparities. Any critique of this community's efforts must acknowledge the important and unprecedented (at least for the United States) vision and scope of this work on a statewide level. As the foregoing discussion makes clear, significant efforts are under way to use this knowledge to inform current and future public health work. Many of the greatest challenges for this work, however, lie ahead.

As the SCHAT realized, a focus on social and economic conditions means that many of the strategies for addressing health needs transcend conventional notions of what constitutes appropriate public health practice. This suggests that for the public health community to be responsive to evolving understandings of health, it will need to transform itself in significant ways. To some extent, public health actors will need to educate themselves in a variety of policy and programmatic areas beyond the scope of their work and make difficult decisions about allocating resources among established and emerging public health priorities. As the *Call to Action* observes and experiences with the Eliminating Health Disparities Initiative and community health services planning demonstrate, fully realizing the implications of this new approach to health will also require a restructuring of funding and implementation methods for health initiatives. Setting discrete goals in narrowly defined areas will impede efforts to address broader health determinants and limit successes even in priority areas.

Advancing health through social and economic change will also require an examination of the ways in which public health agencies work with organizations and agencies in other fields. As the *Call to Action* makes clear, healthy policy spans a multitude of issues, including economic development, housing, and education. As discussed earlier, MHIP and MDH have deliberately included representatives of agencies that deal with such issues as planning, housing, welfare, and employment within MHIP itself and on the work groups and action teams charged with identifying effective strategies for the public health community to pursue. Thus revamping the public health sector in response to the effects of social and economic conditions on health outcomes cannot alone remedy the health inequities that exist in Minnesota. Pursuing these strategies will require that the interaction between these agencies and the health community become bidirectional and that health considerations inform policymaking. To be successful, the public health community must develop a strong case for why such collaborations are mutually advantageous.

Ultimately, to maximize effectiveness and to create sustainable change will require that these new focuses and new relationships become institutionalized. Pursuing this end will require Minnesota's public health community to consider its role as an advocate for health and for healthy public policy. Although the goals established by the Minnesota Health Improvement Partnership are explicitly designed to "inspire voluntary action," the work of the Social Conditions and Health Action Team and the recommendations that it made question whether voluntary action will be sufficient. To a large extent, the persistence of racial disparities is not the result of a lack of information about how to remedy them but rather the result of a lack of political will and commitment. If remedying racial and ethnic disparities in health is a priority that requires action in areas such as housing, education, and employment, experiences in addressing racism in the United States also cast doubt on the sufficiency of voluntary efforts. Voluntary attempts to remedy affordable housing shortages, desegregate neighborhoods and schools, and address discrimination in the workplace and other areas do not have a successful track record in general or when compared to policies and programs that mandate racially just actions.

The future of the *Call to Action* will depend in large part on how we meet these challenges. At the time of this writing, some immediate obstacles and uncertainties exist in Minnesota, including a budget crisis. Accomplishing the goals of the *Call to Action* is a long-term effort that must transcend immediate impediments, requiring continued labors over many years. It will also require winning new converts and developing new allies at the local, state, national, and even international levels. If we succeed, our initial efforts described in this chapter will have played a small role in a much larger story.

Notes

1. I was a member of the Social Conditions and Health Action Team and of one of its progeny, the Health Impact Assessment Action Team. I am one of the parties outside the conventional health sector who has been engaged in this work. In writing this chapter, I have attempted to capture the broader context in which these groups fall but feel the need to acknowledge that this narrative and my criticisms are informed and perhaps limited by these perspectives.

2. A list of the members of MHIP is available at http://www.health.state.mn.us/divs/chs/mhip/mhipmember.htm.

3. Minnesota Health Improvement Partnership, "2001–2002 Purpose and Charge," http://www.health.state.mn.us/divs/chs/mhip.

4. Urban Coalition and Minnesota Department of Health. Populations of Color Health Status Report, 1997.

5. Minnesota Department of Health. "Healthy Minnesotans: Public Health Improvement Goals 2004," http://www.health.state.mn.us/divs/chs/phg/intro.html.

6. Ibid.

7. For general information on the SCHAT, go to http://www.health.state.mn.us/divs/chs/mhip/schteam.htm.

8. http://www.health.state.mn.us/divs/chs/mhip/mhipplan.htm.

9. http://www.health.state.mn.us/divs/chs/mhip/civiccharge.htm.

10. The materials developed by the work group can be found at http://www.health.state.mn.us/communityeng/index.html.

11. http://www.health.state.mn.us/divs/chs/mhip/hiacharge.htm.

12. The literature review, annotated bibliography, and screening tools can be accessed at http://www.health.state.mn.us/divs/chs/mhip/hiateam.htm.

13. Minnesota Statute 145.928. For general information on the initiative, go to http://www.health.state.mn.us/ommh/aboutehdi.html.

14. http://www.health.state.mn.us/ommh/legrpt012103.pdf.

15. Minnesota Statute 145A. Completion of this plan is mandatory for local agencies receiving community health services subsidies from the state.

CHAPTER TWENTY-SEVEN

The Role of Mass Media in Creating Social Capital

A New Direction for Public Health

Lawrence Wallack

In the summer of 1999 the East Coast was suffering through a terrible heat wave, and deaths were mounting (Barstow, 1999). New York City sagged under the oppressive weight of the heat, and city officials were struggling to address the crisis. The apparent cause of death for those who died was the physical effects of the heat. However, the underlying cause simply may have been fear and isolation, in part the consequence of not being connected to a broader community. One news report related the observation of emergency workers, who said "an alarming number of city residents without air-conditioning keep their windows shut because they fear becoming victims of crime, and instead became patients" ("Stifling Heat Retains Grip on East Coast," 1999, p. A1). An earlier heat wave had killed over 700 in Chicago (Semenza and others, 1996). Of course, these deaths were not random occurrences; those most likely to die

I want to express my special gratitude to Ray Catalano, Lori Dorfman, Arthur Kellerman, Linda Nettekoven, Esther Thorson, and Katie Woodruff, whose comments helped shape this work. In addition, Tony Chen, Rachel Dresbeck, Michael Antecol, and Raquel Bournhonesque provided editing, referencing, and other assistance. I also want to express my appreciation to the Institute of Medicine, Committee on Capitalizing on Social Science and Behavioral Research to Improve the Public's Health, for commissioning me to write this chapter. Finally, I would like to especially acknowledge Professor S. Leonard Syme, committee chair. I learned much from him as his student and continue to benefit from his wisdom as his colleague.

were isolated, disconnected, and likely to live in high homicide areas (Shen and others, 1995). A lower risk of death was associated with "anything that facilitated social contact, even membership in a social club" (Semenza and others, 1996, p. 90).

Heat waves provide a useful reference for thinking about the role of media in public health. It is a seemingly simple matter to reduce personal risk by opening a window or going out to a cooling station. Yet people's behavior is strongly influenced by the social, economic, and political context of the larger community. Failure to account for the influence of community forces on behavioral choices will lead to narrowly focused media approaches that perilously ignore significant determinants of health.

The media matter in public health. But just how they matter is often a contentious issue. The way media matter is based on how we conceptualize the nature of public health issues and hence their solutions—and this is often controversial. If public health problems are viewed as largely rooted in personal behaviors resulting from a lack of knowledge, then media matter because they can be a delivery mechanism for getting the right information to the right people in the right way at the right time to promote personal change. If, on the other hand, public health problems are viewed as largely rooted in social inequality resulting from the way we use politics and policy to organize our society, then media matter because they can be a vehicle for increasing participation in civic and political life and social capital to promote social change. Of course, media matter in both these ways and other ways as well.

The central argument of this chapter is that mass media approaches to improving the public's health need to be rethought in light of recent developments in social epidemiology, political science, sociology, and mass communication. Of particular importance is how these findings relate to social capital and population health. Traditional behavioral oriented media campaigns, while useful, have been limited in creating significant behavior change and improvements in health status (e.g., McGuire, 1986). While there are many reasons for these modest results, this may be due in part to the failure of these campaigns to adequately integrate fundamental public health values related to social justice, participation, and social change—values made more important by the increasing research on the relationship between social inequality and health inequality.

There is an expanding science base for understanding public health as a product of social and political arrangements rather than of primarily personal behaviors. This is not to say that individual actions and personal responsibility are not important but only to emphasize that behavior is inextricably linked to a larger social, political, and economic environment. Attempting to address public health problems without attending to the context in which they exist inevitably produces, at best, limited solutions. An important part of that context may be the range of opportunities for people to participate in the life of the community. The importance of involvement in civic life may well be a fundamental characteristic of socially and economically healthy communities (e.g., Sampson, Raudenbush, and Earls, 1997; Gittell and Vidal, 1998). Thus, future media approaches must focus on skill development for participation in the social change process rather than primarily on information for personal change. Civic or public journalism, media advocacy, and photovoice are particularly well suited to this task and will be explored in this chapter.

This chapter will provide a framework for understanding the role of media in advancing public health and social goals. It will briefly review the implications of recent social-epidemiological and political science research for developing mass media interventions, the limits of previous public health efforts to use mass communication strategies, and prospects for a new public health media of engagement and participation.

SOCIAL INEQUALITY AND HEALTH

There is a long history establishing the role of social status, measured in various ways, as a strong determinant of health (Anderson and Armstead, 1995; Adler and others, 1993, 1994; Haan, Kaplan, and Syme, 1989; Haan and others, 1989; Kaplan, 1995; Marmot and Mustard, 1994; Blane, 1995; Lantz and others, 1998). This extensive body of research indicates that social class differences exist for virtually every type of adverse health outcome and for treatable as well as non-treatable diseases. Rather than this being a rich/poor dichotomy or a factor just of poverty, the distribution of disease follows a gradient. This means that even among those in the upper quadrant of income or education levels in the society, those lower in the quadrant have poorer health. These findings are robust and appear consistent over time and across Western industrialized countries. The health differences cannot be explained by traditional risk factors or access to health care. So access to health care is not the defining factor for population health status. The explanation for the social gradient is unclear. A wide range of material (physical resources) and non-material (psychosocial) factors has been suggested.

More recently, this line of research has focused on the specific issue of income inequality as a property of the larger social system. This research suggests that it is not the individual's absolute level of resources which matters as much as one's position relative to everyone else (Wilkinson, 1992, 1996; Duleep, 1995; Kaplan and others, 1996; Smith and Egger, 1992; Navarro, 1997; Kennedy, Kawachi, and Prothrow-Stith, 1996). The central concept is that up to a point the level of absolute income or resources in a society contributes to increasing health status. After that point, however, the way that the resources are distributed has the greatest impact on health: "In the developed world, it is not the richest countries which have the best health, but the most egalitarian" (Wilkinson, 1996, p. 3).

WHAT IS SOCIAL CAPITAL?

Social capital appears to be an umbrella concept that includes anything that helps to remove the barriers to collective action in communities. The general concept is certainly not foreign to the social and community emphasis of public health and is related to various concepts such as collective efficacy, psychological sense of community, neighborhood cohesion, and community competence (Lochner, Kawachi, and Kennedy, 1999). Specifically, Gittell and Vidal (1998) define social capital as "the resources embedded in social relations among persons and organizations that facilitate cooperation and collaboration in communities" (p. 16). Social capital seems rather like a glue made from various ingredients that holds communities together and allows them to better work together to achieve common goals. It is a component of social cohesion that includes social trust and civic participation (Putnam, 1993). Coleman (1990) explains that social capital is defined by its function—what it does rather than what it is: "It is not a single entity, but a variety of different entities having two characteristics in common: They all consist of some aspect of a social structure, and they facilitate certain actions of individuals who are within the structure. . . . Unlike other forms of capital, social capital inheres in the structure of relations between and among persons" (p. 302).

However, there are specific things that appear to be markers for higher levels of social capital. These include increased social trust, generalized norms of reciprocity, group membership, interdependence, and networks or social organizations through which the cooperation of individuals can be facilitated toward action (Putnam, 1993, 1995a; 1995b; Coleman, 1990). In addition, there is an important prescriptive norm associated with social capital that calls on people to "forgo self interests to act in the interests of the collectivity" (Coleman, 1990, p. 311). In sum, social capital is marked by norms, skills, or other individual characteristics, and structures that facilitate groups of people working toward the collective or community good. Civic engagement, when combined with social trust and facilitated by social connectedness, creates social capital (Putnam, 1995b).

Social capital, then, generates new opportunities for communities to participate in civic life. It allows groups to work together toward shared goals that create mutual benefits, and it smooths the process because high levels of trust and connectedness help to overcome the traditional obstacles to collective action

(Putnam, 1993, 1995b)—social capital allows groups to achieve ends that otherwise would be beyond their capacity (Coleman, 1990). Importantly, social capital is cumulative and generalizable. It can be created for one purpose and used for other purposes. For example, a group working to increase the responsiveness of a local school board to community concerns might also be effective in mobilizing people to change the way police interact with the neighborhood.

Another important aspect of social capital is that it is not "owned" by any individual. A community with higher levels of social capital creates benefits for all of those in the community whether they helped create the social capital or not. Consider the East Coast heat wave: if communities had stronger social cohesion—marked, perhaps, by neighborhood watch groups—then individuals might be more likely to open their windows or go to a cooling station regardless of whether they participated personally in a neighborhood watch group.

Social capital, of course, can also be used for ends that many might not view as socially desirable. For example, youth gangs might be seen as reservoirs of social capital for young people in certain communities, and hate groups might flourish because of the social capital generated by the trust, norms, and dense quality of group membership. Thus, from a public health perspective, social capital should have a social justice criterion: Does it contribute to a fairer, more equitable, and more just society? (Chapter Ten).

SOCIAL CAPITAL: A SIGNIFICANT PATHWAY

Drawing on research from political science and sociology (Putnam, 1993, 1995a, 1995b; Coleman, 1990), public health research has now moved beyond identifying the relationship between social inequality and health inequality. It has begun to identify potential explanations for the relationship and implications for the design of public health interventions. The work of Kawachi and Kennedy and their colleagues (Kawachi and Kennedy, 1997; Kawachi, Kennedy, and Lochner, 1997; Kennedy and others, 1998; Kawachi and others, 1997) and others (Wilkinson, 1996; Lynch and Kaplan, 1997) is especially important in that it has identified lower levels of social capital as a pathway that may channel income inequality into increased mortality. For example, higher overall mortality and rates for most major causes of death were associated with lower measures of social capital as measured by group membership, voting levels, and social trust across 39 states in the United States (Kawachi and Berkman, 1998). Kennedy et al. (1998) reported that the depletion of social capital was strongly associated with homicide and violent crime, even when controlling for poverty and access to firearms. Also, self-reported health status, a strong indicator of actual health (Idler and Benyamini, 1997), is significantly related to the amount of social capital at the state level (Kawachi and Berkman, 1998).

There are various ways that social capital might influence population health. For example, areas with higher levels of social inequality may "systematically underinvest in human, physical, health and social infrastructure" (Lynch and Kaplan, 1997, p. 306). Also, lack of social capital might inhibit the flow of health information through populations, could make it less likely that communities band together for collective action to ensure basic health and social services, and might influence psychosocial processes that increase the sense of isolation and low sense of self efficacy of those living in less cohesive communities (Kawachi and Berkman, 1998).

Social capital appears to be an "elastic" commodity in the economic sense. That is, small increases in various components of this public good can result in significant benefits. For example, a 10 percent increase in the level of social trust, a marker of social capital, could result in an 8 percent reduction in overall mortality (Kawachi and others, 1997). Addressing a related concept, Sampson, Raudenbush, and Earls (1997) found that a two standard deviation increase in collective efficacy—a community's willingness to intervene in community life that is linked to social trust and solidarity—was associated with an almost 40 percent reduction in the expected homicide rate.

PUBLIC HEALTH, MASS MEDIA, AND SOCIAL CAPITAL

The mass media are a significant part of the environment in which the pursuit of public health goals occurs. The mass media facilitate the pursuit of public health goals in some ways and obstruct it in other ways. On the one hand, large-scale, mass mediated educational programs to inform the public about health threats have long been a staple of public health practice (Wallack, 1981). Over the years these campaigns have become increasingly sophisticated, with new standards set for the integration of research, theory, planning, and evaluation by the Stanford Heart Disease Prevention Program in the 1970s (Farquhar, Maccoby, and Solomon, 1984; Flora, Maccoby, and Farquhar, 1989; Farquhar, Fortmann, and Flora, 1990; Fortmann and others, 1990). Current programs involve much greater levels of resources and a strong focus on high impact advertising. Nonetheless, current efforts, like previous efforts, have generally been limited in achieving the goals for which they were designed.

On the other hand, the public health community has long been concerned about the mass media as a source of problems. Various types of advertising and the portrayal of health-compromising behaviors and products in the media have been identified as promoting disease rather than health. The potential influence of movies, advertising media, and television programming has been considered in regard to alcohol, tobacco, and other drug use, violence, nutritional behavior, sexual behavior, traffic safety, and various other public health threats (e.g., Kunkel and others, 1999; Kilbourne, 1999; Strasburger, 1995; Strasburger and Comstock, 1993; Gerbner, 1990; Signorielli and Staples, 1997; Centerwall, 1992). Over the years various interventions have been developed to influence the producers, directors, and writers of television series to change or include specific information on various health topics such as alcohol, tobacco, immunization, drunk driving, emergency contraception, and other topics (e.g., Montgomery, 1989; Breed and De Foe, 1982; De Jong and Wallack, 1992; Glik and others, 1997; Langlieb, Cooper, and Gielen, 1999).

The research on social capital has significant implications for developing media strategies in public health. It expands our attention to whether the very nature of the structure and organization of the media might build or destroy social capital, might add to or detract from public health. It suggests that broader issues must be addressed—the nature of commercialism rather than advertising about a specific product, the impact of television on social relations rather than on specific behaviors—but public health has not raised these issues in a substantive way. The introduction of social capital as a concept that cuts across many categories of public health threats demands consideration of the broader effect of media on our social fabric rather than just on our specific behaviors.

The rugged individualism inherent in American society is one of the major barriers to collective action and a cornerstone of a market system that generates excess public health casualties (Chapter Ten, Beauchamp, 1981, 1988; Bellah and others, 1986). Technological trends will likely increase individualism and further undercut the foundation for the type of social cohesion necessary for a civil society (Putnam, 1995a; McChesney, 1999). Hypercommercialism, the commodification and marketing of virtually everything, cuts across all media and into all aspects of everyday living. Hypercommercialism may well increase a sense of hyperindividualism and contribute to a focus on increasing personal accumulation rather than enhancing social participation. This has serious implications for social capital and creates urgency for innovative media approaches to build social capital.

There are various ways that mass media may inhibit the formation of, or reduce, the stock of social capital in the society. If the concept of social capital and civic engagement is broadened to political participation, its potential effects can expand considerably. From a public health perspective, increasing engagement in community health issues is likely to lead to increased participation in the political process. Those working to prevent alcohol problems, limit availability of handguns, prevent tobacco use, improve nutrition in schools, or prevent unsafe sexual activity quickly find themselves moving from simply working with others to confronting political institutions and interest groups on policy issues.

Undermining Social Capital: The Role of the Media

If social capital is the glue that helps communities work effectively on collective issues, then it is important that the media do not dissolve the bonding capacity of the glue. Unfortunately, television, and mass media in general, may function to reduce rather than reinforce or nurture social capital. Putnam (1995a) asserts that there has been a significant decline of social capital in the United States and attributes a substantial part of the blame to television. Both these claims have been disputed, with Ladd (1999) arguing that social capital, far from declining, is being generated at levels beyond anything in the past, and others questioning the focus on television as a significant variable (Schudson, 1996). However, for purposes of this chapter my concern is whether social capital is related to indicators of public health and whether mass media might influence the level of civic participation from a public health perspective.

Television viewing contributes to lower levels of group membership and civic trust—two key components of social capital (Putnam, 1995a). This occurs because the time spent watching television displaces time that might be allocated to other activities related to civic life. Further, increased television viewing may lead to higher levels of pessimism and cynicism about the world.

George Gerbner and his colleagues (1994) have argued that television cultivates a very distorted perception of the world in heavier viewers. For example, these heavy viewers score low on social trust and are less accepting of norms of reciprocity. When compared with lighter viewers, heavier viewers are more likely to believe that most people "cannot be trusted" and are "just looking out for themselves" (p. 30). Further, compared with lighter viewers, they are more likely to overestimate their chances of being victimized by crime or violence, believe that their neighborhood is unsafe, and assume crime is rising regardless of the actual facts. Television "facts" become the basis for making judgments about the real world. Not surprisingly, heavier viewers are more likely to express "gloom and alienation" and "express a heightened sense of living in a mean world of danger, mistrust, and alienation" (Gerbner, Morgan, and Signorielli, 1994, p. 9). So not only do people have less time to participate in civic activities, but their level of fear, mistrust, and alienation would hardly make such participation inviting.

Another issue raised by Putnam (1995a) is that of the passivity-inducing role of television. Indeed, Postman (1985) argues that television, and the media in general, provide an information glut that trivializes public discourse, distracts people from substantive issues, and renders the population passive. The issue of passivity draws us to the broader issue of the structure and function of the mass media. Writing before the diffusion of television, Lazarsfeld and Merton ([1948] 1975) worried that the mass media inhibited social change and suggested that they might contribute to a population that was "politically apathetic and inert" (p. 501). Similar to Postman who followed, they were concerned that the flood of information from a mass media motivated primarily by profit rather than public interest would "narcotize rather than energize the average reader or listener" (p. 502). Schiller (1973) picks up this theme and argues that it is in fact the aim of the mass media to lessen rather than raise concern about social issues.

The primary source of news for people is local television, though newspaper reading is more strongly associated with voting (Stempel and Hargrove, 1996). Journalism, in general, has been severely criticized for its contribution to the trivialization of public discourse and the alienation of the public from the political process (e.g., Fallows, 1997; McChesney, 1999). Part of the reason for this is the way that the news fragments issues and thus obscures the connections among them (Schiller, 1973). Iyengar (1991) argues that television news overwhelmingly frames social issues episodically in concrete, individual, personal stories that communicate personal responsibility rather than social accountability. The result is that viewers are more likely to "blame the victim" for the cause and solution of the problem rather than hold public officials or institutions accountable. He explains, "Because television news generally fails to activate (and may indeed depress) societal attributions of responsibility, . . . it tends to obscure the connections between social problems and the actions or inactions of political leaders. By attenuating these connections, episodic framing impedes electoral accountability" (Iyengar, 1991, pp. 141–142).

Most recently, McChesney (1997, 1999) has argued that the very nature of the media system in the United States "undermines all three of the meaningful criteria for self-government" (1997, p. 7). These criteria are lack of significant disparities in wealth, a sense of community and acceptance of the idea that one's well being is linked to the larger well being, and an effective system of political communication that engages citizens. He argues that the mass media, through corporate concentration, conglomeration, and hypercommercialism, create a depoliticized, passive citizenry who are largely cynical and apathetic (Iyengar, 1991).

In sum, the mass media may adversely affect the development or maintenance of social capital in the United States. A fundamental question is whether the media relate to people as consumers or citizens (Burns, 1989). If they are valued only as a demographic that is more or less likely to consume various types of products, then media will offer little effort to build social capital. If, on the other hand, the media relate to people as citizens who are valued for their potential participation, then media may well offer much support for building social capital. An equally important issue is how people relate to the media.

Public Health Mass Media Campaigns: Building Human Capital

If you ask a group of public health practitioners whether improvements in health status will come about *primarily* as a result of people getting more information about their personal health habits or of people getting more power to change the social and environmental conditions in which they live, they will inevitably voice the latter belief. Because many people enter the public health profession motivated by the opportunity for contributing to social change, and because practitioners are closely connected to people with the problems, they either bring or quickly develop an understanding of social causation of disease. However, when asked where most of their work effort is focused, they explain that they spend most of their time trying to change personal health behaviors, not social factors.[1] The practice of public health, and certainly conventional health education, has to a great extent been the practice of building human capital— providing people with the tools for good health—in this case, health information.

James Coleman (1990) distinguishes between human and social capital, a distinction that is fundamental to understanding the role of public health media campaigns to improve health. He explains, "Human capital is created by changing persons so as to give them skills and capabilities that make them able to act in new ways. Social capital, in turn, is created when the relations among persons change in ways that facilitate action" (p. 304). The history of media campaigns shows that they try to increase human capital, not promote collective action. These campaigns provide individuals with knowledge about risks such as alcohol, tobacco, sedentary lifestyles, diet, unsafe sex, and the like in the hope that they will change the way they act. Sometimes such campaigns might attempt to link people, such as the recent $2 billion anti-drug campaign that tries to get parents to talk to their children about drugs, but for the most part they simply provide people with health information (De Jong and Wallack, 1999). These campaigns are governed by the idea that people need more and better personal information to navigate a hazardous health environment rather than that people need skills to better participate in the public policy process to make the environment less hazardous.

Mass mediated health communication efforts generally flow from a pragmatic logic that assumes an information gap in individuals—if people just knew and understood that certain behaviors were bad for them and others good, then these people would change to the behaviors that benefited their health. Filling the information gap becomes the purpose of the campaign; if enough people changed their behavior, then this would lead to a healthier society. The problem is operationally defined as people just not knowing any better. The goal, then, is to warn and inform people so they can change. In order to make this happen, campaigns focus on developing the right message to deliver to the largest number of people through the mass media. Finding the right message is central to the campaign and extremely important. The message, however, is always about personal change rather than social change or collective action.

Better health communication campaigns are characterized by at least three important factors. First, these campaigns are more likely to use mass communication and behavior change theory as a basis for campaign design. This means using a variety of mass communication channels, making sure the audience is exposed to the message, and providing a clear and specific action for the individual to take. Second, they are more likely to use formative research such as focus groups in order to develop messages and inform campaign strategy. Many better-designed interventions also include various social marketing strategies such as market segmentation, channel analysis, and message pretesting (Lefebvre and Flora, 1988). Third, they are more likely to link media strategies with community programs, thus reinforcing the media message and providing local support for desired behavior changes (Wallack and De Jong, 1995).

While there are many ways that a well-designed campaign can increase the potential for success, meaningful success itself has been elusive. In a comprehensive review of communication campaigns, Rogers and Storey (1987) noted, "The literature of campaign research is filled with failures, along with qualified successes—evidence that campaigns *can* be effective under certain conditions" (italics in original, p. 817). This review, more optimistic than some and slightly more pessimistic than others, generally echoed previous reviews (Wallack, 1981, 1984; Alcalay, 1983; McGuire, 1986) and anticipated later reviews (Salmon, 1989; Brown and Walsh-Childers, 1994; Wallack and De Jong, 1995; De Jong and Winsten, 1998).

Over-reliance on public education campaigns constitutes a barrier to the accomplishment of public health goals. First, such an emphasis conflicts with the social justice ethic of public health, which calls for a fair sharing of the burden for prevention (Chapter Ten). At worst, such campaigns may contribute to the problem they seek to address. This happens when the narrow behavioral focus of the campaign deflects our attention away from social and structural determinants of health by focusing exclusively on the behavior of individuals— in effect blaming the victim for the problem and placing the sole burden for change on him or her (Ryan, 1976; Wallack, 1989, 1990; Dorfman and Wallack, 1993).

Second, participation in civic life is generally not advanced by most of these campaigns, since they tend to focus on personal behaviors that individuals can take on their own behalf in order to improve their health. Public policy or social action is seldom, if ever, a focus of public health media campaigns because these campaigns are usually supported with public money that makes advocacy for specific policies problematic. Also, many media outlets will not accept public service announcements or even paid advertisements that are considered controversial—and policy issues that inevitably confront corporate interests are inherently controversial.

Third, such actions may be necessary or desirable but do not appear to be sufficient for improving the health of populations. Lomas (1998) argues that individual risk factor modification, an approach at the core of most mass media campaigns, has been "spectacularly unsuccessful" (p. 1183).

Finally, it is not possible to define a problem at the community or societal level and then focus primarily on solutions at the personal or individual level. There are many definitions of public health, but one clear thread running through these is the fundamental idea that the primary focus must be on the health and well-being of communities or populations, not individuals (Rose, 1985, 1992; Mann, 1997). It does not follow then that applying primarily individual level solutions can effectively address public health problems.

MEDIA STRATEGIES THAT BUILD SOCIAL CAPITAL

The Institute of Medicine suggests a broad vision of the mission of public health, explaining that it requires creating the conditions in which people can be healthy. It goes on to say, "Clearly, public health is 'public' because it involves organized community effort" (Institute of Medicine, 1988, p. 39). Social capital is a fundamental fuel for generating the kind of collective action that is required for public health to adequately pursue its mission. The crucial issue, then, is what kinds of media approaches can increase the capacity of groups, and broader communities, to act on matters related to public health that potentially benefit the entire society.

Developing media strategies to build social capital has two significant public health implications. First, in general, by increasing the level of social capital in the community, there may be benefits to the public's health in the form of lower overall mortality rates. Second, by increasing the level of social capital, groups may become more effective in advancing policies that may help to build a more egalitarian society and protect health (e.g., early childhood education). In addition, the skills and social structures associated with social capital can be put to use for other issues that might appear less central to health but nonetheless are still central to strong communities.

There are at least three promising media approaches that have the potential to build social capital and thus contribute to public health. These approaches are civic or public journalism, media advocacy, and photovoice.

Civic Journalism

Public health and journalism at their best hold an important value in common: attention to and concern for the well being of the public. The former seeks to create the conditions in which people can be healthy (Institute of Medicine, 1988), and the latter seeks to create the conditions in which people can be good citizens (Merritt, 1995). It is now clear that these "conditions" are inextricably linked through the concept of social capital.

In the late 1980s and early 1990s journalism was in crisis. There was great concern about the loss of public civility and the decline of public life. The 1988 presidential campaign had the lowest voter turnout since 1924, and journalism was being blamed for citizen apathy and cynicism. In 1994 a Times Mirror poll reported that 71 percent of national respondents agreed that "the news media gets in the way of society solving its problems" (Merritt, 1995). The public was alienated from the political process; there was a sense that public life, politics, and journalism all seemed to be caught in a downward spiral (Fallows, 1997, Merritt, 1995, Clark, 1993).

Journalism in general, and newspapers in particular, began a process of soul searching about whether they might do a better job in serving the democratic process. What evolved in the early 1990s was the controversial concept of public journalism (Rosen, 1991, 1993; Merritt, 1995), and soon the term *civic journalism* was being used interchangeably with it (Rosen, 1994).[2] It was not long before interesting collaborations among local newspapers, television stations, and radio stations were developing around the country.

Civic journalism projects seek to engage the community in the process of civic life by providing information and other forms of support to increase community debate and public participation in problem solving. Jay Rosen, an academic, and Davis Merritt, a long-time print journalist, are among the best-known architects of civic journalism. They argue that civic journalism represents a fundamental shift in thinking by the journalist. This shift requires the journalist to be attached to community life rather than maintain the traditional pose of detachment (Rosen, 1994). They argue that journalists have a greater responsibility than just reporting the news. They have a responsibility to help the community work better. The purpose of civic journalism is to create a process by which citizens can participate in the life of the community through public discussion, deliberation, collective problem solving, and ongoing involvement. By the end of the twentieth century, there were approximately 300 civic journalism projects in cities of varying sizes around the country (Friedland, Sotirovic, and Daily, 1998). These projects have addressed a diverse set of issues, including race relations, crime and violence, juvenile delinquency, alcohol, land use planning, domestic violence, economic development, community leadership, and voting participation.

Civic journalism projects are themselves quite diverse, employing a wide range of approaches. Generally, these projects are initiated by newspapers and involve television and radio stations as partners. They are generally based on three broad activities undertaken by civic journalists:

1. There is an extensive information development and data gathering process. This can take the form of in-depth coverage of an issue, where teams of reporters, rather than just one or two, are put on the story. In addition, in an effort to develop more insight into the community, special polls, focus groups, interviews, and other techniques are used (Wiley, 1998). Reports for various neighborhoods might be produced based on polling data, follow up interviews by journalists with poll respondents, dialogues at town meetings, and detailed analyses of crime data.

2. There is far more extensive news coverage of the issue than is commonly seen and the coverage is coordinated with other media outlets. This serves to increase visibility, legitimacy, and urgency of the issue and set the public and policy agenda.

3. There are structures developed to ensure that information and community concern are translated into action. Substantial efforts are often made to insure community participation and are facilitated through various means. In some cases a person is hired by the newspaper to coordinate the process. The Poverty Among Us project in St. Paul, Minnesota, provided money for childcare and translators to remove barriers to participation in community discussions.

Civic journalism is still at an early stage and the evaluation of projects is moving from case studies to more sophisticated survey research and statistical modeling analyses. Case studies provide an impressionistic view of problems, processes, challenges, and successes. For the most part the news is encouraging (Ford, 1998; Pew Center for Civic Journalism, 1997). High levels of media coverage of significant local problems are being generated, and participation in the projects seems extensive. In Charlotte, North Carolina, the *Observer* ran a front-page story on crime and violence that was augmented with four inside pages. The following month the *Observer* provided almost seven pages to exploring life in the community. A local television station and two radio stations followed up with round tables and call in shows focused on solutions to the crime and violence problem (Pew Center for Civic Journalism, 1995). Subsequently, more than 700 groups and individuals volunteered to work on various community needs. The city responded by razing dilapidated buildings, clearing overgrown lots, and opening parks and recreation facilities. Local law firms got involved by providing pro bono services to close crack houses.

In Peoria, Illinois, several hundred people met to develop a citywide action plan known as the Leadership Challenge. New leaders emerged and the shape of city government changed when a person who had been influenced by the project ran for mayor and won. In Springfield, Missouri, the *News-Leader*'s Good Community program focused on juvenile crime. One event attracted 700 people who pledged 13,000 hours to community service. After three years the project is continuing and "crime is down in Springfield and public involvement is up" (Ford, 1998, p. 15).

In Binghamton, New York, the *Press* and *Sun Bulletin* convened a town meeting and devised 10 action teams on topics important for economic development. In addition to hiring a former city official to find discussion leaders for the teams, the newspaper provided special group process training for the team leaders. More than 100 meetings were held, and more than 300 people participated in the team meetings. The media partners in the project covered recommendations of the teams. This particular project, Facing Our Future, continued on to become the Building Our Future program (Ford, 1998). More rigorous evidence is now available to support these anecdotal claims of effectiveness.

The most extensive evaluations of civic journalism have examined five projects in four cites. The first project, Taking Back Our Neighborhoods, addressed crime and violence in parts of Charlotte, North Carolina. The second and third projects, We the People, focused on land use issues and juvenile delinquency in Madison, Wisconsin. The fourth project, Voice of the Voter, tried to increase the vote among low turnout groups in a mayoral election in San Francisco, California, and the final project, Facing Our Future, in Binghamton, New York, sought to stimulate citizen involvement in finding solutions to economic decline.

A series of evaluation studies provide encouraging findings on the effects of the civic journalism efforts (Chaffee, McDevitt, and Thorson, 1997; Ognianova, Thorson, and Mendelson, 1997; Thorson, Mendelson, and Ognianova, 1997; Denton and Thorson, 1998). In general, the survey evaluations focused on outcomes as well as theoretical pathways and found promising results for the hypothesis that the news media can enhance the democratic process by increasing involvement (Denton and Thorson, 1998). It was fairly clear that interest and discussion in civic issues could be attributed to the civic journalism projects (Madison). More importantly, the projects were associated with increased participation in neighborhood problem solving (Charlotte, Madison, San Francisco) and increased voting in groups with usually low turnout (San Francisco) (Chaffee, McDevitt, and Thorson, 1997). Chaffee and his colleagues were encouraged by their findings and concluded that civic journalism programs "appear from our evidence to be effective" (p. 26).

While finding evidence of success, Chaffee and his colleagues were concerned that selective exposure might explain their findings. This would mean that people already interested in the issues and perhaps predisposed to civic participation sought the programs rather than being stimulated by the programs. In a related study which also included the Binghamton site, Ognianova, Thorson, and Mendelson (1997) tested whether the civic journalism project leads to increased concern about issues and civic involvement (media stimulation of involvement) or whether existing involvement leads people to be aware of the civic journalism project (selective exposure). Their conclusion was that awareness of the project led to concern, knowledge, and subsequent involvement: "Analyses of the two alternative models with data from four different cities in the United States showed clear and consistent support for the media stimulation model" (p. 21). Other work on all four cities (Thorson, Mendelson, and Ognianova, 1997) explored the potential of a two-step model of civic journalism where awareness of projects helps to shift attitudes and leads to subsequent increases in civic involvement. This research concluded that indeed civic journalism was an effective means for reconnecting citizens to public life.

Media Advocacy

Media advocacy is the strategic use of mass media in combination with community organizing to advance healthy public policies. The primary focus is on the role of news media with secondary attention to the use of paid advertising (U.S. Department of Health and Human Services, 1988; Wallack, 1994; Wallack and Dorfman, 1996; Wallack and Sciandra, 1990; Wallack and others, 1993, 1999; Winett and Wallack, 1996). Media advocacy seeks to raise the volume of voices for social change and shape the sound so that it resonates with the social justice values that are the presumed basis of public health (Chapter Ten; Mann, 1997). It has been used by a wide range of grassroots community groups, public health leadership groups, public health and social advocates, and public health researchers (Wallack and others, 1993, 1999).

The practical origins of media advocacy can be traced to the late 1980s. It grew from a collaboration of public health groups working on tobacco and alcohol issues with public interest and consumer groups also working on these or similar issues. The public interest and consumer groups brought a new array of strategies and tactics that were more familiar to a political campaign than a public health effort. The public health people provided a clearer understanding of the substantive scientific issues and the importance of theory in creating change. The result has been an approach that blends science, politics, and advocacy to advance public health goals.

From a theoretical perspective, media advocacy borrows from mass communication, political science, sociology, and political psychology to develop strategy. Central to media advocacy are the concepts of agenda setting (McCombs and Shaw, 1972; Deering and Rogers, 1997) and framing (Iyengar, 1991; Gamson, 1989; Ryan, 1991). From a practical perspective, media advocacy borrows from community organizing, key elements of formative research (i.e., focus groups and polling), and political campaign strategy (e.g., application of selective pressure on key groups or individuals) (Wallack and others, 1993). Blending theory with practice provides an overall framework for advocacy and social change.

Media advocacy differs in many ways from traditional public health campaigns. It is most marked by an *emphasis* on:

- Linking public health and social problems to inequities in social arrangements rather than to flaws in the individual,
- Changing public policy rather than personal health behavior,
- Focusing primarily on reaching opinion leaders and policy makers rather than on those who have the problem (the traditional audience of public health communication campaigns),

- Working with groups to increase participation and amplify their voices rather than providing health behavior change messages;
- Having a primary goal of reducing the power gap rather than just filling the information gap

Media advocacy is generally seen as a part of a broader strategy rather than as a strategy per se. One of the fundamental rules of media advocacy is that it is not possible to have a media strategy without an overall strategy. Media advocacy is part of the overall plan, but is not the plan, for achieving policy change. For example, a group in Oakland, California, effectively used media advocacy to advance a city ordinance to place a tax on liquor stores and institute a moratorium on new licenses in the city (Seevak, 1997). The effort took four years to implement, starting at the local zoning commission and ending up in the California State Supreme Court. Over that period, the group used media advocacy to provide legitimacy to the issue, to increase the credibility of their position and add urgency to the problem, and to let politicians know that the community was very involved in the issue and would be following all votes. To achieve this, they used a variety of tactics to generate news coverage and discussion on the editorial pages. This increased the effectiveness of the grassroots coalition advancing the policy but would have made little difference if the coalition did not have strong community support (resulting in large turnouts at key meetings and hearings and visits and calls to politicians), a clear and reasonable policy, and research to back up its claims. The group might have failed lacking any one of the ingredients for change: a reasonable policy goal that could make a difference, an issue that the community supported and was willing to work for, and a media strategy to advance the policy and support community organizing.

Media advocacy focuses on four primary activities in support of community organizing, policy development, and advancing policy:

1. *Overall strategy development.* Media advocacy uses critical thinking to understand and respond to problems as social issues rather than personal problems. Following problem definition, the focus is on elaborating policy options, identifying the person, group, or organization who has the power to create the necessary change, and identifying organizations that can apply pressure to advance the policy and create change (for example, in the Oakland illustration above, various elements of the community were organized to apply pressure on the zoning commission, mayor's office, city council, and state legislature, which were all targets at various points in the campaign). Finally, various messages for the different targets of the campaign are developed.

2. *Setting the agenda.* Getting an issue in the media can help set the agenda and provide legitimacy and credibility to the issue and group. Media advocacy involves understanding how journalism works in order to increase access to the news media. This includes maintaining a media list, monitoring the news media, understanding the elements of newsworthiness, pitching stories, holding news events, and developing editorial page strategies for reaching key opinion leaders.

3. *Shaping the debate.* The news media generally focus on the plight of the victim, while policy advocates emphasize social conditions that create victims. Media advocates frame policy issues using public health values that resonate with broad audiences. Some of the steps include "translat[ing] personal problems into public issues" (Mills, 1959); emphasizing social accountability as well as personal responsibility; identifying individuals and organizations who must assume a greater burden for addressing the problem; presenting a clear and concise policy solution; and packaging the story by combining key elements such as visuals, expert voices, authentic voices (those with experience of the problem), media bites, social math (creating a context for large numbers that is interesting to the press and understandable to the public), research summaries, fact sheets, policy papers, etc.

4. *Advancing the policy.* Policy battles are often long and contentious, and it is important to make effective use of the media to keep the issue on the media agenda. The Oakland effort took four years and now must focus media attention to ensure that the policy is properly implemented. Thus, it is important to develop strategies to maintain the media spotlight on the policy issue on a continuing basis. This means identifying opportunities to reintroduce the issue to the media such as key anniversaries of relevant dates, publication of new reports, significant meetings or hearing, and linking the policy solution to breaking news.

Media advocacy has been applied to a number of public health and social issues, including affirmative action, child care, alcohol, tobacco, childhood lead poisoning, health promotion, violence, handgun control, and suicide prevention, as well as others. To date, most evaluations of media advocacy have been case studies (Wallack and others, 1993, 1999; Wallack and Dorfman, 1996: Woodruff, 1996; Jernigan and Wright, 1996; De Jong, 1996). These case studies have shown that community groups trained in media advocacy can effectively gain access to the news media and enhance their participation in the process of public policy making. In California, for example, media advocacy training, follow-up, and support were provided to hundreds of community activists, researchers, service providers, and others working on violence prevention. These skills were used in the process of passing substantial numbers of local ordinances limiting the availability of firearms and ultimately passing statewide legislation banning the manufacture and sale of Saturday-night specials or "junk guns" (Wallack, 1997, 1999). Nonetheless, media advocacy can be controversial, and there are risks to the organizations that use it as part of their strategy (De Jong, 1996).

In a more systematic evaluation of the role of media advocacy in a controlled study designed to advance community policies to reduce drinking and driving, Holder and Treno (1997) concluded that media advocacy was effective in several areas and "an important tool for community prevention" (p. S198). For example, local people trained in media advocacy were able to increase local news coverage in television and newspapers and presumably frame it around policy issues. Holder and Treno suggest that results of the media advocacy component of the intervention "can focus public and leader attention on specific issues and approaches to local policies of relevance to reducing alcohol-involved injuries" (p. S198). Another evaluation looked at the effects of media advocacy in the Stanford Five City Heart Disease Prevention Project (Schooler, Sundar, and Flora, 1996). Dependent variables included coverage of the issue, prominence of the article, framing of the article (e.g., prevention versus treatment), and the impact on the media agenda (i.e., ratio of locally generated articles on heart disease versus other health issues). The study concluded that "media advocacy efforts can be successful" (p. 361) but found that maintenance of the effects was weak. In both of these evaluation studies (particularly Schooler, Sundar, and Flora, 1996), it was unclear whether there was a focus on advancing public policies or whether, like many media efforts, the focus was more related to increasing awareness. Also, it was unclear as to whether a comprehensive media advocacy approach was implemented as was found in the case studies on limiting alcohol outlets in Oakland or banning junk guns in California.

Photovoice

Photovoice, a relatively new concept, is the use of photography for social change by marginalized and traditionally powerless groups. It has deep roots in documentary photography, feminist theory, empowerment theory, and participatory research (Wang and Burris, 1994, 1997; Wang, Burris, and Xiang, 1996; Wang, Yuan, and Feng, 1996; Wang, Cash, and Powers, 1999; Wang and Pies, 1999; Wang and others, 1998). Photovoice is "designed to enable people to create and discuss photographs as a means of catalyzing personal and community change" (Wang, Cash, and Powers, 1999, p. 4). Much health education and health promotion have at their core a great passion for community participation and social change (e.g., Minkler, 1997), and photovoice is a media approach designed to increase the likelihood of this occurring by "engaging the community to act on its own behalf" (Wang and Burris, 1994, p. 182).

Photovoice focuses on grassroots involvement and attempts to increase the participation of marginalized groups in the policy process. Various projects have been implemented with women in rural China (Wang and Burris, 1994, 1997; Wang, Burris, and Xiang, 1996; Wang, Yuan, and Feng, 1996; Wang and others, 1998), homeless men and women in Ann Arbor, Michigan (Wang, Cash, and Powers, 1999), and people recruited from public health and social service sites in Contra Costa County, California (Wang and Pies, 1999). The goals of these projects are quite similar and clearly reflect the theory and values of the approach:

1. To understand local issues and concerns through the perspective of specific groups of people. This means seeing health, work, and community issues through the eyes of the participants and those most affected by the problems rather than just the usual experts.

2. To promote knowledge and critical discussion about significant community issues. This involves group discussion among participants regarding their photographs.

3. To reach policy makers and others who can be mobilized to create change. This means finding ways to translate and make visible the "data" in the photographs so that others can be enlisted in the social change process.

The photovoice process has been documented in a series of articles by Wang and her colleagues. Once a project is defined, a target audience of policy makers or community leaders is identified and participate in the planning process. Its primary role is to serve as a group with the political will to put participants' ideas and recommendations into practice (Wang, 1999). At the same time, facilitators are trained. This involves grounding in the process of photovoice, including ethical issues such as privacy and power, which might arise in the process of taking pictures. Technical knowledge about cameras and photography is provided, as are basic group process skills for leading discussion.

Trainers or facilitators then recruit participants through a variety of means, depending on the project. (For example, in the Language of Light homeless project participants were recruited through shelters and provided with cameras and small stipends.) Participants, in turn, attend a series of workshops to learn about the methods of photovoice, the technical aspects of using and caring for a camera, and the safety and privacy issues that might arise from using a camera in public or social service settings. After the first workshop, the meetings are used for group discussion and feedback on the pictures. Participants who wish to write about their photographs may follow a series of "root-cause questions" similar to those used in discussion.

In the final stage of the project, facilitators and participants select pictures to share with journalists and policy makers in order to move the documentation process to the action process. Each of the projects achieved some success in reaching broader audiences and policy makers. In China, project facilitators organized a slide show that attracted some of the most powerful policy makers in the province. Three policy decisions—regarding day care for toddlers, training programs for midwives, and educational scholarships for girls—were enacted as a result of facilitators' and participants' advocacy using the photovoice process. The participating Chinese village women highlighted each of these issues through their photographs and stories (Wang, Burris, and Xiang, 1996).

In Ann Arbor, the Language of Light project provided pictures and captions for a series of articles in local newspapers, a gallery exhibition, and a major public forum. These activities communicated concerns of the homeless to a broader population and also put a human face on the issue. The public forum was attended by several hundred people and allowed the project to provide input to policy makers on a proposal to build a new homeless shelter that would have resulted in major disadvantages to the homeless population (Wang, Cash, and Powers, 1999).

The Picture This project in Contra Costa County held exhibitions of its pictures at the County Office of Maternal and Child Health and the state capitol during a statewide meeting. In addition, more than a full page in the local newspaper was provided to show pictures and report on the project. Several stories of change came out of the project, including one resulting from a picture of a closed hospital with a caption complaining about inadequate health services for low income people: "The picture and other complaints prompted the county to improve care at its Pittsburg clinic" (Spears, 1999, pp. A1, A32).

Photovoice, though a new concept that has not been subject to rigorous evaluation, appears to have promise for increasing community involvement. The use of pictures in addition to words may well increase the power of local groups to effectively press their case for social change. Perhaps most important is that this approach may be a particularly useful tool for those who find the usual means of participation in community discussion to be a foreign and unfriendly process that seems to uphold the views of those who already make the decisions.

A NOTE ON THE INTERNET

The Internet promises to provide people with unprecedented access to information about the kinds of factors that affect their health and affords health educators the opportunity to use this medium to design interventions to change health behavior (e.g., Cassell, Jackson, and Cheuvront, 1998). An estimated 33.5 million adults seek out medical information on the Internet (Davis and Miller, 1999) and many others use the Internet to find social support (Bly, 1999). Also, Cart (1997) has discussed the potential of the Internet for local communities to organize, gain immediate access to critical facts, and increase their power as citizens to effectively participate in policy debates. She also suggests that on-line networks have "the potential to bring back 'communities that disappeared with front porches'" (p. 328).

The Internet has the potential to supplement and possibly increase the value of any media approach used. Mass media campaigns that can direct people to the Internet for more detailed and personalized information, as well as social support, will no doubt increase their potential to help people. Civic journalism projects that use the Internet will make it easier for people to participate in a more informed way. For the media advocate, the Internet allows fast and easy access to policy information that was simply unavailable in the past, as well as specialized information and strategic help from colleagues on the other side of the world as easily as from those down the street. This will help increase the potential contribution of media advocacy and other activist approaches because it will build social capital by providing one of the basic elements for effective collective action—easy, fast, and direct communication.

McChesney (1999), however, raises an important question about the Internet: "Cannot the ability of people to create their own 'community' in cyberspace have the effect of terminating a community in the general sense?" (p. 146). Just as the Internet will speed many desirable aspects of our society along, so will it likely accelerate the path to hyperindividualism and hypercommercialism that McChesney warns about. From a social capital perspective, this would not be a welcome direction because of the potential adverse effects of the corporate dominance of media technologies on citizen activism (McChesney, 1997, 1999).

Another important Internet issue is the amount and quality of information. While more people have access to unprecedented amounts of information, the quality of such information is uneven. Those seeking cancer information, for example, could easily end up at sites that might offer information that was potentially damaging to their health. The flood of health and medical advice without some added ability to critically assess accuracy could have significant unintended consequences for consumers of health information.

Finally, access to the Internet is very much influenced by economic status. Efforts to promote universal access have largely faltered, raising the possibility of information "haves" and "have nots" and further increasing the effects of income inequality.

DISCUSSION

Recent research points to the urgency of rethinking the role of mass media to advance the public's health. Research strongly suggests that media approaches should focus on increasing the reservoir of social capital by engaging people and increasing their involvement and participation in community life. This, per se, may have a positive generalized effect on the population's health. In addition, because public health seeks to "create the conditions in which people can be healthy" (Institute of Medicine, 1988), mass media strategies should also provide citizens with the skills to better participate in the policy process to create these conditions. Furthermore, it is crucial that social capital not be seen as a substitute for the kinds of policies that are important to reduce social inequality but as a foundation that makes policy change possible. Social capital then is a prerequisite for policy change and a consequence of the process of generating that change (Putnam, 1993).

In the new century sophisticated versions of the classic mass mediated public health campaigns will play a role in increasing awareness, providing knowledge, and shifting attitudes. However, these campaigns have not had a significant impact on the health of populations and should be a relatively small part of a comprehensive strategy. Public health should not be seduced by a primarily information-based approach that focuses on the individual and ignores more potentially effective but controversial approaches emphasizing policy or political participation.

Civic journalism, media advocacy, and photovoice have been presented as promising approaches, but this is not the same as suggesting that these are successful approaches. Early evaluations are indeed promising, but more important is the set of values underlying these approaches. The goal of these approaches is to engage people in the process of improving their communities through deliberation about problems, discussions about solutions, and participation in the processes that lead to social or political change. They seek to give people a voice rather than leave them with a message, and they point people to solutions that benefit the entire community, not just the individual. Their goal is nothing short of making democracy work better and by doing so affecting the public's health on the most global level.

As a society we exalt the person that can "beat the odds" and succeed against adversity (Schorr, 1988). This "triumphant individual" story is in fact one of the dominant parables that guide political thought, rhetoric, and policy development in our society (Reich, 1988). Public health is a profession that should work to reduce the odds so that more people can succeed, not a profession that simply provides information, services, and encouragement to people so they might be among the few lucky ones to beat the odds (Beauchamp, 1981).

In considering media approaches we must select the kinds of strategies that have the long-range potential to change the odds. The income gap between the rich and the poor has more than doubled in the past 20 years. Currently, 20 percent of the population earns more than one-half of all the income in America. The 20 percent with the lowest income earns only 4.2% of all the income (Johnston, 1999). This inequality gap is bad for society overall and not just those on the bottom rungs, and the public health body count will be one tragic indicator of this. Building social capital is not a panacea, but it can make an important contribution to changing the odds.

Developing media approaches that can enhance social capital and level the playing field is important for the future of public health. There are a number of questions that must be addressed in considering the selection of media strategies:

1. Does the approach increase the capacity of individuals or small groups to participate in collective action by providing participatory skills or creating a structure or network through which individuals, groups, and organizations can act?

2. Does the approach connect the problems or issues to broader social forces?

3. Does the approach increase the community's capacity to collaborate and cooperate by strengthening existing groups (create bonding capital) or connecting various groups (create bridging capital)?

4. Does the approach reflect a social justice orientation—the idea that "each member of the community owes something to all the rest, and the community owes something to each of its members" (Etzioni, 1993, p. 263)?

The greater the degree that a media approach can affirmatively respond to these questions, the more likely it is to build social capital. The public health profession should support such approaches even though in some cases the link to public health might seem tenuous.

The research on the effects of these approaches on public health outcomes is limited, and more comprehensive and systematic evaluations are necessary. One of the problems in determining effects is that these approaches must be seen as supporting and advancing larger interventions for policy change. Civic journalism, media advocacy, and photovoice are likely a means to increase social capital and enhance the capacity of communities to act. This should, if the social epidemiological research is on the right track, lead to improved health across a number of areas. Isolating and linking the contribution of specific media approaches to this kind of social and policy change will be very difficult. Nonetheless, increased participation at the local school board may well result in lower activity at the local hospital.

Public health is, at its core, a political process, and one of our best strategies is to use the democratic process to advance public health goals and objectives. Social and political participation are important, and it is necessary that we develop media strategies that foster community participation rather than just inform personal behavior. The safe and familiar path of mass media campaigns has not been sufficient for change. It is time to travel a new path—even if its terrain is not well mapped and its specific direction must still be clearly marked.

Notes

1. I have asked this question at many professional meetings over the years, and the response is very consistent. Usually, at least 90 percent of the respondents believe that social conditions are the major determinants of health, but fewer that 10 percent ever say that their work focuses on the social-structural aspects of public health.

2. The concept is controversial because many journalists feel it changes the traditional role of the journalist from reporting the news to participating in the news. Some were concerned that the new concept was simply a marketing tool to stem the decline in newspaper readership. Others felt it trampled on the core journalistic value of objectivity by associating journalists with various solutions to community problems. Still others felt that it gave away the power and responsibility of journalists to community people who lacked any special training or insight, particularly as it related to covering political campaigns. Many simply dismissed the more innovative examples of civic or public journalism as good journalism that they were already doing or that they would do if sufficient resources were available. See Black (1997) for an extensive review of this debate.

References

Adler, N. E., and others. "Socioeconomic Inequalities in Health." *Journal of the American Medical Association,* 1993, *269,* 3140–3145.

Adler, N. E, and others. "Socioeconomic Status and Health." *American Psychologist,* 1994, *49,* 15–24.

Alcalay, R. "The Impact of Mass Communication Campaigns in the Health Field." *Social Science and Medicine,* 1983, *17,* 87–794.

Anderson, N. B., and Armstead, C. A. "Toward Understanding the Association of Socioeconomic Status and Health." *Psychosomatic Medicine,* 1995, *57,* 213–225.

Barstow, D. "A Heat Wave Sizzles." *New York Times,* July 7, 1999, p. A1.

Beauchamp, D. "Lottery Justice." *Journal of Public Health Policy,* 1981, *2,* 201–205.

Beauchamp, D. *The Health of the Republic.* Philadelphia: Temple University Press, 1988.

Bellah, R., and others. *Habits of the Heart: Individualism and Commitment in American Life.* New York: HarperCollins, 1986.

Black, J. (ed.). *Mixed News.* Mahwah, N.J.: Erlbaum, 1997.

Blane, D. "Social Determinants of Health." *American Journal of Public Health,* 1995, *85,* 903–906.

Bly, L. "A Network of Support." *USA Today,* July 14, 1999, pp. D1–D2.

Breed, W., and De Foe, J. R. "Effecting Media Change: The Role of Cooperative Consultation on Alcohol Topics." *Journal of Communication,* 1982, *32,* 88–99.

Brown, J. B., and Walsh-Childers, K. "Effects of Media on Personal and Public Health." In J. Bryant and D. Zillmann (eds.), *Media Effects: Advances in Theory and Research.* Mahwah, N.J.: Erlbaum, 1994.

Burns, K. "Moyers: A Second Look—More Than Meets the Eye." *New York Times,* May 14, 1989.

Cart, C. U. "Online Computer Networks." In M. Minkler (ed.), *Community Organizing and Community Building for Health.* New Brunswick, N.J.: Rutgers University Press, 1997.

Cassell, M. M., Jackson, C., and Cheuvront, B. "Health Communication on the Internet: An Effective Channel for Behavior Change?" *Journal of Health Communication,* 1998, *3,* 71–79.

Centerwall, B. S. "Television and Violence." *Journal of the American Medical Association,* 1992, *267,* 3059–3063.

Chaffee, S., McDevitt, M., and Thorson, E. "Citizen Response to Civic Journalism." Paper presented at the annual meeting of the Association for Education in Journalism and Mass Communication, Chicago, Aug. 1997.

Clark, R. P. "Foreword." In J. Rosen, *Community Connectedness Passwords for Public Journalism.* St. Petersburg, Fla.: Poynter Institute for Media Studies, 1993.

Coleman, J. *Foundations of Social Theory.* Cambridge, Mass.: Belknap Press, 1990.

Davis, R., and Miller, L. "Millions Scour the Web for Medical Information." *USA Today,* July 14, 1999, pp. A1–A2.

Deering, J. W., and Rogers, E. M. *Agenda-Setting.* Thousand Oaks, Calif.: Sage, 1997.

De Jong, W. "MADD Massachusetts Versus Senator Burke: A Media Advocacy Case Study." *Health Education Quarterly,* 1996, *23,* 318–329.

De Jong, W., and Wallack, L. "The Role of Designated Driver Programs in the Prevention of Alcohol-Impaired Driving: A Critical Reassessment." *Health Education Quarterly,* 1992, *19,* 429–442.

De Jong, W, and Wallack, L. "A Critical Perspective on the Drug Czar's Antidrug Media Campaign." *Journal of Health Communication,* 1999, *5,* 155–160.

De Jong, W., and Winsten, J. A. *The Media and the Message.* Washington, D.C.: National Campaign to Prevent Teen Pregnancy, 1998.

Denton, F., and Thorson, E. "Effects of a Multimedia Public Journalism Project on Political Knowledge and Attitudes." In E. B. Lambeth, P. E. Meyer, and E. Thorson (eds.), *Assessing Public Journalism.* Columbia: University of Missouri Press, 1998.

Dorfman, L., and Wallack, L. "Advertising Health: The Case for Counter-Ads." *Public Health Reports,* 1993, *108,* 716–726.

Duleep, H. O. "Mortality and Income Inequality Among Economically Developed Countries." *Social Security Bulletin,* 1995, *58*(2), 34–50.

Etzioni, A. *The Spirit of Community.* New York: Simon & Schuster, 1993.

Fallows, J. *Breaking the News.* New York: Vintage Books, 1997.

Farquhar, J. W., Fortmann, S. P., and Flora, J. A. "Effects of Communitywide Education on Cardiovascular Disease Risk Factors: The Stanford Five-City Project." *Journal of the American Medical Association,* 1990, *264,* 359–365.

Farquhar, J. W., Maccoby, N., and Solomon, D. "Community Applications of Behavioral Medicine." In W. Gentry (ed.), *Handbook of Behavioral Medicine.* New York: Guilford Press, 1984.

Flora, J. A., Maccoby, N., and Farquhar, J. W. "Communication Campaigns to Prevent Cardiovascular Disease." In R. E. Rice and C. K. Atkin (eds.), *Public Communication Campaigns.* (2nd ed.) Thousand Oaks, Calif.: Sage, 1989.

Ford, P. *Don't Stop There!* Washington, D.C.: Pew Center for Civic Journalism, 1998.

Fortmann, S., and others. "Effect of Long-Term Community Health Education on Blood Pressure and Hypertension Control." *American Journal of Epidemiology,* 1990, *132,* 629–646.

Friedland, L., Sotirovic, M., and Daily, K. "Public Journalism and Social Capital." In E. B. Lambeth, P. E. Meyer, and E. Thorson (eds.), *Assessing Public Journalism.* Columbia: University of Missouri Press, 1998.

Gamson, W. A. "News as Framing: Comments on Graber." *American Behavioral Scientist,* 1989, *33,* 157–162.

Gerbner, G. "Stories That Hurt: Tobacco, Alcohol, and Other Drugs in the Mass Media." In U.S. Department of Health and Human Services, *Youth and Drugs: Society's Mixed Messages.* Rockville, Md.: U.S. Department of Health and Human Services, 1990.

Gerbner, G., Morgan, M., and Signorielli, N. *Television Violence Profile No. 16: Turning Point.* Philadelphia, Pa: Annenberg School for Communication, 1994.

Gerbner, G., and others. "Growing Up with Television: The Cultivation Perspective." In J. Bryant and D. Zillmann (eds.), *Media Effects: Advances in Theory and Research.* Mahwah, N.J.: Erlbaum, 1994.

Gittell, R., and Vidal, A. *Community Organizing: Building Social Capital as a Development Strategy.* Thousand Oaks, Calif.: Sage, 1998.

Glik, D., and others. "Health Education Goes Hollywood: Working with Prime-Time and Daytime Entertainment Television for Immunization Promotion." *Journal of Health Communication,* 1997, *3,* 263–282.

Haan, M. N., Kaplan, G. A., and Syme, S. L. "Socioeconomic Status and Health: Old Observations and New Thoughts." In J. P. Bunker, D. S. Gomby, and B. H. Kehrer (eds.), *Pathways to Health: The Role of Social Factors.* Menlo Park, Calif.: Henry J. Kaiser Family Foundation, 1989.

Haan, M. N., and others. "Recent Publications on Socioeconomic Status and Health." In J. P. Bunker, D. S. Gomby, and B. H. Kehrer (eds.), *Pathways to Health: The Role of Social Factors.* Menlo Park, Calif.: Henry J. Kaiser Family Foundation, 1989.

Holder, H. D., and Treno, A. J. "Media Advocacy in Community Prevention: News as a Means to Advance Policy Change." *Addiction,* 1997, *92*(Suppl. 2), S189–S199.

Idler, E. L., and Benyamini, Y. "Self-Rated Health and Mortality: A Review of Twenty-Seven Community Studies." *Journal of Health and Social Behavior,* 1997, *38,* 21–37.

Institute of Medicine. *The Future of Public Health.* Washington, D.C.: National Academy Press, 1988.

Iyengar, S. *Is Anyone Responsible?* Chicago: University of Chicago Press, 1991.

Jernigan, D. H., and Wright, P. A. "Media Advocacy: Lessons from Community Experiences." *Journal of Public Health Policy,* 1996, *17,* 306–330.

Johnston, D. "Gap Between Rich and Poor Substantially Wider." *New York Times,* Sept. 5, 1999.

Kaplan, G. A. "Where Do Shared Pathways Lead? Some Reflections on a Research Agenda." *Psychosomatic Medicine,* 1995, *57,* 208–212.

Kaplan, G. A., and others. "Inequality in Income and Mortality in the United States." *British Medial Journal,* 1996, *312,* 999–1003.

Kawachi, I., and Berkman, L. F. "Social Cohesion, Social Capital, and Health." In L. F. Berkman and I. Kawachi (eds.), *Social Epidemiology.* New York: Oxford University Press, 1998.

Kawachi, I., and Kennedy, B. P. "Health and Social Cohesion: Why Care About Income Inequality?" *British Medical Journal,* 1997, *314,* 1037–1039.

Kawachi, I., Kennedy, B. P., and Lochner, K. "Long Live Community: Social Capital as Public Health." *American Prospect,* Nov.-Dec. 1997, pp. 56–59.

Kawachi, I., and others. "Social Capital, Income Inequality, and Mortality." *American Journal of Public Health,* 1997, *87,* 1491–1499.

Kennedy, B. P., Kawachi, I., and Prothrow-Stith, D. "Income Distribution and Mortality: Cross-Sectional Ecological Study of the Robin Hood Index in the United States." *British Medical Journal,* 1996, *312,* 1003–1007.

Kennedy, B. P., and others. "Social Capital, Income Inequality, and Firearm Violent Crime." *Social Science and Medicine,* 1998, *47,* 7–17.

Kilbourne, J. *Deadly Persuasion: Why Women and Girls Must Fight the Addictive Power of Advertising.* New York: Free Press, 1999.

Kunkel, D., and others. *Sex on TV: A Biennial Report to the Kaiser Family Foundation.* Menlo Park, Calif.: Kaiser Family Foundation, 1999.

Ladd, E. C. *The Ladd Report.* New York: Free Press, 1999.

Langlieb, A. M., Cooper, C. P., and Gielen, A. "Linking Health Promotion with Entertainment Television." *American Journal of Public Health,* 1999, *89,* 1116–1117.

Lantz, P. M., and others. "Socioeconomic Factors, Health Behaviors, and Mortality." *Journal of the American Medical Association,* 1998, *279,* 1703–1708.

Lazarsfeld, P., and Merton, R. "Mass Communication, Popular Taste, and Organized Social Action." In W. Schramm (ed.), *Mass Communications.* Urbana: University of Illinois Press, 1975. (Original work published 1948)

Lefebvre, C., and Flora, J. A. "Social Marketing and Public Health Intervention." *Health Education Quarterly,* 1988, *15,* 299–315.

Lochner, K., Kawachi, I., and Kennedy, B. P. "Social Capital: A Guide to Its Measurement." *Health and Place,* 1999, *5*(4), 259-270.

Lomas, J. "Social Capital and Health: Implications for Public Health and Epidemiology." *Social Science and Medicine,* 1998, *47,* 1181–1188.

Lynch, J. W., and Kaplan, G. A. "Understanding How Inequality in the Distribution of Income Affects Health." *Journal of Psychology,* 1997, *2,* 297–314.

Mann, J. M. "Medicine and Public Health, Ethics and Human Rights." *Hastings Center Report,* 1997, *27*(3), 6–13.

Marmot, M. G., and Mustard, J. F. "Coronary Heart Disease from a Population Perspective." In R. G. Evan, M. L. Barer, and T. R. Marmor (eds.), *Why Are Some People Healthy and Others Not? The Determinants of Health of Populations.* Hawthorne, N.Y.: Aldine de Gruyter, 1994.

McChesney, R. *Corporate Media and the Threat to Democracy.* New York: Seven Stories Press, 1997.

McChesney, R. *Rich Media, Poor Democracy.* Urbana: University of Illinois Press, 1999.

McCombs, M., and Shaw, D. "The Agenda-Setting Function of Mass Media." *Public Opinion Quarterly,* 1972, *36,* 176–187.

McGuire, W. "Myth of Massive Media Impact: Savagings and Salvagings." In G. Comstock (ed.), *Public Communication and Behavior.* San Diego, Calif.: Academic Press, 1986.

Merritt, D. *Public Journalism and Public Life.* Mahwah, N. J.: Erlbaum, 1995.

Mills, C. *The Sociological Imagination.* New York: Oxford University Press, 1959.

Minkler, M. *Community Organizing and Community Building for Health.* New Brunswick, N.J.: Rutgers University Press, 1997.

Montgomery, K. *Target: Prime Time.* New York: Oxford University Press, 1989.

Navarro, V. "Topics for Our Times: The 'Black Report' of Spain: The Commission on Social Inequalities in Health." *American Journal of Public Health,* 1997, *87,* 334–335.

Ognianova, E., Thorson, E., and Mendelson, A. "What Makes an Active Citizen? Do the Media Play a Role?" Paper presented to the Communication Theory and Methodology Division of the Association for Education in Journalism and Mass Communication, Washington, D.C., Aug. 1997.

Pew Center for Civic Journalism. *Taking Back our Neighborhoods: A Joint Report by the Pew Center for Civic Journalism and The Poynter Institute for Media Studies.* Philadelphia: Pew Center for Civic Journalism, 1995.

Pew Center for Civic Journalism. *Civic Lessons: Report on Four Civic Journalism Projects.* Philadelphia: Pew Center for Civic Journalism, 1997.

Postman, N. *Amusing Ourselves to Death.* New York Viking Penguin, 1985.

Putnam, R. D. "The Prosperous Community." *American Prospect,* Spring 1993, pp. 35–42.

Putnam, R. D. "Bowling Alone: America's Declining Social Capital." *Journal of Democracy,* 1995a, *6,* 65–78.

Putnam, R. D. "Tuning In, Tuning Out: The Strange Disappearance of Social Capital in America." *PS: Political Science and Politics,* Dec. 1995b, pp. 664–683.

Reich, R. B. *Tales of a New America: The Anxious Liberal's Guide to the Future.* New York: Vintage, 1988.

Rogers, E. M., and Storey, J. D. "Communication Campaigns." In C. R. Berger and S. H. Chaffee (eds.), *Handbook of Science Communication.* Thousand Oaks, Calif.: Sage, 1987.

Rose, G. "Sick Individuals and Sick Populations." *International Journal of Epidemiology,* 1985, *14,* 32–38.

Rose, G. *The Strategy of Preventive Medicine.* New York: Oxford University Press, 1992.

Rosen, J. "Making Journalism More Public." *Communication,* 1991, *12,* 267–284.

Rosen, J. *Community Connectedness Passwords for Public Journalism.* St. Petersburg, Fla.: Poynter Institute for Media Studies, 1993.

Rosen, J. "Making Things More Public: On the Political Responsibility of the Media Intellectual." *Critical Studies in Mass Communication,* Dec. 1994, pp. 363–388.

Ryan, C. *Blaming the Victim.* New York: Vintage, 1976.

Ryan, C. *Prime-Time Activism.* Boston: South End Press, 1991.

Salmon, C. *Information Campaigns: Balancing Social Values and Social Change.* Thousand Oaks, Calif.: Sage, 1989.

Sampson, R. J., Raudenbush, S. W., and Earls, F. "Neighborhoods and Violent Crime: A Multilevel Study of Collective Efficacy." *Science,* 1997, *277,* 918–924.

Schiller, H. *The Mind Managers.* Boston: Beacon Press, 1973.

Schooler, C., Sundar, S. S., and Flora. J. A. "Effects of Stanford Five-City Project Media Advocacy Program." *Health Education Quarterly,* 1996, *23,* 346–364.

Schorr, L. *Within Our Reach.* New York: Anchor/Doubleday, 1988.

Schudson, M. "What If Civic Life Didn't Die?" *American Prospect,* Mar.-Apr. 1996, pp. 17–20.

Seevak, A. *Oakland Shows the Way: The Coalition on Alcohol Outlet Issues and Media Advocacy as a Tool for Policy Change.* Berkeley, Calif.: Berkeley Media Studies Group, 1997.

Semenza, J. C., and others. "Heat-Related Deaths During the July 1995 Heat Wave in Chicago." *New England Journal of Medicine,* 1996, *335,* 84–90.

Shen, T., and others. *Community Characteristics Correlated with Heat-Related Mortality.* Springfield: Division of Epidemiological Studies, Illinois Department of Public Health, 1995.

Signorielli, N., and Staples, J. "Television and Children's Conceptions of Nutrition." *Health Communication,* 1997, *9,* 289–301.

Smith, G. D., and Egger, M. "Socioeconomic Differences in Mortality in Britain and the United States." *American Journal of Public Health,* 1992, *82,* 1079–1081.

Spears, L. "Picturing Concerns." *Contra Costa Times,* Apr. 11, 1999, pp. A1, A32.

Stempel, G. H., and Hargrove, T. "Mass Media Audiences in a Changing Media Environment." *Journalism and Mass Communication Quarterly,* 1996, *73,* 549–559.

"Stifling Heat Retains Grip on East Coast." *New York Times,* July 6, 1999, pp. A1, A19.

Strasburger, V. C. *Adolescents and the Media.* Thousand Oaks, Calif.: Sage, 1995.

Strasburger, V. C., and Comstock, G. A. *Adolescent Medicine: State of the Art Reviews.* Philadelphia: Hanley and Belfus, 1993.

Thorson, E., Mendelson, A., and Ognianova, E. "Affective and Behavioral Impact of Civic Journalism." Paper presented to the Mass Communication and Society, Division of the Association for Education in Journalism and Mass Communication, Washington, D.C., Aug. 1997.

U.S. Department of Health and Human Services. *Media Strategies for Smoking Control.* Rockville, Md.: U.S. Department of Health and Human Services, 1988.

Wallack, L. "Mass Media Campaigns: The Odds Against Finding Behavior Change." *Health Education Quarterly,* 1981, *8,* 209–260.

Wallack, L. "Drinking and Driving: Toward a Broader Understanding of the Role of Mass Media." *Journal of Public Health Policy,* 1984, *5,* 471–498.

Wallack, L. "Mass Communication and Health Promotion: A Critical Perspective." In R. E. Rice and C. K. Atkin (eds.), *Public Communication Campaigns.* (2nd ed.) Thousand Oaks, Calif.: Sage, 1989.

Wallack, L. "Improving Health Promotion: Media Advocacy and Social Marketing Approaches." In C. K. Atkin and L. Wallack (eds.), *Mass Communication and Public Health: Complexities and Conflicts.* Thousand Oaks, Calif.: Sage, 1990.

Wallack, L. "Media Advocacy: A Strategy for Empowering People and Communities." *Journal of Public Health Policy,* 1994, *15,* 420–436.

Wallack, L. "Strategies for Reducing Youth Violence: Media, Community and Policy." In University of California and California Wellness Foundation, *1997 Wellness Lectures.* Berkeley: Regents of the University of California, 1997.

Wallack, L. "The California Violence Prevention Initiative: Advancing Policy to Ban Saturday Night Specials." *Health Education and Behavior,* 1999, *26,* 841–857.

Wallack, L., and De Jong, W. "Mass Media and Public Health." In U.S. Department of Health and Human Services, *The Effects of Mass Media on the Use and Abuse of Alcohol.* Bethesda, Md.: National Institutes of Health, 1995.

Wallack, L., and Dorfman, L. "Media Advocacy: A Strategy for Advancing Policy and Promoting Health." *Health Education Quarterly,* 1996, *23,* 293–317.

Wallack, L., and Sciandra, R. "Media Advocacy and Public Education in the Community Trial to Reduce Heavy Smoking." *International Quarterly of Community Health Education,* 1990, *11,* 205–222.

Wallack, L., and others. *Media Advocacy and Public Health: Power for Prevention.* Thousand Oaks, Calif.: Sage, 1993.

Wallack, L., and others. *News for a Change. An Advocates Guide to Working with the Media.* Thousand Oaks, Calif.: Sage, 1999.

Wang, C. C. "Photovoice: A Participatory Action Research Strategy Applied to Women's Health." *Journal of Women's Health,* 1999, *8*(2), 185–192.

Wang, C. C., and Burris, M. A. "Empowerment Through Photo Novella: Portraits of Participation." *Health Education Quarterly,* 1994, *21,* 171–186.

Wang, C. C., and Burris, M. A. "Photovoice: Concept, Methodology, and Use for Participatory Needs Assessment." *Health Education Quarterly,* 1997, *24,* 369–387.

Wang, C. C., Burris, M. A., and Xiang, P. Y. "Chinese Village Women as Visual Anthropologists." *Social Science and Medicine,* 1996, *42,* 1391–1400.

Wang, C. C., Cash, J. L., and Powers, L. S. "Who Knows the Streets as Well as the Homeless?" *Health Promotion Practice,* 1999, *1*(1), 81-89.

Wang, C. C., and Pies, C. A. "Family, Maternal, and Child Health Through Photovoice." *Maternal and Child Health Journal,* Oct. 1999.

Wang, C. C., Yuan, Y. L., and Feng, M. L. "Photovoice as a Tool for Participatory Evaluation." *Journal of Contemporary Health,* 1996, *4,* 47–49.

Wang, C. C., and others. "Photovoice as a Participatory Health Promotion Strategy." *Health Promotion International,* 1998, *13,* 75–86.

Wiley, S. "Civic Journalism in Practice." *Newspaper Research Journal,* 1998, *19,* 16–29.

Wilkinson, R. G. "National Mortality Rates: The Impact of Inequality?" *American Journal of Public Health,* 1992, *82,* 1082–1084.

Wilkinson, R. G. *Unhealthy Societies: The Afflictions of Inequality.* New York: Routledge, 1996.

Winett, L., and Wallack, L. "Advancing Public Health Goals Through the Mass Media." *Journal of Health Communication,* 1996, *2,* 173–196.

Woodruff, K. "Alcohol Advertising and Violence Against Women: A Media Advocacy Case Study." *Health Education Quarterly,* 1996, *23,* 330–345.

NAME INDEX

SUBJECT INDEX